Bennett G. Zier, M.D.
Professor and Chairman
Department of Internal Medicine
California College of Podiatric Medicine
San Francisco, California

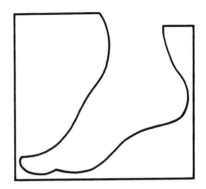

ESSENTIALS OF INTERNAL MEDICINE IN CLINICAL PODIATRY

1990
W.B. SAUNDERS COMPANY
Harcourt Brace Jovanovich, Inc.
Philadelphia   London   Toronto
Montreal   Sydney   Tokyo

W. B. Saunders Company
Harcourt Brace Jovanovich, Inc.

The Curtis Center
Independence Square West
Philadelphia, PA 19106

Library of Congress Cataloging-in-Publication Data

Essentials of internal medicine in clinical podiatry / [edited by]
    Bennett G. Zier.
            p.   cm.
    ISBN 0-7216-1400-0
    1. Internal medicine. 2. Podiatry. I. Zier, Bennett G.
    [DNLM: 1. Internal Medicine. 2. Podiatry. WB 115 E78]
    RC46.E885   1990
    616—dc20
    DNLM/CLC
                                                            89-10052

Editor: William Lamsback
Designer: Maureen Sweeney
Production Manager: Bill Preston
Manuscript Editor: Ellen Thomas
Mechanical Artist: Arlette Ramphal
Illustration Coordinator: Brett MacNaughton
Indexer: Julie Palmeter

Essentials of Internal Medicine in Clinical Podiatry   ISBN 0-7216-1400-0

Printed in the United States

Last digit is the print number: 9   8   7   6   5   4   3   2   1

*To my wife, Cynthia Stange, and sons,
Lucas and Travis, whose love and
companionship made this possible.*

*And to my parents, Herman and Helen,
who instilled in me a love for learning and
a desire to teach.*

CONTRIBUTORS

STEVEN BAKER, M.D.

Assistant Clinical Professor of Dermatology, University of California School of Medicine–San Francisco, San Francisco, California. Assistant Professor of Dermatology, California College of Podiatric Medicine, San Francisco, California.
Dermatology

STEPHEN BECKER, M.D.

Associate Professor of Medicine, California College of Podiatric Medicine, San Francisco, California. Assistant Clinical Professor of Medicine, University of California School of Medicine–San Francisco, San Francisco, California.
Postoperative Assessment

MICHAEL S. COHEN, M.D.

Assistant Clinical Professor of Neurology, University of California School of Medicine–San Francisco, San Francisco, California. Chief of Neurology, Seton Medical Center, Daly City, California. Active Staff, Peninsula Hospital and Medical Center, Burlingame, California.
Neurology

JAMES A. DAVIS. M.D.

Associate Clinical Professor of Medicine, University of California School of Medicine–San Francisco, San Francisco, California. Assistant Chief of Medicine, Mount Zion Hospital and Medical Center, San Francisco, California. Director, Rheumatology Clinic, California College of Podiatric Medicine, San Francisco, California.
Rheumatology

GREG FITZ, M.D.

Associate Professor of Medicine, Duke University Medical Center, Durham, North Carolina.
Gastroenterology

JULIE L. GERBERDING, M.D.

Assistant Professor of Medicine, University of California School of Medicine–San Francisco, San Francisco, California. Physician Specialist, San Francisco General Hospital, San Francisco, California.
Infectious Disease

GAIL M. GRANDINETTI, D.P.M., M.S.

Assistant Professor of Medicine, Departments of General Medicine and Podiatric Medicine, California College of Podiatric Medicine, San Francisco, California. Pacific Coast Hospital, San Francisco, California.
Hematology and Oncology; Metabolic Bone Disease; Peripheral Vascular Disease

ARLENE F. HOFFMAN, D.P.M., PH.D.

Professor, Departments of Basic Medical Sciences and Podiatric Medicine, California College of Podiatric Medicine, San Francisco, California. Chief, Noninvasive Vascular Laboratory, Pacific Coast Hospital and Clinics, San Francisco, California.
Peripheral Vascular Disease

WESLEY H. JAN, M.D.

Assistant Clinical Professor of Medicine, University of California School of Medicine–San Francisco, San Francisco, California. Active Staff, Mount Zion Hospital and Medical Center and Chinese Hospital, San Francisco, California. Courtesy Staff, Saint Francis Memorial Hospital, Pacific Presbyterian Medical Center, and Children's Hospital, San Francisco, California.
Renal Disease

JONATHAN LEVIN, M.D.

Assistant Professor of Medicine, California College of Podiatric Medicine, San Francisco, California. Chief, Vascular Surgery Clinic, Pacific Coast Hospital and Clinics, San Francisco, California. Attending Physician, Mount Zion Hospital and Medical Center, San Francisco, California.
Peripheral Vascular Disease

JAY LUXENBERG, M.D.

Assistant Clinical Professor of Medicine, University of California School of Medicine–San Francisco, San Francisco, California. Associate Medical Training Director, San Francisco Institute on Aging, Mount Zion Hospital and Medical Center, San Francisco, California.
Geriatrics

RICHARD B. ODOM, M.D.

Clinical Professor of Dermatology, University of California School of Medicine–San Francisco, San Francisco, California. Professor of Dermatology, California College of Podiatric Medicine, San Francisco, California.
Dermatology

JOAN OLOFF-SOLOMON, D.P.M., F.A.C.F.S.

Assistant Professor, Departments of Podiatric Medicine and Podiatric Surgery, California College of Podiatric Medicine, San Francisco, California. Active Staff, Good Samaritan Hospital, San Jose, California; El Camino Hospital, Mountain View, California; and Pacific Coast Hospital, San Francisco, California.
Metabolic Bone Disease

ROBERT A. SANDHAUS, M.D., PH.D., F.C.G.P.

Assistant Professor of Medicine, University of Colorado Health Sciences Center, Denver, Colorado. Staff Physician, Porter Memorial Hospital, Denver, Colorado; Swedish Medical Center and Craig Hospital, Englewood, Colorado; and Littleton Hospital, Littleton, Colorado. Consulting Staff, National Jewish Center for Immunology and Respiratory Medicine, Denver, Colorado.
Pulmonology

ROBERT SHAPS, M.D.

Assistant Clinical Professor of Dermatology, University of California School of Medicine–San Francisco, San Francisco, California. Assistant Professor of Dermatology, California College of Podiatric Medicine, San Francisco, California.
Dermatology

LEON SMITH, M.D.

Clinical Professor of Pediatrics, University of California School of Medicine–San Francisco, San Francisco, California. Attending Physician, University of California, San Francisco Medical Center, Pacific Coast Hospital, San Francisco, California; and Marin General Hospital, Greenbrae, California. Consulting Physician, Children's Hospital, San Francisco, California.
Pediatrics

ROBERT B. TELFER, M.D.

Associate Professor of Clinical Neurology, University of California School of Medicine–San Francisco, San Francisco, California. Medical Advisor for Neurology and Active Staff Member, Peninsula Hospital and Medical Center, Burlingame, California. Active Staff Member, Seton Medical Center, Daly City, California.
Neurology

BENNETT G. ZIER, M.D.

Professor and Chairman, Department of Internal Medicine, California College of Podiatric Medicine, San Francisco, California. Associate Clinical Professor of Internal Medicine, University of California School of Medicine–San Francisco, San Francisco, California.
Cardiology; Endocrinology; Hematology and Oncology; Neurology; Peripheral Vascular Disease; Preoperative Assessment

FOREWORD

Most podiatrists function to some extent within the confines of allopathic medicine. As with all generalists and specialists within this environment, general medical knowledge is a prerequisite. Certainly, podiatry is no exception to this rule. This fact has always been emphasized by our teachers and is best exemplified by the statement that the foot is connected to a person. The question is no longer whether a podiatrist needs a working knowledge of general medicine, but rather how much.

At long last there is an authoritative medical text specifically designed for the podiatrist. I feel that this text serves as testimony to our profession's growth over recent years. The subject matter is covered in a concise fashion, blending together the necessary academics and clinical realities that confront podiatrists on a daily basis. Dr. Zier's long-standing intimate relationship with podiatry has given him the insight to establish starting parameters for the medical subject matter. Most of the book is organized on the traditional system-oriented format for medical texts. Its unique characteristics become apparent with the inclusion of chapters requiring greater emphasis, such as those chapters devoted to Perioperative Assessment. This text is designed to serve as an appropriate starting point in general medicine for our students as well as an excellent review for podiatrists. Traditional internal medicine textbooks can be used to clarify more esoteric matters.

Dr. Zier and the distinguished list of contributors that he has gathered should be congratulated for this long overdue project. Dr. Zier should be additionally commended for the creation of a text that can be utilized by the practitioner and the student alike. I know that it will prove to be a valuable addition to my own library.

Lawrence Oloff, D.P.M.

Dean, Academic Affairs
Associate Professor, Department of Surgery
Co-Director, Special Problems Clinic
California College of Podiatric Medicine
San Francisco, California
Clinical Assistant Professor
Stanford University School of Medicine
Stanford, California

PREFACE

As a specialist in general internal medicine who has been intimately involved with clinical podiatry as well as undergraduate and postgraduate podiatric education, I have seen podiatry evolve in enormously positive directions during the past 15 years. Allopathic physicians are increasingly utilizing podiatrists as specialist-consultants for surgical and medical foot problems. The podiatrist has been an important figure in providing care in the burgeoning area of sports medicine. Postgraduate-level podiatric training exemplifies these and other changes. Residency training in allopathic as well as podiatric hospitals is the rule rather than the exception. Podiatry residents now train alongside internal medicine and general surgical residents on busy clinical services. Their medical and surgical knowledge base is expected to be at a level that allows them to function as productive members of the ward team providing care to patients with a wide variety of medical and surgical illnesses. The sum of these changes is that the podiatric physician is increasingly perceived as the preeminent specialist in diseases and surgery of the foot. This is extremely gratifying to the faculty at the California College of Podiatric Medicine, who have labored long and hard to fashion a well-trained podiatric physician who can assume his or her rightful place as a specialist in foot care.

The foundations of this text date back to 1976, when I was appointed Chairman of the Department of General Medicine at the California College of Podiatric Medicine. Before that time I had been a full-time faculty member in the Department of Internal Medicine at the University of California School of Medicine–San Francisco and had taught podiatry students during their clinical rotations in the ambulatory medical clinics. During my early encounters with podiatry students, I was struck with their enthusiasm for learning general medicine and their determination to apply that knowledge to their chosen specialty of podiatry. When I accepted the chairmanship of CCPM, my objective was to update and expand the curriculum in general medicine and make it relevant to the clinical practice of podiatry. Accomplishing this objective has not been an easy task as the scope of clinical podiatry has broadened considerably during the past 15 years. This growth has mandated an ever-increasing database in general medical knowledge as it relates to podiatry. It is now quite clear that podiatrists utilize an enormous amount of general medicine data in their everyday clinical work. The assessment of a patient's general health is crucial to preoperative evaluation; so too is the postoperative assessment of myriad general medical problems presented to podiatrists who do rearfoot as well as forefoot surgeries. Information relating to pediatrics, geriatrics, dermatology, neurology, ethics and general internal medicine are all an integral part of a podiatric physician's knowledge base. Our curriculum at the California College of Podiatric Medicine reflects this.

This text represents what I believe to be the essentials of general medicine relevant to the undergraduate and graduate podiatrist. In addition to chapters reflecting the organ systems classically associated with internal medicine, specific chapters in pediatrics, geriatrics, dermatology, neurology, peripheral vascular diseases, preoperative assessment, and postoperative assessment have been written to emphasize those areas of general medicine that the practicing podiatrist encounters more frequently than physicians in other specialties. As the specialty of podiatric medicine and surgery continues to grow and further define its clinical interests and responsibilities, it is my hope that future editions will reflect the evolution of podiatric practice as it relates to general medicine.

Finally, this entire project was in many ways generated by the motivation and dedication of all the students who matriculated through the general medicine curriculum during the past 15 years. Their enthusiasm and desire to be as complete a physician as possible made this work so personally fulfilling. It has been a privilege for me to know these students and an honor to be their instructor.

Bennett G. Zier, M.D.

San Francisco, California
September, 1989

ACKNOWLEDGMENTS

I am deeply indebted to a great number of people whose support and encouragement made this book possible. There are a number of faculty at the California College of Podiatric Medicine who were instrumental in teaching me about the profession of podiatry and about podiatric medical education. Joshua Gerbert is a leading educator in the field of undergraduate and graduate podiatry and was constantly helpful and supportive. Paul R. Scherer, Albert E. Burns, Joel R. Clark, Bruce Dobbs, William M. Jenkin, Steven J. Pallodino, Thomas Melillo, Ronald L. Valmassy, Christopher E. Smith, Jack L. Morris, Howard Sokoloff, William T. Stewart, James W. Stavosky, Barbara M. Kriz, Hugh Ribeiro, Maureen Sass, Stephen L. Becker, Emil Smetko, Arlene F. Hoffman, and Irma Walker-Adamé are among the many faculty and friends who helped educate me.

I wish to thank the contributors for their effort and tolerance. Their willingness to attempt a venture at defining a general medicine database pertinent to podiatry is extremely gratifying. To each and every one of them I want to express my most sincere appreciation for their work in transmitting their special experience and knowledge to the podiatric profession.

A special note of thanks to Larry Oloff, Dean of Academic Affairs at the California College of Podiatric Medicine, and Richard Lanham, President of the California College of Podiatric Medicine, who care deeply about the future of podiatric medical education and were extremely supportive of this project.

Fern Youngswick, my departmental administrative assistant, is another special individual who always lent a helping hand and, more importantly, just listened.

This project could never have happened without the excellent editorial assistance from my dear colleagues at W. B. Saunders Company. William Lamsback, Medical Editor, always believed in this project, and for this I am deeply grateful. Ellen Thomas, Copy Editor, was always so very kind and responsive in her management of the innumerable details this venture necessitated.

This book would not have been possible without the help of one individual who shared my most difficult moments. I want to express my deepest gratitude to Gail Grandinetti, who shared these times and helped me fit all the pieces of this puzzle into a whole.

Finally, I want to let my wife, Cynthia Stange, know that I could never have accomplished this without her encouragement, support, and caring.

CONTENTS

PART |*II*|

PART 1

SYSTEMS IN GENERAL MEDICINE

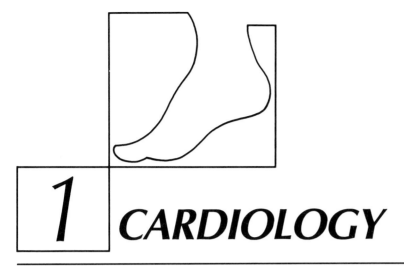

1 CARDIOLOGY

BENNETT G. ZIER

OVERVIEW

Regardless of subspecialty orientation, a physician in any active clinical practice requires a thorough understanding of cardiovascular disease evaluation. The cardiovascular system is an extremely important functional entity, vital for homeostasis of nearly every other anatomic unit in the body. Effective podiatric practice is concerned with foot function in the context of other physiologic and anatomic systems and their possible contributions to foot pathology. Podiatric surgery necessitates a clear understanding of the presence of cardiovascular diseases and surgical outcomes.

Certain cardiovascular problems such as hypertension have immediate as well as long-term consequences on a patient's health. Other problems such as rheumatic heart disease, ischemic heart disease, and congestive heart failure have definite implications in assessing a patient's suitability for surgery.

Although the study of cardiovascular disease is quite extensive and ever expanding, there is a finite body of knowledge that is a necessary part of each clinical practitioner's armamentarium. An understanding of the preoperative assessment of the hypertensive patient is part of this knowledge base as is an understanding of rheumatic heart disease and its association with endocarditis.

The purpose of this chapter is to present concepts of cardiovascular diagnosis, evaluation, and treatment relevant to podiatric medical and surgical practice.

PATHOPHYSIOLOGY

The function of the heart is to keep blood flowing through the circulatory system. The heart has two separate pumps. One pumps blood from the systemic circulation into and through the lungs, and the other pumps blood from the lungs through the remainder of the body and back again to the heart. Blood that enters the right atrium from the venous system is forced by atrial contraction through the tricuspid valve into the right ventricle. The right ventricle pumps blood through the pulmonary valve into the pulmonary artery, into the lungs, and finally into the pulmonary veins to the left atrium. Left atrial contraction then forces the blood through the mitral valve into the left ventricle from where it is pumped through the aortic valve into the aorta and then through the systemic circulation (Fig. 1–1).

In order to pump blood, the heart must alternately relax and contract, allowing blood to enter its chambers during the diastolic or relaxation phase and forcing it out during the systolic or contraction phase. This alternating systolic-diastolic cycle is integrated into cardiac function by an inherent rhythmicity of the cardiac muscle itself. The sinoatrial (S-A) node is the pacemaker of the heart because this is where the impulse begins. The impulse is transmitted from the S-A node, into the atria, then into the atrioventricular (A-V) node, and then finally through Purkinje's network to all parts of the ventricles (Fig. 1–2).

The four valves of the heart are all oriented so that blood never flows backward but always forward when the heart contracts (Fig. 1–3). The tricuspid valve prevents backflow or regurgitation from the

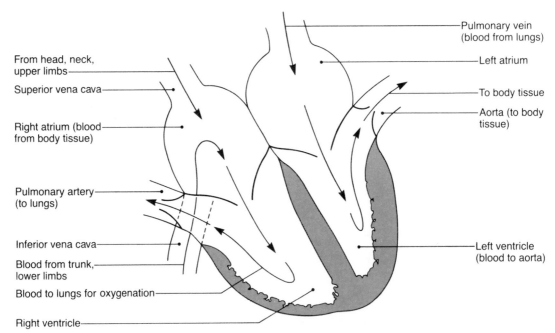

Figure 1–1. The heart as a pump. (Redrawn from McNaught J, Callander M: Nurses' Illustrated Physiology, 3rd ed. New York: Churchill Livingstone, 1975.)

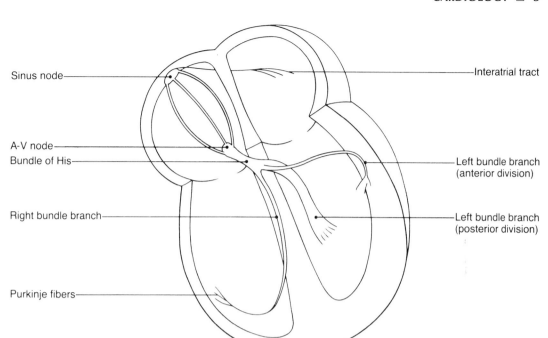

Figure 1–2. The conductive system. (Redrawn from Conover, MH, Zalis EG: Understanding Electrocardiography: Physiological and Interpretive Concepts, 2nd ed. St Louis: CV Mosby Co, 1976.)

right ventricle into the right atrium, and the mitral valve prevents regurgitation from the left ventricle into the left atrium. The pulmonary and aortic valves prevent backflow into the right and left ventricles, respectively, from the pulmonary and systemic arterial systems. These valves have the same function as valves of any type of

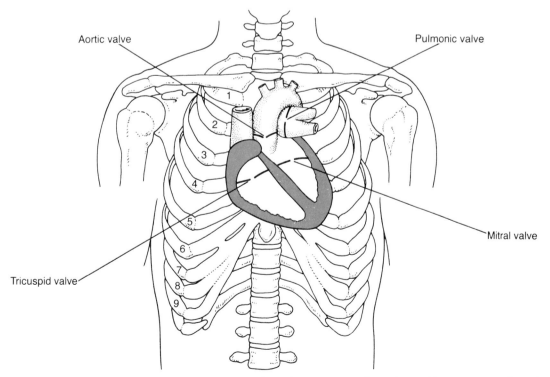

Figure 1–3. Anatomical locations of the heart valves. (Redrawn from Burns KR, Johnson PJ: Health Assessment in Clinical Practice. Englewood Cliffs, NJ: Prentice-Hall, Inc, 1980, p. 172.)

compression pump; no pump of this type can operate if fluid is allowed to flow backward during the filling cycle.

The amount of blood pumped by the heart is determined by the amount of blood flowing from the veins into the right atrium. The heart is a four-chambered pump that continues to pump all the time; whenever blood enters the right atrium, it is pumped on through the heart. There is a maximum rate at which the heart can pump. Within physiologic limits, the heart pumps all the blood that flows into it without excessive damming of the blood in the veins. However, if the heart is damaged, even normal quantities of blood returning to the heart cannot be pumped with ease. Thus the blood begins to dam up within the veins of either the lungs or the systemic circulatory system. The heart becomes congested and is said to be failing; this leads to congestive heart failure.

Arterial blood pressure is regulated by the combined effects of cardiac output and peripheral resistance. Hypertension is due to an increase in peripheral vascular resistance or an increase in cardiac output. Blood pressure determines the average rate at which blood flows through the systemic vessels. If arterial pressure equals cardiac output times peripheral resistance either a generalized constriction of all blood vessels or an increase in cardiac output raises the arterial pressure.

PRESENTING FEATURES

Although the study of cardiovascular disease can be quite far ranging and complex, there are certain key concepts that are basic to an understanding of its presence. Proper history and physical examination data as well as basic information on common diseases can help the clinician in differential diagnosis regardless of his or her particular subspecialty.

Symptoms

During the initial assessment of any patient, whether in an ambulatory or hospital setting, certain symptoms when elicited may be indicative of underlying cardiovascular pathology.

Chest Pain. Perhaps the most important cardiovascular symptom to elicit because of its far-ranging complications is that of chest pain. The differential diagnosis of chest pain includes far more than simply ischemic heart disease (Table 1–1). However, it behooves the clinician to prove that the patient's chest pain is not myocardial ischemia because once this is established, the fear of an immediate clinical crisis is alleviated.

The typical pain of myocardial ischemia, angina pectoris, is described as being a heavy pressurelike, tight, or squeezing sensation usually located in the substernal region. Characteristically, it is precipitated by exertion and relieved by rest. Angina pectoris can also be provoked by emotion, cold, meals, or sexual activity. Although angina usually begins substernally, it often radiates to the arms, neck, jaws, shoulders, and back. Variations in location and character of the pain may occur, so it is important not to rule out angina simply because of an atypical location, especially if the pain is related to exertion. Angina typically persists for 1 to 5 minutes. Chest pain that lasts only a few seconds is unlikely to be angina. Conversely, pain that lasts longer than 20 minutes may indicate myocardial infarction. Angina can occur at rest, usually at night; this variant type of angina is called Prinzmetal's angina.

The pain of myocardial infarction is similar to that of angina pectoris in location and radiation but is more intense and lasts longer (from 30 minutes to 2 to 3 hours). It is also more frequently associated with constitutional symptoms such as nausea, vomiting, and diaphoresis.

Chest pain may be indicative of pericarditis (inflammation of the sac surrounding the heart). The pain in pericarditis is usually pleuritic in nature and is typically relieved by the patient's sitting up.

Chest pain may indicate aortic dissection. In aortic dissection, the chest pain is sudden and excruciating, peaking immediately and often radiating to the interscapular area.

Other pathologic processes cause chest pain. Lung diseases (pneumonia, pleurisy), gastrointestinal diseases (esophagitis, ulcers, cholecystitis), rheumatologic diseases (arthritis, bursitis, costochondritis), and psychoneurotic conditions (hy-

Table 1-1. HOW VARIOUS CAUSES OF CHEST PAIN DIFFER

	Myocardial Infarction	Pericarditis	Angina	Pleuropulmonary	Esophagogastric	Musculoskeletal
Onset	Sudden	Sudden	Build-up of intensity (crescendo), or sudden	Gradual or sudden	Gradual or sudden	Gradual or sudden
Location	Substernal; anterior chest and midline	Substernal, to left of midline or precordial only	Substernal, not sharply localized; anterior chest	Over lung fields to side and back	Substernal, anterior chest; midline	To side of midline
Radiation	Down one or both arms to jaw, neck, or back	To back or left supraclavicular area	To back, neck, arms, jaw, and occasionally upper abdomen or fingers	Anterior chest, shoulder, neck	To upper abdomen, back, or shoulder	
Duration	At least 30 min; usually 1–2 hrs; residual soreness 1–3 days	Continuous; may last for days, residual soreness	Usually less than 15 min and not more than 30 min (average: 3 min)	Continuous for hours	Continuous for short or longer intervals, or intermittent	Continuous or intermittent
Quality-Intensity	Severe, "stabbing," "choking," "squeezing," "viselike"; intense pressure, deep sensation	Sharp, "stabbing," "knifelike"; moderate to severe or only an "ache"; deep or superficial	Mild to moderate, heavy pressure, "squeezing," "viselike"; vague, uniform pattern of attacks, deep sensation, tightness	Sharp, "ache," not severe; "knifelike," "shooting"; deep; crushing	Sneezing, "heart burn"	Soreness
Signs and Symptoms	Apprehension, nausea, dyspnea, diaphoresis, dizziness, weakness, pulmonary congestion, increased pulse, decreased BP, gallop heart sound, fatigue	Precordial friction rub, muscle movement, and inspiration causes increased pain; pain decreases on sitting or leaning forward, increases when on left side, laughing, or coughing	Dyspnea, diaphoresis, nausea, desire to void; associated with belching, apprehension, or uneasiness	Dyspnea; tachycardia; apprehension; increasing pain with coughing, on inspiration and on movement; pain decreased on sitting; pleural rub; fever	Dysphagia, belching, diaphoresis, reflux esophagitis; pain decreases on sitting or standing; vomiting	Pain increases with movement
Precipitating Factors	Not necessarily anything; may occur at rest or with increased physical or emotional exertion	Not induced with effort	Exertion; stress; eating; cold or hot, humid weather; recumbency; micturition or defecation	Pneumonia or other respiratory infection	Food intake, recumbency, alcohol ingestion, highly seasoned foods, history of GI problems	History of previous neck and arm pain

(Modified from Cheney DL (ed): Assessing Vital Functions Accurately. Horsham, Penn: Intermed Communications, 1977.)

7

perventilation) all may cause episodic chest pain.

Dyspnea. Another extremely important cardiovascular symptom is that of shortness of breath, or dyspnea. Pulmonary disease also causes dyspnea, and it may be difficult to differentiate between cardiovascular and pulmonary disease by history alone. Cardiac dyspnea usually has a more acute onset than pulmonary dyspnea and is often related to exertion. Cardiac dyspnea is an early sign of heart failure.

Orthopnea is dyspnea that occurs when the patient is lying supine and is relieved by the patient sitting upright with the aid of pillows. Paroxysmal nocturnal dyspnea is characterized by acute dyspneic episodes that usually awaken the patient from sleep; the patient must sit up or stand to become comfortable. Besides cardiac- and pulmonary-induced dyspnea, one other cause of dyspnea is hyperventilation syndrome. It is not uncommon for patients who experience incapacitating dyspnea, with or without chest pain, to have a negative diagnostic work-up; they are often somatizing personal life stresses and tensions.

Palpitations. Another major cardiovascular symptom is that of palpitations. A patient who is experiencing palpitations describes an awareness of forceful, pounding, irregular, or rapid heartbeat. Although these symptoms suggest a cardiac arrhythmia, they may also be psychoneurotic in origin. At the very least, one must make the assumption that the complaint of palpitations may be indicative of a significant cardiac arrhythmia, possibly leading to severely compromised cardiac function.

Edema. Patients may also complain of edema. A patient with cardiac-induced edema usually presents with dependent bilateral lower extremity swelling, which worsens at the end of the day. In the bedridden patient, cardiac edema may be found in the sacral area. When the patient is supine, the presacral area is most dependent and therefore most liable to exhibit edema. This is an extremely important clinical finding to recognize in nonambulatory patients.

Syncope. Syncope refers to a transient loss of consciousness. Cardiac arrhythmias as well as certain cardiac abnormalities (e.g., aortic stenosis) can cause syncope by decreasing cerebral blood supply.

Nonspecific Symptoms. There are a number of nonspecific constitutional symptoms, such as fatigue, decreased exertional tolerance, and recurrent pulmonary infections, that may be indicative of underlying cardiovascular disease.

Family History. Family history plays an important role in cardiovascular risk assessment (Table 1–2). A history of early death or sudden death in a patient's relatives should bring to mind the issue of familial hyperlipidemic states, which would account for early, accelerated atherosclerosis, leading to coronary thrombosis and myocardial infarction at an early age. If a patient has a positive family history for sudden death and myocardial infarction, clearly a coronary risk lipid profile or lipoprotein electrophoresis should be obtained.

Signs

Blood Pressure. Objective parameters of cardiac disease include certain key physical signs that aid in diagnosis. Perhaps the most important of these is blood pressure determination. Hypertension and hypotension are important in assessing a patient's suitability for surgery as well as in providing some measure of cardiac function and state of hydration during the perioperative period.

The proper equipment and technique are needed for measuring blood pressure. One must be aware of any past medical history that alludes to hypertension. With the patient supine and quiet, a sphygmomanometer is expanded to the point at which

Table 1–2. CARDIAC RISK FACTORS

Nonmodifiable Risk Factors	Modifiable Risk Factors
	Major
Age	Elevated serum cholesterol and
Sex	triglycerides
Familial history	Habitual diet high in total calories, fats, cholesterol, carbohydrates, and salt
	Hypertension
	Cigarette smoking
	Carbohydrate intolerance
	Minor
	Obesity
	Sedentary living
	Personality type
	Psychosocial tensions

the brachial artery pulse disappears on palpation. This ensures that a gap in auscultation is not missed, which can occur when one tries to measure systolic pressure by auscultation alone. Approximately 10% of hypertensive patients have a silent region in the midst of the systolic pressure recording. If this silent period or "gap" occurs, one may miss the systolic pressure above this region; blood pressure may be recorded as 140/80, when in actuality it is 190/80 with a silent period from 190 to 140. After the brachial artery pulse disappears, the diaphragm of the stethoscope is placed in the medial part of the antecubital fossa, with the patient's arm held at the level of the heart. The sphygmomanometer is slowly released. Systolic pressure is recorded at the appearance of sound, and diastolic value is recorded at the muffling or disappearance of sound. Systolic or diastolic blood pressure readings less than the values listed below are accepted as being within normal limits in adults.

Age (Years)	Systolic/Diastolic
Over 45	160/95
Under 45	140/90

Orthostatic hypotension refers to a situation in which blood pressure is normal in the recumbent position, but when the patient arises, the systolic and diastolic pressures fall to levels that produce faintness. This particular measurement of hypotension is of crucial importance in assessing the state of hydration as well as rate of blood loss that leads to decreased blood volume.

Pulse Rate and Rhythm. Determination of pulse rate and rhythm is another important measure of cardiovascular function. The pulse can be palpated in any accessible artery. Carotid, brachial, and radial pulses are the most often used sites. Because vigorous pressure on the carotid artery may cause bradycardia and asystole, the radial pulse area is better utilized. For the purpose of this discussion, the essential information to record from pulse palpation is pulse rate and rhythm. Arterial rate is counted by measuring the number of beats in 15 seconds and then multiplying by four. Normal resting values range from 50–100; >100 = tachycardia and <50 = bradycardia.

Pulse rate must be viewed in the context of the patient's medical condition. Athletes involved in aerobic sports traditionally have low resting pulse rates, sometimes as low as 40 beats/minute. The same pulse rate in a geriatric patient who complains of dizziness may be indicative of a heart block. Conversely, rapid heart rates may reflect hypovolemia, in which case the heart is trying to augment its output by increasing its contractions over unit time. Tachycardia may also be indicative of congestive heart failure. In this case, stroke volume is diminished because of a failing myocardium; the compensatory mechanism is to increase the heart rate in order to maintain cardiac output.

After assessing heart rate, the clinician should check for the presence of an irregularity of rhythm. When irregularities are found, attempts should be made to relate the rhythm to respiratory movements or other stimuli, such as caffeine, nicotine, and certain medications (e.g., antiasthmatic drugs and cardiac drugs).

Venous Pressure. After examining blood pressure and pulse, the clinician next evaluates the patient's jugular veins for any evidence of elevated central venous pressure, indicating right-sided heart failure. The patient is instructed to lie supine, and the neck is raised to a 45°-angle position. The head is tipped slightly away from the neck area so as to better observe the external jugular vein. If venous pressure is normal, the top of the venous pulsation is less than 3 cm above a perpendicular line that the clinician mentally draws from the jugular vein to the area where the clavicle meets the sternum (Fig. 1–4). Any venous pulsation above this level is indicative of right-sided heart failure. The right-sided heart chambers are failing, causing backflow of blood into the venous system, producing elevated neck veins even in a gravity-dependent position.

Pulmonary Auscultation. Following evaluation of venous pressure, the clinician systematically listens to both lung fields. Pulmonary auscultation should be performed in a systematic fashion over both lungs, always comparing one side with the other. Wheezing can occur with cardiovascular disease but is more likely indicative of bronchospasm secondary to asthma. Rales, however, are a cardinal sign

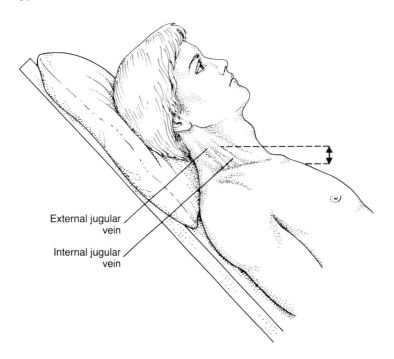

Figure 1–4. Estimation of jugular venous pressure. (1) Identify the external jugular veins. (2) Note the pulsations of the internal jugular vein. (3) Note the highest point at which it is possible to visualize the pulsations of the internal jugular vein. (4) Measure the vertical distance between this point and the sternal angle. (5) If the internal jugular pulsations cannot be visualized, locate the point above which the external jugular veins appear to be collapsed. (6) Record the vertical distance ascertained by either method in centimeters above the sternal angle together with the angle at which the patient is lying (e.g., at a 45-degree angle, as in this figure). (Redrawn from Bates B: A Guide to Physical Examination. Philadelphia: JB Lippincott Co, 1974.)

External jugular vein

Internal jugular vein

of congestive heart failure. In early or mild failure, rales are located at both bases, whereas in severe failure, rales may be located all over both lung fields. Rales arise from fluid in the alveoli, and their sound is simulated by rubbing hairs between the thumb and forefinger near the ear. A failing left ventricle causes backflow pressure on blood that enters the left side of the heart, pushing this blood back into the lungs. Pressure keeps increasing in the pulmonary blood vessels, resulting in transudation of fluid from the vessels into the alveoli, which leads to rales.

Cardiac Auscultation

Heart Sounds. Auscultation of the heart can be quite complex. However, if the clinician keeps in mind certain key principles, cardiac auscultation can be rewarding. First, one should listen in all four listening areas, known as the aortic, mitral, tricuspid, and pullmonic areas (Fig. 1–5), with the patient supine and sitting. The following should be noted:

1. The first heart sound (S_1) is the closure of the A-V valves (tricuspid and mitral).

2. The second heart sound (S_2) is the closure of the semilunar valves (aortic and pulmonic).

The interval between S_1 and S_2 is the systolic cycle and physiologically represents the ejection of blood from both ventricles into the pulmonary and systemic arterial circulation. Physically, one can time the systolic interval by placing one finger on the carotid artery, located at the angle of the jaw. The carotid impulse is due to blood being expelled from the left ventricle into the carotid system and is therefore indicative of the systolic time interval. The impulse begins with S_1 and ends in S_2. In this way, systole and diastole can be timed (Fig. 1–6).

$$S_1\text{———————}S_2$$
carotid impulse

The first heart sound is best heard over the mitral area with the diaphragm. The second heart sound is best heard over the base of the heart (aortic and pulmonic areas), again with the diaphragm, and is normally louder than S_1. Gallop sounds are the third and fourth heart sounds (S_3 and S_4), both of which are extra heart sounds that occur in diastole; diastole can be timed from the carotid impulse. The third heart sound is an early diastolic sound and is heard best with the bell of the stethoscope in the mitral area (Fig. 1–7).

$$S_1\text{————}S_2\text{————}S_3\text{————}S_1$$
systole   diastole

The third heart sound is considered an extra sound in children and young adults.

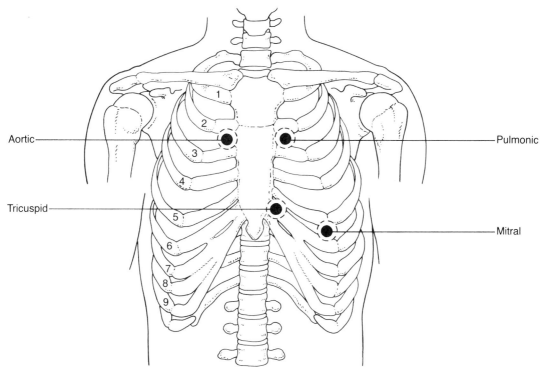

Aortic

Tricuspid

Pulmonic

Mitral

Figure 1–5. Cardiac auscultatory sites. (Redrawn from Burns KR, Johnson PJ: Health Assessment in Clinical Practice. Englewood Cliffs, NJ: Prentice-Hall, Inc, 1980, p. 172.)

If heard in an older person, it is considered to be a sign of left ventricular failure, probably due to blood slapping against the wall of a noncompliant ventricle during diastolic filling. The fourth heart sound is a late diastolic sound and is heard best with the bell of the stethoscope just medial to the mitral area.

$$S_1\text{————}S_2\text{————}S_4\text{————}S_1$$

An S_4 is commonly called an atrial gallop sound. It is due to atrial contraction that the listener appreciates because the atria have enlarged in "sympathy" with the left ventricle, which needs help in pushing blood through a high pressure head in the aorta. Therefore, the most common cause of an S_4 gallop is hypertension, although aortic stenosis and coronary artery disease may also cause this sound.

Heart Murmurs. Heart murmurs are of longer duration than heart sounds (Fig. 1–8). They may originate within the heart itself or within one of its great vessels. Heart murmurs can be caused by

1. Flow across a partial obstruction (i.e., aortic stenosis).

2. Increased flow through normal structures (i.e., exercise).

3. Backward (regurgitant) flow across an incompetent (insufficient) valve (i.e., mitral regurgitation).

4. Shunting of blood out of a high pressure chamber or artery through an abnormal passage (i.e., congenital ventricular septal defect).

Heart murmurs may be related to diseases of heart valves (Fig. 1–9). There are many different types of murmurs, and it can be very demanding to try to correlate murmurs with specific lesions. An ex-

Figure 1–6. The cardiac cycle. (From Burns KR, Johnson PJ: Health Assessment in Clinical Practice. Englewood Cliffs, NJ: Prentice-Hall, Inc, 1980, p. 173.)

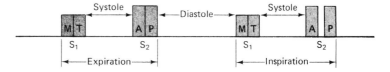

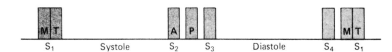

Figure 1–7. Graphic illustration of the relationship of heart sounds S_3 and S_4 to S_1 and S_2. (From Burns KR, Johnson PJ: Health Assessment in Clinical Practice. Englewood Cliffs, NJ: Prentice-Hall, Inc, 1980, p. 173.)

tremely helpful rule of thumb is to distinguish between pathologic and innocent (functional, benign, or organic) murmurs.

Pathologic murmurs, by and large, originate within the heart itself. They can occur within the systolic or diastolic cycle. Murmurs in the systolic cycle may be either pathologic (e.g., aortic stenosis, pulmonic stenosis, mitral regurgitation, tricuspid regurgitation) or innocent. In contrast, diastolic murmurs are always pathologic. Hence it is valuable to time abnormal sounds to the carotid pulse so that the sound can be placed in either systole or diastole. Pathologic murmurs are indicative of abnormal cardiac anatomy. Once a murmur is classified as pathologic, there are very real implications relating to potential cardiac failure, arrhythmias, and microbial endocarditis.

Innocent murmurs are of little significance and are called benign (functional, physiologic, or nonpathologic). The criteria that follow define an innocent murmur:
1. The murmur is always in systole, *never* in diastole.
2. The patient is asymptomatic.
3. The murmur is practically always heard along the left sternal border with no radiation.

4. The loudness of the murmur varies with respiration (i.e., louder on inspiration, softer on expiration).
5. The loudness of the murmur is never greater than grade IV/VI.
   I. A murmur heard only with greatest difficulty (barely appreciated).
   II. A murmur heard on careful listening.
   III. Obvious murmur.
   IV. A very loud murmur.
   V. A murmur that is appreciated on barely touching the stethoscope to the cardiac listening area.
   VI. A murmur heard without use of the stethoscope.

If the clinician appreciates a murmur on auscultation, the important questions to ask are:
1. Is this a systolic or diastolic murmur?
2. If systolic, does it meet the criteria for an innocent murmur? (See Table 1–3.)

Laboratory and Physiologic Data

Cardiac Enzymes

Certain enzymes liberated from necrotic myocardial cells are quite sensitive and

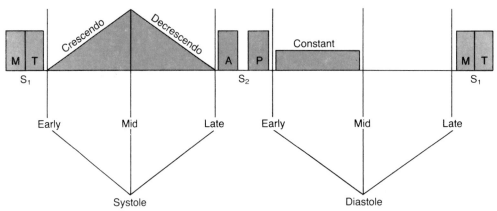

Figure 1–8. Graphic illustration of cardiac murmurs. Systole and diastole can be divided into three phases of early, mid, and late. Murmur duration is described using these phases, such as early-to-mid, mid-to-late, early-to-late, or pansystolic. Murmur intensity is described as crescendo, decrescendo, or of constant intensity. (Redrawn from Burns KR, Johnson PJ: Health Assessment in Clinical Practice. Englewood Cliffs, NJ: Prentice-Hall, Inc, 1980, p. 174.)

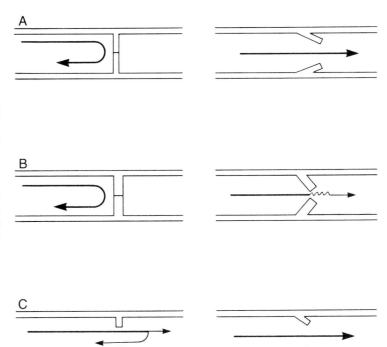

Figure 1–9. Diseases of heart valves. *A,* Normal valve: closes "watertight" (*left*); opens widely for free blood flow (*right*). *B,* Stenosis or narrowing: thickened, bound down by scarring (*left*); opens only part way, hinders flow (*right*). *C,* Regurgitation or leaking: valve leaflets are puckered and pulled apart by scar tissue and cannot close; blood leaks back into the chamber it has just left. (Redrawn from Phibbs B: The Human Heart: A Guide to Heart Disease, 3rd ed. St Louis: CV Mosby Co, 1975.)

specific indicators of myocardial infarction (Table 1–4). Creatinine phosphokinase (CPK) may appear in serum as early as 4 hours after a myocardial infarction. It is the first enzyme to become abnormal. Because CPK is liberated in injured tissue from brain, liver, thyroid, striated muscle, and smooth muscle cells, elevated CPK must be fractionated into different bands. A myocardial band (MB) of CPK can be detected by electrophoresis. If the CPK-MB exceeds 5% of the total CPK, myocardial cell damage can be assumed.

The CPK level usually returns to normal within 4 to 6 days. Serum glutamic-oxaloacetic transaminase (SGOT) rises 6 to 12 hours after myocardial infarction and re-

turns to normal 5 to 7 days later. Serum glutamic-oxaloacetic transaminase elevation is less specific than CPK-MB, as it may occur in patients with liver disease, skeletal muscle disease, and pulmonary embolism and in patients who are receiving intramuscular injections. Lactate dehydrogenase (LDH) is the last enzyme to appear elevated in serum after myocardial infarction, rising 48 hours after the infarction and remaining elevated for approximately 9 days. Lactate dehydrogenase is also liberated in large amounts in hemolysis, megaloblastic anemia, shock, skeletal muscle disease, and myocardial inflammation. Similar to CPK, LDH has an isoenzyme, hydroxybutyrate dehydrogenase (HBDH),

Table 1–3. INNOCENT AND ORGANIC HEART MURMURS

	Innocent (Benign, Functional)	Organic (Pathologic)
Timing	Usually early systolic	Systolic or diastolic at any point during or continuous
Location	Second or third intercostal space along left sternal border	May be heard in any listening area
Position in which heard	Usually supine	Heard in all positions
Duration	Short	Longer
Quality	Soft and musical	Louder, blowing, harsh, rumbling
Intensity	Soft (grades I, II)	Loud (grades III, IV, V)
Affected by exercise	Yes	Constant

Table 1–4. ENZYMES IN MYOCARDIAL INFARCTION

Enzyme	Normal Value Per Ml*	Elevation in Myocardial Infarction	Elevation in Other Diseases
SGOT (serum glutamic-oxaloacetic transaminase)	12–40 units	Occurs about 6 hrs after infarction; in 24–48 hrs reaches peak that is 2 to 15 times normal value; usually returns to normal after 3 to 4 days	Occurs in acute pericarditis, congestive heart failure, coronary insufficiency, and hepatocellular disease
LDH (serum lactic dehydrogenase)	150–300 units	Occurs 6–12 hrs after infarction; in 48–72 hrs reaches a peak that is 2 to 8 times normal; usually returns to normal 5–6 days later, but may persist to tenth day	Occurs in variety of muscle, renal, neoplastic, hepatic, and hemolytic diseases as well as in number of pulmonary conditions simulating myocardial infarction
CPK (creatine phosphokinase)	6–30 units	Increases within 2–5 hrs after acute myocardial infarction; peak value during first 24 hrs; 5 to 15 times normal; returns to normal by second or third day	Elevated in muscle disease, brain damage, and hypothyroidism

* May vary with different laboratory determinations.

that is more specific for myocardial cell infarction. The amount of enzyme liberation, regardless of whether it is CPK, SGOT, or LDH, can grossly quantify the size of an infarction.

Electrocardiography

The data derived from electrocardiography provide extremely important information about cardiovascular function. Although electrocardiographic reading requires detailed knowledge of electrocardiographic principles as well as vast and continual experience in actual electrocardiogram (ECG) interpretation, it is clearly within the scope of the podiatric physician to be able to interpret the type of data that the ECG can provide. Most podiatric physicians have not had the training or experience in interpreting ECGs as part of their clinical work; however, podiatric physicians should be able to utilize ECG data in three areas: (1) to interpret conduction abnormalities and arrhythmias in the operating room, (2) to recognize electrocardiographic representation of myocardial ischemia, and (3) to correlate the electrocardiographer's report with the patient's clinical presentation.

The ECG is nothing more than a recording of the heart's electrical activity (Table 1–5, Fig. 1–10). Cardiac cells in their resting state are electrically polarized. The insides of the cardiac cells are negatively charged with respect to their outsides. The cardiac cells lose their internal negativity in a process called depolarization. Depolarization is then propagated from cell to cell and across the entire heart, representing a flow of electrical current that can be detected by electrodes placed on the surface of the body. Once depolarization is complete, the cardiac cells restore polarity through a process called repolarization. All the different currents seen on an ECG are manifestations of depolarization and repolarization. The heart is a three-dimensional organ, and its electrical activity must be understood in three dimensions as well. The standard ECG consists of 12 leads, with each lead determined by the placement and orientation of various electrodes on the body. Each lead views the heart at a unique angle, resulting in twelve views of the heart. (see Fig. 1–17). During myocardial depolarization and repolarization, deflection or waves are inscribed on the ECG. By convention, positive forces (electrical forces directed toward the ECG lead) produce upright deflection, and negative forces (electrical forces directed away from the ECG lead) are represented by downward deflection. The distances between deflection and waves are called segments and intervals, respectively. The most important data derived fall into one of the following categories: (1) cardiac rate, (2) cardiac rhythm, (3) chamber size, (4) myocardial ischemia, (5) myocardial necrosis, (6) electrolyte disturbances, and (7) pericardial inflammation.

Table 1–5. WAVES IN A TYPICAL ELECTROCARDIOGRAM

Wave	Significance	Time Span	Abnormalities
P wave	Signifies depolarization and contraction of the atria	0.08 sec	Abnormal or absent P waves: another area of the heart muscle is acting as pacemaker instead of the SA node
PR interval	Signifies time it takes impulse to pass from atria to ventricles	Average time = 0.16 sec; usually less than 0.20 sec	Prolonged PR interval: impulse conducted more slowly than normal through AV node Shortened PR interval: impulse conducted over a shortened abnormal route from atria to ventricles
QRS complex	Depolarization and contraction of ventricles	0.06–0.12 sec	Prolonged QRS complex signifies abnormal conduction or delay of conduction through the ventricles
ST segment	Period following completion of depolarization of ventricles and preceding repolarization of ventricles	0.12 sec	Elevation or depression of ST segment indicates ischemia or infarction of the heart muscle
T wave	Repolarization of ventricles following contraction	0.16 sec	Inverted T wave: implies ischemia or infarction of heart muscle

(Data from Luckmann J, Sorensen KC: Medical-Surgical Nursing: A Psychophysiological Approach, 2nd ed. Philadelphia: WB Saunders Co, 1980.)

As an introduction to electrocardiograph reading, it is important to know that the heart is divided into two primary areas: the upper atria and the lower ventricles. The electrical wave from the S-A node spreads throughout the two atria, causing them to contract. At the lower part of the atrium, there is another node of specialized tissue, the A-V node, which is stimulated by the electrical waves spreading through the atria. The A-V node then relays the electrical wave to the ventricles. The pathway to the ventricles is the bundle of His, which separates into two divisions, the right and left bundle branches. Each bundle breaks up into an interlacing system called Purkinje's network, which spreads outward to the ventricular musculature. The electrical wave is brought to the ventricles through this specialized conduction network, causing ventricular contraction.

This sequence of electrical events is recorded by the ECG machine as a series of waves or deflections. Each deflection corresponds to a particular part of the heart cycle (Fig. 1–11). The P wave is atrial contraction. The P-R interval is from the beginning of the P wave to the beginning of the QRS complex; this is the time it takes from the beginning of atrial contraction to the beginning of ventricular contraction. The QRS complex is the contraction (depolarization) of both ventricles. The T wave represents the ventricular recovery (recharging or repolarization).

In terms of actually performing an ECG, the points of electrical contact (electrode positions) are the four limbs together with specific positions on the thorax (Fig. 1–15, p. 18). The limb leads are arranged so as to provide an analysis of the sum of the electrical forces arising in the heart (Fig. 1–16, p. 18). The standard limb leads are

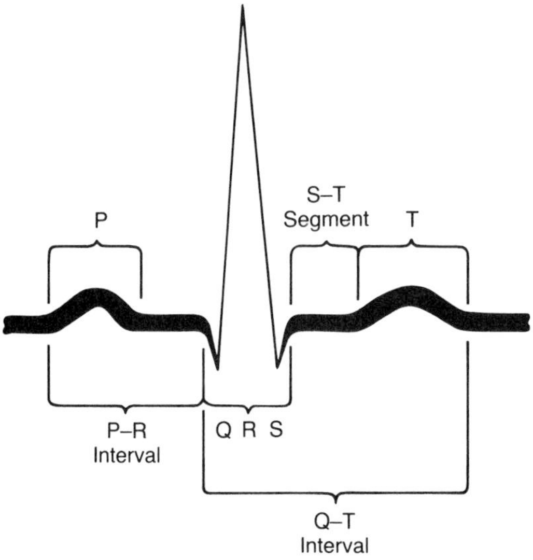

Figure 1–10. The ECG complex. See table and text on this page for discussion of waves and their meaning.

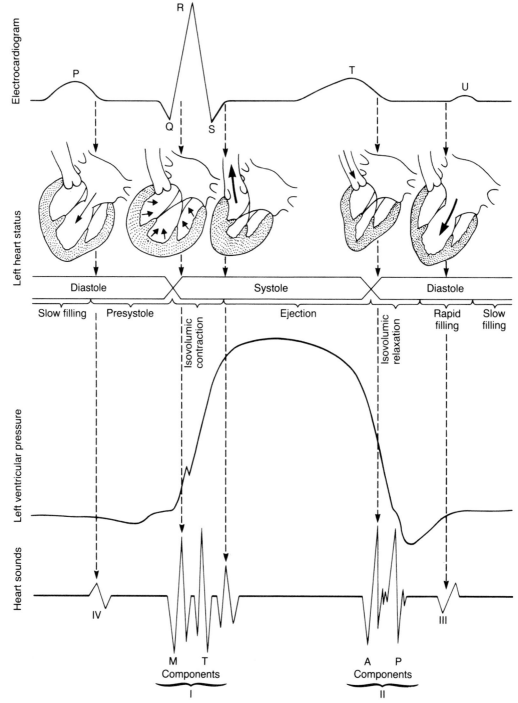

Figure 1–11. Events in the cardiac cycle. (Redrawn from Youkman FY (ed): The Ciba Collection of Medical Illustrations, vol 5. Ciba Publications Dept, 556 Morris Ave, Summit, NJ 07901, 1969.)

as follows:

Bipolar

    Lead I, right arm–left arm

    Lead II, right arm–left leg

    Lead III, left arm–left leg

Unipolar

    AVR, right arm

    AVL, left arm

    AVF, left foot

The standard placements of the chest leads

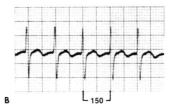

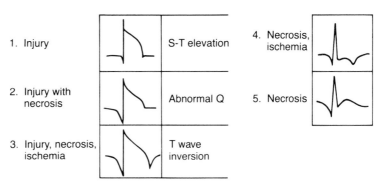

Figure 1–12. *A*, Calculating heart rate by determining the distance between the R waves. If there are two large squares between the R waves, the rate is 150; if three large squares, the rate is 100; and so on. *B*, Since there are two large squares between the R waves, the rate is 150. (*A* From Luckmann J, Sorensen KC: Medical-Surgical Nursing: A Psychophysiological Approach, 2nd ed. Philadelphia: WB Saunders Co, 1980. *B* from Phillips RE, Feeney MK: The Cardiac Rhythms. Philadelphia: WB Saunders Co, 1973.

A   per minute

B   └─ 150 ─┘

Figure 1–13. ECG changes in acute myocardial infarction. (From Vinsant MO, Spence MI: Commonsense Approach to Coronary Care: A Program, 5th ed. St Louis: CV Mosby Co, 1989.)

1. Injury		S-T elevation
2. Injury with necrosis		Abnormal Q
3. Injury, necrosis, ischemia		T wave inversion

| 4. Necrosis, ischemia | |
| 5. Necrosis | |

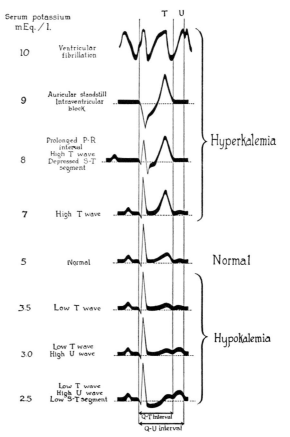

Figure 1–14. Effects of extra-cellular fluid potassium-ion concentration on the electrocardiogram. (From Burch GE, Winsor T: A Primer of Electrocardiography, 6th ed. Philadelphia: Lea & Febiger, 1972.)

Serum potassium mEq. / l.

10	Ventricular fibrillation	Hyperkalemia
9	Auricular standstill Intraventricular block	
8	Prolonged P-R interval High T wave Depressed S-T segment	
7	High T wave	
5	Normal	Normal
3.5	Low T wave	Hypokalemia
3.0	Low T wave High U wave	
2.5	Low T wave High U wave Low S-T segment	

Q-T Interval
Q-U interval

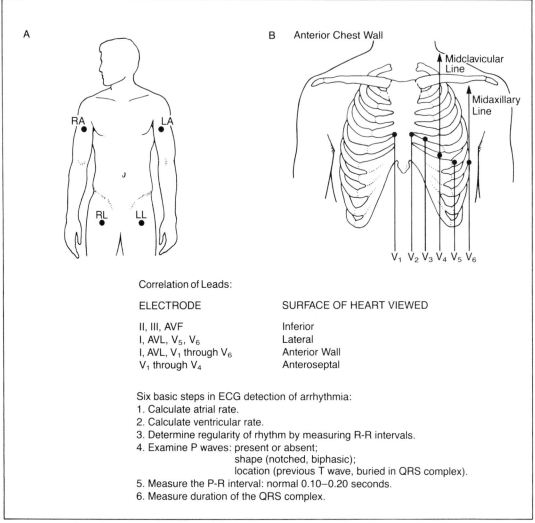

Correlation of Leads:

ELECTRODE	SURFACE OF HEART VIEWED
II, III, AVF	Inferior
I, AVL, V_5, V_6	Lateral
I, AVL, V_1 through V_6	Anterior Wall
V_1 through V_4	Anteroseptal

Six basic steps in ECG detection of arrhythmia:
1. Calculate atrial rate.
2. Calculate ventricular rate.
3. Determine regularity of rhythm by measuring R-R intervals.
4. Examine P waves: present or absent;
    shape (notched, biphasic);
    location (previous T wave, buried in QRS complex).
5. Measure the P-R interval: normal 0.10–0.20 seconds.
6. Measure duration of the QRS complex.

Figure 1–15. Electrode position. Derivation of leads for ECG tracings: *A,* limb leads; *B,* chest leads. (Redrawn from Vinsant MO, Spence MI: Commonsense Approach to Coronary Care: A Program, 5th ed. St Louis: CV Mosby Co, 1979.)

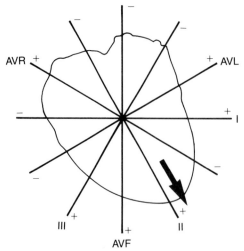

Figure 1–16. Electrical forces of the heart. (From Vinsant MO, Spence MI: Commonsense Approach to Coronary Care: A Program, 5th ed. St Louis: CV Mosby Co, 1979.)

are shown in Figure 1–17. Leads II, III, and AVF record changes from the lateral border of the heart; the chest leads overlie the interventricular septum in the interior wall of the left ventricle (Fig. 1–17).

CONDUCTION ABNORMALITIES*

It is important to relate the deflections of the ECG to their origins in the heart. Conduction abnormalities disrupt the normal P-QRS-T sequence.

First Degree Heart Block. The normal P-R interval is less than 0.2 second. In first degree heart block, there is a delay in the

* ECG strips from Johnson R, Swartz MH: A Simplified Approach to Electrocardiography. Philadelphia: WB Saunders Co, 1986. Sinus arrest ECG strip from Stein E: The electrocardiogram. Philadelphia: WB Saunders Co, 1976.

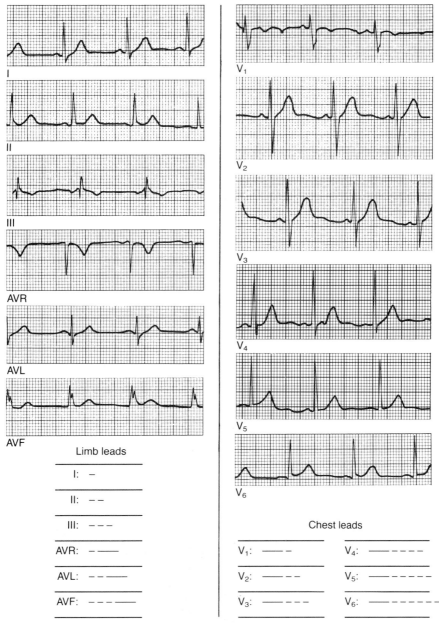

Figure 1–17. Standard 12 lead electrocardiogram. (From Dubin D: Rapid Interpretation of EKG's; A Programmed Text, 3rd ed. Tampa: COVER Publishing Co, 1974.)

transmission of the electrical impulse from the atria to the ventricles. It is characterized by a prolongation of the P-R interval beyond 0.2 second; despite this delay, all the impulses from the atria are conducted to the ventricles.

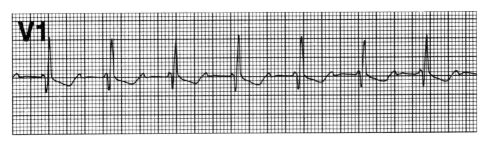

Second Degree Heart Block. This is a situation in which not all atrial impulses are conducted to the ventricles. Type I (Wenckebach's) second degree A-V block is present when atrial impulses encounter progressive delays in conduction to the ventricles, resulting in eventual failure of conduction of an impulse. Type II (Mobitz's) second degree A-V block is present when atrial impulses fail to be transmitted to the ventricles without prior progressive delays in conduction.

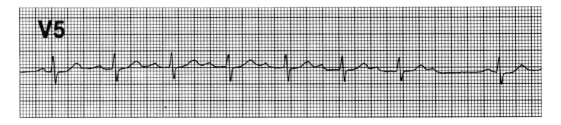

Third Degree (Complete) Heart Block. In complete heart block, none of the atrial impulses are transmitted to the ventricles. On the ECG, the ventricles contract at a rate independent of the atrial rate.

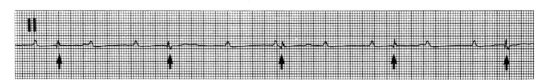

In essence, A-V conduction delays imply a disturbance in conduction of sinus or atrial impulses to the ventricles. The more common causes of A-V block include the use of cardiac drugs and ischemic heart disease. First degree A-V block is relatively benign. It is usually the result of degenerative changes in the A-V conducting system caused by aging. Digitalis, exaggerated vagal tone (as seen in athletes), and myocardial ischemia are also common causes. Second degree A-V block is more ominous than first degree block. Again, degenerative changes in the A-V node, digitalis toxicity, and myocardial ischemia may be causes. Type II (Mobitz's) second degree block is of much greater concern than type I because it frequently progresses to complete heart block.

Third degree A-V block is the most malignant type of heart block. Degenerative changes in the conducting system that result from aging and acute myocardial infarction are the most common causes. Complete A-V block is usually a signal that large amounts of myocardial tissue have been damaged. In this situation, early recognition is important because a pacemaker is usually required.

Bundle-Branch Block. In bundle-branch block, there is an interruption of

Table 1–6. ARRHYTHMIAS SUMMARY

Disorders arising in the sinoatrial node
  Sinus tachycardia
  Sinus bradycardia
  Sinus arrhythmia
  Sinus arrest
Disorders arising in the atria
  Premature atrial contractions (PAC)
  Paroxysmal atrial tachycardia (PAT)
  Paroxysmal atrial tachycardia with AV block
  Atrial flutter
  Atrial fibrillation
Disorders arising in the AV junction
  Disorders in which the AV junction takes over the role
    of pacemaker
      Junctional rhythm
      Premature junctional contractions (PJC)
      Paroxysmal junctional tachycardia (PJT)
  Disorders of conduction through the AV node
      First degree heart block
      Second degree heart block
      Third degree heart block
Disorders arising in the ventricles
  Disorders caused by ventricular irritability
      Premature ventricular contractions (PVC)
      Ventricular tachycardia
      Ventricular fibrillation
  Disorders of conduction
      Right bundle branch block (RBBB)
      Left bundle branch block (LBBB)

(Data from Luckmann J, Sorensen KC: Medical-Surgical Nursing: A Psychophysiological Approach, 2nd ed. Philadelphia: WB Saunders Co, 1980.)

one of the bundle branches, causing delayed conduction to one ventricle. The QRS duration is greater than 0.12 second. For example, if the left bundle is interrupted, conduction to the left ventricle is delayed, and it becomes activated after right ventricular conduction has occurred. Right bundle-branch blocks can be caused by diseases of the conduction system, such as ischemia and infarction. However, a right bundle-branch block can be a fairly common occurrence in an otherwise healthy heart. Left bundle-branch block rarely occurs in normal hearts and almost always reflects significant underlying heart disease, such as degenerative disease of the conduction system and coronary artery disease.

ARRHYTHMIAS

Because the ECG provides a record of both atrial excitation and ventricular excitation, the ECG is extremely helpful in analyzing cardiac arrhythmias.

The podiatric physician is expected to be able to determine heart rate from an ECG recording because this is the very first step in determining the heart's rhythm.

The horizontal axis on an ECG represents time. The distance between each light line (one small square or 1 mm) equals 0.04 second, and the distance between each heavy line (one large square or 5 mm) equals 0.2 second. Five large squares represent 1 second. A cycle that repeats itself every five large squares represents one beat per second (60 beats/minute).

The simplest method for calculating heart rate (Fig. 1–12, p. 17) is:

1. Find an R wave that falls on or nearly on one of the heavy lines.

2. Count the number of large squares until the next R wave.

3. Determine the rate in beats per minute by dividing 300 by the number of large squares between R waves (e.g., 300 ÷ 5 squares = 60).

Arrhythmias may be divided into atrial arrhythmias and ventricular arrhythmias. (Table 1–6).

Atrial Arrhythmias

Sinus Arrest. Sinus arrest occurs when the sinoatrial node stops firing. If this malfunction is not corrected, the ECG shows a flat line without any electrical activity. Prolonged electrical activity is called asystole.

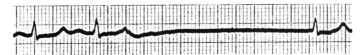

Sinus Bradycardia. All impulses originate in the S-A node. All complexes are normal, and the rate is less than 50 beats/minute.

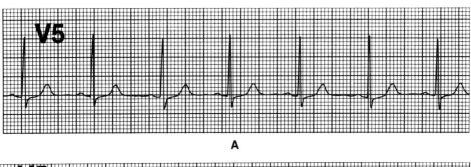

A

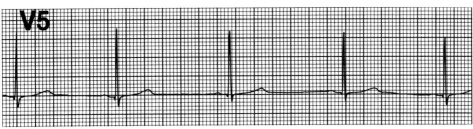

B

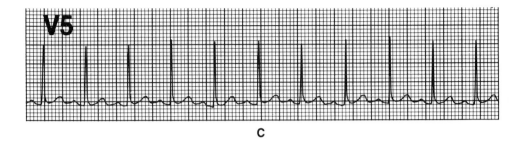

c

Sinus Tachycardia. Impulses originate at the S-A node. All complexes are normal and are greater than 100 beats/minute.

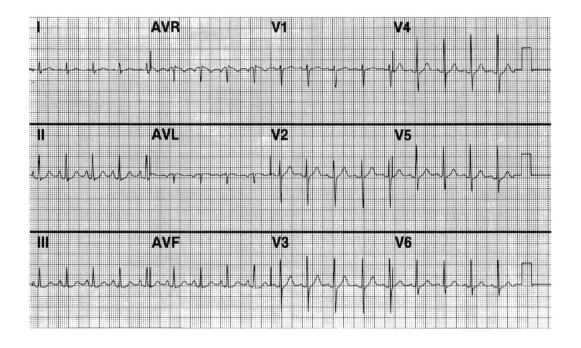

Premature Atrial Contraction (PAC). This occurs when some focus in the atrium other than the S-A node depolarizes prematurely.

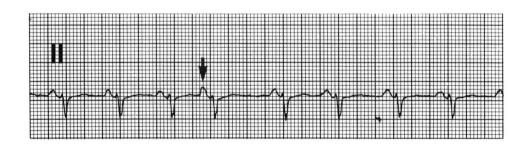

Paroxysmal Atrial Tachycardia (PAT). A focus in the atrium other than the S-A node gives rise to a series of rapid heart beats at a regular rate of between 150 and 220 beats/minute.

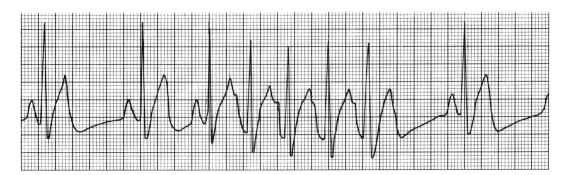

Atrial Flutter. This is due to a rapid firing of an ectopic atrial focus. The atria depolarize at a rate of 250 to 300 beats/minute. Only some of the atrial beats pass through the A-V node to the ventricles, resulting in a ventricular rate of 150 beats/minute or less. This characteristically appears as a "Sawtooth" pattern.

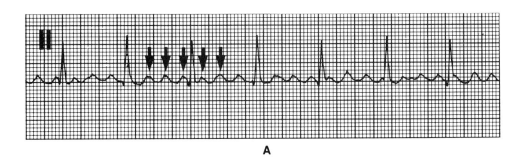

A

Atrial Fibrillation. This is the result of multiple atrial foci that discharge chaotically in excess of 300 beats/minute. Only a small number of atrial impulses pass through to the ventricles, producing a classic "irregularly irregular" rhythm.

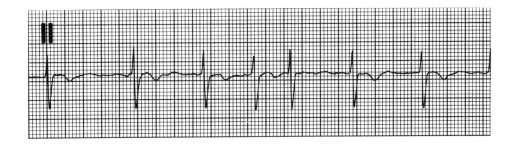

Ventricular Arrhythmias
Premature Ventricular Contraction (PVC). This arises from an ectopic focus in any portion of the ventricular myocardium. PVCs may occur in normal individuals with ECGs that reveal less than five PVCs/minute from a single ectopic focus. However, frequent PVCs (greater than five to ten/minute) or PVCs arising from different foci are of serious concern because they can degenerate into life-threatening ventricular tachycardia or ventricular fibrillation.

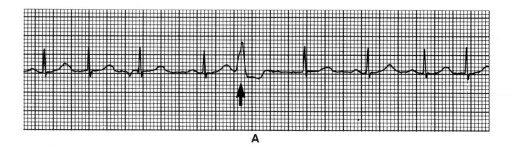

A

Ventricular Tachycardia. This is a sustained arrhythmia that originates in the ventricular tissue. The rate usually ranges from 120 to 220 beats/minute. This rhythm usually has serious hemodynamic consequences and frequently degenerates into ventricular fibrillation.

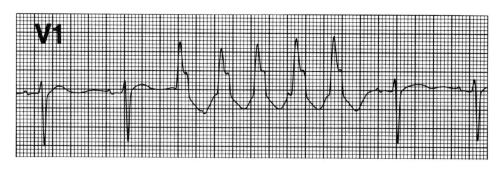

Ventricular Fibrillation. This is a rapid, irregular, disorganized ventricular rhythm that results in lack of cardiac output and absent pulse and blood pressure.

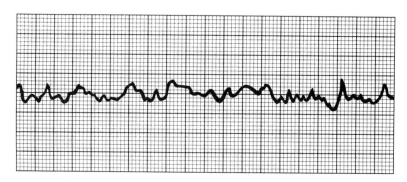

Dangers of Cardiac Arrhythmias. Cardiac arrhythmias are dangerous for three reasons: (1) rhythm too slow or potentially too slow, (2) rhythm too rapid or potentially too rapid, and (3) serious ventricular irritability.

Bradycardia is present when the heart rate is less than 60 beats/minute. Sinus bradycardia is an expected normal finding in young healthy adults and athletes; however, in the elderly or those with heart disease, sinus bradycardia may seriously decrease cardiac output. Sinus bradycardia is abnormal in the presence of congestive heart failure, pain, or exercise. It may normally accompany the administration of drugs such as beta-blocking agents, morphine, and digitalis. Sinus bradycardia may also be a consequence of acute inferior myocardial infarction. If bradycardia is accompanied by hypotension, it may be treated by cautious administration of small (0.4 mg) doses of atropine.

Rhythms that are associated with A-V block are dangerous because of their potential for severe bradycardia. Type II (Mobitz's) second degree A-V block can potentially lead to complete heart block, resulting in a ventricular escape rhythm with a very slow heart rate; third degree A-V block may lead to asystole or ventricular tachycardia.

The danger from rapid heart rates depends on age and extent of cardiac disease. Infants and children commonly have high heart rates. In older people who may have heart disease, tachycardia can be quite dangerous because it can lead to myocardial ischemia.

Arrhythmias in which the atrial rate is extremely rapid but some degree of A-V block maintains an effectively slower ventricular rate are dangerous because of their potential for severe tachycardia. If the A-V block decreases, the ventricular rate may increase and may lead to clinically dangerous tachycardia. Atrial flutter and atrial fibrillation cause these problems.

Finally, ventricular irritability is of major concern. In most cases, sudden cardiac arrest is caused by ventricular fibrillation. Some ventricular arrhythmias have the potential to degenerate into ventricular fibrillation. Ventricular tachycardia is in this category. Two to three PVCs in a row, or even large numbers of single PVCs, are associated with an increased risk of ventricular fibrillation.

MYOCARDIAL INFARCTION

Myocardial infarction alters the ECG by the successive production of abnormalities in the S-T segments, the development of Q waves, and T wave inversion (Fig. 1–18). Within the first 2 hours of an infarction, the ECG may be virtually normal. Subsequently the S-T segments become raised. In a few days, the T waves become inverted. The S-T segment gradually returns to the baseline, taking several weeks to do so. T-wave inversion may eventually return to normal, but some inversion usually persists. Abnormal Q waves are usually permanent.

MALIGNANT RHYTHMS

There are four rhythms that it is imperative that the podiatrist recognize. These rhythms are malignant in the sense that if they go unrecognized or untreated patients die of cardiac arrest. In these instances, basic cardiopulmonary resuscitation (CPR) must be begun by the health care personnel who are present. During this time, arrangements must be made to have the patient triaged to an intensive care setting for advanced cardiopulmonary life support, which often includes antiarrhythmic pharmacologic therapy. Those rhythms considered to be malignant are

1. Sinus arrest with asystole (prolonged electrical inactivity).

2. Ventricular tachycardia without a palpable pulse or blood pressure measurement.

3. Ventricular fibrillation.

4. Electromechanical desiccation. An organized rhythm may be seen on the ECG, but there is no palpable pulse or blood pressure. The most common forms of electromechanical desiccation are bradyarrhythmias, primarily of ventricular origin.

ELECTROCARDIOGRAPHIC INTERPRETATION

The most important point to keep in mind when receiving ECG data about a patient is that clinical correlation with observed ECG patterns is absolutely essential. Abnormal ECGs may be found in patients without cardiovascular disease. Indeed, in one study, findings of abnormal ECGs in normal individuals included first degree A-V block, PACs, and PVCs greater

Figure 1–18. Myocardial infarction. Frame 1 shows a normal ECG. In frame 2, hours after an infarction, the ST segment has become elevated. In frame 3, hours or days after an infarction, the T wave is inverting and the Q wave is becoming larger. In frame 4, days or weeks after an infarction, the ST wave is almost back to normal, but the T wave remains inverted. In frame 5, weeks to months after an infarction, the T wave has become upright again, and the only residual of a myocardial infarction may be an abnormally large Q wave.

than six complexes/minute. However, certain abnormalities should alert the podiatrist who is assessing the patient from a preoperative standpoint.

The finding of nonspecific S-T segment changes in a preoperative patient is an extremely common problem. One study noted that nonspecific S-T segment changes and flat or inverted T waves were associated with increased postoperative cardiac mortality. The patient should be carefully assessed preoperatively for ischemic or valvular heart disease and possible electrolyte disturbances. Following surgery, the patient should be monitored for possible postoperative myocardial infarction or congestive heart failure.

The finding of ECG changes consistent with a myocardial infarction of an indeterminate age in the asymptomatic preoperative patient is another common problem. It is important to try to determine the age of this myocardial infarction with a careful review of old ECGs. The age of infarction is crucial in view of studies that document the high cardiovascular risk accompanying surgical procedures performed in the first 3 to 6 months following a myocardial infarction. If no older ECG tracings can be found, it is prudent to delay elective surgery a minimum of 6 months.

Electrocardiography encompasses many areas, including electrolyte disturbances (Fig. 1–14, p. 17), pericardial inflammation, left ventricular hypertrophy, and others. It is beyond the scope of this discussion to elaborate on these areas. Any complete textbook of medicine will have appropriate information regarding the previously mentioned areas.

Echocardiography

Echocardiography has assumed a leading role in cardiac diagnosis because highly significant information can be derived without the use of invasive techniques in the patient. Echocardiography, otherwise known as cardiac ultrasonography, employs high-frequency sound waves directed toward various parts of the heart. These waves are reflected from different cardiac structures and are recorded on an oscilloscope (Fig. 1–19). Echocardiographic interpretation is a function of the anatomic relationships of cardiac structures. The complexity and wide variety of

heart diseases commonly encountered makes echocardiography applicable to a large variety of situations. The following are general disease states or situations in which echocardiography is helpful:

1. Ventricular diseases.
2. Valvular diseases.
3. Pericardial diseases.
4. Congenital heart diseases.
5. Arrhythmias and conduction diseases.
6. Tumors and masses of the heart.
7. Surgical monitoring.
8. Functional evaluation of the heart.

Podiatrists may utilize echocardiography in two situations. The first is to gain objective data in a noninvasive manner about the etiology of a cardiac murmur. Such information may indicate that the patient does indeed have objective evidence of valvular heart disease and may require endocarditis prophylaxis. The second situation in which the podiatrist may utilize echocardiography is in the diagnosis of infective endocarditis. The aortic valve is the one most commonly involved in infective endocarditis. Vegetations, which are sites of bacterial deposition on deformed heart valves, may be visualized with the use of echocardiography if they are in excess of 2 to 3 mm in diameter. A normal echocardiogram does not rule out the presence of infective endocarditis because vegetations smaller than 2 mm may not be detected.

Cardiac Radiology

Cardiovascular pathologic processes are often accompanied by changes in the cardiac silhouette, the appearance of the great vessels, and the characteristic patterns of pulmonary vascular distribution. The most important area of cardiac radiology for the podiatrist is the utilization of the chest radiograph to diagnose congestive heart failure (Figs. 1–20 and 1–21). In left-sided heart failure, the left side of the heart is unable to push blood out into the systemic circuit. The increased hydrostatic pressure in the left ventricle is transmitted backward into the left atrium and causes increased hydrostatic pressure in the pulmonary vessels, leading to a leak of fluid into the interstitial tissues of the lungs. The chest radiograph in congestive heart failure shows diffuse multichamber enlargement. In the normal individual, the upper

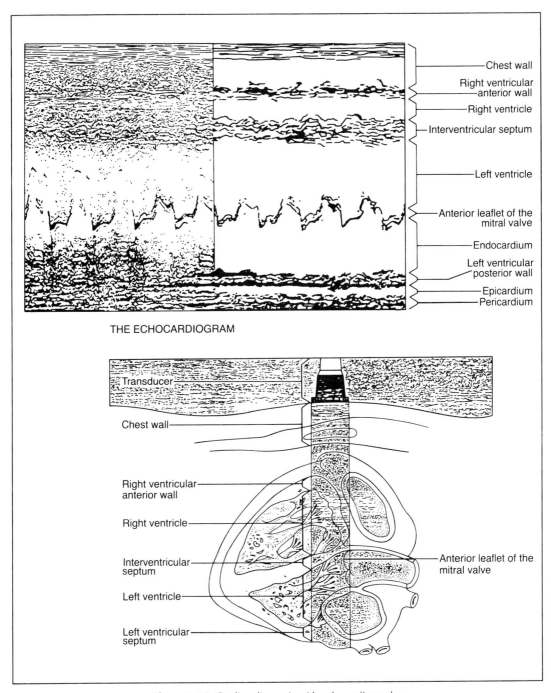

THE ECHOCARDIOGRAM

Chest wall
Right ventricular anterior wall
Right ventricle
Interventricular septum
Left ventricle
Anterior leaflet of the mitral valve
Endocardium
Left ventricular posterior wall
Epicardium
Pericardium

Transducer
Chest wall
Right ventricular anterior wall
Right ventricle
Interventricular septum
Left ventricle
Left ventricular septum
Anterior leaflet of the mitral valve

Figure 1–19. Cardiac diagnosis with echocardiography.

lobe vessels are distinctly smaller than those at the bases. However, when left atrial pressure increases, the lower lobe vessels constrict and the upper lobe vessels increase in caliber. As congestive heart failure worsens and left atrial pressure rises, transudation of fluid occurs into the lung interstitium, thickening the alveolar walls and interlobular connective tissues. This action results in multiple linear densities, known as Kerley's lines. These lines are short, thin, transverse lines best seen laterally near the *costophrenic* angles.

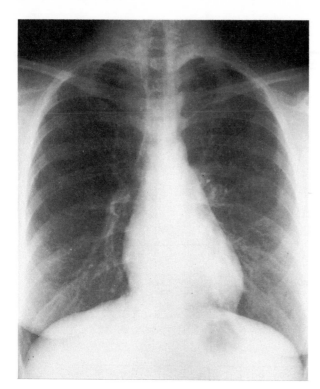

Figure 1–20. A normal chest radiograph. (From Weinberger SE: Principles of Pulmonary Medicine. Philadelphia: WB Saunders Co, 1986.)

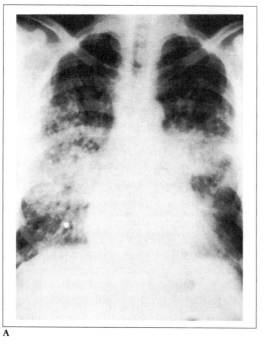

A

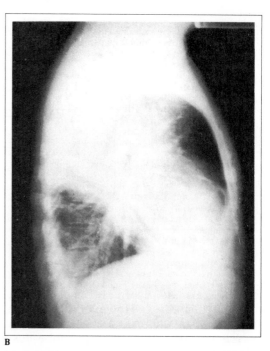

B

Figure 1–21. Posteroanterior (*A*) and lateral (*B*) chest radiographs of patient in heart failure. There is cardiac enlargement, which on the lateral projection is seen to be primarily left ventricular. Lung fields demonstrate the typical "butterfly" pattern of pulmonary edema. (From Stein JH (ed): Internal Medicine. Boston: Little, Brown & Co, 1983.)

CARDIOVASCULAR DISEASES

Hypertension

Hypertension is the most common cardiovascular problem of patients encountered by podiatrists. It is important for the clinician to be aware of the magnitude of this problem and to have an understanding of the associated pathophysiology and clinical features. Furthermore, the podiatrist must be knowledgeable about antihypertensive treatment so that proper precautions are taken when hypertensive patients receive podiatric care. Podiatric physicians encounter hypertensive patients in a variety of clinical situations:

1. Detecting hypertension for the first time in a patient during a routine blood pressure check
2. Rendering podiatric care to the hypertensive patient in the office
3. Providing invasive surgical care to the hypertensive patient in the operating room
4. Treating the podiatric manifestations of hypertensive disease (i.e., peripheral vascular disease).

Pathophysiology

Hypertension is a function of mean arterial pressure, which itself is a function of cardiac output times peripheral resistance. Therefore, the mechanism of hypertension is related to two important hemodynamic factors: increases in cardiac output and increases in peripheral vascular resistance. Increased cardiac output leads to hypertension due to increased blood volume or hypervolemia, caused by deficient renal sodium excretion. Elevations in peripheral vascular resistance result from vasoconstriction of vascular smooth muscle. Thus the pathophysiology of hypertension may be viewed as a problem of either volume or vasoconstriction.

Etiology

Clinically, the etiology of more than 95% of cases of hypertension is unknown. This is called essential or primary hypertension, which is probably a function of hypervolemia and vasoconstriction. A positive family history of hypertension, increased salt intake, obesity, and stressful occupation are all factors in patients with essential hypertension.

Secondary hypertension refers to hypertension caused by specific known disorders. These disorders account for less than 5% of all hypertensive disease but are of great importance because they are curable. Therefore, the physician should exclude all causes of secondary hypertension before accepting primary hypertension as the diagnosis. Certain clinical clues point to secondary hypertension as a diagnostic possibility: new onset of hypertension in the young (less than 25 years of age) or old (greater than 65 years of age), hypertension refractory to conventional treatment, and severe or accelerated states of hypertension.

The most important disorders causing secondary hypertension are as follows:

1. Renal artery stenosis. This leads to decreased renal blood flow, which activates the renin-angiotensin-aldosterone system, leading to salt retention, which in turn causes hypervolemia.
2. Diseases of the adrenal gland.
   A. Adrenal cortex. Excess aldosterone is produced by hyperplastic or adenomatous areas of the zona glomerulosa, leading to salt retention, which causes hypervolemia.
   B. Adrenal medulla. A tumor in this region produces excess catecholamines, leading to vasoconstriction.
3. Coarctation of the aorta (a congenital constriction of the aorta). It is unclear why this causes hypertension. Clinically, it produces delayed and diminished pulses in the lower extremities as compared with the upper extremities.

Diagnosis and Treatment

It is of utmost importance to control hypertension. Hypertension, both systolic and diastolic, is a risk factor for many life-threatening illnesses including angina, myocardial infarction, congestive heart failure, aortic dissection, renal failure, and stroke. The aim of treatment is to reduce the likelihood of these complications.

Most patients with hypertension are asymptomatic and are detected only on routine examination. Other patients, usually those with severe hypertension, may present with headaches, shortness of breath, or blurred vision. There are a small percentage of patients whose first manifestation of long-standing, undetected hypertension is myocardial infarction, congestive heart failure, or stroke.

Systolic or diastolic blood pressure readings above the values listed below are indicative of hypertensive blood pressure readings:

Age (Years)	Systolic/Diastolic
Under 45	140/90
Over 45	160/95

The level of systolic pressure is as important as the level of diastolic pressure in assessing morbidity resulting from hypertension.

The diagnosis of hypertension is generally accepted if the patient's blood pressure is consistently recorded above normal on three separate visits. This eliminates the possibility of blood pressure readings that vary widely with mood and activity.

Antihypertensive treatment may involve many modalities, including diet modification to eliminate salt, weight loss to treat obesity, and biofeedback and psychotherapy to reduce internal and external stress. However, the predominant treatment for hypertension is pharmacologic, with a fairly sophisticated armamentarium of drugs available (Table 1–7). The pharmacology of antihypertension relates directly to the underlying pathophysiology. If the patient is believed to have hypervolemia as the cause of hypertension, a diuretic to increase renal excretion of sodium, and with it water, is the drug of choice. If vasoconstriction is the problem arteriolar dilators and drugs with peripheral sympatholytic or central sympatholytic action are used. Angiotensin converting enzyme (ACE) inhibitors lower blood pressure by decreasing formation of angiotensin II. Calcium channel blockers cause vasodilatation, which decreases peripheral resistance.

Unfortunately, the clinical distinction of hypervolemic and vasoconstrictive hypertension is often difficult. Consequently, most physicians initiate antihypertensive drug regimens with a diuretic and then add other drugs, in a stepwise approach, until control is achieved (Figs. 1–22 and 1–23).

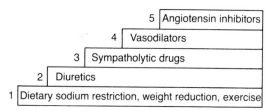

Figure 1–22. Stepped-care approach to treatment of hypertension. (From Stein JH (ed): Internal Medicine. Boston: Little, Brown & Co, 1983.)

Podiatric Implications

When the podiatric physician treats a patient who is hypertensive, the following issues must be addressed:

1. If the podiatrist is the first physician to detect hypertension in a patient, that patient should be referred to another appropriate physician for diagnosis and treatment. Furthermore, the podiatrist should receive some verification that this patient has indeed received antihypertensive intervention. Many patients who are asymptomatic fail to obtain further care because they are not aware of the long-term consequences of untreated hypertension.

2. If the patient is known to be hypertensive and is being treated, the podiatrist should check to see if the hypertension is controlled. Surprisingly, approximately 40% of all treated hypertensive patients are not well controlled because of a variety of factors. Among these are noncompliance, inadequate therapy, and other illnesses that worsen the underlying hypertensive condition. The podiatrist should notify the physician treating such hypertensive patients.

3. When the adequately controlled hypertensive patient is a candidate for surgery, the question arises as to whether the antihypertensive medication should be continued throughout the perioperative period. It is quite clear that antihypertensive medication should not be stopped at any time during the perioperative period. Excellent prospective studies have shown that normotensive and adequately controlled hypertensive patients experience far less cardiovascular morbidity than do poorly controlled hypertensive patients.

There are a number of other points that need to be stressed concerning the hypertensive patient who is to undergo elective

Table 1–7. ANTIHYPERTENSIVE MEDICATIONS

Class	Initial Dose	Range	Adverse Effects
Diuretics			
Hydrochlorothiazide	12.5–25 mg qd	12.5–100 mg	↓K⁺, ↓Mg⁺⁺ glucose
Other thiazides	Various	Various	
Chlorthalidone	12.5–25 mg	12.5–50 mg qd	Rash, impotence, metabolic changes
Metolazone*	2.5 mg	2.5 mg–5 mg qd	
Combination Agents			
Hydrochlorothiazide and triamterene (Dyazide)	1–2 capsules qd	1–4 capsules qd	Same as diuretics plus gastrointestinal disturbances
Hydrochlorothiazide and triamterene (Maxide)	½ tablet qd	½–2 tablets qd	
Moduretic†	½ tablet qd	½–2 tablets qd	
Beta-Blockers			
Propranolol	20 mg bid	20–160 mg bid	Bradycardia, fatigue, sleep disturbance, bronchospasm, cold extremities, impotence, ↓HDL cholesterol, ↑triglycerides
Metoprolol	50 mg bid	50–200 mg bid	
Nadolol	20 mg qd	20–160 mg qd	
Atenolol	50 mg bid	50–200 mg qd	
Timolol	5 mg qd	5–10 mg qd	
Pindolol	5 mg qd	5–20 mg qd	
Labetalol‡	100 mg bid	100–600 mg bid	
Acebutolol	400 mg qd	400–1200 mg in 1–2 doses	
Angiotensin Converting Enzyme Inhibitors			
Captopril	12.5–25 mg bid	50–300 mg in 2–3 doses	Skin rash, taste disturbances, cough, angioneurotic edema, hypotension, renal insufficiency
Enalapril	5 mg qd	5–40 mg in 1–2 doses	
Calcium Blockers			
Verapamil§	240 mg qd	240–480 mg in 1–2 doses	Constipation, headache, edema, bradycardia
Diltiazem	120 mg bid	120–240 mg bid	Headache, eczema, bradycardia
Nifedipine	10 mg tid	10–30 mg bid	Headache, palpitations, edema
Central Sympatholytics			
Methyldopa	250 mg bid	250 mg–1 g bid	Sedation, dry mouth, hemolytic anemia, hepatitis
Clonidine‖	0.1 mg bid	0.1–0.3 bid	Sedation, dry mouth
Guanabenz	4 mg bid	4–16 mg bid	Sedation, dry mouth
Peripheral Sympatholytics			
Prazosin	1 mg bid	1–10 mg bid	Syncope (after first dose) palpitations, headache
Guanethidine	10 mg qd	10–100 mg qd	Orthostatic hypotension, diarrhea
Reserpine	0.1 mg qd	0.1–0.25 mg qd	Depression, peptic disease
Arteriolar Dilators			
Hydralazine	25 mg bid	25–200 mg bid	Gastrointestinal intolerance, headache, tachycardia
Minoxidil	5 mg qd	5–20 mg bid	Headache, fluid retention, hirsutism

* K⁺ replacement often necessary.
† Trade name for amiloride hydrochloride with hydrochlorothiazide.
‡ Combined beta- and alpha-blocker.
§ Slowed-release form.
‖ Rebound hypertension.
Bid, twice a day; HDL, high-density lipoprotein; qd, every day; tid, three times a day.

surgery. Thiazide and related diuretics are the cornerstone of antihypertensive treatment. Because diuretics promote renal excretion of potassium, hypokalemia may be a problem. Patients may present with weakness of the lower extremities, fatigue, or nocturnal leg cramps. Intraoperatively, hypokalemia predisposes a patient to cardiac arrhythmias. It is of utmost importance to check the serum potassium level for any patient receiving diuretics prior to surgery. If the serum potassium level is less than 3.5 mEq replacement in the form of oral potassium should be ordered. In patients who are taking digitalis, glycosides, and diuretics, it is prudent to keep serum

Diastolic Blood Pressure (mm Hg)

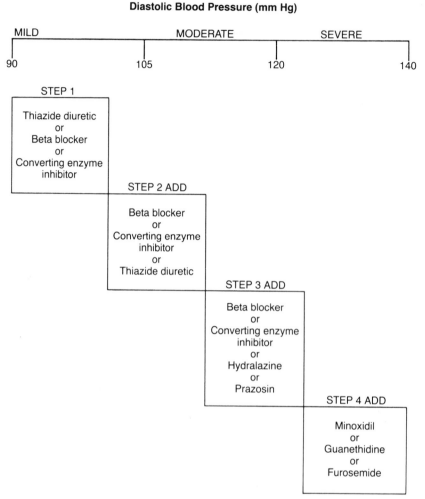

Figure 1–23. A stepped-care general antihypertensive regimen.

potassium levels above 4 mEq/l because hypokalemia predisposes them to digitalis toxicity.

Monoamine oxidase inhibitors are generally used as antidepressant medications. They were used as hypertensive medications before newer agents made them obsolete. It is not uncommon to still find patients being considered for surgery who are on monoamine oxidase inhibitors. These drugs act by blocking catecholamine metabolism, causing the build-up of intracellular amine levels. Because of this effect, these drugs have significant interactions with many drugs that may be given during the perioperative period. Among the most important is the interaction between general anesthetics and monoamine oxidase inhibitors, in which catecholamines may be liberated into the blood stream in excessive amounts, causing a hypertensive crisis. For this reason alone, all monoamine oxidase inhibitors should be discontinued 3 to 4 weeks prior to any elective surgery.

Ischemic Heart Disease

Ischemic heart disease refers to two clinical syndromes, angina pectoris and myocardial infarction. Angina pectoris is pain or discomfort in the chest and adjacent areas caused by relative myocardial ischemia. It is by definition transient and reversible. Conversely, myocardial infarction is irreversible damage to heart muscle that occurs when myocardium is subjected to prolonged ischemia. Angina pectoris and myocardial infarction result from myocardial oxygen demand exceeding oxygen supply.

Angina Pectoris

The diagnosis of angina is best made by obtaining a history. The pain is most frequently substernal, although it may be in the neck, lower jaw, arm, or hand. In some instances, the pain may be in the neck, lower jaw, arm, or hand areas without substernal chest pain. The pain is often characterized by discomfort and may be described as squeezing or bandlike choking or smothering. Angina is usually related to exertion, and often patients may stop whatever they are doing to relieve the pain. The typical attack is 1 to 3 minutes; it almost always lasts less than 10 minutes but longer than 1 minute. In addition to exertion or emotion causing the pain, cold weather, large meals, and sexual activity may also precipitate angina. It is alleviated by rest, cessation of activity, and often by ingestion of nitroglycerin. There may be associated symptoms such as dyspnea, nausea, dizziness, and diaphoresis.

Myocardial Infarction

Myocardial infarction lasts longer than 10 minutes and may last up to 2 to 3 hours. Pain is the most common symptom, often accompanied by nausea, vomiting, anxiety, and diaphoresis. There is often a history of angina. Of myocardial infarctions, 15 to 20% are painless. These silent myocardial infarctions are more common in diabetic and elderly patients. In both angina and myocardial infarction, risk factors play an important role in terms of diagnostic evaluation. A family history of arteriosclerotic heart disease, myocardial infarction, angina, or premature death in male relatives is an important risk factor. Other extremely important risk factors are hypertension and smoking. Secondary risk factors include diabetes mellitus, lipid disorders, and obesity.

Although the diagnosis of angina is best made by history, the diagnosis of myocardial infarction depends on meeting two of three criteria. The first criterion is typical pain, described earlier. The second is ECG changes, which appear almost immediately after pain begins. There is a classic sequence of evolution on the ECG, consisting of S-T segment elevation, T wave inversion, and development of Q waves. The third criterion is serum enzyme changes. The CPK and isoenzymes specific to cardiac muscle (CPK-MB) are released when damage occurs to the myocardium. This is a quite specific indication of myocardial damage.

Podiatric Implications

Podiatrists should be aware that patients with coronary artery disease, whether it be angina or myocardial infarction, have an increased risk over the general population in terms of perioperative morbidity and mortality when undergoing anesthesia and surgery. The administration of anesthetics and the performance of surgery clearly place increased amounts of stress on the myocardium. In general, elective surgery should be delayed in any patient who has had a myocardial infarction in the past 6 months. Elective surgery should also be delayed several months in patients with unstable angina. The unstable angina should be treated medically or, if necessary, the coronary artery anatomy should be studied to give a better indication of the patient's risk.

When the patient with ischemic heart disease undergoes elective surgery, the patient's antianginal medication should be continued throughout the perioperative period. When the order for the patient is nothing by mouth (NPO), either sublingual long-acting nitrates or nitroglycerin preparations for use on the skin may be used. Beta-blockers such as propranolol should be given throughout the preoperative and perioperative periods when they are being used for control of angina.

Congestive Heart Failure

Congestive heart failure is a clinical syndrome that results from the inability of the heart to deliver a supply of oxygenated blood sufficient to meet the demands of the metabolizing tissues. The causes of congestive heart failure may be classified into the following six areas:
1. Systemic hypertension.
2. Valvular heart disease.

3. Myocardial disease.
4. Pericardial disease.
5. Pulmonary hypertension.
6. High output states such as thyrotoxicosis or anemia.

In the aforementioned situations, there is either increased cardiac work or decreased myocardial function. In either case, there is decreased pumping effectiveness of the heart, which results in the inability to pump adequate quantities of blood to the tissues. When it is primarily the left side of the heart that is failing, the right side continues to pump blood into the lungs normally, but the left side of the heart is unable to push the blood on into the systemic circulation. The resulting accumulation of blood in the lungs increases the pressures in all the pulmonary vessels and engorges them with blood, allowing the leakage of fluid into the lung tissues, which results in pulmonary edema. If the right side of the heart fails, right atrial pressure rises, causing most of the blood attempting to return to the heart to be backed into the peripheral veins. As a result, the pressures throughout the entire venous system rise; neck veins become greatly distended; venous reservoirs in the liver and spleen become engorged with blood; and eventually lower extremity edema occurs, as the entire venous circulatory system causes leaking into the tissue spaces (Table 1–8).

Clinical Manifestations

The clinical manifestations of left-sided congestive heart failure include dyspnea, orthopnea, paroxysmal nocturnal dyspnea, and acute pulmonary edema. In all these situations, there is a congestion of blood in the lungs resulting from back-up of blood from the left atrium. The most prominent physical findings in left-sided congestive heart failure are moist rales in the lungs, tachypnea or rapid breathing, and an extra mid-diastolic sound known as the S_3 gallop. The S_3 gallop indicates a failing left ventricle. Clinical manifestations of right-sided congestive heart failure are dependent edema in the lower extremities and distended neck veins.

Diagnosis and Treatment

Ancillary data that are useful in diagnosing congestive heart failure include the chest radiograph. The earliest radiographic sign of congestive heart failure is distention of the pulmonary veins of the

Table 1–8. EFFECTS OF HEART FAILURE

Backward Effects	Forward Effects
Failure of the Left Ventricle	
Decreased emptying of left ventricle	Decreased cardiac output
Increased volume and pressure in left ventricle	Decreased perfusion of body tissues
Increased volume and pressure in left atrium	Decreased blood flow to kidneys and glands
Increased volume in pulmonary veins	Increased secretion of sodium- and water-retaining hormones
Increased volume in pulmonary capillary bed	
Transudation of fluid from capillaries to alveoli	Increased reabsorption of sodium and water
Rapid filling of alveolar spaces	Increased extracellular fluid volume
Pulmonary edema	Increased total blood volume
Decreased emptying of right ventricle	
Sometimes referred to as congestive theory or backward theory of heart failure	Sometimes referred to as low output theory or forward theory of heart failure
Failure of the Right Ventricle	
Decreased emptying of right ventricle	
Increased volume and increased end-diastolic pressure in right ventricle	
Increased volume (pressure) in right atrium	
Increased volume and pressure in great veins	
Increased volume in systemic venous circulation	Decreased volume from right ventricle to lungs
Increased volume in distensible organs (liver, spleen)	Decreased return to left atrium and subsequent decreased cardiac output
Increased pressure at capillary line	
Hepatomegaly, splenomegaly	All forward effects of left-sided heart failure
Dependent edema and serous effusion	Expansion of blood volume

(From Groer ME, et al.: Basic Pathophysiology: A Conceptual Approach. St. Louis: CV Mosby Co, 1979.)

upper lobe in an upright chest film. In addition, there may be interstitial pulmonary edema appearing as septal edema, known as Kerley's lines. Electrocardiographic findings are generally not helpful in the diagnosis of congestive heart failure.

The therapy for congestive heart failure includes correction of any reversible factors such as cardiac arrhythmias, anemia, thyrotoxicosis, and hypertension. Surgical correction of significant valvular or congenital cardiac lesions may be indicated in specific situations. Congestive heart failure that persists after correction of reversible causes is best treated with a combination of salt restriction, digitalis glycosides, and diuretics. Although diuretics and digitalis are the cornerstones of therapy, they are often inadequate in treating patients with severe disease. This is particularly true in elderly patients with other chronic diseases, among whom the incidence of congestive heart failure is relatively high. Consequently, adjunctive pharmacologic therapy with venous and arterial dilators is increasingly utilized in severe congestive heart failure. These dilators relieve dyspnea as well as symptoms of low cardiac output.

Angiotensin converting enzyme inhibitors have been widely used to treat chronic congestive heart failure that has not responded adequately to digitalis and diuretics. Adding an ACE inhibitor to digoxin and a diuretic may be the optimal treatment for some patients with chronic congestive heart failure.

Finally, bed rest is also extremely helpful as a treatment modality because it mobilizes fluid from the peripheral circulation and increases venous return to the heart. Bed rest reduces metabolic demands and, therefore, diminishes blood flow requirements, allowing the heart to work less hard.

Podiatric Implications

In terms of podiatric concerns, two issues should be addressed. First, if a patient has signs or symptoms of congestive heart failure and it appears that the patient's symptoms are acute or may be under poor control, the patient should be referred immediately for evaluation of management of congestive heart failure before any podiatric treatment is rendered. Second, if a patient with congestive heart failure is being treated with diuretics and is being assessed preoperatively, it should be determined that he or she does not have electrolyte disturbances induced by diuretics, mainly hypokalemia. Also, the podiatrist should be aware that if the patient is being treated with digitalis glycosides, he or she may conceivably have symptoms indicative of digitalis overdose, such as gastrointestinal symptoms of anorexia, nausea, and vomiting; visual disturbances of blurring or green or yellow tinting of images; or life-threatening arrhythmias.

Congestive heart failure when controlled is not a contraindication to elective surgery. However, if the patient clearly has poorly controlled congestive heart failure manifested by symptoms of shortness of breath, orthopnea, and expressing signs such as neck vein distention while supine and an S_3 gallop or rales on auscultation of the lungs, it is well advised to have the patient treated for the congestive heart failure before embarking on elective surgery.

Bacterial Endocarditis

Infective endocarditis is a microbial infection of the heart valves or endocardium. Two conditions must be met before bacterial endocarditis can occur. First, there must be an underlying cardiac lesion or deranged blood flow. Such lesions may be artificial heart valves or deformed heart valves secondary to rheumatic fever or congenital heart disease. Second, the infecting organism must have a portal of entry into the blood stream and must establish a bacteremia. Although transient bacteremia is usually asymptomatic, those patients with valvular heart disease are notable exceptions. Bacteria introduced into the blood stream are clumped by circulating antibodies and deposited on these pre-existing lesions. Fibrous vegetations may then separate and be propelled as emboli into the systemic or pulmonic circulation or both, producing bacterial abscesses in such organs as the brain, spleen, kidney, and lungs.

Clinical Manifestations and Physical Findings

Although patients with infectious endocarditis may present clinically in many different ways, there are certain symptoms and signs that are present (Fig. 1–24). A patient suffering from subacute infectious endocarditis may present with complaints such as "I am just not myself" or "I find I get tired so easily." This feeling of malaise and tiredness may have been present for several months before the patient sought any medical attention. A patient may complain of anorexia and weight loss. Some patients complain of a low-grade fever but only those who are conscious of a slight rise in temperature. Often the patient may complain of aching joints. Polyarthritis is one of the most common complaints.

The traditional acute form of bacterial endocarditis is a rapidly progressive, destructive lesion to the heart valves and endocardium by a highly virulent organism, most commonly *Staphylococcus aureus*. Surgery of infected tissue or bone, intravenous drug abuse, and insertion of a prosthesis are risk factors for this type of endocarditis. The patient usually presents with more abrupt and remarkable symptoms; he or she may complain of a sudden onset of high fever, shaking, chills, and profound weakness. The patient often states that he or she felt quite well until the onset of the illness and can frequently remember to the date when symptoms began.

Physical findings of infectious endocarditis include petechiae on the conjunctivae, buccal cavity, and skin, especially over the trunk. Painful fingertips (Osler's nodes) and painless erythematous lesions usually on the palms of the hands or soles of the feet (Janeway's lesions) along with splinter hemorrhages of the nails are also common physical signs. Fever, splenomegaly, and anemia may be present.

One of the most common clinical findings in patients at risk for endocarditis or with active endocarditis is a pathologic heart murmur. Abnormal heart sounds or murmurs are produced by excessive blood flowing through a normal valve or by blood flowing through a damaged valve. Either situation has a high risk for endocarditis. There are certain criteria that distinguish an innocent or benign murmur from a pathologic murmur (see Table 1–3). With an increase in the amount of surgery that is performed in the physician's office, the importance of the podiatrist's listening to the heart for abnormal sounds is obvious. If a pathologic murmur is heard, the patient should be referred to an internist for eval-

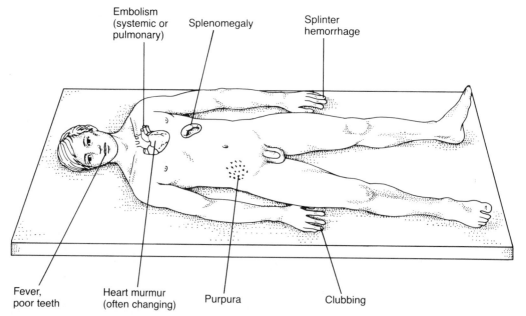

Figure 1–24. Clinical features of subacute bacterial endocarditis. (Redrawn from Hull D, et al.: Essentials of Paediatrics. London: Churchill Livingstone, 1981.)

uation. In most cases, these patients then undergo echocardiography.

Diagnosis

A blood culture is the most important laboratory test for diagnosis. This is because of the constant shedding of bacteria from the valvular site into the systemic circulation. Suspicion of infective endocarditis should be followed up by obtaining six blood cultures, preferably at different fever spikes. Within 2 to 7 days of incubation, 80 to 90% of these cultures grow organisms and permit specific drug selection. A complete blood count (CBC) is helpful in diagnosing significant leukocytosis and anemia. Leukocytosis is caused by bacterial systemic infection, whereas anemia is caused by relative bone marrow suppression by the infection. Echocardiography may show the presence of bacterial clumps known as vegetations on affected heart valves. Electrocardiograms and chest radiographs are not helpful for this diagnosis.

Podiatric Implications

The actual risks of developing endocarditis with a specific cardiac lesion following a particular procedure are unknown. A previous episode of infective endocarditis and a history of rheumatic valvular disease are both high risks for developing endocarditis infections. Patients with congenital heart lesions also warrant prophylactic antibiotic consideration before undergoing a podiatric procedure. Patients with prosthetic valves present a very high risk of incurring infection, probably as a result of the colonization of the prosthesis or the site of attachment of the prosthesis during transient bacteremia. Another subset of patients who must be considered for endocarditis prophylaxis are those patients with prolapsed mitral valves. In studies of apparent failure of endocarditis prophylaxis, mitral valve prolapse was found to be the most common underlying cardiac lesion. It is recommended that a patient with a prolapsed mitral valve associated with mitral valve regurgitation be given prophylactic antibiotics when undergoing surgery. It is not necessary to give prophylactic treatment to patients with mitral valve prolapse that is not associated with regurgitant flow.

There are certain podiatric surgical procedures that warrant consideration for prophylaxis in a high-risk patient. Included among these are surgery of any infected or contaminated tissues; operative procedures, regardless of whether they are forefoot or rearfoot, lasting longer than 90 minutes, especially if a tourniquet is used; and procedures associated with a high morbidity, for example, major foot reconstruction or excessive tissue dissection. Prosthetic implantation in the foot is another clean surgery in which prophylaxis is indicated in patients at risk for endocarditis.

When choosing the proper antibiotic for endocarditis prophylaxis, one must remember that the most common bacterial organisms are S. aureus, coagulase-negative staphylococci, lipophilic diphtheroids, and Propionibacterium. The most common organism found in podiatric infections is S. aureus. Therefore, the proper antibiotic for prophylaxis is assumed to be cephalosporin or penicillinase-resistant penicillin (Table 1–9).

The concept of antimicrobial prophylaxis and bacterial endocarditis is eminently reasonable. However, it has not been possible to perform prospective clinical studies to demonstrate the efficacy of any antimicrobial regimen in the prevention of endocarditis. The most widely quoted recommendations for antimicrobial prophylaxis have been those of the Committee on Rheumatic Fever and Infective Endocarditis, sponsored by the American Heart Association. These recommendations are updated every year and are available in pamphlets and abbreviated wallet-card forms from the American Heart Association. Every clinical podiatrist should become familiar with the latest American Heart Association statement about endocarditis prophylaxis.

CARDIAC MEDICATIONS IN CLINICAL PODIATRY

Perhaps the most common group of drugs encountered by the podiatrist are those used to treat cardiovascular diseases. Hypertension, ischemic heart disease, and congestive heart failure are very common,

Table 1–9. CURRENT RECOMMENDATIONS FOR TREATMENT OF BACTERIAL ENDOCARDITIS

Organism	Preferred Antibiotics in Order of Preference	Dosage	Route	Duration (wk)	Exceptions and Comments
Streptococcus fecalis (enterococcus)	1. Penicillin	20 mU/d*	IV	4–6	Some would use ampicillin, but no evidence of superiority available
	and Streptomycin	500 mg q12h	IM	4–6	
	2. Penicillin	20 mU/d*	IV	4–6	Recommended by some if organism resistant to streptomycin (MIC >2000 µg/ml)
	and Gentamicin	1 mg/kg q8h	IM	4–6	
	3. Vancomycin	0.5 g/q6h	IV	4–6	Allergy to penicillin—watch carefully for renal toxicity or ototoxicity; follow vancomycin blood levels (peak <30 and trough <10 µg/ml)
	and Streptomycin	500 mg q12h	IM	4–6	
Viridans streptococci (i.e., penicillin-sensitive oral streptococci, including *S. bovis*)	1. Aqueous crystalline penicillin G	10–20 mU/d*	IV	2	Primarily for patients <65 yr old with normal renal and VIIIth nerve function and uncomplicated disease
	and Streptomycin	10 mg/kg body wt (not >500 mg) q12h	IM	2	
	or Procaine penicillin G	1.2 mU/q6h	IM	2	
	and Streptomycin	10 mg/kg body wt (not >500 mg) q12h	IM	2	
	2. Aqueous crystalline penicillin G	10–20 mU/d*	IV	4	Preferred in most patients >65 yr old or with impairment of renal or VIIIth nerve function, which serve as relative contraindications to the use of streptomycin
	3. Aqueous crystalline penicillin G	10–20 mU/d*	IV	4	Recommended for patients with shock, extracardiac foci of infection, prosthetic valve endocarditis, or when infected with nutritionally deficient variants of viridans streptococci
	and Streptomycin	10 mg/kg body wt (not >500 mg) q12h	IM	2	
	4. Vancomycin	10 mg/kg body wt (not >500 mg) q6h	IV	4	Allergy to penicillin and cephalosporin; VIIIth nerve toxicity, and, occasionally, nephrotoxicity may occur
	5. Cephalothin	2.0 g q4h	IV	4	Allergy to penicillins
	or Cefazolin	1.0 g q6h	IV or IM	4	

Organism	Drug(s)	Dosage	Route	Duration (wk)	Comments
	6. Aqueous crystalline penicillin G	20 mU/d*	IV	4	If resistant to penicillin G (MIC >0.2 µg/ml)
	and				
	Streptomycin	10 mg/kg body wt (not >500 mg) q12h	IM	2–4	Should omit aminoglycoside when renal or otic impairment present. Prosthetic valve should be treated 6 wk
Staphylococcus aureus	1. Nafcillin	1.5 g q4h	IV	4	
	and				
	Gentamicin or tobramycin	1 mg/kg q8h	IM or IV	(3–5 days)	
	2. Nafcillin (Methicillin) (Oxacillin)	1.5 g q4h	IV	4	Allergy to penicillins and cephalosporins
	3. Vancomycin	0.5 g q6h	IV	4	Allergy to penicillins—other cephalosporin may be substituted
	4. Cephalothin	1.5–2 g q4h	IV	4	If tolerant strain isolated
	5. Vancomycin	0.5 g q6h	IV	4	
	and				
	Rifampin	300 mg q12h	PO	4	
Staphylococcus epidermidis or *Corynebacterium* species (diphtheroids) infection on prosthetic cardiac valve	1. Vancomycin	500 mg q6h	IV	6	Ideal initial treatment pending results of sensitivity testing
	and				
	Rifampin	300 mg q12h	PO	6	
	and				
	Gentamicin	1 mg/kg q8h	IM or IV	1	
	2. Penicillin	20 mU/d	IV	6	If organism shows by tube sensitivity testing it is sensitive to penicillin or nafcillin or cephalothin (others may be as good)
	or				
	Nafcillin	1.5 g q4h	IV	6	
	or				
	Cephalothin	1.5 g q4h	IV	6	
	and				
	Rifampin	300 mg q12h	IV	6	
	and				
	Gentamicin	1 mg/kg q8h	IM	1	
	3. Either of above for 6 wk followed by rifampin, 300 PO q12h for 6 mo, and cloxicillin or an oral cephalosporin, 500 mg PO q6h for 6 mo				If complication develops or relapse from initial infection (surgical removal may also be necessary)

* Constant IV infusion preferred, but q4h bolus probably as good.
MIC, Minimal inhibitory concentration; mU, million units.
(From Anderson GS, Katz JH, Zier BG: Bacterial endocarditis: Clinical considerations and prophylaxis. J Am Podiatr Med Assoc 76(6):332, 1986.)

and drugs used to treat these entities must be considered in the course of preoperative evaluation as well as in nonoperative clinical settings. Many cardiac drugs have utility in more than one disease. For example, diuretics are used to treat hypertension as well as congestive heart failure. An overview of the more common cardiac drugs and their implications for podiatric practice is presented (Table 1–10).

Diuretics

Diuretics are used to treat hypertension, congestive heart failure, and less commonly venous insufficiency and lymphedema. Diuretics are classified into three main groups: thiazide-type diuretics, loop diuretics, and potassium-retaining diuretics.

Thiazide-type diuretics have traditionally been the first drug used for the treatment of hypertension. Much concern has been raised regarding the hypercholesterolemic effect of thiazides because thiazides increase serum low-density lipoprotein cholesterol and triglyceride concentrations. This effect has been linked to atherosclerosis and ischemic heart disease. Consequently the use of thiazide-type diuretics as first-line drugs for hypertension is diminishing in favor of beta-blockers and ACE inhibitors. Thiazides can also cause hyperglycemia and hyperuricemia. These drugs are a causative factor in acute gouty attacks, although thiazide-related gout is rare. Probably the most important and frequent adverse effect of thiazides is hypokalemia. Preoperative patients taking thiazides should have serum potassium levels checked because hypokalemia can predispose to intraoperative cardiac arrhythmias.

Loop diuretics, such as furosemide, bumetanide, and ethacrynic acid, are used in hypertensive patients with fluid retention refractory to thiazides and in patients with impaired renal function. Loop diuretics are also used in patients with severe heart failure refractory to thiazides. Besides hypokalemia and hyperuricemia, these medications can cause dehydration and circulatory collapse because they have a more rapid onset of action and are more potent than thiazides. Preoperative potas-

Table 1–10. CARDIAC MEDICATIONS IN CLINICAL PODIATRY

Diuretics

Thiazides
Chlorothiazide (Diuril)
Hydrochlorothiazide (Esidrex)
Polythiazide (Renese)
Chlorthalidone (Hygroton)

Loop Diuretics
Bumetanide (Bumex)
Furosemide (Lasix, others)

Potassium-Retaining
Amiloride (Midamor, others)
Spironolactone (Aldactone, others)
Triamterene (Dyrenium)

Combinations
Aldactazide (Hydrochlorthiazide and spironolactone
Hydrochlorothiazide and triamterene (Dyazide, Maxide)
Hydrochlorothiazide and amiloride (Modiuretic)

Beta-Adrenergic Blocking Drugs

Acebutolol (Sectral)
Atenolol (Tenormin)
Metoprolol (Lopressor)
Nadolol (Corgard)
Propranolol (Inderal)

Angiotensin Converting Enzyme Inhibitors

Captopril (Capoten)
Enalopril (Vasotec)
Lisinopril (Prinivil)

Calcium-Entry Blockers

Diltiazem (Cardizem)
Verapamil (Calan, Isoptin)

Central Sympatholytic Drugs

Clonidine (Catapres, Catapres Trandemal, others)

Nitrates

Nitroglycerin Sublingual Tablets
Nitroglycerin Transdermal System
Nitroglycerin Sustained Oral Release Tablet
Nitroglycerin Ointment
Intravenous Nitroglycerin
Isosorbide Dinatrate (Isordil, Sorbitrate)

Digitalis Glycosides

Digitoxin
Digoxin (Lanoxin)

Cardiac Arrhythmia Drugs

Acebutolol (Sectral)
Disopyramide (Norpace)
Flecanide (Tambocor)
Lidocaine (Xylocaine, others)
Procainamide (Pronestyl, others)
Propranolol (Inderal, others)
Quinidine (many brands)
Verapamil (Isoptin, Calan)

sium levels must be checked and careful attention paid to perioperative fluid balance.

Potassium-retaining diuretics, such as spironolactone and aldactone, are used mainly with other diuretics to prevent or correct hypokalemia. These diuretics can cause life-threatening hyperkalemia if used in patients with unsuspected renal impairment.

Beta-Adrenergic Blocking Drugs

Beta-adrenergic blocking drugs are often used for the initial treatment of hypertension. These drugs are effective in hypertension because they decrease heart rate and cardiac output as well as decrease renin release. Beta-adrenergic blockers also prevent angina by reducing myocardial oxygen requirements during exertion and stress. Consequently these drugs are often used for long-term therapy to prevent angina. Beta-adrenergic blockers can cause fatigue, bradycardia, decreased exercise tolerance, and congestive heart failure. Beta-adrenergic blockers can also precipitate bronchial asthma in predisposed patients. The podiatrist must recognize that beta blockers can precipitate Raynaud's phenomenon and aggravate existing peripheral vascular arterial disease.

Angiotensin Converting Enzyme Inhibitors

Angiotensin converting enzyme inhibitors are being increasingly used in mild to moderate hypertension, often as a first-line drug. These agents act by inhibiting the renin-angiotensin-aldosterone system. Angiotensin converting enzyme inhibitors are effective vasodilators for the treatment of congestive heart failure. These agents can produce significant hypotension in some patients with congestive heart failure, particularly after initial dosing. These agents can also exacerbate or cause renal insufficiency owing to inadequate renal perfusion pressures. Other side effects include skin rashes, taste alterations, and chronic cough.

Calcium-Entry Blockers

Calcium-entry blockers cause vasodilatation, which decreases peripheral resistance and lowers blood pressure. Calcium-entry blockers are sometimes used as a first-line drug for hypertension. These drugs also inhibit coronary artery vasospasm and therefore play a role in treating unstable myocardial ischemia. Calcium-entry blockers can adversely effect A-V conduction and should be used with caution in patients with congestive heart failure.

Clonidine

Clonidine is a centrally acting sympatholytic drug used primarily for its antihypertensive effect. The central actions of clonidine result in reduced plasma concentrations of norepinephrine with a resulting decrease in systolic and diastolic blood pressures and heart rate. Clonidine is usually used as a second-line drug in treating hypertension, usually in combination with a diuretic or beta-blocker. Other uses include migraine prophylaxis, treatment of dysmenorrhea, and opiate and alcohol withdrawal. The podiatrist must be aware that a severe rebound in blood pressure may occur if the drug is discontinued abruptly, especially after high dose, long-term therapy, or use with a concomitant beta-blocker. For patients undergoing surgery, the last dose of clonidine is usually given 4 to 6 hours before scheduled surgery. Patients may be given a parenteral antihypertensive if necessary until oral medication can be resumed.

Nitrates

Nitrates are potent venodilators with antianginal, anti-ischemic, and antihypertensive effects. The action of nitrates is to relax vascular smooth muscle with resulting vasodilatation of peripheral blood vessels. Nitrates are used mainly for prophylaxis, treatment, and management of angina pectoris. Intravenous nitroglycerin is used to control blood presssure in perioperative hypertension and hypertension associated with congestive heart failure due to acute myocardial infarction.

Nitrates can commonly cause headache, weakness, dizziness, postural hypotension, and tachycardia. Transdermal preparations can cause contact dermatitis, and nitroglycerin ointment can cause topical allergic reactions.

Patients who are hospitalized for elective podiatric surgical procedures may be allowed to keep sublingual nitroglycerin tablets at their bedside to be taken if substernal chest discomfort occurs. At the same time, this chest discomfort must be carefully assessed to rule out significant cardiac ischemia or arrhythmias. Patients receiving long-acting nitrates who are to take nothing by mouth can be switched to equivalent doses of nitroglycerin ointment or transdermal preparations so as to continue prophylaxis for myocardial ischemia. Patients receiving nitrate preparations should have frequent assessment of blood pressure and pulse in supine and sitting positions to guard against hypotension and tachycardia.

Digitalis Glycosides

Digitalis was once the mainstay of treatment in congestive heart failure. However, there is increasing evidence that patients with underlying coronary artery disease are at greater risk of death when treated with digitalis. In addition, the availability of potent diuretics and vasodilators that more consistently relieve the symptoms of heart failure have relegated digitalis to a more secondary role in the drug therapy of heart failure. The therapeutic-to-toxic ratio of digitalis is quite narrow. Consequently digitalis toxicity is a common problem. Symptoms of digitalis toxicity include anorexia, nausea, vomiting, headache, visual changes, and disorientation. Cardiac arrhythmias may also reflect digitalis toxicity. Serum digoxin assays are readily available and can help to make the diagnosis of digitalis toxicity. The podiatrist should realize that hypokalemia predisposes to digitalis toxicity. If a podiatrist has need to prescribe diuretics in a patient already receiving digitalis, serum potassium levels must be monitored. In addition, preoperative patients receiving diuretics and digitalis should have potassium levels assessed.

Drugs for Cardiac Arrhythmias

The most common antiarrhythmic agents encountered by the podiatrist include digitalis, for atrial fibrillation and atrial flutter; verapamil, for supraventricular tachycardia; lidocaine, for ventricular premature contractions, ventricular tachycardia, and ventricular fibrillation; procainamide, for chronic therapy of ventricular premature contractions; propranolol, for controlling ventricular rate in atrial tachyarrhythmias; and quinidine, for atrial fibrillation and ventricular premature contractions.

Podiatric considerations regarding the use of antiarrhythmic agents are mainly directed toward two clinical situations. One is the treatment of acute-onset arrhythmias in the intraoperative period. The decision to use antiarrhythmic agents in this setting is one that is reached after consultation with anesthesia or internal medicine specialists. The role of the podiatrist should be to institute basic cardiopulmonary resuscitation while triaging the patient to an intensive care setting for definitive diagnosis and therapy. The second consideration regarding antiarrhythmic therapy has to do with patients presenting preoperatively who are taking long-term antiarrhythmic agents. As mentioned previously, patients taking digitalis need to have serum digitalis assays measured as well as potassium levels assessed. Patients taking digitalis, procainamide preparations, quinidine, and beta-blockers should have these drugs continued throughout the perioperative period. Obviously any patient with a history of cardiac arrhythmia or palpitations or who is taking an antiarrhythmic agent should have a preoperative ECG performed as a reference.

PODIATRIC SURGERY IN THE CARDIAC PATIENT

Approximately 10% of people in the United States have some form of cardiovascular disease. Because of the frequency with which cardiovascular disease occurs, the patient must be evaluated very carefully when podiatric surgery is considered to determine whether such disease is present. Significant cardiovascular disease in an individual patient may not be obvious. The podiatrist must evaluate all pertinent aspects of the patient. The preoperative evaluation should include a careful history and physical examination, a chest x-ray study if the patient has not had a chest x-ray in the posteroanterior plane since the age of 16, documentation of an old or new ECG in patients over the age of 40, and any pertinent laboratory blood chemistry data.

Risk Factors. Several classifications have been used in an attempt to categorize cardiac risk factors in all potential surgical patients. In 1977 and 1978, Goldman and associates produced an excellent study, reporting on 1001 consecutive patients, all age 40 or over, who underwent noncardiac operations. Table 1–11 lists in decending order the approximate risk ratio to determine for perioperative cardiac death. Because optimum management of complications is predicated on identifying high-risk patients, such a table allows one to screen an individual patient and to see what risk factors he or she has and how much each risk factor is increased as compared with the normal patient. A history of myocardial infarction within 3 months, jugular venous distention or S_3 gallop, cardiac rhythm other than sinus, age over 70 years, an emergency operation, the presence of a significant aortic stenosis, and ventricular arrhythmias are all high-risk factors for myocardial infarction and cardiac death after noncardiac surgery. One other important consideration is the reversibility of some of these risk factors, such as timing of elective surgery following a prior myocardial infarction, correction of congestive heart failure, medical management of a serious cardiac arrhythmia, and special cautions in patients over the age of 70.

Drug Therapy. Finally, one other point involves the issue of preoperative cardiac drug therapy. For the most part, drugs used to control cardiovascular disorders should not be withdrawn before surgery. Drugs used for the treatment of hypertension, arrhythmia, cardiac failure, and angina pectoris can usually be given with a sip of water on the day of surgery, and therapy can be continued orally the next day. Alternatively, these drugs can usually be given parenterally. There are specific hazards to withdrawing abruptly some drugs; for example, withdrawing clonidine hydro-

Table 1–11. CARDIAC RISK FACTORS FOR PATIENTS UNDERGOING SURGERY*

Criteria	Finding	Points
History	Age over 70	5
	Myocardial infarction in previous 6 months	10†
Physical examination	S_3 or jugular venous distention	11†
	Significant aortic stenosis	3
Electrocardiogram	*Any* rhythm other than normal sinus	7
	Premature atrial contractions on last preoperative ECG	7†
	More than 5 premature contractions per minute on *any* previous ECG	7
General status	Po_2 less than 60 mm Hg, Pco_2 greater than 50 mm Hg	
	K^+ less than 3.0 mEq/L, HCO_3 less than 20 mEq/L	
	BUN greater than 50 mg/dl, creatinine greater than 3.0 mg/dl	
	Abnormal SGOT or signs of chronic liver disease	3†
Operation	Emergency surgery	4†
	Intraperitoneal, thoracic, or major vascular procedure	3

* For clinical purposes, each finding is assigned a point value. Cardiac risk index is noted by the total number of points assigned to a particular patient.
Class I = 0–5 points
Class II = 6–12 points
Class III = 13–25 points
Class IV = >26 points
There is a statistically significant increase in cardiac risk in the progression from risk class I to risk class IV.
   † Risk factors that may be altered by preoperative intervention or delay of surgery.
   BUN, Blood urea nitrogen; HCO_3, the bicarbonate radical Pco_2, carbon dioxide partial pressure or tension; Po_2, partial pressure of oxygen; SGOT, serum glutamic-oxalacetic transaminase.
   (Adapted from Goldman L, Caldera DL, Nussbaum SR, et al.: Multifactorial index of cardiac risk in noncardiac surgical procedures. N Engl J Med 297:845, 1977.)

chloride may cause rebound hypertension, and withdrawing propranolol hydrochloride may cause a myocardial oxygen supply-demand imbalance.

As mentioned previously in the section on endocarditis, patients with valvular heart disease or with prosthetic valves are at risk of developing infective endocarditis during many forms of noncardiac surgery. The American Heart Association recommends antibiotic prophylaxis to be used in those patients when undergoing surgery or instrumentation of the upper respiratory, gastrointestinal, and genitourinary tracts or when having dental procedures likely to cause gingival bleeding. The American Heart Association guidelines should also be followed in podiatric surgery in which the surgical site is infected or in which the procedure involves the rearfoot or requires a prolonged operating time (longer than 1 hour).

In the operating room, prevention of regional myocardial oxygen imbalance in patients with coronary artery disease and ventricular dysfunction in all patients with cardiac disease is of paramount concern. Tachycardia must not be allowed to persist in patients with known coronary artery disease. In addition, blood pressure should not be allowed to remain in an extremely labile state. Episodes of hypertension during surgery are common, particularly during maintenance anesthesia. Swings in blood pressure are more marked in hypertensive patients and are more likely, in surgery, to be associated with cardiovascular complications. Antihypertensive medications should be continued up to the time of surgery because blood pressure during surgery is more stable when the patient is receiving treatment. Adverse interactions between anesthetic agents and antihypertensive medications are mild.

Finally, postoperative pain management should be effected, especially in the cardiac patient, in order to lessen any undue anxiety and tachycardia.

Bibliography

Anderson JL, Mason JW: Testing the efficacy of antiarrhythmic drugs. N Engl J Med 315:391, 1986.

Barnett PA, et al.: The frequency and prognostic significance of electrocardiographic abnormalities in clinically normal individuals. Prog Cardiovasc Dis 23:299, 1981.

Bigger JT: Definition of benign versus malignant ventricular arrhythmia. Am J Cardiol 52:47C, 1983.

Bor DH, Himmelstein DU: Endocarditis prophylaxis in patients with mitral valve prolapse. Am J Med 76:711, 1984.

Clemens JD, Ransohoff DF: A quantitative assessment of predental antibiotic prophylaxis for patients with mitral valve prolapse. J Chron Dis 37:531, 1984.

Colucci WS, Wright RF, Braunwald E: New positive inotropic agents in the treatment of congestive heart failure. N Engl J Med 314:349, 1986.

Cranley JJ, et al.: The diagnosis of deep venous thrombosis, fallibility of clinical signs and symptoms. Arch Surg 11:34, 1976.

Dustan HP: Nutrition and hypertension. Ann Intern Med 98:660, 1983.

Everett ED, Hirshman JV: Transient bacteremia and endocarditis prophylaxis: A review. Medicine, 56:61, 1977.

Fairbairn JF II, et al. (eds): Clinical Manifestations of Peripheral Vascular Disease, 5th ed. Philadelphia: WB Saunders Co, 1980.

Goldmann DR, et al. (eds): Medical Care of the Surgical Patient: A Problem-Oriented Approach to Management. Philadelphia: JB Lippincott Co, 1982.

Goodreau JK, Creasy JK, Flanigan DP, et al.: Rational approach to the differentiation of vascular and neurogenic claudication. Surgery 84:749, 1978.

Graboys TB: The treatment of supraventricular tachycardias. N Engl J Med 312:43, 1985.

Hallet JW Jr, et al. (eds): Foot Care Manual of Patient Care in Vascular Surgery. Boston: Little, Brown & Co, 1982.

Harrison DC, Fitzgerald MD, Winkle RA: Ambulatory electrocardiography for diagnosis and treatment of cardiac arrhythmias. N Engl J Med 294:373, 1976.

Huisman MV, Buller HR, et al.: Serial impedance plethysmography for suspected deep venous thrombosis in outpatients. N Engl J Med 314:823, 1986.

Hurst JW (ed): Medicine for the Practicing Physician. Boston: Butterworth Publishers, 1983.

Kammerer WS, Gross RJ: Medical Consultation. Baltimore: Williams & Wilkins, 1983.

Lewis HD, Davis JW, Archibald DG, et al.: Protective effects of aspirin against acute myocardial infarction and death in men with unstable angina. N Engl J Med 309:396, 1983.

McKee PA, et al.: Natural history of congestive heart failure: The Framingham study. N Engl J Med 285:1444, 1971.

Molitch ME: Management of Medical Problems in Surgical Patients. Philadelphia: FA Davis Co, 1982.

Pollock ML, Wilmore JH, Fox SM: Exercise in Health and Disease. Philadelphia: WB Saunders Co, 1984.

Porter JM, Baur GM: Pharmacologic treatment of intermittent claudication. Surgery 92:966, 1982.

Rubenstein E, Federman DD (eds): Scientific American Medicine. New York: Scientific American, Inc, 1987.

Ruschhaupt WF: Differential diagnosis of edema at the lower extremities. Cardiovasc Clin 13:307, 1983.

Wyngaarden JB, Smith LH: Cecil Textbook of Medicine, 17th ed. Philadelphia: WB Saunders Co, 1984.

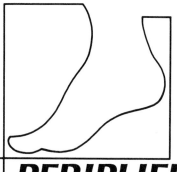

2 PERIPHERAL VASCULAR DISEASE

JONATHAN LEVIN, BENNETT G. ZIER, GAIL M. GRANDINETTI, and ARLENE F. HOFFMAN

Common Venous Disorders
    Venous Obstruction or Insufficiency
    Deep Venous Thrombosis
    Superficial Thrombophlebitis
    Chronic Venous Insufficiency

Therapeutic Approaches to Venous
    Diseases
Common Lymphatic Disorders
    Lymphedema
    Lymphangitis

OVERVIEW

Diseases of the peripheral vascular system are very common and may involve the arteries, veins, and lymphatics. It is essential that the podiatric physician become familiar with the circulation and its incumbent abnormalities in the lower extremity. In order to manage vascular problems with predictable, successful outcomes, one not only depends on his or her own skill and knowledge but also on the body's ability to heal, no matter what interventional measures are taken. The most important factor determining whether or not healing will take place is the degree of blood supply to the operated or affected area. Many other factors are also involved in wound healing, and, in some cases, there is less than optimal healing even in the presence of an adequate blood supply. An intact transport system, the components of which are the heart, blood vessels, and lymphatics, is essential. Any alterations in the function of any of these components affect delivery of nutrients, oxygen, and other substances to various parts of the body.

The objective of this chapter is to provide a basic working knowledge of diseases in the vascular system with particular attention to lower extremity problems and their therapeutic management. The diseases include aortoiliac, femoropopliteal, and aortic occlusive and aneurysmal disorders. The two most important pathologies of the peripheral arteries are atherosclerosis of the larger arteries and microvascular disease.

Although one would presume that age and arterial occlusive disease go hand in hand, there are certain diseases in which arterial occlusions exist at an earlier age. These diseases include diabetes mellitus, hypercholesterolemia, hypertriglyceridemia, and accelerated hypertension. Therefore the possibility of diagnosis of arterial insufficiency in a youthful patient should not be precluded simply because of age. However, incidence of arterial occlusive disease does increase with age, and manifestations may be present in patients in their 40s. Men over 40 years of age are the most commonly affected.

Atherosclerosis tends to be a generalized disease, with some involvement of all major vessels and affecting the medium-sized and large-sized vessels of the extremities. The narrowing and occlusion of the vessel with a decreased blood supply, resulting in ischemia, is the most common manifestation. Atherosclerosis may also manifest itself by aneurysmal dilatation of the arterial segment. Risk factors include hypercholesterolemia, diabetes mellitus, smoking, and hypertension. Obese patients do not necessarily carry an increased risk for atherosclerosis, although increased dietary cholesterol and fat do appear to lead to increased low-density lipoprotein (LDL) in plasma, which has been postulated to be atherogenic.

Microvascular arterial disease occurs in patients with diabetes mellitus. Changes develop in the small arterioles and medium-sized arteries that impair circulation to the skin or nerves, especially of the lower extremities, producing symptoms of ischemia.

A less common arterial disease that must be considered is arteritis of both large and small arteries.

Peripheral venous disease often progresses to venous stasis and thrombotic disorders. One of the dread complications of thrombotic disease is pulmonary embolism.

STRUCTURES AND PHYSIOLOGY

The blood is pumped by the right side of the heart to the pulmonary circulation, where it is oxygenated and then pumped out by the left side of the heart into the systemic circulation, where it delivers oxygen and nutrients to the tissues, removes the metabolic waste products, and carries various substances throughout the body. The blood vessels must be intact and functioning for this to occur.

The vascular system is a series of distensible conduits that subdivide into arterial (Fig. 2–1), venous (Fig. 2–2), and capillary components. The lymphatic system performs a complementary function to the circulatory system and must be considered when discussing this system. Large-

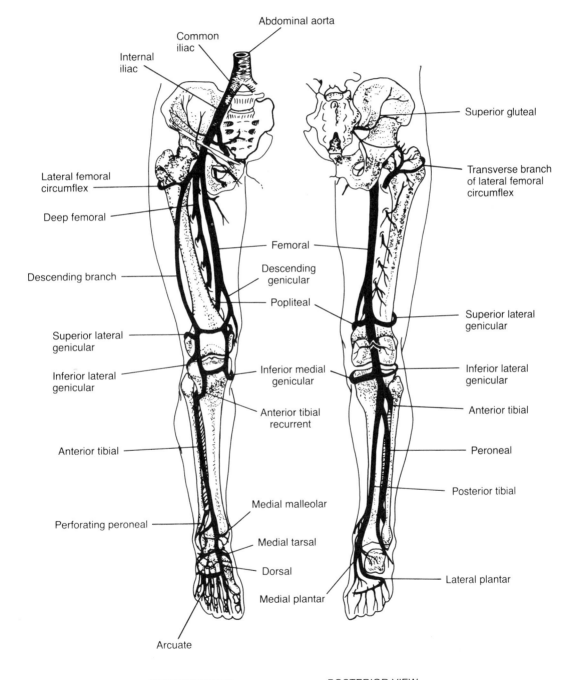

ANTERIOR VIEW   POSTERIOR VIEW

Figure 2–1. Arteries of the lower extremity.

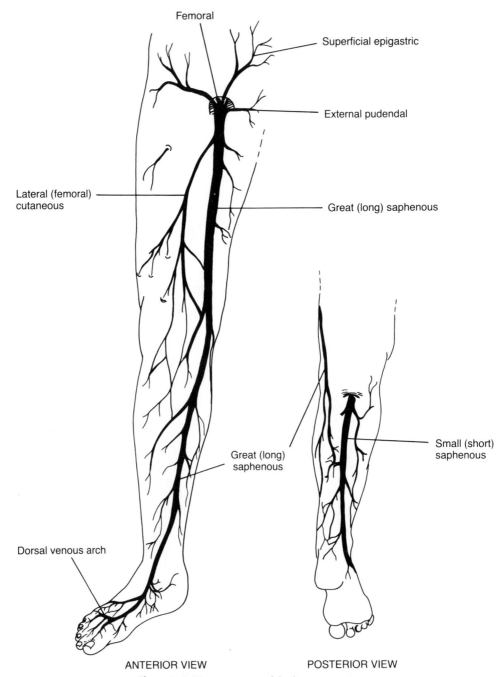

Figure 2–2. Venous system of the lower extemity.

diameter arteries, such as the aorta and its main branches, have a high elastic fiber content that converts the intermittent cardiac stroke volume to an even steady flow. These arteries are distensible, which allows accommodation for significant changes in pressure. This distensibility, along with the high resistance offered by the terminal arterioles, constitutes a hydraulic filtering system, which converts intermittent blood flow to a continuous flow to the capillaries. Blood flow during systole is the result of cardiac contraction, and blood flow during diastole is the result of the elastic recoil of the arteries as they discharge the blood that has caused their distention during systole. Reduced distensibility of the arteries results in less efficient flow during systole, reduced capillary blood flow during diastole, and increased cardiac work load.

As a result of sympathetic innervation, the vascular tone of the arterioles can be altered to increase or decrease their diameter and hence resistance to blood flow. These arterioles regulate volume and pressure in the arterial system and blood flow to the capillary bed. The arterioles, capillaries, and venules constitute the microcirculation.

Capillary distribution varies among the different types of tissues present in the body. Metabolically active tissue, such as skeletal muscle, has a relatively greater concentration of capillaries than does metabolically inactive tissue, such as cartilage. True capillaries are under neural, local, and humoral control. Changes in capillary diameter are passive and caused by changes in precapillary and postcapillary resistance.

The arterioles and precapillary sphincters are sympathetically innervated and respond to sympathetic stimulation. The capillary membrane is highly permeable to the various substances dissolved in the plasma and tissue fluids with the exception of relatively large particles, such as the plasma proteins.

Similar in appearance and closely aligned to the capillaries and tissue cells are the terminal lymphatic vessels. The vessels are more permeable to large particles than the capillaries as a result of absence of a basement membrane and presence of loose junctions between endothelial cells. The lymphatics remove excess fluid and larger-sized particles from interstitial spaces and return them to the venous circulation. The lymph vessels have valves to prevent reflux and movement of fluid within them as a result of milking action transmitted from neighboring arteries and muscles. The lymph system is the only means by which proteins that have left the intravascular compartment can be returned to it. The lymphatics are richly supplied with lymphatic tissue. Lymph nodes, many of which are located between major proximal skeletal joints, aid in filtering the lymphatic fluid before it enters the blood. The most important clinical symptoms of lymphatic obstruction are lymphedema and lymphangitis.

The venules form as the capillary network coalesces and converges to form veins of progressively larger diameter. The efficiency of the veins' returning blood to the heart depends on patency of the veins, competent valves within the veins, and adequate pumping action of the muscles that surround the veins. The veins also have valves to prevent reflux. The action of the muscles exerts a milking action, promoting venous return. Blood flow through the veins can be slowed by defective valves, which may be a result of stretching or inflammation (phlebitis) of the veins. Varicose veins and venous insufficiency are secondary to these conditions.

PATHOPHYSIOLOGY

Arterial disorders may be the result of two mechanisms: obstruction and generalized constriction or dilation of the vessels. Exposure to freezing temperatures may also impair arteriole circulation through the mechanisms of vasoconstriction and thrombosis.

Venous disorders may be the result of obstructive or nonobstructive processes. Varicose veins and chronic venous insufficiency, the sequelae of obstruction, and the resultant valvular incompetence, may result in serious damage to the skin and soft tissue.

The occlusive process reduces the lumen diameter and includes atherosclerosis, thrombus formation, and embolism. Signs of insufficiency depend on the vessel system affected.

Atherosclerosis refers to a thickening and hardening of the arteries. Muscles and elastic tissue are replaced with fibrous tissue. Calcification may occur. The ability of the arteries to change the lumen size is reduced. Atherosclerotic plaques in these arteries often give rise to thrombus formation.

Most, if not all, the ischemic problems that the podiatrist encounters are due directly or indirectly to the effects of atherosclerosis. Clinically recognizing characteristics of blood flow through nondiseased arteries is essential in assessing the blood flow in a person who has atherosclerosis. Blood flow through normal vessels requires less energy than turbulent blood flow through atherosclerotic vessels. Normal blood flow is laminar, is fairly rapid, and progresses down the artery in a pulsatile fashion with both forward and backward flow. The lumen is not narrowed by atheroma, and there is elastic recoil of the wall of the artery. As a result, assuming normal blood pressure to be 120/80, a pulse pressure of 40 mm Hg is usually sufficient to propel the blood.

Blood flow in atherosclerotic vessels differs from that in normal vessels owing to the specific changes that occur in the vessels in this disorder. In atherosclerosis, the endothelium of the intima becomes disrupted and invaded with lipids, primary cholesterol, and macrophages. This invasion represents an early lesion. As atherosclerosis progresses and becomes symptomatic, fibrous plaques with lipid cores appear. These plaques are located primarily at arterial bifurcations. As the disease progresses, necrosis of the plaque leads to ulceration of the lumen. Thrombi form at these ulceration sites. The elasticity of the arterial wall is lost as local accumulations of calcium occur. As the atherosclerotic process continues, the lumen becomes progressively narrowed.

The spectrum of atherosclerotic involvement of arteries in the lower extremities includes three groups: the aortoiliac, femoropopliteal, and tibioperoneal arteries. In many patients, there is overlap with respect not only to atherosclerotic narrowing and occlusion but also to the clinical presentation. The patient's blood pressure is a clinical measurement that allows an objective picture of the degree to which atherosclerosis is affecting arterial vascular function.

To better envision the difficulty that blood has in flowing through atheromatous vessels as compared with normal vessels, think of how much harder it is to skate on a bumpy surface as compared with a smooth surface. In a similar fashion, it requires much more energy to propel blood through a vessel the endothelium of which is no longer smooth and intact. More energy is required to propel blood through an inelastic vessel, the lumen of which is narrowed by atheromatous material. Poiseuille's equation describing fluid dynamics illustrates this fact by showing that blood flow varies directly with the pressure and indirectly with the resistance, with resistance varying directly as the radius taken to the fourth power. Flow varies, therefore, indirectly as the radius taken to the fourth power. Thus much more energy is required to propel blood through narrowed, rigid atheromatous vessels. The body provides this energy by increasing the pulse pressure. Eventually the pulse pressure can no longer be increased. When this limit occurs, first the velocity of blood flow and then the actual volume of blood flow decrease.

These changes result first in the loss of backward flow. As atherosclerosis progresses, the second change noticed is the slower velocity of blood flow and the last is the decreased volume of the flow.

Because of changes that the body can make, such as increasing pulse pressure (e.g., 160/85), blood flow and pressure are not significantly decreased until there is approximately a 50% reduction in the lumen diameter. Therefore the disease is fairly advanced by the time blood flow to an extremity is decreased. However, the characteristics of the blood flow are abnormal even before symptoms are noticed.

As atherosclerosis progresses, the atheromatous material narrows the lumen more and more. Eventually the resistance encountered by blood flow through this lumen becomes so high and the pressure to propel this blood so excessive that alternate pre-existing narrow-diameter vessels called collateral vessels begin to open up and carry blood around the obstructed vessel. Even if a major vessel, whether the superficial femoral artery or the posterior tibial artery, were to become totally occluded by atheromatous material, blood would be carried around this obstruction by collateral blood vessels. Sometimes collateral blood flow is quite adequate to maintain function in tissues that were fed by the obstructed vessel. However, sometimes this flow is not adequate.

Healing requires many factors, some recognized and identified, others not. In the elderly, tissues change. It is quite probable that the elderly do not have the same substances needed for healing and tissue repair as they did when they were younger. As a result, poor appearing tissue that is difficult to heal results. This type of tissue is often referred to as "tired tissue." Extreme caution must be exercised when assessing whether surgery should be performed on this type of tissue.

ASSESSMENT

The podiatric physician should be able to decide whether the patient is at risk for developing complications based on arterial and venous insufficiency to the tissues of the foot. However, it must be stressed that the vascular examination is only a part of the overall clinical evaluation of the patient and must be considered in context with the remainder of the history and physical examination. The decision that the patient has arterial insufficiency should be made only after a well thought out, deliberate, and compulsive evaluation of each patient. Again, all the integral parts of the history and physical examination as well as diagnostic and therapeutic maneuvers must be used, with consideration of the patient as a whole rather than small parts of the patient to be treated.

It is of primary importance to be able to recognize the presence of atherosclerosis and to assess its severity. More specifically, the podiatrist should be able to evaluate whether there is sufficient blood flow entering the foot and leg to maintain its normal nutrition, to heal, and to sustain nutrition following surgery. If it is judged that the blood flow is severely diminished, the podiatrist should refer the patient to a vascular surgeon to determine whether reconstructive vascular surgery may be performed. The probability for healing following elective podiatric surgery must be ascertained as being as close to 100% as possible, and the podiatrist must evaluate arterial flow, using very stringent criteria. A thorough and compulsive evaluation of the patient, with accurate documentation, is imperative. As atherosclerotic disease unremittingly progresses, the clinician will want to make comparisons over time and note changes, not only in the history but also in the physical examination.

History

In most instances, the patient's history reveals whether there is an ischemic problem (Table 2–1). Like a good detective, the clinician must be trained to ask the correct questions to reveal the presence of pathology. It is imperative that the clinician not ask the patient leading questions. For example, one should not ask "Do you experience more pain while walking up a hill?" Instead questions should be posed without stating an expectation. An example is "Is there any difference in your pain when you walk either up a hill or down a hill?" Pain is the principal symptom of atherosclerosis and other peripheral vascular diseases. The mode of onset, characteristics, chronologic sequence, associated symptoms, and progression of pain are historical clues that are invaluable in determining the involved vessels and severity of the disease process.

If the chief complaint or presenting complaint is gangrene of a toe or some other obvious classic ischemia-related symptom, it can be quite easy to make the diagnosis. However, oftentimes the chief complaint is not related to ischemia, and further questions must be asked. The symptoms of lower extremity arterial insufficiency are pain, numbness, coldness, burning, pallor (also a sign), tingling, and paresthesias. Most of these symptoms could be due to other disorders as well, and further clarification of the nature of the symptoms must be undertaken.

Many patients with peripheral vascular disease are asymptomatic. However, the following symptoms are manifestations of vascular disease in some patients, and questioning during the history should be focused on these specific common findings.

Pertinent Symptoms

PAIN

Pain is an extremely important symptom. The location, intensity (sharp, dull, aching), duration, exacerbating and alleviating factors, and other associated considerations must be delineated. When a patient complains of pain in the calf, arch, thigh, hip, or buttocks while walking, peripheral vascular disease of the arteries must be considered.

Ischemic Pain. Ischemic pain in muscle occurs when the metabolic demands of the tissues are not met by the energy sup-

Table 2–1. PATIENT HISTORY FOR THE PERIPHERAL VASCULAR SYSTEM

General History

1. Ask the correct questions to reveal presence of the pathology
   a. Do not ask leading questions, e.g., "Do you experience more pain while walking uphill?"
   b. Pose questions without stating an expectation, e.g., "Is there any difference in your pain when you walk either up a hill or down a hill?"
2. Chief complaint or presenting complaint
   a. An ischemic problem; classic related symptom, gangrene of a toe, easy to diagnose
   b. Complaint is not related to ischemia; further questions must be asked
   c. Patient may be asymptomatic
3. Symptoms of lower extremity arterial insufficiency
   a. Pain
   b. Numbness
   c. Coldness
   d. Burning
   e. Pallor
   f. Tingling
   g. Paresthesias
4. Differentiate symptoms from other disorders; elucidate nature of symptoms
5. History questioning should be focused on most common findings in peripheral vascular disease

Pain

1. Mode of onset
2. Characteristics
3. Chronologic sequence
4. Associated symptoms
5. Progression
6. Body location
7. Duration
8. Intensity (sharp, dull, ache)
9. Exacerbating and alleviating factors; other associated considerations
10. Pain on flat walking surface or hills
11. Distant walk
12. Relieved by rest or exercise, elevation or dependent position

Ischemic Pain

1. Ischemic complaints in order of frequency are pain, numbness, coldness, tenderness, burning, fullness, and pallor, more severe during exercise
2. Ask questions to discern differential diagnosis; i.e., neuropathy, arthritis, anemia, trauma
3. Ask about joint pain, lower back pain, specific positional pain, unequal leg length
4. Document if pain is as severe at rest as during exercise to rule out ischemic origin
5. Confirm intermittent claudication if ischemia is suspected

Intermittent Claudication

1. Inquire about pain, tightness, pressure cramp, ache, or deep pulling that is reproducible with specific activity, e.g., walking
2. How long has the intermittent claudication been present?
3. Inquire about the changes and establish progression in the symptoms that have occurred since the patient first noticed the intermittent claudication
4. How many blocks could the patient walk when the intermittent claudication was first noticed?

5. How far can the patient go now before symptoms occur (quantify distance in flat city blocks)?
6. Ask if recovery from the symptoms occurs with rest and recurs or if symptoms improved
7. Confirm if intermittent claudication occurs during exercise and if involves the buttocks, thigh, and calf areas.
8. If a male patient complains of buttock or thigh pain while walking, inquire about impotence
9. Ulcers or gangrene is usually absent unless there is femoropopliteal or tibial involvement
10. Include questions to differentiate venous claudication; shin splints; tendonitis; Morton's neuralgia; vitamin B_1 deficiency; metabolic disorders, such as McArdle's disease; and pseudoclaudication of spinal stenosis
11. Determine smoking history and level of daily activity

Rest Pain

1. Determine if onset is insidious or acute
2. Ask patient to describe and give location and time of day most noticed
3. Ask if ever awakened by this pain, and if pain is aggravated by cool temperature and elevation
4. Is pain improved by walking?

Edema

1. When was the swelling first noted, are both legs swollen equally, was it sudden swelling, is it worse at any particular time of day, and does it disappear after a night's sleep?
2. Is swelling painful or does it feel like a "heaviness" of the extremity?
3. Is swelling symmetric edema of the lower extremities that worsens as the day progresses?
4. Ask about shortness of breath and fatigue to help differentiate the source of edema

Color and Temperature Changes

1. To rule out vasospastic disorders, ask if hands and feet ever change color and what provokes these color changes
2. Does cold or heat aggravate the problem?
3. Type of pain present
4. What relieves the pain?
5. Ask about connective tissue disease; patients with connective tissue disease are more likely to have problems healing

History of Emboli

1. Ask about a history of emboli, venous stasis, prolonged bed rest, congestive heart failure, obesity, pregnancy, cancer, and use of oral contraceptives
2. History of leg ulcers, including presentation, cause, rapidity of progression, pain, treatment, occurrence
3. Symptoms secondary to emboli, such as shortness of breath, abdominal pain, neurologic symptoms, extremity pain

Ability to Heal

1. Ask about anemia, alcoholism, connective tissue disease (rheumatoid arthritis, systemic lupus erythematosus, scleroderma, Sjögren's syndrome, mixed connective disease), vasospastic disorders, poor nutrition, and "tired tissue"
2. Inadequate nutrition, such as lack of protein intake, citrus fruits, and B vitamins

Table 2–1. PATIENT HISTORY FOR THE PERIPHERAL VASCULAR SYSTEM *Continued*

3. Polycythemia or sickle cell anemia 4. Ask the patient how he or she heals when cut or bruised.	**Social Factors** 1. Cigarettes 2. Stress
Past Medical History 1. Ten risk factors have been associated with atherosclerosis: chronic cigarette smoking, hypertension, diabetes mellitus, hypercholesterolemia, hyperlipidemia, obesity, stress, lack of exercise, age, and genetic inheritance. 2. Conditions associated with atherosclerosis or embolic disease include myocardial infarction, angina, valvular heart disease, atrial fibrillation, aneurysms, and stroke. 3. Previous vascular surgeries or vascular-related hospitalizations	**Pertinent Review of Systems** *Pulmonary* 1. Heavy smoker presently or in the past *Cardiovascular* 1. Angina pectoris, coronary artery disease, myocardial infarction, valvular disease, cerebrovascular disease, peripheral vascular disease, hypertension, history of endocarditis, history of congenital heart disease
Family History 1. Hypertension, diabetes mellitus, stroke, myocardial infarction, arterial disease, hyperlipidemia, peripheral vascular disease	*Gastrointestinal* 1. Postprandial symptoms (postprandial abdominal pain) *Endocrine* 1. Diabetes mellitus, obesity, menopause, estrogen therapy, impotence
Medications 1. Medications the patient is taking currently and took in the recent past 2. Allergies	*Neurologic* 1. Impotence, stroke (cerebrovascular accident), dizziness, and changes in consciousness, contralateral hemiplegia, contralateral sensory deficits, and dysphasia.
Medical Care 1. Currently under care of internist, for what problems, last visit, health maintenance	2. Vertebrobasilar disease: diplopia, cerebellar dysfunction, changes in consciousness, facial paresis, lower extremity paresthesia, numbness, tingles, and "pins and needles" sensation.

ply. Muscle uses sugar, fat, and protein as well as oxygen as substrates for energy. The by-products of metabolism (lactate, CO_2, and other substances) accumulate and may be involved in the generation of pain and ischemic muscle. It is unknown, however, why ischemic muscle is painful. Whatever the exact reason for muscular pain in a chronically ischemic setting, the circumstances in which it arises are often similar to those that follow.

Ischemic complaints usually appear (in order of frequency) as pain, numbness, coldness, tenderness, burning, fullness, and pallor. Because these complaints are also signs of neuropathy, arthritis, anemia, trauma, and musculoskeletal abnormalities, it is important to be able to ask questions to discern the differences. Ischemic pain is more severe during exercise. The pain is located in muscles. Arthritic pain is localized in joints. Pain of neurologic origin probably correlates with lower back pain, and the pain is noticed in specific positions. Individuals with unequal leg length may be more likely to present with neurologic pain. If the presenting problems are just as severe at rest as at exercise, the complaint, most likely, is not of ischemic origin. If the patient's chief complaint is due to ischemia, the patient most likely has intermittent claudication, that is, muscle pain of ischemic origin brought on by exercise.

Intermittent Claudication. Intermittent claudication occurs during exercise. When taking the history, the physician finds the majority of these patients to have pain involving the buttocks, thigh, and calf areas. If a male patient complains of buttock or thigh pain while walking, the interviewer should inquire about impotence. Leriche's syndrome is chronic aortoiliac obstruction. The patient presents with intermittent claudication and impotence. In this syndrome, the terminal aorta and iliac arteries are involved by severe atherosclerosis at the aortic bifurcation. Distal tissue loss in the form of ulcers or gangrene is usually absent unless there is concomitant femoral popliteal or tibial involvement. Questions should be directed toward establishing the progression of the patient's symptoms, because the disease may be stable or decompensating owing to occlusion. However, symptoms may improve as collateral arteries develop and enlarge with exercise.

In the lower extremities, for example, exercising muscles call for greater blood supply. When there is no extra blood forthcoming, certain symptoms commonly occur. These symptoms are usually described as pain, tightness, pressure cramp, ache, and a deep pulling that comes on reproducibly with specific activity, most commonly walking. Obviously, the patient must be able to ambulate in order to develop these symptoms. The patient may be able to tell the physician exactly how far he or she can walk before symptoms occur. It is reasonable to attempt to quantify this distance in flat city blocks. These symptoms are known as intermittent claudication, intermittent because they occur with exercise and claudication from the Latin "to limp." To be classic intermittent claudication, there must be recovery from the symptoms described by the patient with rest, with recurrence only if the patient resumes the same activity. During this period, presumably the by-products of metabolism are cleared, and the metabolic needs of the exercising tissue decrease so that the symptoms abate. Intermittent claudication can occur at any site where there is diminished blood flow to the muscle. Thus foot, thigh, and buttock claudication are also seen. Generally with arterial blockage, the lesion occurs one joint or level above the muscle group in which the symptoms manifest. Superficial femoral artery occlusion may manifest with calf claudication. The differential diagnoses of intermittent claudication encompass musculoskeletal disorders; venous claudication; shin splints; tendonitis; Morton's neuralgia; vitamin B_1 deficiency; metabolic disorders, such as McArdle's disease; and pseudoclaudication of spinal stenosis. However, careful questioning usually will differentiate these conditions from true intermittent claudication.

Intermittent claudication generally is not an indication for reconstructive surgery, unless the symptoms are debilitating and, for example, do not allow the patient to pursue his or her livelihood. The symptoms that usually stabilize are improved if the patient stops smoking and begins exercising. Studies show that the need for revascularization is less than 5% for cases of intermittent claudication. Years ago many more patients were operated on for intermittent claudication.

When normal muscles are exercised, metabolic by-products are released. The metabolites directly cause relaxation of smooth muscle in the arterioles, venules, and precapillary sphincters. As a result, resistance in the vessels greatly decreases. Because flow is inversely proportional to resistance, blood flow through normal exercising muscles may increase 10 to 20 times. This amount of blood is required to remove the build-up of noxious metabolic waste products. When someone with atherosclerosis of the lower extremity exercises, relaxation of the smooth muscle in the vessels occurs. However, because the lumen of the atherosclerotic vessel is greatly narrowed and uneven, the volume of blood that can flow through this lumen is limited. The vessel is not then able to provide the increased volume of blood that the exercising muscle requires. Metabolic waste products build up within the muscle and produce pain. More exercise results in more waste products and increased pain. Once a person stops exercising, the rate of metabolism decreases, and the flow into the muscle gradually removes the previous built-up waste products. When enough products are removed, not only does pain decrease, but also tone increases in the smooth muscle, and blood flow into the muscle decreases.

It is therefore essential to ask the patient about how far he or she can walk and what stops him or her. It might be found that walking is limited by shortness of breath or by cardiac palpitations and not by true intermittent claudication. If the patient has intermittent claudication the onset of pain is faster if the patient walks faster or up hills. The pain usually is so severe that the patient cannot continue to walk with the pain. The patient needs to rest several minutes before being able to resume ambulation. The localization of the pain generally correlates with where the obstruction is located. The pain is usually perceived one segment distal to the obstruction. Toe pain generally reflects an occlusion in the midfoot, arch pain an occlusion in the ankle or distal leg, calf pain an occlusion in the knee or distal thigh, and so forth.

History should be correlated with physical findings; that is, the patient's information should be used to help find where the occlusion is located. For example, if the patient states that he or she has calf pain when walking and a significant occlusion in the popliteal or distal superficial femoral artery region cannot be demonstrated, non-invasive testing should be repeated after having performed an exercise test on the patient. The physician should inquire about the changes in the symptoms that have occurred since the patient first noticed the intermittent claudication. Questions that should be asked include how long the intermittent claudication has been present, how many blocks the patient could walk when the intermittent claudication was first noticed, and what changes have occurred since that time. For example, a patient who has had intermittent claudication after 4 blocks for 5 years without change would probably be a better surgical risk than someone who first developed intermittent claudication after 6 blocks 1 year ago, noticed that it progressed to intermittent claudication after 5 blocks 6 months ago, and currently experiences it after walking 4 blocks.

Patients occasionally complain of bilateral leg pain or numbness occurring while walking as well as at rest. This condition is termed pseudoclaudication and is a symptom of musculoskeletal or neurologic disease in the lumbar area.

Rest Pain. As the disease and ischemic changes progress, the patient characteristically develops rest pain, usually insidious in onset. Rest pain is associated with multilevel occlusive disease. This pain is often described as a burning or painful sensation in the foot, instep, or heel that is most noticeable at night. The pain may be present during the day, but the patient generally notes the symptom at night when there are no distractions. It is important to ask the patient about the presence of pain at night when he or she is sleeping or at rest.

Rest pain is another symptom of ischemic disease and reflects severe ischemia. The pain is produced by the body's shunting blood from the periphery to a more central circulation when the person is sleeping. When atherosclerosis is severe, the resistance in the atherosclerotic vessels in the lower extremity is extremely high. Slight diversion of blood to a central system results in a greatly decreased volume of blood going to the muscles at the lower extremity. As a result, metabolic waste products begin to build up in the muscles, and pain is elicited.

The patient with rest pain is generally awakened by it. This pain is often severe and aggravated by cool temperature and elevation. Physiologically the awakening of the patient causes blood to be shunted back to the periphery. This flow is assisted by gravity when the person sits and dangles the feet over the bed. Hence waking up, sitting up, and dangling the feet make it easier for more blood to enter into the ischemic muscle, and therefore the pain goes away.

In some cases, the patient sleeps seated with the legs hanging down over long periods of time, developing edema in the dependent tissues, and this may confuse the physician as to the nature of the primary problem, which is arterial insufficiency. There are, of course, many other causes of edema in the lower extremities, such as congestive heart failure, hypoalbuminemia, lymphatic abnormalities, infection, and venous insufficiency. One must be aware that these problems may co-exist with arterial insufficiency. Rest pain is an indication for diagnostic work-up, including angiography, and the appropriate reconstructive operation if warranted.

If the patient describes calf pain when sleeping that is relieved by walking the pain cannot be of ischemic origin because exercise should only make the pain worse. Causes of night calf pain made better with exercise are low potassium levels, insufficient stretching of muscles, and venous insufficiency. Rest pain reflects severe ischemic disease. Elective podiatric surgery should not be considered.

EDEMA

Patients who present with lower extremity edema should be asked the following questions:

1. When was the swelling first noted?
2. Are both legs swollen equally?
3. Was it sudden swelling?
4. Is the swelling worse at any particular time of day?
5. Does the swelling disappear after a night's sleep?

Because lymphedema is usually painless, the only symptom is "heaviness" of the extremity. Swelling of the legs, a form of dependent edema associated with congestive heart failure, is symmetric edema of the lower extremities that worsens as the day progresses. Inquiries should be made regarding shortness of breath and fatigue to help differentiate the source of this edema.

COLOR AND TEMPERATURE CHANGES

To rule out the presence of vasospastic disease, the clinician should ask the patient whether the hands and feet ever change color and what causes these color changes. Does cold or heat aggravate the problem? What type of pain is present? Does anything make the pain resolve? Individuals with connective tissue disease are more likely to have problems healing postsurgically because of potential vasospasm or vasculitis. Before considering surgery on any of these patients, the physician must be assured that if vasospasm or vasculitis occurs there is more than adequate blood flow and collateral vessels to compensate for potential problems. Patients who are vasospastic should be identified prior to any podiatric surgery, and steps should be taken postsurgically to minimize any tendency toward vasospasm. This tendency can be minimized by the administration of local anesthesia or by the application of heat distal to the surgical site.

History of Emboli

ARTERIAL EMBOLI

Arterial emboli should be suspected whenever there is a sudden and marked decrease in circulation to an extremity. Along with thrombotic occlusion, embolus is the most common cause of arterial insufficiency. The source of arterial embolus is the heart in over 90% of cases. In young patients with known rheumatic heart disease, atrial fibrillation or prosthetic cardiac valves, the cause of acute arterial insufficiency is fairly clear. However, in older patients in whom atherosclerosis may exist, the cause of arterial insufficiency is more difficult to ascertain. Mitral stenosis, acute myocardial infarction, ventricular aneurysm, intracardiac tumors, bacterial endocarditis, and prosthetic valves all predispose to emboli. Embolic material lodges at branch points of the arterial system. Most

lodge in arteries supplying the lower extremities: 46% in the femoral arteries, 18% in the iliac arteries, and 11% in the popliteal-tibial tree. Emboli to the upper extremities and cerebral, renal, and mesenteric arteries are less frequent.

VENOUS EMBOLI

The venous circulation is subject to emboli whenever venous thrombi form. Prolonged bed rest, congestive heart failure, surgery, obesity, local trauma to veins, pregnancy, oral contraceptive use, and cancer have all been associated with venous thrombus formation and subsequent pulmonary emboli.

Ability to Heal

It is important to be able to predict how well a person will heal, particularly if elective surgery is being contemplated. Usually adequate blood flow correlates with ability to heal. There are, however, conditions in which the presence of adequate blood flow does not correlate with the ability to heal. These conditions include anemia; alcoholism; connective tissue disease, such as rheumatoid arthritis, systemic lupus erythematosus, scleroderma, Sjögren's syndrome, and mixed connective tissue disease; vasospastic disorders; polycythemia; sickle-cell disease; poor nutrition; and "tired tissue." If the patient has any of these conditions the podiatrist must be extremely cautious before performing elective surgery because the presence of such conditions exacerbates the problems caused by arterial disease. If the podiatrist believes that a person with any of these conditions is able to heal, the measured blood flow in such a patient must be much better than adequate before surgery is performed. In addition, there must be excellent documentation of existing factors that suggest healing will occur.

Conditions associated with inadequate nutrition may similarly cause poor healing. It can be hypothesized that with inadequate nutrition, there is a lack of factors, such as albumin and red blood cells, essential for healing. Poor nutrition is frequently found in the elderly and in alcoholics. Individuals with anemia similarly heal poorly. Poor healing may result from nutritional deficiencies, especially the B vitamins, or from inadequate tissue oxygenation. Individuals with anemia frequently complain of tiredness.

Healing is poor in individuals with untreated polycythemia or sickle cell anemia because of changes in the red blood cells. In polycythemia, the increased number of red blood cells greatly increases the viscosity of the blood. As a result, blood flow through narrow-diameter vessels, such as capillaries, becomes most difficult. Blood flows much more slowly (as molasses would), and eventually coagulation and thrombosis occur within capillaries. In sickle cell anemia, flow through capillaries greatly decreases. In this instance, the flow is not decreased because of viscosity changes but instead is affected because of the altered shape of the red blood cell. The result is the same, that is, capillary obstruction and decreased nutrition to the tissues.

It is essential for the podiatrist to recognize the presence of any condition that can adversely affect healing. In addition to specifically asking about the presence of the aforementioned conditions, the podiatrist should also ask the patient how he or she heals when cut or bruised. The patient's answer should be correlated with the condition of the patient's skin. If the skin appears to heal poorly, unless proved otherwise, elective surgery should be deferred.

Medical History

Ten risk factors have been associated with atherosclerosis. The three major risk factors are long-term cigarette smoking, hypertension, and diabetes mellitus. The other risk factors are hypercholesterolemia, hyperlipidemia, obesity, stress, lack of exercise, age, and genetic inheritance. Conditions associated with atherosclerosis or embolic disease include myocardial infarction, angina, valvular heart disease, atrial fibrillation, aneurysm, and stroke. A history about any of these factors should be obtained. In younger patients, it should be determined whether a family history of hypertension, diabetes mellitus, stroke, myocardial infarction, or arterial disease exists. The podiatrist should always inquire about what medications the patient is taking. The patient should be asked when he or she last saw a physician, when the physician wants to see the patient again, and why the patient is being treated by the physician.

Pertinent Review of Systems

PULMONARY DISEASE

Patients who have lung disease often have been heavy smokers in the past. Smoking has been known to be related to atherosclerosis for a number of years.

CARDIOVASCULAR DISEASE

Patients with cardiac disease generally have diseased arteries in other parts of the body. There is a high incidence of concomitant cardiac, cerebrovascular, and peripheral vascular disease.

GASTROINTESTINAL DISEASE

Abdominal complaints may or may not be related to circulatory abnormalities. Disease entities to be kept in mind are mesenteric vascular occlusive disease, which may lead to postprandial symptoms of arterial insufficiency (postprandial abdominal pain), and certain acute disorders related to embolic phenomena.

NEUROLOGIC DISEASE

Impotence may be secondary to vascular insufficiency to the tissue composing the autonomic nervous system that is responsible for genital response. This symptom must be ascertained when taking a thorough vascular history. Cerebral occlusive disease causes many neurologic symptoms, including stroke (cerebrovascular accident), dizziness, and changes in consciousness. Occlusion of the internal carotid artery produces a syndrome of contralateral hemiplegia, contralateral sensory deficits, and dysphasia. Vertebrobasilar disease is associated with diplopia, cerebellar dysfunction, changes in consciousness, and facial paresis. Paresthesia complaints in the lower extremity may also be secondary to vascular insufficiency. The patient complains of numbness, tingles, and "pins and needles" sensation.

Physical Examination

A thorough physical examination is essential to the proper workup of the patient. One can perform the vascular examination as a unit or as part of the overall procedure, looking at each level as it is incorporated into the whole (Table 2–2). For example, the head and neck portion of the physical examination would include auscultation of carotid arteries, funduscopic vasculature, and jugular venous evaluation.

The extremities are readily accessible to examination. Usually a correct clinical diagnosis can readily be made with findings from pertinent history, physical examination, and special techniques. The physical examination of the peripheral vascular system includes measuring the blood pressure and assessing integrity of accessible arteries and veins, using standard methods and special techniques. All these techniques are usually integrated with the rest of the examination in a systematic approach. The patient's history should provide documentation for the presence or absence of arterial disease. The history should be closely correlated with the findings of the physical examination. Any discrepancies that exist between the history and the findings of the physical examination should be double-checked.

General Appearance of Lower Extremities

Skin

General Appearance. On inspection of both legs from the groin to the toes, the physician should note symmetry in size, color, and texture of skin; nailbeds; condition of nails; hair presence and distribution on the lower legs, feet, and toes; pigmentations; rashes; scars; ulcers; edema; venous pattern; and venous enlargement. The patient should be evaluated for hydration; turgor and elasticity; and lesions, including color, size, location, type, grouping, and distribution. Arterial ischemic disease in the legs often causes hair loss; dystrophic nails; and dryness, which may appear as pruritus. Lymphedema over several years causes the skin to thicken and take on a rough consistency similar to pigskin. Tissue that is adequately nourished looks healthy. If blood flow is inadequate the temperature of the skin decreases, and, in several months, the appearance of the skin and nails changes. More specifically, tone decreases, skin appears thin and atrophic, texture becomes dry and scaly, hair is absent on the digits, and nails look uniformly dystrophic. The physician should look for the presence of bruises, scars, and ulcers. The patient's appearance should be correlated with the history and the physician's subsequent estimation of blood flow. With chronic occlusive disease, it may take several months for the appearance of the pedal skin to change. In spite of normal-appearing skin, vascular ischemia of recent origin might be present. Therefore any discrepancies that might exist between the temperature and the appearance of the skin must be noted and correlated with the patient's symptoms.

Venous Patterns. The physician should ask the patient to stand for a more thorough evaluation of varicosities. The varicose veins in the areas around the proximal femoral ring and distal portion of the legs are not always seen in the supine position. The saphenous system should be inspected for varicosities. If varicosities are present the physician should look for redness or discoloration and palpate for tenderness or cords. Redness and tender cords over the region of the femoral vein suggest phlebitis. Trendelenburg's test is used to evaluate the competency of valves in the great saphenous vein and in the communicating veins between the superficial and deep venous systems. (See Special Techniques and Tests for the Lower Extremity).

Color. Color changes are common with vascular disease. Chronic arterial insuffi-

---

Table 2–2. PHYSICAL EXAMINATION OF THE LOWER EXTREMITY PERIPHERAL VASCULAR SYSTEM

Vital Signs

Blood pressure, pulse: rate and rhythm

Skin

General appearance, texture, turgor, hair distribution, ulceration: ischemic, venous, gangrene

Vascular Signs

Arterial pulses: femoral, posterotibial, dorsal artery of the foot; SPVPFT, pallor on elevation, venous patterns, color, temperature, edema, bruits: carotid, abdominal, femoral, calf pain

Lymphatics

Edema

Neurologic Signs

Sensory: sharp-dull, hot-cold, vibratory, proprioception, protective threshold, deep tendon reflexes: Achilles, patellar

SPVPFT, Subpapillary venous plexus filling time.

ciency produces a pale extremity. If chronic arterial insufficiency is suspected the 5-minute reactive hyperemia test may be useful. The degree of erythema that develops is correlated inversely with the degree of decreased circulation (see Noninvasive Diagnostic Tests for the Arterial System).

With chronic venous insufficiency, stasis changes produce increased pigmentation, swelling, and an "aching" or "heaviness" in legs. The leg becomes erythematous, and erosions produced by excoriations result. These changes are characteristically in the lower third of the extremity and are more prominent medially. In deep vein thrombosis, secondary inflammation of the tissue surrounding the vein produces redness, a sign of inflammation.

The color of the skin is important especially when it is correlated with temperature. Pale-colored, cool skin usually is associated with lack of blood. Bluish cool skin implies more blood flow than in pale-colored skin, but there is still less than normal flow. The blue color results from slow-flowing blood. There is more time to extract oxygen from the hemoglobin molecule. Greater amounts of reduced hemoglobin cause the bluish tinge to the skin. Erythematous warm skin is caused by increased blood flow. Infected skin is not always red and warm. If severe organic disease exists there might not be enough blood able to flow into the skin to make it red and warm. Skin that is red (ruborous) and cool is the most ominous. This is the appearance of skin just before the onset of gangrene and is caused by ischemic changes in the subpapillary venous plexus and the venules. Because there is limited arterial inflow, the skin is cool. The ischemic changes cause relaxation of smooth muscle, and venous blood backs up into the subpapillary venous plexus, giving the skin a ruborous appearance. In this instance, the reddish blue coloration reflects the beginning of tissue necrosis.

Temperature. The temperature of the skin is important to ascertain. The physician should palpate to determine symmetry in temperature by using the back of the hands, evaluating comparable areas of each extremity at the same time. Warmth is correlated with blood flow through the capillaries and the arteriovenous shunts. The physician should look for temperature gradations. Are these changes symmetric?

Sympathetic tone is high in the pedal skin and particularly in the toes. Therefore normal functional vasoconstriction might exist in the toes or distal foot. If coolness is noted it must be discerned whether the cause is vasospasm (a functional problem) or arterial occlusion (an organic problem). The 5-minute reactive hyperemia test described subsequently can readily differentiate between these two possibilities. The temperature is cool in arterial insufficiency. Chronic venous insufficiency produces a warmer than normal extremity. Patients with deep vein thrombosis have secondary inflammation of the tissue surrounding the vein. Deep vein thrombosis produces signs of inflammation, including warmth, redness, and edema.

Edema. The physician should determine if edema is pitting or nonpitting. The physician should press firmly with the thumb for at least 5 seconds behind the medial malleolus, on the dorsum of the foot, and over the shins. How proximal the edema extends within the lower extremity should be recorded. When venous insufficiency occurs, edema of dependent areas results. Swelling is the most reliable symptom and sign associated with venous obstruction. This finding is indicative of severe deep venous obstruction because the superficial veins of the lower extremity carry only 20% of the total drainage and are not associated with swelling. The extremities should be compared, and a difference in circumference of 2 cm at the ankle or midcalf should be considered significant. Lymphedema results from either a primary abnormality in the development of the lymphatic system or an acquired obstruction to flow. Whether one is dealing with the congenital or the acquired form of lymphedema, the net result is stasis of lymph fluid in the tissues, producing a firm, nonpitting edema.

Ulcerations

Ischemic Ulceration. Persistent ischemia of a limb is associated with ischemic ulceration and gangrene. Ulceration related to arterial insufficiency occurs as a result of trauma and pressure to the toes and heel. These ulcers are painful; have discrete edges, producing a "punched-out" appearance; and are often covered with crust.

Venous Ulceration. In contrast to ulcers caused by arterial insufficiency, ulcers caused by venous insufficiency are not painful. These ulcers are usually localized to the ankle area or lower leg just above the malleolus. The classic presentation is a diffusely reddened, thickened area over the medial malleolus. The skin has a cobblestone appearance, which has resulted from fibrosis and venous stasis. Ulceration occurs with the slightest trauma. Rapidly developing ulcers are commonly arterial, whereas slowly developing ulcers are usually venous.

Gangrenous Ulceration. Ulceration associated with gangrene is often described as wet or dry. Gangrenous tissue that is accompanied by drainage or liquefaction usually implies an infectious element. Dry gangrene cannot help but be contaminated with bacteria. What is actually described in differentiating wet versus dry gangrene is the host's response to the devitalized and contaminated tissue. Gangrene that is well contained has normal-appearing tissue proximal to the involved area with adequate blood supplies, so that the physical examination of the normal-appearing tissue reflects the blood supply (Table 2–3).

Arterial Pulses

The peripheral arterial pulses routinely evaluated are the radial, brachial , femoral, popliteal, dorsal artery of the foot, and posterior tibial. These pulses should be palpated and graded. The symmetry of the pulses is evaluated for rhythm, which should be regular, and amplitude, which should not vary from beat to beat. Amplitude does vary with size of artery. Pulse character should neither be bounding nor thready. The description of the amplitude of the pulse is most important. The following is the most accepted grading system: 0 = absent, 1 = diminished, 2 = normal, 3 = increased, and 4 = bounding. The following grading system can also be used: N = normal, D = diminished, A = not palpated (or absent), and B = bounding.

The timing of the femoral and radial pulses is important. Normally these pulses peak either at the same time or with the femoral pulse preceding the radial pulse. To evaluate, the physician places one hand on the femoral artery and the other on the radial pulse. The peaking of each pulse is determined. Any delay of the femoral pulse is suggestive of coarctation of the aorta, especially in hypertensive individuals. Diminished or absent pulse may suggest arterial insufficiency. If a pulse is absent in a vessel but present proximally occlusion of the vessel has occurred. Just because the vessel is occluded, blood flow distally is not necessarily inadequate. The collateral blood flow, which carries blood around the obstruction, might be sufficient to provide for distal tissue nutrition. Similarly the presence of pedal pulses does not necessarily indicate adequate pedal flow because occlusion distal to the palpation sites might exist.

Bruits

CAROTID BRUITS

The carotid artery supplies the brain and is an important part of vascular evaluation because it is helpful in determining if atherosclerotic changes may be occurring. The carotid arterial pulse is localized; strong; thrusting; and unchanged by inspiration, expiration, and changes in position. Normally either nothing or transmitted heart sounds are heard. Occasionally loud heart murmurs are transmitted to the neck and must be differentiated from a bruit, which is an adventitious sound of venous or arterial origin heard on auscultation. The carotid pulse should be examined one side at a time by gently palpating the artery in the lower half of the neck. Both carotid arteries should be equal in pulse rate, rhythm, strength, and elasticity. Decreased or absent carotid pulse suggests

Table 2–3. DIFFERENTIAL DIAGNOSIS OF THE MAIN VASCULAR DISEASES CAUSING GANGRENE

Feature	Diabetes Mellitus	Atherosclerosis	Thromboangiitis Obliterans	Raynaud's Disease	Arterial Insufficiency
Age (years)	>60	>40	<40	<40	Any
Sex	Either	Either	Male	Female	Either
Onset	Gradual	Gradual	Gradual	Gradual	Sudden
Pain	Moderate	Moderate	Severe	Moderate	Often severe
Distal pulses	May be absent	May be absent	May be absent	May be absent	May be absent

arterial narrowing or occlusion. To evaluate for a bruit, the physician listens to the carotid arteries with the diaphragm of the stethoscope while the patient holds his or her breath during auscultation.

ABDOMINAL BRUITS

If the femoral pulses are also absent the physician should listen for bruits in the abdomen. The patient should be lying supine. The examiner should place the diaphragm of the stethoscope midline about 2 inches above the umbilicus and listen carefully for the presence of an aortic bruit. The presence of a bruit may indicate aortoiliofemoral disease.

FEMORAL BRUITS

If all pulses below the femoral artery are diminished or absent the physician should listen over the femoral arteries for bruits. The diaphragm of the stethoscope is placed over the femoral artery. The presence of a femoral bruit may also indicate obstructive aortoiliofemoral disease. A localized systolic bruit may indicate the point of partial arterial occlusion.

Calf Palpation

Calf palpation involves squeezing of the calf muscle against the tibia, noting any tenderness, increased firmness, or tension in the muscle. Any tenderness, increased firmness, or tension suggests phlebitis in the calf. Calf pain, soreness, or increased muscular resistance on dorsiflexion of the foot suggests thrombophlebitis. Unfortunately thrombophlebitis frequently exists without any physical signs. Further diagnostic studies are always needed to confirm this suspicion.

Lymphatics

For evaluation of the lymphatics, the physician should palpate the superficial inguinal lymph nodes, both horizontal and vertical groups. The size, consistency, tenderness, mobility, and skin color or texture change over an enlarged node should be noted. Tenderness suggests lymphadenitis. Lymph nodes should be described as painless or tender and single or matted. Physical signs of lymphatic disease include palpable lymph nodes, lymphangitis, and lymphedema. Generalized lymphadenopathy is the presence of three or more palpable lymph node chains and suggests a different diagnosis than localized lymphadenopathy. Generalized lymphadenopathy differential diagnosis includes lymphoma; leukemia; collagen vascular disorders; and systemic bacterial, viral, and protozoal infections. Localized lymphadenopathy is usually the result of localized infection or neoplasm. Lymphangitis is lymphatic spread manifested by thin red streaks on the skin. Obstruction to lymphatic flow produces lymphedema, which is not always easy to distinguish from other types of edema.

Neurologic Sensory Assessment

Sensory response should be present and symmetric over all dermatomes and peripheral nerves. Light touch, temperature, superficial and deep pain, position, protective threshold, and vibratory senses should be tested. The large nerve fibers are often affected early in the course of peripheral neuropathy. Protective threshold is a quantitative measure of the extent of sensory loss in the lower extremity. Usually a 35 mm–long nylon monofilament with a 5.07-g force is used to evaluate sensitivity threshold level. This filament exerts a consistent force on the skin when the filament buckles and allows for a qualitative measurement. If the patient is unable to feel 5.07-g force or greater in three of six plantar sites, it is speculated that he or she is at an increased risk for plantar ulceration. This speculation is helpful in explaining the degree of sensory change and in establishing a risk factor for the patient.

Noninvasive Diagnostic Tests for the Arterial System

Subpapillary Venous Plexus Filling Time Test

The subpapillary venous plexus filling time (SPVPFT) test is performed by raising the digit to or slightly above the heart level, milking any congested venous blood flow out of the digit and then briefly pressing hard on the digital pulp to create an area of pallor. The time it takes arterial blood to completely fill the site of pallor is recorded. Normal SPVPFT is less than 3 seconds. A time of more than 10 seconds reflects the presence of significant organic disease, whereas a time of 4 to 9 seconds might reflect either functionally constricted vessels (i.e., the person is cold or scared and has sympathetic vasoconstriction) or organic disease. Although this test is simple to perform, two errors in performance do exist: the digit was below heart level and the venous blood was not adequately removed. Hence what is measured is actually venous backflow and not arterial inflow. If this test shows prolonged filling, unless proved otherwise, the 5-minute reactive hyperemia test should be performed.

Elevation-Dependency Test (Pallor on Elevation Technique)

To perform the elevation-dependency test, the foot and leg are raised at 60 degrees and kept elevated for one minute. The observer records whether there is pallor in the pedal skin and the approximate time it took to appear. After one minute, the foot and leg are put in a dependent position (that is, the patient sits up), and the time it takes for the previously elevated foot to display erythema is noted. In a normal foot, pallor on elevation and erythema on dependency are not observed. Although this sounds like a simple test, many observers record incorrect findings. The major cause for these errors is that the observers record color changes caused by venous blood flow and not arterial blood flow. That is, observers note a sudden pallor in the legs when they are raised, and the change is mistakenly recorded as pallor. In dependency, observers record the sudden return of venous blood as representing arterial inflow. To avoid this mistake, if the observer thinks that there is pallor immediately on elevation he or she should perform the SPVPFT test with the leg raised. If actual inflow is noted pallor does not exist and the color change was caused by lack of venous blood. When the foot is in dependency, there has to be an inverse correlation between the time for pallor and the time for color return. If there is an immediate return of color when the foot is dependent, there should be minimal

pallor on elevation. If both pallor and color return occur quickly, the test must be repeated because it was performed incorrectly and venous blood flow distorted the findings.

It is easy to understand the concept of the elevation-dependency test. If organic disease (such as atherosclerosis) exists there is narrowing of the vessels leading to the foot and hence increased vessel resistance. With the foot in an elevated position, because of gravity, it becomes even more difficult to pump blood into the foot, and the skin appears to have pallor. The greater the resistance of the occlusive disease, the faster the time of pallor. In contrast, there is no pallor on elevation when a leg without organic occlusion is raised because the body is able to continue pumping blood into the elevated leg. A foot that has shown pallor on elevation is an ischemic foot that has metabolites building up that vasodilate vessels (mentioned previously). As a result, when the foot is placed in a dependent position (with gravity now helping and not opposing the flow) with a minor obstruction, much blood can flow into the foot, and erythema is noted to occur quickly. If the organic occlusion is severe blood flow through the obstructed arteries is greatly restricted, and erythema may not be observed.

The 5-Minute Postocclusive Reactive Hyperemia Test

The 5-minute reactive hyperemia test visually indicates whether an obstruction exists in the distal foot. The test differentiates between organic and functional obstruction. This test shows the adequacy of collateral flow and gives an estimation of the maximal flow that can enter the foot. The 5-minute reactive hyperemia test should be performed on any person with questionable flow who is being considered for podiatric surgery.

The 5-minute reactive hyperemia test is performed by having the subject lie supine. The leg is raised 30°, and the foot is dorsiflexed and plantarflexed several times. Flexing the foot empties the venous blood from it and makes subsequent color changes easier to observe. An ankle blood pressure cuff is inflated to 100 mm Hg above the ankle pressure. If the ankle pressure has not been determined (see Segmental Pressures subsequently) the cuff is inflated to 100 mm Hg above brachial systolic pressure. The foot is placed at heart level. After 5 minutes, the cuff is quickly deflated, and the time it takes for color to return to the foot is noted. It should be noted whether color return is uniform or is delayed in certain regions of the foot. After noting the time for color to return to different regions of the foot, the degree of erythema present should be assessed. Is the foot markedly erythematous? Is the erythema uniform? Can the erythema be seen? After what period of time is a decrease in the erythema noticed?

In normal individuals, the return of color to the entire foot and toes is almost instantaneous, maximum erythema occurs at approximately 1 minute, and the foot is noticeably uniformly erythematous. In vasospastic individuals with no organic disease, the return of color to the foot is uniform but slightly delayed, especially in the toes. A return of color time to the toes of approximately 5 to 8 seconds is representative. Time for maximum erythema is longer than normal, being approximately 2 minutes. A hallmark for functional disease is that the foot and toes get markedly erythematous. In individuals with severe organic occlusion, the return of color to the foot and toes is not uniform and requires at least 15 seconds to reach the toes, maximum erythema takes longer than 2 minutes, and the amount of erythema is less than normal. In particularly severe cases, erythema may never be noted. Elective podiatric surgery should not be considered on anyone with a return of color to the toes of 15 seconds or more, unless other contradictory data are available.

The pathophysiology of the 5-minute reactive hyperemia test is simple. For reasons described previously, when blood flow into the foot is stopped, vasodilatory metabolites accumulate and cause relaxation of the smooth muscle in the arterioles, venules, and precapillary sphincters. As a result, resistance in these vessels decreases. As resistance decreases, blood flow into the foot should increase. If, however, there is significant organic occlusion in the foot or proximal to it, even though resistance has decreased in the foot, the volume of blood that can flow past the obstruction per unit of time is limited. Hence it takes longer for the blood to flow distally.

If the obstruction is severe the volume of blood that flows past the obstruction is greatly decreased compared to normal blood flow. If the volume is so greatly decreased that blood cannot fill all those "open capillaries" erythema of the skin of the foot may never be noticed following the postocclusive reactive hyperemia test. Therefore by observing how quickly color returns to the foot and toes and how erythematous the skin appears, it is possible to get a qualitative appreciation of the increased volume that is able to enter the foot.

The 5-minute postocclusive reactive hyperemia test can be used to aid the differentiation of vasospastic (functional) foot disease from organic disease. In vasospastic disease, blood flow is limited by the increased tone of the smooth muscles that surround the blood vessels. In organic disease, the blood flow is limited by the material clogging the lumen of the vessels. The metabolic build-up that occurs overrides the constriction caused by the vasospasm. Therefore blood flow into a foot with vasospastic disease greatly increases. No significant increase is noted when the pathology is caused by organic disease. The 5-minute reactive hyperemia test also can be used to overcome effects of increased sympathetic tone. Overcoming such effects is useful if one wants to assess blood flow into the foot of a patient who is anxious or cold or who is in pain. The test can also be used to predict how successful a contemplated sympathectomy to increase pedal skin blood flow would be.

Trendelenburg's Maneuver (Retrograde Filling Test)

Trendelenburg's maneuver evaluates for retrograde filling of the superficial venous system. The patient's leg is elevated to 90° to empty its venous blood, and a tourniquet is placed around the upper thigh tight enough to occlude the great saphenous vein. The physician should have the patient stand and observe the time it takes for the saphenous vein to fill from below (normal time is about 30 to 35 seconds). The tourniquet should be released at 60 seconds. No sudden increment in venous filling should occur if saphenous vein valves are competent. Any sudden filling indicates incompetent saphenous vein valves.

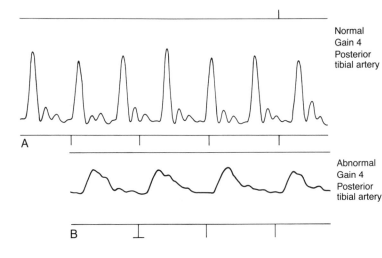

Normal
Gain 4
Posterior
tibial artery

Abnormal
Gain 4
Posterior
tibial artery

Figure 2–3. Doppler signal. *A,* Normal flow is represented by a triphasic form. Note the full, sharp-peaked waves, reflecting high velocity and normal volume. *B,* Abnormal flow is represented by a monophasic form. Note the low amplitude and broad waves, reflecting lower velocity and decreased volume.

Doppler Signal

All podiatrists should become familiar with the use of a hand-held Doppler device. The Doppler device is an ultrasonic flow detector. The Doppler probe emits a beam of a certain frequency (5 mHz in venous studies, 8 to 10 mHz in arterial studies). The frequency of the emitted beam is altered by any object moving faster than 6 cm/second (e.g., blood flow in a vessel). The reflected beam is received by the probe and compared with the emitted beam. An amplifier filters the sound and gives a flow signal (sound) or a tracing that is proportional (e.g., to the blood flow velocity). The slower the flow, the lower the pitch.

If waveforms are being recorded the faster the blood can flow, the steeper is the recorded waveform.* There are two types of continuous wave Doppler signals: unidirectional and bidirectional. The sounds produced by each Doppler signal are identical. The difference between them is that the unidirectional Doppler signal records both forward and backward flow as waveforms going above the baseline, whereas the bidirectional Doppler signal records the forward flow above the baseline and the backward flow below the baseline. Unidirectional Doppler signals should be more than adequate for podiatric assessment.

The qualitative audible Doppler signal, when made into a tracing, shows that the normal arterial pattern is a triphasic picture (Fig. 2–3). The monophasic sound denotes collateralized flow. The differences between the two extremes can usually be picked up by the examiner's ear with practice. When a tracing is not available, as when using the hand-held Doppler device, the qualitative nature of the signal should be appreciated by the examiner. This information factored into the clinical impression of the status of the vascular supply is extremely helpful in terms of assessment. Obviously when more sophisticated equipment is used to determine the nature of the arterial tree with noninvasive modes, the information is more quantitative than qualitative, but nevertheless the examining physician should be able to determine the qualitative nature of the Doppler signal without difficulty.

As explained in the beginning of this chapter, blood flow is usually pulsatile and flows both forward and backward. Because of their small diameter, only digital arteries have forward flow alone. In the absence of organic disease, blood flows at a high velocity because proximal arteries are smooth, elastic, and unobstructed. If one were to listen to normal arteries with a Doppler device two distinct and brief sounds would be produced. The first sound represents forward flow, and the second sound represents backward flow. In normal arteries, a third sound may also be heard. The etiology of the third sound is not definitely known. In organic occlusive disease, the intima is disrupted, the lumen is narrowed, and the vessel is calcified. As a result, blood flows slower, and

---

* By convention, the Doppler signal is recorded on paper moving at 25 mm/second.

backward flow may not occur because of the higher resistance encountered. When the flow through this type of vessel is heard with a Doppler device, the pitch is lower, and one sound is heard. If the disease is severe a less distinct sound or "longer swish" sound is heard. If waveforms are being recorded normal flow appears as a narrow first peak followed by one or two smaller peaks (a biphasic or triphasic recording). Flow through organically occluded vessels is recorded as a single broader and flatter curve (a monophasic recording).

Three illustrations are as follows:

1. All pedal vessels are heard as having two clear quick sounds. The recording is clearly biphasic. It therefore can be assumed that there is no significant proximal occlusion.

2. The posterior tibial artery is not heard. The popliteal artery is heard as having two quick sounds. In this instance, it seems obvious that the posterior tibial artery is totally occluded.

3. The posterior tibial artery has one low-pitched slow sound. The popliteal artery has two quick sounds. In this instance, there is more blood flowing through the dorsal artery of the foot than the posterior tibial artery, the posterior tibial artery is either totally occluded and supplied with minimal collateral blood flow or is greatly stenotic, and the dorsal artery of the foot is probably stenotic.

Segmental Pressures

To further characterize the flow through the vessels, it is necessary to record the pressure of the vessel. To do this for pedal arteries, a blood pressure cuff is placed around the ankle of a patient lying supine with the foot at heart level.* The correct cuff is imperative to the accuracy of pressures. The cuff should be the same width or 25% larger than the part it is encircling. If too narrow a cuff is used a falsely elevated pressure is recorded. The sounds through a pedal vessel are first obtained. The cuff is inflated so that the sounds are no longer audible. The cuff is slowly de-

flated until a sound is heard with the Doppler device. The pressure in the ankle cuff is recorded when the sound first becomes audible. This sound represents the pressure of the artery where the cuff is located. The process is repeated so that the pressures of all three pedal arteries are recorded. The correct-sized cuffs should be placed below the knee, above the knee, and high thigh levels. Pressures are recorded in each segment. The process for recording these segmental pressures is similar to that discussed previously. The Doppler device produces the best-sounding pedal vessel and should be used. While listening to this pedal vessel, the segmental cuff is inflated until no sound is heard. The cuff is then deflated, and the pressure in the segmental cuff is recorded when the pedal artery sound is first heard. A pressure gradient of more than 20 mm Hg between cuff levels suggests a hemodynamically significant occlusive lesion in the intervening segment. A contralateral pressure difference of more than 20 mm Hg similarly suggests the presence of a significant occlusive lesion.

Segmental leg pressures can be misleading. Collateral blood flow may be so well developed that a 20-mm pressure drop does not occur across a significant occlusive segment and severely calcified vessels. Such a misleading pressure reading is observed particularly in individuals with diabetes mellitus and in the elderly. A rigid, calcified vessel may not be compressible and therefore gives a falsely elevated leg pressure. The limitations of segmental leg pressure emphasize that results must be combined with physical findings. Exercise testing, pulse-volume recordings, and Doppler analysis add important information to the evaluation.

Digital Doppler Studies

Unlike the other arteries, only one sound is heard in the digital vessels. Just one sound is heard because of the small diameter and high resistance of digital vessels. The number of digital arteries heard in representative toes should be recorded. The pitch should be listened for because it correlates with velocity of flow. Normally each toe contains two plantar and two dorsal digital arteries. To hear the digital arteries, the Doppler probe should be

---

* Even though it is commonly stated that the pressure of the dorsal artery of the foot is recorded, in reality, the pressure of the anterior tibial artery underlying the ankle cuff is recorded.

held at 90° to the toe and lightly placed at the medial and lateral base, both plantarly and dorsally. One must be extremely careful not to move the toe being examined because the resulting slight pressure might be sufficient to occlude flow in the digital artery. If one or two digital arteries are audible in the toe functional causes, such as vasospasm secondary to temperature, fear, anxiety, caffeine, and nicotine, must be differentiated from organic causes. The 5-minute reactive hyperemia test provides data to differentiate functional from organic disease. Because this test affects flow dynamics, it should be performed after all proximal arteries are examined and segmental pressures recorded. The number of digital arteries present and the quality of the sounds should be recorded both before and after hyperemia.

The following example illustrates a functional problem. One digital vessel is heard before reactive hyperemia. After the reactive hyperemia test, digital vessels are clearly audible, color returns to the toes in less than 3 seconds, and the foot is noted to become markedly erythematous.

The following example illustrates organic disease. One digital vessel is noted before reactive hyperemia. After the reactive hyperemia test, one or two digital vessels are audible, each having a low-pitched sound. Color returns to the toes in 10 seconds, and the foot is noted to only become mildly erythematous. In the presence of organic disease, the number of digital arteries audible with a Doppler device may actually decrease following the reactive hyperemia test.

Arm-Ankle Index

This index has many synonyms, including ischemic index, ankle-brachial pressure ratio, and ankle-wrist ratio. The index is obtained by dividing the brachial artery systolic pressure into the systolic pressure of one of the pedal arteries.

Unfortunately the early literature tried to generalize about the meaning of the arm-ankle index. It is commonly noted in the literature that an arm-ankle pressure of 1.0 or greater indicates the absence of organic disease. In limbs with one primary arterial occlusion, the index is usually 0.5 to 0.8. An index of less than 0.5 usually indicates multilevel occlusive disease, reflecting severe pathology, and, until proven otherwise, no elective podiatric surgery should be contemplated. These guidelines fail to consider the effects of calcification within the vessel. It is impossible to interpret the meaning of an arm-ankle index that is above 0.5 by looking solely at the number.

Falsely elevated arm-ankle indexes can occur in processes that stiffen vessels. In arteries of diabetic individuals, a condition called medial calcinosis, or Mönckeberg's sclerosis, is commonly noted. This condition is associated with calcification forming within the media. Unlike atherosclerosis, this calcification does not narrow the lumen of the artery. Similar to atherosclerosis, this condition causes stiffening of the artery. The arteries of individuals who have atherosclerosis, particularly diabetics, are therefore likely to be quite stiff because of calcification not only in the lumen but also in the media of the artery. If a pressure were recorded for this stiff vessel it would not reflect the pressure of the blood in the lumen but instead would reflect the ability of the wall to resist compression. The pressures recorded for the individuals would be falsely elevated because they reflected arterial wall stiffness and not blood pressure.

To understand why this pressure is misleading, the reader should consider the following. We have two vertical tubes containing a fluid. We wish to record the pressure of the fluid within these tubes. Tube A is thin flexible vinyl, and tube B is a lead pipe. Blood pressure cuffs are placed around each tube, and both cuffs are inflated until the walls of the tubes are almost touching (our analogy for taking blood pressure). If we stated that the pressure of the fluid in tube B equaled the recorded pressure in the cuff around B, it would seem extremely naive. It can easily be seen that the measured pressure reflects the strength of the walls of the lead pipe and not the fluid pressure.

By similar analogy, in people with stiff vessels, especially diabetics, the pedal systolic pressure might be better correlated with the stiffness of the vessels rather than the blood pressure within the lumen. In those individuals, the arm-ankle pressure index is misleading and falsely elevated. The question of when can the systolic pressure recorded for pedal vessels be believed is then raised. The pressure can be believed when it meaningfully correlates with the velocity indicators (pitch and waveform morphology) recorded for that artery. To illustrate, two distinct quick sounds are heard in the posterior tibial vessel. Brachial pressure is 120 mm Hg. Recorded pressure of the posterior tibial artery is 140 mm Hg. The arm-ankle index is 140/120 or 1.2. The quality of the sounds is characteristic for normal velocity blood flow. The index is "within normal limits." Since both the sounds and the velocity of blood flow are consistent with the arm-ankle index, this number may be considered accurate and not misleading.

In another example, the recorded pressures were similar to those mentioned previously. The posterior tibial artery pressure is 140 mm Hg, and the brachial pressure is 120 mm Hg. When the posterior tibial vessel is heard with a Doppler device, one low-pitched "long swish" sound is heard. As previously discussed, this sound is representative of slow-flowing blood. Therefore a significant proximal occlusion or stenosis is probably present. The arm-ankle index of 1.2 is obviously misleading and falsely elevated.

The patient's resting blood pressure may also be another indicator to help assess the validity of the arm-ankle index. Previously in the chapter, the reasons why some people with atherosclerosis have elevated pulse pressures were discussed. It was stated that these pressure alterations were caused by the presence of stiff, inelastic vessels. Therefore, on the one hand, if a patient has a blood pressure of 160/85 it is possible that he or she may have stiff vessels and that the arm-ankle index may be falsely elevated. On the other hand, if a patient has a blood pressure of 110/70 his or her vessels are probably elastic, and the arm-ankle index is less likely to be falsely elevated. Fear, anxiety, cold, and discomfort may all elevate pulse pressures and give the false impression of the presence of atherosclerosis. Conversely, individuals who may have elevated pulse pressure can be taking medications that lower the pulse pressure. These individuals may appear to have normal pulse pressures only because they are taking hemodynamically active medications. With these exceptions in mind, the systemic blood pressure can provide a clue as to whether the arm-ankle index is falsely elevated. There have been a number of methods tried to determine tissue viability. These methods include xenon wash out, arm-ankle index, thermography, and measurement of transcutaneous oxygen and carbon dioxide levels.

Exercise Test

If there is doubt about whether the arm-ankle index is falsely elevated the modified exercise test of Carter can be utilized. This test has been selected because it is simple; requires no extra equipment; and, unlike treadmill testing, has never been associated with a fatality. To perform the test, the pressures of the best two pedal arteries are recorded. The patient's leg is then raised 30°. Against a slight resistance, the foot is dorsiflexed and plantarflexed for 1 minute at a rate of one cycle/second. After 1 minute, the foot is returned to heart level, and the pressures of both pedal arteries are recorded at 30 and 60 seconds after exercise and then at 1-minute intervals. If there is significant proximal occlusion the ankle pressures fall more than 20% and do not return to normal within the first 2 minutes following the exercise. By recording these pressure changes, falsely elevated arm-ankle indices may be unmasked.

The following example illustrates why the pressure falls. There is a significant stenosis in the distal superficial femoral artery, and collateral vessels cannot sufficiently bypass this stenosis. As described previously, exercising muscle requires many times the normal volume of blood flow. Because of metabolic build-up, the resistance within the exercising muscle is low. Blood entering the leg preferentially goes into these low-resistance vessels. In other words, blood is shunted into the exercising muscle. Since the stenosis is severe because of high resistance and turbulent flow, the volume of blood that is capable of flowing through the stenosis, or the smaller-diameter collateral vessels, is limited. As a result, most of the blood flows into the exercising muscles, leaving a lowered pressure at the level of the ankle. The greater the occlusion, the lower the ankle pressure. By following the pressure in the ankle after the leg is exercised, one can get a feeling for the ability of the body to deliver blood into the leg.

The exercise test should be utilized if a patient reports having intermittent claudication and if other tests do not reveal the pathology. The exercise test, however, cannot be used to tell the podiatrist about blood flow in the foot. The test reveals only pressure changes at the ankle level. Therefore the exercise test would not be useful if one wanted to know whether there was sufficient blood flow to perform lower extremity surgery.

Photoplethysmography

Photoplethysmography is a modality used to provide an indication of skin blood flow. The photoplethysmograph sensor emits a beam of near infrared frequency. The emitted beam is reflected by hemoglobin molecules located in the cutaneous microcirculation. A photoelectric detector measures this reflected beam, and the signal is transformed to be displayed as a recorded waveform. This waveform is representative of pulsatile flow in the subpapillary venous plexus of the skin. Photoplethysmography should be used to record skin arterial blood flow both before and after vasodilation. Photoplethysmography should also be used to record skin flow around ulcerations. By adding a digital

blood pressure cuff, digital pressures can be recorded. Because photoplethysmography is a measurement of skin blood flow, it is essential that this modality be utilized if one is considering doing lower extremity surgery. Photoplethysmography waveform morphology of plantar tufts of digits have markedly increased vasculature when compared with other places on the skin. Therefore the waveforms recorded from the plantar tufts of the digits are much larger than those recorded from other places on the skin. The photoplethysmography waveform reflects the characteristics of the red blood cell flow through the subpapillary venous plexus.

When there is normal flow and no organic occlusion, red blood cells flow quickly and in a forward direction only. Therefore the recording looks like a narrow teepee. Occasionally digital arteries are wide enough not to dump out backward flow quickly through the subpapillary venous plexus. In this instance, most of the flow is in a forward direction, and a large narrow teepee is recorded (Fig. 2–4). The lesser backward flow appears as a second, much smaller peak on the downslope of the first. The notch between the two peaks is

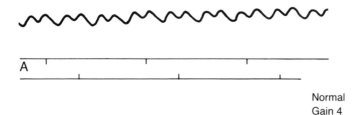

Abnormal
Gain 4
Hallux

A

Normal
Gain 4
Hallux

B

Figure 2–4. Photoplethysmography. *A,* Note the igloo waveform, representing slow flow and decreased volume. *B,* Note the teepee waveform, representing normal rapid flow.

called the dicrotic notch. Dicrotic notching is therefore noticed in any blood that flows in a forward and backward fashion. The appearance of waveforms with dicrotic notching implies that there is no significant obstruction in any proximal connecting artery.

Because skin vessels are so small, unlike other places in the body, dicrotic notching might be absent, yet flow can still be normal. In organic disease, blood flows slower through the digital vessels into the subpapillary venous plexus. A photoplethysmography waveform should be correlated with digital Doppler results. If there are any discrepancies between the two (e.g., dicrotic notching noted on photoplethysmograph waveforms but only one sound heard in each of the digital arteries), both tests should be repeated.

Digital Blood Pressure

Digital blood pressure is obtained by placing an appropriate-sized cuff (i.e., one that is 1.0 to 1.25 times the width of the digit) around the digit. Care should be taken to avoid placing the cuff around a joint because false pressures are obtained. After obtaining several waveforms from the photoplethysmography sensor on the distal plantar aspect of the digit, the cuff is inflated until a straight line recording is obtained. The cuff is then deflated until a small deflection is first noticed. After recording photoplethysmography waveforms and correlating them with Doppler signals, the digital blood pressure is obtained by inflating the digital cuff until a straight line recording is obtained. The digital cuff is then deflated until a very small deflection is recorded by the photoplethysmography sensor. The pressure where this deflection first occurs represents the systolic pressure of the digital arteries. Because of variances caused by sympathetic tone, digital blood flow and pressure in normal vessels can vary tremendously. Therefore waveform morphology that looks like flattened igloos may be obtained. To minimize this variance of sympathetic tone, blood flow studies should best be done after the patient has rested. The patient should also be told to avoid any vasoactive substances, such as alcohol, coffee, and cigarettes, for at least 2 hours prior to the examination. The results of digital flow, pressure, and number of digital arteries heard with a Doppler device should be evaluated and cross checked. If sympathetic tone is high, as it is in vasospastic disease and patient anxiety, the 5-minute reactive hyperemia test must be performed.

In normal digits without any pathology, one would expect to record the presence of four digital arteries. Pressure generally is between 70 and 110 mm Hg, and waveforms look more like teepees than igloos. In the presence of vasospasm or proximal organic occlusive disease, frequently no digital arteries are audible with a Doppler device, and photoplethysmography waveforms are quite flattened (reflecting low-velocity flow) and have low pressures (below 50 mm). To differentiate vasospasm from organic occlusive disease, the 5-minute reactive hyperemia test must be performed. If vasospasm is present the skin becomes red, more digital arteries are heard with a Doppler device, and the pitch reflects faster flow. Photoplethysmography tracings become larger, and pressures rise.

In severe organic occlusive disease, the skin may not become erythematous, the number of digital vessels audible may decrease, photoplethysmography tracings are smaller and look more like igloos, and pressure falls. To illustrate the differential diagnosis of vasospastic from organic disease, let us consider two patients, A and B. Both patients have organic occlusive disease. Both patients wish to have an arthroplasty of the second digit. Before the reactive hyperemia test, both patients had two digital arteries out of four recorded by a Doppler device. Both patients had identical digital skin flow, as measured by photoplethysmography, and both had identical digital surgery pressures of 50 mm Hg. Following the reactive hyperemia test, color returned to the second digit of A in 5 seconds, and color returned to the second digit of B in 20 seconds. The number of second toe digital arteries heard with a Doppler device was four in A and one in B. Pressure after dilation was recorded as 80 mm Hg for A and 25 mm Hg for B. Digital skin flow in A tripled, whereas digital skin flow in B greatly diminished. The second toe of A appeared quite erythematous, with maximum erythema occurring within the first minute. The second toe of B became only slightly erythematous, and maximum color occurred in approximately $2\frac{1}{2}$ minutes. In the case of A, blood flow into the second toe was not greatly limited by organic occlusion. With B, however, it appears that following the reactive hyperemia test, flow actually decreased.

Blood flow decreased because the volume of incoming blood was limited by the presence of organic occlusion. Following the reactive hyperemia test, this limited flow into the foot encountered many more functioning capillaries. Flow therefore was first diverted to the proximal tissue, and blood took a longer time to reach the distal tissue. By the time the flow reached the second digit, the volume was minimal, pressure was low, and velocity was slow. Hence the number of digital arteries heard with a Doppler device and toe pressure decreased. If surgery were performed A would have a better chance of healing than B. Therefore because vessels must be cut when surgery is performed, in the opinion of the authors, any person with decreased pedal circulation should have the 5-minute reactive hyperemia test performed prior to having surgery. This test gives the observer an idea as to whether the body can effectively increase flow into the foot if it were to be required following surgery.

It is prudent to reconsider elective podiatric surgery if dilated toe pressures fall below 40 mm Hg, if the toes remain blanched for 10 to 15 seconds or more, or if both situations occur. Because shoe pressure exerts approximately 20 to 30 mm Hg pressure on a digit, digital pressure necrosis is expected if toe pressures fall below this level. In cases of skin ulcerations, photoplethysmography recordings both before and after reactive hyperemia provide useful information regarding healing probability. If flow does not increase appreciably following hyperemia one can assume that sympathectomy similarly would not help the patient.

Volume Plethysmography

Pulse volume recording, as may be inferred from the name, reflects the volume of blood that pulses under a sensor cuff. Pulse volume recordings are obtained by placing cuffs filled to 60 mm Hg pressure around the parts to be measured. Most often these parts would be the toe, midfoot,

ankle, below the knee, above the knee, and high thigh regions. When blood pulses under the air-filled cuff, the volume of the part under the cuff expands. This expansion causes changes in the air-filled cuff, which are recorded on a strip recorder. The resulting waveform that is produced reflects the arterial pulse under the cuff. The pulse volume recording closely corresponds to direct intra-arterial recordings at that level. The pulse volume recording is a qualitative not quantitative representation of arterial flow. The authors are continually astounded by both the sensitivity and the simplicity of this machine.

The waveforms produced reflect the general principles described previously. Specifically normal flow is recorded as two superimposed curves, the first representing forward blood flow, the second backward flow. The notch between the two peaks is called the dicrotic notch. Flow that is fast is recorded as a narrow teepee; flow that is slow is recorded as an igloo. The pulse volume recordings should be correlated with Doppler device findings.

If the volume plethysmography waveforms recorded for the foot look essentially like a straight line there is minimal pedal flow, and no lower extremity surgery should be contemplated. The patient needs to be referred to a vascular surgeon for possible reconstructive surgery. The waveforms obtained are for high thigh, above the knee, below the knee, ankle, and foot levels. Changes in waveform morphology between segments reflect severe stenoses or occlusions. As an example, a recording might be obtained at the above the knee level that looked like a narrow teepee, whereas that obtained at the below the knee level looked like a small igloo (Fig. 2–5). Since the above the knee level is a "narrow teepee" with no backward flow, as would be reflected by the presence of dicrotic notching, it can be assumed that there is some proximal blockage. However, because the waveform morphology is that of a narrow teepee, it can be inferred that flow is fast, the volume is adequate. Conversely the below the knee waveform morphology is similar to a small igloo; that is, flow velocity is slow, and volume is small. Therefore it can be concluded that there is organic obstruction in the region between the two cuffs and that collateral flow is not adequate.

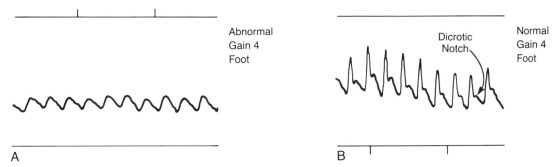

Figure 2–5. Volume plethysmography. *A,* Note the igloo appearance of the waveform. This appearance represents slow flow and low volume, implying that there is organic obstruction. *B,* Note the teepee appearance of the waveform. Normal flow is recorded as two superimposed curves. The first curve is forward flow, and the second curve is backward flow. The notch between the two peaks is known as the dicrotic notch.

The waveform morphology should be analyzed for changes between segments and for differences existing between right and left segments. If waveform morphologies obtained from both right and left high thigh areas are equally altered to show only forward flow with slow flow and the recordings appear similar, it is probable that a lesion exists that is equally affecting flow in both extremities. Such a lesion would probably be located in the distal aorta, most likely at the aortoiliac bifurcation. Alterations of volume plethysmographic waveforms should correlate with alterations noted in segmental pressures. Pulse volume recordings provide a visual reference for checking flow characteristics through both extremities. The flatter the curve, the slower the flow and the less the volume. Occasionally when there is a discrete stenosis, turbulence can be recorded.

Invasive Diagnostic Tests for the Arterial System

Special instrumentation and angiography are rarely necessary to diagnose arterial insufficiency. These tests are helpful to document the location and extent of disease if surgical correction is contemplated. Invasive tests should not be ordered unless confirmatory findings are first obtained in noninvasive vascular tests.

Among the major advances enabling surgeons to perform revascularization procedures are the development of safe diagnostic techniques to evaluate the vascular circuit, the development of safe anticoagulants, and the development of suitable bypass conduits. The 1930s and 1940s saw the development of safe arteriography, which set the stage for the remainder of the advancements to occur. There has been continued improvement over the years in terms of the safety of the procedure as well as the use of arteriographic modality in terms of pressure measurement and percutaneous transluminal angioplasty (PTA) and laser angioplasty. The technologic advances have allowed less use of contrast material and better visualization of the vascular tree (e.g., digital subtraction arteriography). The basic technique of the arteriogram is to isolate the vessel to be used for placement of the arteriogram catheter. This vessel is commonly the femoral artery. If the iliac system is patent on the side of the arterial puncture the catheter can be advanced into the aorta to give bilateral runoff arteriograms or even advanced into the contralateral iliac and thus femoral system and below to give more selective views. If the femoral artery cannot be used for some reason, such as occlusion, the axillary artery can be used for placement of the catheter, or, although not as commonly employed today as in the past, a translumbar arteriogram can be performed.

Typical aortogram pictures of the aortoiliac, femoral, popliteal, and distal circulation are shown in Figure 2–6. As already stated, intra-arterial pressure measurements can be made at the time of arteriography. Therapeutic dilations using the balloon and laser can be undertaken as well. Figure 2–6 shows the basic technique of PTA. The laser application today involves the opening of a stenotic or occluded area in an artery, followed by a balloon dilation. Developments in laser technology are researched in order to allow

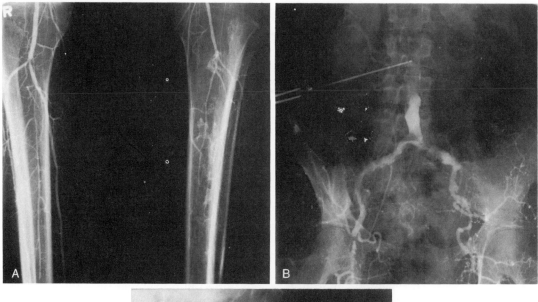

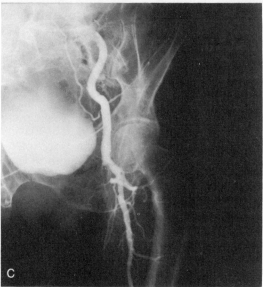

Figure 2–6. *A*, A 56-year-old man with a history of type I diabetes mellitus. The patient presented with gangrene of the left third and fourth digits. The arteriogram reveals occlusion of the left anterior and posterior tibial arteries as well as occlusion of the left peroneal artery. *B*, A 74-year-old smoker with a history of hypertension and atherosclerotic coronary artery disease. The patient presented with severe intermittent claudication. The arteriogram reveals bilateral occlusion of the iliac vessels and collateralization. *C*, An 84-year-old man who presented with gangrene of the left fifth toe. The arteriogram reveals occlusion of the left superficial femoral artery at origin.

vaporization of atherosclerotic lesions without damage to the arterial tissue.

Complications with arteriography, other than those associated with balloon or laser angioplasty, have dropped dramatically from years past. The more common complications seen today are dye reactions, contrast-induced changes in renal function, and localized hematoma.

Noninvasive Evaluation of the Venous System

Impedance Plethysmography

Impedance plethysmography is based on the principle that during the respiratory cycle there are changes in the venous volumes of the lower extremity. These volume changes cause concomitant changes in electrical impedance in accordance with Ohm's law (voltage = resistance × current). The cuff occlusion technique is used, which is performed by placing a pressure cuff around the thigh and inflating it to a pressure between arterial and venous pressures, approximately 50 to 60 mm Hg. The outflowing venous blood from the lower extremity is translated into an electrical tracing, which shows a gradual rise in volume of the leg and, when the cuff is released, a rapid fall in volume. With obstruction of the venous system, this fall is of smaller magnitude and less rapid than in the normal situation. Impedance plethysmography is a good test for screening patients for suspected deep venous thrombosis.

Segmental Plethysmography

With segmental plethysmography, the principles are generally the same as impedance plethysmography, but the changes in limb volumes and pressures are detected by pneumatic bladders and strain gauges, which are placed around the leg at usually more than one level. Impedance plethysmography is in general usage today and has a high accuracy rate for thromboses in the more proximal venous system but has been criticized as not being accurate for below-knee thrombi.

Phleborheography

Phleborheography is a technique using pneumatic cuffs at various levels, including the foot, three areas on the calf, and the thorax. Respiratory variations are measured. The cuffs can be used interchangeably as occluding and measuring modes. This test is said to be accurate when compared with venography in detection of deep venous thrombosis but is used less commonly than impedance plethysmography in the clinical situation because it is a more complicated test to perform.

Doppler Ultrasonography

Doppler ultrasonography is used for detection of venous problems as well as arterial problems. A probe that can detect flow in both directions is placed over the veins at certain locations. The quality of the signal gives valuable information for detecting obstruction. There are five facets to the Doppler signal that are evaluated: spontaneity, phasicity, augmentation, competence, and pulsatility. The accuracy of this examination in many ways is dependent on the experience of the person performing it. Spontaneity refers to flow signals in the veins that are present all the time, and absence of these signals represents venous obstruction. Phasicity refers to the changes in the flow signal with respiration. With inspiration, venous flow decreases, and with expiration, venous flow increases. With venous obstruction, this respiratory variation decreases. Augmentation refers to changes in the venous flow by compression of the tissue proximal and distal to the examining probe. These changes disappear with venous obstruction. Competence refers to the state of the venous valves in relationship to flow signals and the various maneuvers that are entailed in the examination. For example, when the venous valves are incompetent, Valsalva's maneuver shows augmentation of retrograde flow. Pulsatility refers to situations, such as congestive heart failure, in which with elevated venous pressure, the venous sounds may be difficult to distinguish from arterial sounds, and, instead of varying with the respiratory cycle, pulsations can be appreciated.

Diagnostic tests for varicose veins are primarily used to delineate primary from secondary varicose veins, referring to deep and communicating venous incompetence. Usually there is associated deep venous obstruction. Venography may be used for this purpose, but Doppler ultrasonography and other noninvasive modalities, including outflow plethysmography, have been used reliably to make the distinction.

I^{123} Fibrinogen Leg Scanning

I^{123} fibrinogen leg scanning depends on incorporation of labeled fibrinogen into a developing thrombosis. The accuracy of this method in the diagnosis of deep venous thrombosis formation exceeds 90%. Readings over both legs are recorded as a percentage of activity over the sternum. Venous thrombosis is suggested by an increase in the reading value of greater than

20% at any point along the vein when compared with the value in contiguous points on the same leg at the same point and the value on the day before and the same area on the other leg. The diagnosis is considered definite if the value recorded for the scan remains abnormal and persists for more than 24 minutes. This test is not sensitive to thrombin in the pelvic veins and common femoral veins because of high background radioactivity in the bladder and pelvic vessels. False-positive results are often encountered.

Invasive Evaluation of the Venous System

Peripheral Venography

Venography of the extremities is an extremely important examination for the di-

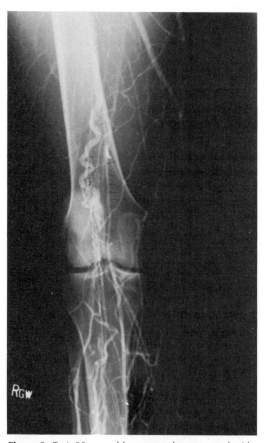

Figure 2–7. A 29-year-old woman who presented with significant edema of the right lower extremity below the knee. The patient had a history of oral contraceptive use over 4 years. The venogram demonstrates total occlusion of the left popliteal vein.

agnosis of suspected thrombophlebitis. The basic principle of this examination is to fill as many of the patent deep veins as possible. Peripheral venography is usually performed by radiologists, and good technique is essential to ensure a valid study. Venography is the most reliable and specific test for the diagnosis of deep vein thrombosis. A definite filling defect that appears in an otherwise opacified vein would be accepted as evidence for venous thrombosis (Fig. 2–7). Additional findings, such as altered flow pattern and presence of collateral vessels, are suggestive but not absolutely definitive. The technique of venography involves radiation exposure and continuous flow. Venography can cause discomfort to the patient, and there are occasional problems due to allergy and sensitivity to contrast material. There is also a slight risk of thrombosis secondary to the use of contrast material. However, a properly performed venogram confirms or disproves the presence of disease. Venography remains the standard of comparison for all other aids in the diagnosis of deep venous thrombosis.

PERIPHERAL VASCULAR DISORDERS

Arterial Occlusive Disorders

Arterial Insufficiency

The clinical presentation of distal arterial occlusion is usually more severe than claudication and includes pain and tissue loss with ischemic ulcers and gangrene. In the chronic state, there may be loss of sensation and atrophy of muscles, skin adnexa, nails, and subcutaneous tissue. Examination reveals no pedal pulses. Because this pattern of involvement is often coupled with proximal disease, the pulse examination above the calf is included. Patients with distal arterial occlusion are extremely sensitive to minor trauma and infections in the feet and toes, which so often tragically lead to major amputation. Rest pain, ischemic ulcers, and gangrene usually lead to major amputation unless an effective vascular reconstructive operation to bring blood to the affected part is undertaken.

The progress of occlusive disease ultimately involves tissue or limb loss. In the absence of normal skin temperature, capillary refill, presence of skin appendages, and normal Doppler arterial signals, the patient is usually at risk for limb loss unless new circulation can be brought to the involved part. Encompassed in this situation, ischemic ulcers, fissures, gangrene, and nonhealing wounds can be found. The podiatrist at times is the first to see these problems. Unquestionably this type of pathology represents the tip of an iceberg in terms of associated systemic disease. Half the patients who present with these changes are able to relate exactly how the problem began.

AORTOILIAC DISEASE

Physical examination of patients with aortoiliac disease reveals a diminished femoral pulse often with bruit. With exercise, the femoral pulse may disappear or a bruit may be auscultated though absent in the resting state. Distal leg pulse may be present but often disappears with exercise as well. Nutrition of the tissue of the leg and foot is usually normal. Trophic changes are generally absent. Elevation pallor may be absent but may appear with prolonged elevation (2 minutes) of the foot.

Aortoiliac atherosclerosis has been known to cause the majority of atheroarterial embolic events, that is, embolization from one artery to another artery. Ulcerated plaques in the aorta may liberate small pieces of debris, calcified plaque, thrombus, or fibrin platelet complex, which, when lodged distally in the arterial tree, cause ischemia distal to the point of lodgment. This process can cause necrosis of tissue and has been described as the "blue toe" syndrome. Recognition of this disorder should alert the practitioner to the possibility of aortoiliac atherosclerosis. Aortoiliac atherosclerosis is characterized by Leriche's syndrome. This syndrome is described as stenosis or occlusion at the aortic bifurcation with resultant claudication, impotence, and absence of gangrene in male patients.

Generally patients with predominant involvement of the aorta and iliac arteries are in their 40s, 50s, or 60s, and their symptoms are mild. This is due to the propensity for development of collateral vessels of moderate size. Narrowing at the aortic, iliac, and femoral bifurcations leads to occlusion with propagation of thrombus in the aortic, iliac, and common femoral arteries. Rarely does this process extend cephalad beyond the renal arteries or lower than the deep femoral artery. Thus arterial reconstruction is possible in the majority of these patients, usually with an aortofemoral bypass. In this patient population, there is often coronary and carotid system atherosclerotic involvement. Results of operation for patients exhibiting claudication with aortoiliac involvement are almost universally good in terms of relieving symptoms. Gangrene usually but not always requires a secondary, distal operation for correction.

Femoropopliteal Disease

Occlusion of the superficial femoral artery produces claudication in most instances. Depending on the patency and degree of stenosis to the major collateral artery of the thigh, the deep femoral artery, symptoms may stabilize or gradually improve with exercise and cessation of smoking as new and larger collateral circulation develops. In a small number of patients, gangrene develops at a rate of 1% per year, with superficial femoral artery as the sole arterial abnormality.

TIBIOPERONEAL DISEASE

Tibioperoneal disease is most commonly seen in diabetic patients. In such patients, the anterior and posterior tibial arteries are obliterated, often with preservation of the peroneal artery, which unfortunately does not extend directly to the foot. Why this pattern so commonly occurs in diabetics is unknown. Thromboangiitis obliterans (Buerger's disease) and other collagen vascular disorders, such as scleroderma, may occlude the distal arterial tree. The "blue toe" syndrome, that is, emboli emanating from proximal arterial surfaces, also may obliterate distal vessels.

Arteriosclerosis Obliterans

Arteriosclerosis obliterans is caused by narrowing or obstruction of large-sized and medium-sized arteries supplying the extremities. Symptoms and signs are produced by ischemia. Arteriosclerosis obliterans is the leading cause of obstructive arterial disease of the extremities after age 30. The lower extremities are involved most commonly. The superficial femoral artery is affected by stenosis or obstruction in approximately 90% of the cases. The aortoiliac and popliteal areas are the next most common sites. The greatest incidence of superficial femoral artery and more distal arterial disease occurs in the 70s, but aortoiliac disease has its peak a decade earlier. The disease is more common in men than in women, especially before menopause. The ratio is about 9 to 1. Patients with diabetes mellitus develop arteriosclerosis obliterans more frequently and at an earlier age than patients without this disease. Diabetics have the same incidence of femoropopliteal disease but a greater frequency of vessel involvement between the knee and ankle than nondiabetics. High plasma cholesterol and total lipid concentrations are frequent findings in patients with isolated aortoiliac disease.

The pathologic process is usually segmental. The intima displays widespread arteriosclerotic changes proximal and distal to the segmental lesion. Although the occlusive or stenotic lesions causing symptoms are usually proximal to the knee, the incidence of concomitant lower leg arterial occlusions is as high as 45% in some surveys and rises with age. The posterior tibial artery is the calf vessel most often affected.

Symptoms and signs are produced by inadequate oxygenation of the tissues distal to the arterial lesion, secondary to the decrease in blood flow or pressure at rest or during exercise. Large-sized and medium-sized arteries must have a decrease in cross-sectional area of 70 to 90% before a decrease in blood flow at rest or during exercise. A 69% decrease may suffice. Decreased flow and pressure are also dependent on the velocity of flow and therefore the peripheral resistance. The length of stenotic segment has a lesser effect. Although all vessels of a system contribute to its total resistance, the arterioles and precapillary sphincters are of greatest importance. Peripheral resistance is regulated reflexively by the sympathetic nervous system and locally by the formation of vasodilator metabolites. Activity of the sympathetic nervous system causes cutaneous vasoconstriction, increasing peripheral resistance.

Patients who develop ischemic symptoms only during exercise may have normal calf blood flow at rest. However, during exercise, the blood flow may stop or be abnormally slow. The decreased blood pressure in the arterial vasculature distal to the obstructive lesion allows the contracting muscles to obstruct arterial flow partially or completely during exercise. If reactive hyperemia (full vasodilation) is produced in an involved limb the total blood flow is usually much less than in the normal limb. Reflex vasoconstriction, when the extremity is exposed to cold, can be harmful to an ischemic extremity. Removal of vasoconstrictor activity in an extremity results in vasodilation. Blood vessels in skeletal muscle also are affected by sympathetic activity but only to a very limited extent during exercise when vasodilator metabolites are active.

Blood supply to the limb distal to an obstructing or stenotic arterial lesion is via collateral blood vessels. Most of these collateral vessels are present in the normal limb but unused until an obstruction occurs. Many collateral vessels appear almost immediately after an acute arterial occlusion, but others form more gradually over a period of months.

Thromboangiitis Obliterans (Buerger's Disease)

Thromboangiitis obliterans involves the intermediate small-sized arteries and veins of the extremities and usually occurs in 30- to 40-year-old men who have a smoking history. Because both arterial and venous areas are involved, it was postulated that these patients have abnormal hypercoagulable properties of their blood. In fact, an increased platelet adhesiveness has been reported that disappears with cessation of smoking. The increased association of human leukocyte antigens (HLAs) A9 and B5 has been noted. There may be a vasospastic component to the disorder, which disappears with cessation of smoking. There is a distinct male predominance in the disease. Intermittent claudication is the most common initial symptom. Eventually a majority of patients have involvement of their upper extremities as well. The disorder is generally limited to the extremities, but cerebrovascular, cardiac, and visceral problems exist in these patients. In contrast to the other inflammatory disorders, typical nonspecific inflammatory symptoms, such as fever and malaise, usually are not seen in this disorder.

Laboratory evaluations are nonspecific for thromboangiitis obliterans, and the erythrocyte sedimentation rate (ESR) usually is not elevated. Angiogram is the definitive study for diagnosis in order to delineate the areas of profound involvement. There tends to be more symmetric involvement than is seen in atherosclerotic vascular disease. The pathologic changes seen in the arterial wall go through an acute to chronic process, first involving infiltration of the arterial wall with inflammatory polymorphonuclear neutrophil (PMN) cells and gradually ending up as fibrotic and narrowed or occluded vessels.

The therapy for thromboangiitis obliterans is based primarily on cessation of smoking and approach of the ischemic problems of the extremities in much the same fashion as with arteriosclerosis obliterans. Most operative success has been achieved with bypass of large vessels, such as the iliac arteries. Much less success has been achieved with femoral, popliteal, and distal bypasses. Although most of these patients end up with major amputations of both upper and lower extremities, the arterial reconstructive procedures should be attempted to postpone the inevitable amputation. There is no successful medical therapy for this disorder at the present time.

Arterial Embolus

Acute blockage of a particular artery may or may not represent a surgical emergency. The viability of the tissue distal to the blockage is dependent on the existing or rapidly developing collateral circulation. If, for example, the superficial femoral artery is acutely obstructed, because there are few collateral vessels to the lower leg under normal circumstances at this level, the calf and foot would within 6 hours lose viability. The mandate for acute occlusive changes is immediate attention in terms of diagnosis and treatment.

Arterial embolus refers to matter forming in or breaking off of one structure, being carried in the blood stream, and lodging in a distal vessel the diameter of which is just smaller than the embolic debris. Over 90% of arterial emboli originate in the heart. Emboli or thrombi form in the heart under a variety of conditions, including arterial fibrillation and other arrhythmias, acute myocardial infarction, valvular disease, prosthetic valve, ventricular aneurysm, and atrial myxoma. Obviously the workup for acute ischemic changes in the leg would include the appropriate tests for the above conditions. Emboli may also originate in an atherosclerotic ulcer. Emboli may be formed from atherosclerotic debris as well as platelet and thrombotic material. The larger arteries, the aorta, and the iliac vessels are responsible for the majority of these atheroembolic events. Aneurysms and atherosclerotic ulcers, mostly identifiable on angiogram, liberate embolic material. Paradoxical emboli originate as venous thrombi, pass through a patent foramen ovale in the heart, and enter the arterial circuit.

The untreated course of arterial embolism is variable, depending on its location, collateral development, and degree of thrombosis both proximal and distal to the embolus that occurs. The accompanying thrombosis may actually become more devastating to tissue survival than the original embolic event. Administration of intravenous heparin retards the progression of thrombosis and should be administered as soon as embolism is diagnosed. The clinical presentation is variable, depending on location, collateral development, and degree of thrombosis. Generally the location of an acute embolus is fairly easy to determine, based on the appearance of the tissue distal to it, the loss or absence of pulse and Doppler signal, and the symptoms evoked by the ischemia.

The classic five "P's" have been described over and over in the vascular textbooks pertaining to acute ischemia. The five "P's" are pain, pallor, paresthesias, paralysis, and pulselessness. Pain is usually the first symptom, its onset being acute and severe and occurring distally in the extremity, gradually migrating proximally toward the level of occlusion. Pain is unremitting, constant, and severe. Pallor and coolness then occur as a consequence of the acute blockage. One should compare the involved limb with the other side and, of course, search old charts and office records for changes from previous physical examination (this underscores the need for complete data gathering on every admission history and physical examination form). Coolness occurs somewhat distal to the blocked level that relates to collateral supply. Paresthesias, especially hypoesthesia, occurs as a consequence of sensory nerve damage. Eventually paralysis occurs. Paralysis is manifested as the inability to wiggle toes and move the ankle, which are both ominous signs denoting impending if not actual irreversibility of ischemic changes.

An intense calf pain from infarcted muscle may occur with irreversible ischemia. The classic time limit before irreversibility in the lower extremity is 6 hours after onset of ischemia. However, this time is variable. Emboli tend to lodge at bifurcations, where there is usually a reduction in the caliber of the arterial branches. Areas of stenosis are favored sites for the same reason. The common femoral, common iliac, and popliteal arteries are predisposed for embolic involvement in the lower extremities.

The differential diagnosis of embolism includes arteriosclerotic thrombosis, acute thrombophlebitis, low flow state secondary to poor cardiac output, arterial dissection, vasospasm, aneurysmal thrombosis, and unrecognized trauma. At times, it is difficult, if not impossible, to differentiate from embolism. Acute thrombophlebitis in its early stages may mimic acute embolism, with loss of palpable pulses, pallor, coolness, and pain. However, development of edema and good Doppler signals help in the differentiation. The therapy for this entity is nonsurgical, using thrombolytic agents or anticoagulants. The low flow state may produce cool, cyanotic extremities, but involvement is usually symmetric, and Doppler signals are audible. There may be concomitant congestive heart failure or myocardial infarction.

Management of an embolus is directed at removing the embolus as well as the propagating clot in order to restore blood flow. This should be done as soon as possible. Intravenous heparin is instituted immediately to prevent further propagation of blood clot. Because most of the embolectomy procedures on the lower extremity can be undertaken with local anesthesia, work-up should be limited to chest radiograph, ECG, and laboratory tests. Ob-

viously if a critical accompanying medical illness is suspected this should be expeditiously evaluated. If the leg is viable and the condition of the patient is so dire that operation would be life threatening embolectomy should be delayed until the patient's condition is more optimal. Late embolectomy may be successful but should not be performed in the face of frank gangrene. Needless to say, each case is evaluated individually, and the decision to operate cannot be made in a cookbook-type fashion.

Preoperative angiography is called for if the level of occlusion is questioned. Accurate information about level of occlusion may change the operative plan. For example, general instead of local anesthesia may be employed if more than the femoral operative site is to be used, as might occur with femoral and popliteal embolectomies. If emboli occur in the aorta or iliac arteries a much more extensive operation may not be necessary because transfemoral Fogarty's catheter embolectomy is often successful in extracting the occluding material. However, occasionally transabdominal or retroperitoneal and popliteal procedures are called for. Intraoperative angiography, once the procedure is under way, is an alternative to save time. The role of thrombolytic agents in embolism therapy has not been totally elucidated.

Transfemoral embolectomy is the most common operation for lower extremity embolus. Complete removal of thrombus, however, is usually not possible, and intimal damage occurs with the passage of the catheter. Usually the surgeon continues making passes with the catheter until no further clot is removed. Through a transfemoral approach, aortic, iliac, femoral, popliteal, and more distal emboli may be retrieved.

Systemic heparinization is continued postoperatively, and eventually the patient is converted to warfarin (Coumadin). Postoperative thrombolytic agents may result in complications, especially hemorrhage from the operative site, and are usually not called for. Treatment of an underlying cardiac condition, such as arrhythmia, if present is, of course, attended to in the postoperative period. Close monitoring of pulses and all the described signs and symptoms for reocclusion is undertaken. Results of embolectomy, although a wide range exists in various series, average 63% limb salvage and 28% mortality. Mortality is predominantly secondary to a cardiac cause.

Microembolic atherosclerosis is not only associated with embolic phenomena but also with the presence of microemboli. Microemboli consist of small cholesterol crystals and equally small thrombi. These microemboli originate from atheroma, emboli, and thrombi. Because of their size, microemboli do not obstruct large vessels. Instead very small vessels and even arterioles are blocked. The physician must consider microemboli in the differential diagnosis of small patches of gangrene.

Arterial Thrombosis

Acute arterial thrombosis usually accompanies embolism to some degree, but it is a separate entity, and the therapy is different from that of embolism. The most common cause is simply progression of atherosclerotic disease. An increasingly common source of problems is iatrogenic placement of catheters in arteries for various reasons, such as hemodynamic monitoring and chemotherapy. In hemodynamic monitoring, thrombosis occurs when flow is impeded to such a degree by stenosis or a series of stenoses that blood clots in situ in the vessel or a plaque becomes undermined. Hemorrhage occurs behind the plaque in the wall of the artery, leading to occlusion.

The incidence of embolism and acute thrombosis is approximately even, and the distribution of the two entities is about the same, with embolism being somewhat more common in the aortoiliac segment and acute thrombosis more common in the calf circulation. This distribution would make sense because the caliber of the calf vessels is, of course, much smaller than the more proximal arteries. Diabetics have more distal thrombosis than nondiabetics.

The presentation of acute thrombosis is similar to embolism, especially if the affected artery was widely patent before the event. In vessels with major stenoses, the impetus for collateral formation may well have established an adequate collateral network already, thus diminishing the severity of the presenting signs and symptoms. Pain, pallor, cyanosis, paresthesias, pulse changes, and paralysis are the hall-marks of clinical presentation. Cardiac disease is usually present.

One can easily see how embolism and acute thrombosis can be confused. Nevertheless the overall surgical approach is different. Intravenous heparin is given immediately, as with embolus. However, in acute thrombosis, arteriography plays a much more pivotal role than in embolism because thrombectomy alone is usually not adequate to restore blood flow. Because the chain of events is consistent with those that occur with chronic progression of disease, the therapy is the same. In acute thrombosis, therapy is instituted at an accelerated rate because of the precarious nature of limb viability. Endarterectomy and bypass procedures are indicated in whatever location it takes to restore blood flow. Thrombolysis has been used to advantage in acute thrombosis, but definitive therapy must follow to remove or bypass the cause of the thrombosis. Occasionally this cause is a lesion that is amenable to PTA or laser angioplasty, thus obviating an operation. As already mentioned, embolism and thrombosis may coexist. The advent of thrombolytic therapy has somewhat modified the approach to operation for acute, occluded vessels but is an adjunct to more definitive therapy, such as surgery, balloon angioplasty, and laser angioplasty.

Aneurysm

Aneurysmal disease refers to the dilatation of an arterial segment due to as yet uncharacterized stimuli. Over 9 out of 10 arterial aneurysms today are associated with atherosclerosis, with other causes including mycotic arteritis, trauma, and congenital abnormalities. The most common complications of aneurysmal disease include expansion with rupture, thrombosis of the arterial segment involved, and embolism. There has been some research concerning the etiology of the dilatation process, and there appear to be differences from normal concerning some of the enzymatic components of the arterial wall. There is some evidence that fragmentation and degradation of the elastic lamellae in the media of the arterial wall occur. There may be a difference in the elastase enzymes in aneurysmal arterial wall as compared with normal arterial wall as well. Collagenase activity may be increased in the aneurysmal state, and an imbalance between the reparative and degradative processes in the arterial wall may account for the dilatation that occurs. As dilatation progresses, laminated clot forms on the walls of the artery, and the actual blood flow through the dilated vessel represents only a small portion of the lumen surrounded by this laminated thrombus.

In the aorta, a favored location for aneurysmal formation is between the renal arteries and the bifurcation of the aorta into the common iliac vessels. Rupture of an aneurysm in this location obviously has profound effects on the survival of the patient. It has been shown that once the diagnosis is made of an abdominal aortic aneurysm, there is a significant chance that the patient will, if left untreated, rupture the aneurysm within a relatively short period of time. Specifically of patients less than 60 years of age at the time of diagnosis, 60% rupture the aneurysm within 2 years. The percentage is slightly less for patients over 60 years of age.

The nonruptured abdominal aortic aneurysm is usually discovered serendipitously by a radiographic or ultrasonographic procedure undertaken for some other problem. Computed tomography (CT) scan, ultrasonography, and plain films may disclose the presence of an aneurysm of the aorta quite well. Expanding aneurysms may produce symptoms that are usually described as abdominal pain in the epigastrium and back and less commonly as flank or groin pain. Obviously there are a myriad of causes of the aforementioned complaints, but one should keep in mind this diagnosis when evaluating patients, especially older hypertensive patients who may have evidence of atherosclerotic involvement in other areas, such as cerebrovascular, renal, or extremity problems. Infrequently a patient presents at the office complaining of a pulsatile mass in the abdomen.

On physical examination there is commonly a pulsatile abdominal mass, which may even be visible in the mid upper abdomen in asthenic patients. This mass may be felt above the umbilicus, to the right or left of midline. Over 9 out of 10 abdominal aortic aneurysms begin below the level of the renal arteries. Some confusion may be caused in distinguishing aneurysmal dilatation of the aorta with a tortuous vessel, especially in thin patients. Transmitted pulsations from the aorta through other masses and organs in the abdomen may confuse the examiner as to the exact nature of the size of the aorta. A tender aortic aneurysm is a cause for concern because this may indicate leaking or more rapid enlargement of the structure. The presence of the aneurysm in the aorta does not preclude the presence of femoral pulses. In fact, even with rupture of the aneurysm, the femoral pulses may well be palpable. Auscultation of the abdomen may reveal an abdominal bruit, either related to the aortic aneurysm or stenosis in one of the branches of the aorta, such as the renal arteries.

The next step in identifying the presence of an aneurysm after history and physical examination is radiographic study. Plain films of the abdomen, including a cross table lateral view, may reveal calcification in the wall of the aneurysm and give some ideas as to the size of the structure. Ultrasonography is a noninvasive and inexpensive way to follow aneurysms and is also quite accurate in determining the size. Computed tomography can be used the same way. Computed tomography is more expensive but may reveal the presence of other pathology in the abdomen. Arteriography is an invasive procedure but gives the surgeon exact information concerning the location of the aneurysm and the presence of possible concomitant aneurysmal involvement of the iliac or femoral vessels as well as lower extremity runoff vessels. In addition, the branches of the aorta immediately in and around the area of the aneurysm, such as the renal and inferior mesenteric arteries, are shown to advantage and help in planning the operation. The aortogram is not used in the emergency rupture situation. Frequently with a "leaking" aneurysm and stable patient, a CT or ultrasonography study shows that there is hemorrhage around the aneurysm. With a leaking or rupturing aneurysm, the patient should be taken immediately to the operating room for definitive therapy.

The rupturing aortic aneurysm is a dire surgical emergency. If the patient is conscious he or she usually relates a history of severe abdominal or back pain, acute in onset and perhaps radiating to one of the groin areas. The patient often relates a history of fainting. In the emergency room, the patient may be thought of as having renal colic or some other intra-abdominal catastrophe, and precious time may be lost in pursuing diagnostic tests that are of no help. The most critical factor in determining survival is the amount of time between the rupture of the vessel and the clamp placed on the aorta to control bleeding. If the diagnosis is suspected the patient should be taken to the operating room immediately and resuscitation performed on the operating table as the patient is being prepared for laparotomy. Replacement of an aortic aneurysm has been found to be a durable, life-saving procedure even in its elective form. In the lower extremities, other areas of aneurysmal involvement include the common iliac, hypogastric, common femoral, and popliteal arteries. Common iliac and hypogastric artery aneurysms behave in many ways similar to aortic aneurysms, that is, rupture is more common than thrombosis. Femoral and popliteal aneurysms are more prone to thrombosis than rupture. Thrombosis of an aneurysm is a variation of an acute occlusion with all its concomitant sequelae. With a good collateral bed, viability is maintained, and in the absence of collateralization, the extremity is put at risk.

Resection of common iliac and hypogastric artery aneurysms follows the same principles elucidated in the aortic procedure. The principles include proximal and distal control, systemic heparinization, and replacement of the involved vessel with graft material. Most commonly these aneurysms occur in conjunction with aortic aneurysms but occasionally are found alone.

The popliteal aneurysm is especially problematic because it usually occurs in a younger, more active age group, and when complications occur, the consequences are often dire. Aneurysms at this location much more commonly thrombose than rupture, and because of the paucity of collateral formation at this level, thrombosis can lead to limb loss. Not uncommonly these aneurysms are often bilateral. The operative technique involves a retrogeniculate approach or the standard medial approach both above and below the knee joint. The problem with the retrogeniculate approach is exposure proximally and distally of the inflow and outflow vessels should the need arise to explore and deal with these vessels. The basic operative approach is to exclude the aneurysm from the circulatory tree and to perform a bypass using autogenous vein.

Vasculitis

Vasculitis is an inflammation of blood vessels. In the process of inflammatory disease of blood vessels, the wide clinical spectrum of presentations of vasculitides is dependent on the different areas of the organ systems and regions of the body that are affected by these widely varying inflammatory processes. The original classification of these differing syndromes was based on vessel size and location, type of blood vessel and its infiltrate, and location of the inflammatory response in and around the blood vessel. As new tests became available, there was ongoing redefinition of the vasculitides. This section does not attempt to delve into this subject in depth but to present briefly an overview of vasculitis entities that may affect the lower extremities in relation to circulation.

The important vasculitis entities that affect the circulation in the lower extremities include the giant cell arteritides temporal arteritis and Takayasu's arteritis, which are granulomatous vasculitides of the medium and large-sized arteries, and thromboangiitis obliterans, which is an inflammatory disorder of the intermediate-sized to small-sized arteries and veins of the extremities.

Giant Cell Arteritis (Temporal Arteritis)

Giant cell arteritis can involve any medium-sized or large-sized artery of the body, but the majority of the symptoms resulting from this disease are in branches of the carotid artery. Giant cell arteritis is not a common disorder and mostly affects elderly individuals. The etiology of the disease is unknown. Genetic and environmental factors may be important in the development of the disorder. The most common presenting symptoms are headache, malaise, fatigue, and jaw claudication. Extremity claudication occurs in less than 1 out of 10 patients. Constitutional symptoms of fever, weight loss, malaise, anorexia, and depression are common. Physical findings include tenderness and nodule formation along the course of the superficial temporal artery and can be demonstrated in approximately one half of the cases. Pathologic findings on biopsy of the vessel may be present without these characteristic physical findings. The most dangerous sequela of this disease is visual impairment, which is caused by thrombosis of the optic artery and results in sudden blindness. Visual impairment affects approximately 36% of patients with the disorder. Most patients have other symptoms of the disease prior to the onset of visual changes. However, most of these symptoms are fairly nonspecific. Unfortunately a number of patients present initially with blindness, which is irreversible. Other visual symptoms include diplopia, amaurosis fugax, and blurry vision. Jaw claudication, which is pain or weakness with speaking or chewing, is another unusual symptom that is often related to this disorder.

The laboratory findings in temporal arteritis are fairly nonspecific, but most of the cases are accompanied by an elevated ESR and often abnormal liver function tests, specifically elevated alkaline phosphatase. Because of the risk of sudden blindness from optic neuritis, the clinician should have a high index of suspicion for this disorder. A biopsy of the temporal artery should show the distinctive histopathologic features of giant cells, which may not be found, and an inflammatory reaction with mononuclear, PMN, and eosinophil cells. In addition, often intimal proliferation is seen, which may narrow the lumen of the vessel. The inflammatory reaction in the vessel is usually of a segmental nature. The surgeon performing the vessel biopsy harvests at least 1 cm or 2 cm of vessel because of knowledge of this segmental involvement. Symptoms and findings below the head and neck area are not common with this disorder, but lower extremity claudication due to involvement of the vessels to the leg has been described.

There is an uncertain relationship between polymyalgia rheumatica and giant cell arteritis. Both are diseases of older individuals, and both are frequently seen in the same patient. Of patients with giant cell arteritis, 60% experience polymalgia rheumatica at some time during their illness. As with polymyalgia rheumatica, patients with giant cell arteritis respond well to steroid treatment.

When giant cell arteritis is diagnosed or even suspected, treatment should be started immediately with at least 50 mg of prednisone in order to preserve vision. If the diagnosis is proved by biopsy the dose should be continued for 4 weeks and then tapered to a maintenance dose of 7.5 mg of prednisone daily.

Takayasu's Disease

Takayasu's disease is an inflammatory disorder with resulting stenosis or occlusion of intermediate and large arteries predominantly affecting young women and involving the aortic arch and its various branches. Takayasu, in 1908, first described changes in the retinas of young women, and various workers have more fully characterized the disease over the years. The disorder has been known by a number of different names, the most common of which is pulseless disease. The disease predominantly affects women in their 20s and is marked by acute inflammatory and chronic occlusive phases separated by a number of years. The acute inflammatory phase is heralded by nonspecific constitutional complaints, such as fever, night sweats, myalgias, and arthralgias. The later occlusive phase is associated with signs and symptoms referred to the involved areas with visual and cerebrovascular symptoms and upper extremity findings predominating. Radial pulses are almost uniformly absent, whereas femoral pulses are absent in a small minority of cases (5%). Accompanying bruits of the stenotic vessels are often present. In the lower extremities, intermittent claudication occurs in 3 out of 10 cases. A number of patients describe a "face down" position with flexion of the neck that helps to avoid ischemia to the optic vasculature, which is often exacerbated with the head held up in the extended "face up" position. Patients are often hypertensive on the basis of renal vascular ischemia. Although cardiac and pulmonary complications occur in 30 to 50% of cases, eventually the major cause of mortality with this disorder is congestive heart failure and myocardial infarction.

Laboratory findings are generally nonspecific. However, an elevated ESR is common. Arteriography is the important test in diagnosis. The pathologic finding in the vessels affected is infiltration of all layers of the arterial wall with mononuclear giant cells. Aneurysmal involvement may be seen. The secondary atherosclerotic changes narrowing the vessel are often found as well. The therapy of the disease is steroid suppression of the inflammatory response in its early phases and vascular reconstructive procedures for the chronic stenotic and occlusive arteries. Reconstructive procedures during the inflammatory initial part of the disease are usually not successful. Concomitant therapy of associated medical problems, such as hypertension and hypercholesterolemia, should be undertaken.

Therapeutics in Arterial Vascular Disease

The overriding concern that all physicians have in treating patients is that they "first do no harm" to the patients. Every therapeutic intervention that physicians undertake must be tempered with careful deliberation.

Medical Therapy

The medical treatment of vascular disease is predominantly reduction of the effects of the most important risk factors of development of the diseases; antiplatelet therapy; anticoagulant therapy; thrombolytic therapy; administration of certain drugs; and nonsurgical modalities for dealing with stenotic or occlusive lesions, such as PTA and laser angioplasty techniques.

MAJOR RISK FACTORS

The major risk factors for development of atherosclerosis have been enumerated and include elevated serum lipid levels, cigarette smoking, and hypertension.

Serum Lipids. Elevated LDL (low-density lipoprotein) levels in the serum have been associated with increased development of atherosclerotic disease. Conversely elevated levels of HDLs (high-density lipoproteins) have been thought to be protective for the disorder. Certainly in those disorders that exhibit hyperlipidemia on a congenital basis, the concomitant atherosclerotic changes are obvious. However, there are many patients who present with atherosclerotic disease who have normal levels of lipids in the serum. Nevertheless if such a patient is encountered who does have elevated serum lipid levels, an effort should be made to convince the patient that certain dietary restrictions should be followed in order to bring these values into the normal range. There are innumerable dietary and exercise programs abounding in the medical and lay literature that do achieve more favorable serum lipid levels. These programs have a beneficial effect on the progress and development of atherosclerotic plaques. Reference should be made to any one of many dietary sources in recommending to patients the proper diets to follow.

Cigarette Smoking. The second potent risk factor, which is extremely prevalent in society, is cigarette smoking. The exact mechanism or mechanisms by which cigarette smoking aids and abets the progression of atherosclerotic disease; the earlier failure of vascular reconstructive procedures; and the induced vascular complications other than peripheral vascular problems, such as myocardial infarction and cerebrovascular insufficiency, is unknown. It is known, however, that cigarette smoke increases platelet aggregation, increases vascoconstriction, and decreases HDL. Cigarette smoke is also the most common source of carbon monoxide in the blood. It is the duty of the physician to advise and counsel the patient as to the ills of smoking, not only with respect to vascular disease but also with respect to its well-known effects in other disorders, such as development of cancer.

Hypertension. Hypertension often accompanies atherosclerotic disease and causes many other complications with respect to the vascular system, such as stroke and kidney failure. Hypertension participates in aneurysm formation and in complications associated with vascular reconstructive procedures, such as the development of false aneurysms. The therapy for hypertension is much more widely well received by the patient population than changing diet and smoking habits, however. These risk factors must be well documented in the patient's chart on workup, and attempts by all medical personnel to ameliorate these risk factors should be undertaken until the patient complies.

Vasodilation Therapy

Vasodilation therapy would seem to be a reasonable approach to peripheral vascular insufficiency. Nevertheless medical therapy with vasodilatory agents has not met with success over the years. Generally speaking, the homeostatic mechanisms pertaining to vasodilation have been most likely used to their maximum by the body in the face of arterial insufficiency. Further endeavors to increase the amount of blood flow through dilatation of the vessels by pharmacologic means using a variety of agents, such as tolazoline, papaverine, nitroglycerin and other related compounds, dermal nitroglycerin, and other agents, have not been effective in general in improving the arterial inflow to the lower extremity. Surgical cutaneous vasodilation accomplished with lumbar sympathectomy does have a role in the ischemic lower extremity. Severe vasospastic disorders, such as Raynaud's syndrome, are usually not amenable to pharmacologic manipulation, and sympathectomy either cervical or lumbar for the respective extremity may or may not be successful.

Rheologic Agent

Pentoxifylline (Trental) has been given to patients with complaints of intermittent claudication and rest pain and seems to be successful in improving symptoms in perhaps 15% of the patient population, according to subjective and objective parameters. This drug is a rheologic agent, which allows the red cell membrane to become more deformable and theoretically allows passage of red blood cells through smaller capillaries, thus increasing the amount of oxygen delivered to the tissues. The studies attempting to quantify improvement in the patient population generally relate an improved walking distance capability in those patients who do note improvement. This drug causes gastrointestinal side effects and is expensive. Pentoxifylline certainly is not a panacea for arterial insufficiency but most likely should be tried in selected instances of patients who complain of severe intermittent claudication or in those patients with poor skin flow who are not surgical candidates. The drug has no role in tissue loss situations.

Aspirin is able to decrease platelet aggregation when given in low doses. Many patients are given aspirin, one a day, to take advantage of this property. With respect to the cerebrovascular circulation, it has been shown that patients taking one aspirin a day have fewer transient ischemic attack symptoms but do not have a decreased incidence of stroke. It has not been shown whether patients who are susceptible to developing lower extremity vascular insufficiency benefit by taking aspirin or not.

Anticoagulation Therapy

Anticoagulation therapy includes heparin and warfarin products. Heparin and warfarin are often used perioperatively for arterial operations, but their effectiveness in terms of graft patency and maintaining arterial circulation has not been established in any randomized studies. Nevertheless patients who are considered to be hypercoagulable are often maintained on anticoagulation therapy (patients are first given heparin and then converted to oral warfarin products for a number of months postoperatively). These agents are used in acute arterial insufficiency situations, as explained in sections dealing with those topics. Heparin and warfarin are used with venous thrombotic diatheses. As far as is known, anticoagulants do not affect the development of atherosclerotic lesions one way or the other. Warfarin products have one of the highest rates of outpatient complications for any drug specifically related to bleeding.

Surgical Management

RECONSTRUCTIVE SURGERY

The objective of vascular arterial reconstruction is to restore pulsatile flow to the foot level when possible. Pulsatile flow in short is the most viable way of predicting if wounds will heal and whether symptoms of rest pain and intermittent claudication will be relieved. Generally speaking, patients suffering from intermittent claudication are not operated on today as they have been in the past. For intermittent claudication, exercise programs, cessation of smoking, weight loss, and other conservative measures usually allow the patient to develop collateral circulation, which relieves or improves the claudication. True rest pain is an ominous symptom when it occurs and mandates a vascular work-up and intervention. In the absence of tissue loss situations, such as gangrene or ulcer, reconstructive arterial operations that improve the blood flow to the foot level but do not restore pulsatile flow are generally successful in relieving rest pain.

If gangrene or ulcer exists, with or without infection, the operation should be designed to bring a palpable pulse to the foot whenever possible. This is not to say that a successful reconstructive procedure that improves the blood flow to the most distal levels will not effect healing. Even if the bypass procedure does not remain patent after healing has occurred, many times the healed gangrenous area or ulcer remains healed, and the patient is symptom free. If flow is significantly increased to the most distal part healing may well occur, but the quality of the arteries is such that a palpable pulse is not able to be felt owing to the calcification of the arterial wall. In general, however, the return of a palpable pulse in the foot is the gold standard concerning revascularization procedures.

As stated, there are three general patterns of atherosclerotic involvement concering the blood supply to the foot that can be categorized as aortoiliac, iliofemoral, and femorodistal disease. There is quite a bit of overlap in patients, but these classic forms of atherosclerotic involvement have implications concerning the ultimate perfusion of the tissues of the foot. Aortoiliac involvement, which can be characterized by Leriche's syndrome, concerns occlusion of the distal aorta and proximal iliac vessels. Patients with this problem usually complain of weakness in the legs, and men complain of impotence. However, patients generally do not present with ulcerated or gangrenous problems. Aortofemoral bypass is the operation of choice for this problem.

The diminution of blood flow in the aortoiliac segment constitutes the basic problem of inflow inadequacy to the lower extremity. Inflow to the lower extremity is characterized by the femorotibial vessels. Generally speaking, one should not attempt an outflow revascularization procedure unless the inflow is adequate to maintain the patency of the more distal operations. At times, there may be problems deciding whether the patient's primary problem is an inflow or outflow inadequacy. The history and physical examination as well as noninvasive and arteriographic work-up should answer this question. The pertinent details contained in the history and physical examination that deal with the problem of inflow inadequacy are the presence of buttock and thigh claudication rather than calf claudication, impotence in men, diminished femoral pulse, bruit over the femoral pulse indicating iliac stenosis, and diminution of the femoral pulse with exercise.

With noninvasive examination, segmental arterial pressures may suggest problems with the aortoiliac areas in comparison with arm pressures, and the arteriogram may show high-grade stenoses or occlusion of segments in the aortoiliac region. In addition, it is common practice in performing aortography to measure pressures in the aortoiliac segment, thus determining hemodynamically significant lesions. It is also common practice to dilate focal lesions in the aortoiliac region at the time of aortography, which may improve the inflow to the femoral artery and distal vessels before outflow-type procedures are performed. More and more today infrainguinal PTA and laser angioplasty procedures are undertaken either at the time of initial arteriography or shortly thereafter with moderate success to improve vascular supply to the distal lower extremity.

Before the 1950s, there were generally two types of procedures performed for lower extremity arterial insufficiency: amputation and lumbar sympathectomy. The popularity of lumbar sympathectomy has waned, primarily because of its inability to reverse rest pain and avoid limb loss situations. However, there is clearly a role for this operation even today. The sympathetic denervation causes an increase in the resting blood flow in the cutaneous microcirculation. There is usually no change in the muscular perfusion. It has been noted over the years that this increase in oxygen supply, the effects of which usually last over a 6- to 12-month period, can help in the healing of shallow cutaneous ulcerations. In addition to the increase in cutaneous flow, there is an abolition of the transmission of certain pain stimuli that helps the patient endure some of the ischemia-related pain in the malperfused tissues, with or without ulceration. The indications for this operation are usually situations in which the patient is considered to be inoperable in terms of direct revascularization. In this context, effects of the lumbar sympathectomy usually are not successful in reversing the pain or avoiding limb loss situations. However, in select patients, this operation can achieve success in healing certain ulcerations and in relieving pain either in conjunction with a revascularization procedure or before the revascularization procedure is performed.

Femoropopliteal bypass is usually indicated for rest pain and tissue loss situations of the lower extremity and was quite often performed for intermittent claudication in the past. The success rate in relief of intermittent claudication with femoropopliteal bypass was high. However, it was realized that in the absence of operation for bypass of an occluded superficial femoral artery under certain circumstances, which included increased exercise, smoking cessation, and weight loss, most patients would significantly improve in their walking tolerance. Currently bypass procedures for intermittent claudication, unless the symptom is disabling, are not performed.

Femoral, including deep femoral artery to tibial or pedal arteries, and distal bypass procedures are performed for rest pain and tissue loss situations in an ever-increasing variety. The basic techniques of exposure and anastomosis are the same in all situations. However, the big difference between lower extremity bypass procedures today and in years past is the meticulous attention to detail, with the use of magnifying lenses for precise anastomosis and exposure. The best bypass conduit remains autogenous vein in terms of patency rates, and it should be used exclusively with the more distal bypasses. Patency rates in the larger vessels, such as iliac or superficial femoral bypass above the knee, are as good with Dacron or Gore-Tex as with autogenous vein.

Operations for acute arterial insufficiency may combine some or all of the bypass techniques used for chronic situations as well as the use of thromboembolectomy. The operative procedure includes immediate heparinization on diagnosis of an acute thrombosis or embolus and then thromboembolectomy by exposing the artery at the level of the suspected involvement and using a Fogarty's type balloon-tip catheter to remove embolic and thrombotic material in both antegrade and retrograde directions. Examination of the retrieved material may be able to identify the nature of the initial occluding event, be it thrombotic or embolic, and rarely demonstrates unusual pathology, such as a cardiac atrial myxoma. After reestablishment of flow through the involved vessels, if, in the opinion of the operating surgeon, the resultant flow is inadequate to salvage the more distal portions of the limb a bypass operation may be combined with a thromboembolectomy procedure. In these acute situations, the patient is given heparin postoperatively and then converted to warfarin as an outpatient for 3 to 6 months. This therapy is in contrast to operations for chronic ischemia in which this type of postoperative anticoagulant therapy is usually not employed, although most patients are given aspirin or other antiplatelet medication for chronic situations.

Generally speaking, better results in terms of long-term patency are achieved in situations in which there is good inflow and outflow surrounding the bypass conduit that has been placed. The contribution of antiplatelet and anticoagulant concomitant therapy in conjunction with bypass operations has not truly been assessed. However, most patients today are given at least antiplatelet therapy postoperatively. The bypass of more proximal and hence larger vessels is accompanied by longer patency rates in general. Longer distal bypasses going to small arterial outflow vessels in the foot and in the lower leg do not remain patent as long as the larger more proximal bypass procedures. However, although the goal of vascular reconstructive surgery is to place a graft that in most cases should remain patent, in many situations a bypass procedure is performed, which allows healing of necrotic or gangrenous tissue followed by eventual occlusion of the bypass graft but without deterioration of the distal tissue that has healed and remains stable.

Peripheral Vascular Disease Due to Abnormal Vasoconstriction and Vasodilation

Raynaud's Phenomenon and Disease

Raynaud's phenomenon is a syndrome manifested by attacks of pallor and cyanosis of the digits in response to cold or to emotion. As the attack abates, these color changes are replaced by redness. When the disorder is primary, it is called Raynaud's disease. When the disorder is secondary to another disease or cause, it is called Raynaud's phenomenon. The cause of Raynaud's disease is unknown. Causes of secondary Raynaud's phenomenon include occlusive arterial disease, such as arteriosclerosis obliterans, Buerger's disease, arterial embolism, vasculitis, and arterial thrombus; connective tissue diseases; vascular injury; neurogenic disorders; intravascular coagulation; drugs; and exposure to chemicals.

Although Raynaud's disease can begin at any age, it becomes clinically manifested most commonly between the ages of 20 and 40. Raynaud's disease is much more common in women than in men. The onset of Raynaud's disease is usually gradual. The patient notices an occasional mild and short-lasting attack during winter. Over succeeding years, the severity and duration of the attacks may increase. A wide variation in severity is present. Most commonly, the attacks are provoked by exposure to cold. In some patients, attacks are also precipitated by emotion. The attacks may be terminated by rewarming or may abate spontaneously. Between attacks, the patient is asymptomatic, and physical examination shows no abnormalities. Some patients may complain of chronically cold hands and feet and may have cold fingers with cyanosis on examination.

In a typical attack, the fingers become symmetrically pale with sharply demarcated pallor at the level of the metacarpophalangeal joints, reflecting spasm of the digital arteries. At a later stage, pallor is replaced by cyanosis. The patient may have a feeling of coldness, numbness, and occasional pain. On warming, the cyanosis is replaced by intense redness, and the patient may feel tingling or throbbing. Most commonly, only the hands are affected. In severe, progressive cases, trophic changes may occur. Hair may disappear, and nails may grow more slowly and become brittle and deformed. The skin becomes atrophic, thin, and tight (sclerodactyly). Ulcerations may develop at the fingertips or around the nail bed. These ulcerations heal slowly and may become infected. The ulcerations are extremely painful especially at night and leave small pitted scars when healed.

Diagnosis is usually made on the basis of history. When description of an attack is unclear, provocation of an attack may be helpful. An attack may be provoked by immersing the hands in 10° to 15° C (50° to 59° F) water. A negative result does not exclude Raynaud's phenomenon (Table 2–4). Differentiation from acrocyanosis is usually easy, unless the presentation is atypical. Distinguishing features include the following:

1. The color changes in Raynaud's phenomenon are episodic but are sustained in acrocyanosis.

2. Cyanosis is the more typical color change in acrocyanosis than pallor.

3. In Raynaud's disease, only the digits are involved, and in acrocyanosis, the color changes usually involve the whole hand or foot and sometimes even more proximal portions of the limbs.

4. The skin of the palms is usually dry in Raynaud's disease and is wet and clammy with sweat in acrocyanosis.

5. Acrocyanosis rarely causes trophic changes and ulcerations.

Obstruction in major arteries from arteriosclerosis, angitis, embolism, or thrombosis may lead to color changes in the digits that simulate Raynaud's phenomenon. The distinction is made by the demonstration of changes in arterial pulses and by the fact that the color changes in these disorders are likely to be confined to one limb rather than be symmetric. Arteriography demonstrates the arterial lesion and shows normal major arteries and diffuse spasm of the digital arteries in Raynaud's phenom-

Table 2–4. DIFFERENTIAL DIAGNOSIS OF RAYNAUD'S DISEASE FROM RAYNAUD'S PHENOMENON

Feature	Raynaud's Disease	Raynaud's Phenomenon
Sex	Female	Male
Bilaterality	Present (often symmetric)	± (Asymmetric)
Ischemic changes	Rare	Common
Precipitated by cold	Common	Uncommon
Gangrene	Rare	Common
Underlying condition*	No	Yes

* Scleroderma, systemic lupus erythematosus, dermatomyositis, rheumatoid arthritis.

enon. In Raynaud's phenomenon, the Doppler velocity studies show patent arteries with sharply peaked blood flow velocity patterns in the digits.

The distinction of Raynaud's disease from secondary Raynaud's phenomenon is based mainly on the exclusion of disorders known to cause the phenomenon. The exclusion of obstructive arterial disease, as stated, is by arteriography. Connective tissue disorders, particularly scleroderma, are excluded by absence of arthralgias or arthritis, alterations of esophageal motility, and absence of pulmonary oxygen diffusion defects. The presence of a normal sedimentation rate and the absence of circulating autoantibodies, such as antinuclear antibodies, provide additional reassurance.

A careful occupational history is necessary to exclude Raynaud's phenomenon secondary to minor repetitive trauma. A history of drug ingestion or exposure to chemicals is helpful in identifying drug-induced Raynaud's phenomenon. Neurologic disorders, such as thoracic outlet syndrome, can be recognized by their somatic neurologic manifestations. The presence of intravascular agglutination or coagulation of blood elements may be suspected if in the presence of cyanosis the blood cannot be expelled from vessels by pressure and if there are isolated areas of redness as the attack abates during rewarming. Confirmation is obtained by demonstrating the cold agglutinins or cryoglobulins in the patient's blood. The prognosis of the patient with Raynaud's phenomenon is good. There is no mortality associated with the disease, and morbidity is low. Loss of portions of digits as a result of ulcerations is the most common complication. In about 1% of cases, amputation may be necessary. About 15% of patients with Raynaud's phenomenon develop a connective tissue disorder, most commonly scleroderma. The prognosis in secondary Raynaud's phenomenon depends on the course of the primary disorder. In scleroderma, the prognosis is unsatisfactory particularly when digital ulcerations are part of the presentation. Treatment is tailored to the individual needs of the patient, taking into consideration the frequency and severity of the attacks.

All patients can benefit from reassurance and protective measures against exposure to cold. Patients should limit the duration of exposure to cold and wear heavy clothing that protects not only the hands and feet but also the face and trunk. Exposure to cold of other portions of the body may reflexively induce vasoconstriction in the digits and precipitate Raynaud's phenomenon. Patients should be taught to terminate attacks by returning promptly to a warm environment and placing the hands in warm water (43° C [109° F]) or using a warm-air blow dryer to warm the hands rapidly. Smoking causes cutaneous vasoconstriction and is therefore contraindicated in Raynaud's phenomenon.

Simple measures suffice for infrequent and mild attacks. More frequent and severe attacks, especially with trophic changes and ulcerations, need to be supplemented with drugs. The aim of drug therapy is to induce vascular smooth muscle relaxation, thereby relieving spasm, raising resting blood flow, and limiting the degree of ischemia. The drug of choice is a calcium antagonist. Nifedipine (10 to 20 mg three to four times a day) has been found to be effective in several well-controlled, double-blind studies. Diltiazem (60 mg three or four times daily) may be substituted if nifedipine is not well tolerated or if it causes side effects. Reserpine is the best-studied drug among the group that interferes with the function of the adrenergic nervous system. Reserpine is given by mouth in doses of 0.1 to 0.5 mg daily. In cases with ulcerations, reserpine may be dissolved in sterile normal saline and given by slow infusion over several minutes intra-arterially through the brachial or radial artery.

Acrocyanosis

Acrocyanosis is a rare disorder characterized by persistent cyanosis of the skin of the hands and feet and reduced skin temperature. The cause of this primary disorder is unknown. Acrocyanosis is more common in women than in men. The onset of the disease is usually in young or middle-aged adults. The smaller precapillary vessels (arterioles) are abnormally constricted, causing reduction in blood flow that results in cyanosis and lowered skin temperature. Constriction of the arterioles occurs under normal environmental conditions and becomes more pronounced on exposure to cold because of increased sensitivity of these vessels to the effects of cold. Features of acrocyanosis are reduced venous tone, secondary dilatation, and no venous obstruction. This lack of obstruction can be seen when the affected limb is elevated and the blue color is eliminated and when the color is intensified by placing the limb in a dependent position and overfilling the veins.

Patients with acrocyanosis have persistent blue discoloration of the hands. Less commonly the feet are also involved, and the blue color may extend to more proximal portions of the limbs. The skin is cold and wet and clammy from sweat. No pallor is usually present, but spots of pallor surrounded by confluent cyanosis may be seen. The blue color intensifies by exposure to cold and is converted to purple or red by exposure to heat. There are few accompanying symptoms. The patient has feelings of coldness and occasionally numbness. Ulcerations and other trophic changes are distinctly unusual.

Acrocyanosis and cyanosis related to arterial obstruction can be differentiated on the basis of a normal pulse, by the bilateral and symmetric occurrence of acrocyanosis, and through angiography if necessary. Limitation of the cyanosis to the hands and feet, improvement in warm environment, and absence of reduced arterial blood saturation distinguish acrocyanosis from generalized, systemic cyanosis due to cardiopulmonary problems.

No therapy is usually required because acrocyanosis is a benign disease. Reassurance and protection from cold usually suffice. Drug therapy used in Raynaud's phenomenon may also be used in acrocyanosis, especially with unusually severe symptoms.

Livedo Reticularis

Livedo reticularis is a reticular, bluish discoloration of the skin of the extremities that produces a lacy, irregular appearance that outlines central areas of normal-appearing skin. The disorder usually begins before the ages of 20 and 30, is of unknown etiology, and is equally common in men and women. There may be perivascular infiltrates and proliferative lesions of the skin arterioles and thrombus in the arteriole, leading to cutaneous infarction and

ulceration. Similar changes are seen in the veins. The mechanism is presumed to be constriction of arterioles followed by stasis and dilatation of capillaries and veins. The capillaries are filled with desaturated blood. The reticular appearance of livedo reticularis reflects the anatomic arrangement of the affected vessels. The bluish areas are believed to represent the arborizations of peripheral capillaries from central penetrating arterioles. Blood flow is faster in the central regions closer to the penetrating arteriole, whereas the more distant areas have lower flow, with consequent stasis and cyanosis.

The lower extremities are involved more often than the upper extremities with usually no symptoms. However, patients seek medical attention for cosmetic reasons or concern over bluish discoloration. In some cases, there may be paresthesias or a feeling of coldness. The bluish discoloration becomes more intense on exposure to cold and may disappear in a warm environment. Ulcerations occur rarely and usually appear in winter and heal in summer. Protection from cold and abstinence from smoking may be helpful, and usually no treatment is required. Drugs useful in Raynaud's phenomenon, such as nifedipine and reserpine, may be tried.

Erythromelalgia (Erythermalgia)

Erythromelalgia occurs with episodes of erythema accompanied by increased skin temperature and pain involving the feet and less commonly the hands. This disorder may be primary or secondary to obstructive arterial disease, polycythemia, and hypertension. There is no sex predilection, and the disease may occur at any age. Erythromelalgia is occasionally hereditary. Vasodilation and consequent hyperemia are the usual causes of the rise in skin temperature. However, an increased blood flow is not essential because once symptoms have been induced by heat, they may continue even though blood flow is reduced to zero with a cuff inflated above the systolic pressure levels. These features suggest that the cause of the disorder is abnormal sensitivity of the cutaneous pain fibers to heat or tension from the dilated blood vessels.

The onset of the disease is gradual, but with progression, the frequency and duration of attacks may become more pronounced. Eventually symptoms may become almost continuous and cause total disability. During an attack, complaints include burning pain usually in the balls of the feet and the tips of the toes and less commonly in the corresponding parts of the hands. Pain is aggravated by dependent positions and alleviated with elevation. Exposure to heat aggravates the disorder, whereas cold provides relief. Trophic changes, ulcerations, and gangrene are rare.

Peripheral neuropathy may cause burning pain simulating erythromelalgia. The pain may be accompanied by cutaneous vasodilation. The detection of the associated sensory and motor manifestations of peripheral neuropathy should help distinguish this condition from erythromelalgia. Arteriosclerosis obliterans or thromboangiitis obliterans may also produce localized burning pain and redness. The alteration in the peripheral pulses and the absence of high skin temperature differentiate these disorders from erythromelalgia. Vascular damage from prolonged exposure to cold, as after frostbite, may simulate erythromelalgia. In these cases, the condition is more persistent, and the history of cold exposure should help make the distinction possible.

Treatment includes avoidance of exposure to heat. Elevation of the extremity and application of cold may terminate the attack. Aspirin (650 mg orally) is adequate to relieve the pain in most cases. The response is sometimes so striking it is of diagnostic value. Vasoconstrictive agents, such as methysergide or epinephrine, or beta-adrenergic blocking agents, such as propranolol, have been reported to be effective in some patients. In secondary cases, treatment of the primary disorder may allevaite the attacks.

Peripheral Vascular Disease Related to Cold Exposure

Immersion Foot (Trench Foot)

Immersion foot is characterized by vascular damage resulting from prolonged exposure of the extermities to cold by wearing wet socks or wet footwear. Usually the exposure is for several days at about 0° C (32° F). Dependency of limbs and immobility as well as conditions that lead to general debility, such as lack of sleep and starvation, are major contributing factors. The condition has occurred primarily in soldiers at war and has also been described in survivors of shipwrecks, who were immobilized in crowded small crafts for a long time and exposed to wetness and cold. Maceration of skin with sea water and secondary infection also contribute.

The condition results from vascular injury from the initial effect of cold. Vasoconstriction with loss of heat, facilitated by moisture, results in ischemia with injury to tissues and increased endothelial permeability. There is extensive extravasation of protein and fluid. As a result, there may be increased hematocrit, sludging, and further aggravation of ischemia. In advanced cases, one sees extensive vascular injury and gangrene with periarterial fibrosis and thickening in the small arteries, which may also be occluded. The veins show perivenous fibrosis, inflammatory reaction, and hemorrhage. The nerves may also be affected. In cases of immersion foot at relatively high temperatures, hyperhydration of the plantar stratum corneum may be the only finding.

Three successive stages, each with distinct clinical manifestations, are recognized. The involved extremity, during exposure to a wet, cold environment, becomes pale and cool. The patient has paresthesia and a feeling of coldness. Patients are most commonly observed during the second stage of hyperemia with a red, hot, edematous extremity. There may be pain or paresthesias. The swelling may be aggravated by heat and by placing the limb in a dependent position. Subsequently blebs appear, filled with serous or hemorrhagic fluid. Hemorrhages may occur in the skin and subcutaneous tissue. This stage may persist for several days. In severe cases, gangrene may supervene. The condition may be complicated by lymphagitis, cellulitis, and thrombophlebitis. Mild cases or those treated early may recover after this second hyperemic phase. In other cases, a third late vasospastic phase occurs in which there is increased sensitivity to cold and typical secondary Raynaud's phenomenon, with excessive sweating, pain, and paresthesias of the lower extremities. This phase may persist for years.

Treatment for the initial vasoconstrictive phase includes bed rest with the extremity in the horizontal position and a warm environment. During the hyperemic phase, the extremity should be placed at heart level and kept cool to diminish edema. Local care to keep the foot dry and clean should be instituted to avoid infection. Control of pain may require analgesics or narcotics. Sympathectomy may be helpful in the hyperemic stage and also in preventing the late vasospastic phenomena.

Chilblain (Pernio)

Chilblain is an inflammatory condition of the skin of the extremities that is induced by cold and characterized by erythema, itching, and ulceration. Chilblain is more common in cold, damp climates. This condition affects women more than men and begins before the age of 20 in most patients. The cause is unknown. In chronic cases, the lesions consist of angitis with intimal proliferation, thickening of the arterial wall, and perivascular infiltration with lymphocytes and polymorphonuclear leukocytes. There may be necrosis of the adipose tissue and chronic inflammatory infiltrates in the subcutaneous tissue.

A typical presentation is a young female in winter with bluish red discoloration and edema of the skin of the lower limbs associated with burning and warmth. The lesions are persistent and are associated with itching. These lesions generally last from 7 to 10 days and then resolve, often leaving a residual pigmentation of the skin at the site of involvement. In severe cases, the lesions may become hemorrhagic, blebs may appear, and infection may supervene. With repeated exposure to cold, susceptible persons may develop chronic lesions. Such erythematous, ulcerative, and hemorrhagic lesions begin as raised, red areas 0.5 to 1 cm in diameter. These lesions are then transformed into blebs and finally ulcerate. Healing occurs over the summer, leaving a permanent, pigmented region.

Acute chilblain is distinguished from other forms of dermatitis by its characteristic distribution and by its relationship to cold. Chronic chilblain needs to be distinguished from erythema induratum and erythema nodosum. Erythema induratum affects the upper part of the legs more frequently than the lower part. This condition is caused by *Mycobacterium tuberculosis*. If the infection is active the differential diagnosis can be made by microscopic demonstration or culture of bacteria. The lesions are more nodular, deeper, infiltrative, and more permanent than lesions of chilblain. Erythema nodosum is a more acute process, and it is usually associated with a systemic reaction, consisting of fever, malaise, and arthralgias. There is no seasonal association.

In mild cases of chilblain, treatment consists of protection from the cold, local application of anti-inflammatory ointments, avoidance of scratching, and cessation of smoking. These measures are usually sufficient. In severe cases, drugs that have been found useful in the treatment of Raynaud's phenomenon, such as reserpine, may be effective.

Frostbite

Frostbite is due to freezing of tissues that may result in damage to skin, muscle, blood vessels, and nerves. Superficial freezing begins when the deeper tissues reach about 10° C (50° F). During the Korean War, most cases of frostbite occurred at −6.5° C (21° F) or below after 7 to 18 hours of exposure. Predisposing factors include any type of peripheral vascular insufficiency, improper clothing, exhaustion, and previous cold injury. Blacks are more susceptible than whites to frostbite. Most frostbite is of the slow freezing type, but rapid frostbite occurring in a few minutes takes place at high altitudes with extremely low temperatures and has a predilection for the extremities rather than the face and ears.

Whether actual tissue freezing or decreased blood flow from vasoconstriction, the exact mechanism producing cell injury is unknown. Damage is probably due to a combination of direct freezing with the formation of extracellular ice crystals, inducing dehydration of cells, and intense vasoconstriction. The vasoconstriction is due to direct cold exposure of the tissues but may also involve reflex vasoconstriction from chilling of other body areas. The reduced blood flow leads to capillary stasis and arteriolar and capillary thromboses. Capillary permeability is increased and results in edema formation.

Initially frostbite appears with a sharp, pricking sensation that draws attention to a yellowish white numb area of hardened skin. However, cold itself produces numbness and anesthesia that may allow freezing of tissue without warning. When the freezing is superficial, thawing leads to local reddening and wheal and flare formation. When freezing involves deep tissues, subcutaneous edema occurs with thawing followed by formation of vesicles and bullae. As the edema subsides in a day or two, necrosis and gangrene may become evident. However, it may take 2 to 3 months before final demarcation between viable and dead tissue can be ascertained. In the healing phase, a black eschar usually covers the area. The traditional classification of frostbite has been from first to fourth degree, depending on the depth of tissue injury. Because the true extent of tissue damage cannot be judged on initial examination, a simpler classification of superficial and deep frostbite is practical. The prognosis depends on the depth of freezing because superficial cases usually have no sequelae, whereas deep freezing may end in amputation.

Frostbite is preventable and occurs rarely among those who have been instructed on how to protect themselves. Prophylactic measures include observance of each other for signs of frostbite; wearing adequate, loose-fitting, dry clothing and mittens; exposure for only brief periods when exercise is not possible; and avoidance of smoking before and during exposure. Feet and socks should be kept dry.

Treatment for superficial frostbite includes immediate rewarming. Areas affected with superficial frostbite should not be rubbed with snow or exercised. Treatment of deep frostbite should be delayed until adequate facilities for rewarming are available. It is best to rewarm tissue as fast as possible in 40 to 44° C (104 to 111° F) water. Massage, exposure to too-high temperatures, and reactive hyperemia should be avoided because they tend to increase pain and edema. Analgesics usually are needed during rewarming. After rewarming, which usually requires about 20 minutes, the frostbitten area is exposed to room air at 21 to 26° C (69 to 78° F). Although pressure dressings may be used, the open method with sterile surroundings is usually preferred. Vesicles, bullae, and eschars are left untouched. Antimicrobial drugs are indicated if infection is present. Smoking should be prohibited. Regional sympathectomy has been reported as beneficial both clinically and experimentally if performed at an optimal time of 24 to 48 hours after frostbite occurs. Sympathectomy may conserve tissue and lead to earlier demarcation, cessation of pain, and healing of tissue. Eventual recovery is usually surprisingly good, the black eschar peeling off to leave normal tissue beneath. Sensitivity to cold, paresthesia, and predilection to repeated frostbite and fibrosis of tissue may lead to disability. Gangrenous extremities may require amputation.

Common Venous Disorders

Venous Obstruction or Insufficiency

Venous disorders of the lower extremity have as their etiology either obstruction or insufficiency. The disorders to be discussed that involve obstruction of the venous system include deep venous thrombosis, superficial thrombophlebitis, and iliofemoral venous thrombosis. The insufficiency states include varicose veins, the postphlebitic syndrome with ulceration, and pulmonary embolism. Dangerous pulmonary embolus is not discussed in this section. All these clinical problems may appear at the podiatric clinic.

The frequency of occurrence of varicose veins in the general public is high. The major associated problems include symptomatic pain and leg swelling as well as cosmetic complaints. The obstructive or thrombotic problems associated with the venous system account for common morbidity and mortality in the United States and around the world, and an estimated 200,000 people a year in the United States die from these complications. Autopsy series indeed show that the scope of the problem is far more extensive than was suspected. The increasing usage of cardiac monitoring, dialysis, and pacing devices placed in the upper extremity veins will undoubtedly add to venous-related complications in the future.

There are certain conditions associated with venous thrombosis, and these include hypercoagulable states, malignancy, congestive heart failure, prolonged bed rest and immobility, increasing age, postoperative states, sepsis, injury, and pregnancy. All associated conditions should be thoroughly investigated at the time of initial history and physical examination in a patient presenting with ulceration, deep venous thrombosis of the lower extremity, superficial thrombophlebitis, or iliofemoral venous thrombosis. The history and physical examination of these entities and discussion of the pertinent clinical aspects and therapy are contained in this section.

Deep Venous Thrombosis

Deep venous thrombosis refers to occlusion of the venous outflow channels of the lower extremity due to thrombosis. There is a long list of predisposing factors, some of which include prolonged bed rest, malignancy, use of oral contraceptives, sepsis, and postoperative state (Table 2–5). The pathophysiologic process involves injury to the vein endothelium with deposition of fibrin and platelets and eventually ensuing thrombosis. With propagation of the thrombus, there is deposition of blood clot in the more proximal larger veins and the danger of a free-floating portion of this thrombus, which can travel in the venous system toward the heart, ultimately resulting in the danger of a pulmonary embolus. There is a naturally occurring thrombolytic mechanism in the circulatory system, but in the peripheral veins, this mechanism is not quite as well developed as it is in the lung pulmonary vasculature. Eventually, however, in 2 to 3 weeks after the original insult, the thrombus in the veins may become recanalized. The majority of the time when this process occurs there is destruction of the venous valves, resulting in a vein that is incompetent to resist the forces of gravity. This incompetence may result in postphlebitic syndrome.

The classic symptoms and signs of deep venous thrombosis may not be obvious in as many as half of the patients with the problem. The two symptoms that are most commonly present, edema and pain, can occur with many other problems. Homan's sign, which is tenderness of the calf produced by passive dorsiflexion of the foot, has been touted in the past as a pathognomonic sign of deep venous thrombosis but is in reality very nonspecific for thrombosis. Advanced thrombosis produces phlegmasia alba dolens and phlegmasia cerulea dolens. Deep venous thrombosis produces a moderately painful lower extremity but not the degree of pain associated with arterial insufficiency states. Seen once, deep venous thrombosis is rarely confused with other diagnoses. Phlegmasia alba dolens refers to a situation in which the swelling has impeded the arterial inflow to the lower extremity. Advanced venous occlusion may result ultimately in venous gangrene and loss of the extremity. The differential diagnosis of phlegmasia alba dolens includes edema due to congestive heart failure; lymphatic insufficiency states; compression of the venous outflow by tumor, trauma, or hematoma; cellulitis; and a variety of other conditions, such as ruptured popliteal cyst and prolonged dependency of the lower extremities.

The diagnosis of deep venous thrombosis of the lower extremity utilizes objective tests, such as I^{123} fibrinogen scanning, venography, Doppler ultrasonography, and venous outflow plethysmography. The gold standard examination is venography, which in and of itself may cause the complication of thrombophlebitis in a small percentage of cases. Most commonly, screening techniques using impedance plethysmography and Doppler ultrasonography provide accurate and reliable diagnoses when clinical suspicion is high.

Table 2–5. PRECIPITATING FACTORS IN THROMBOEMBOLISM

Factor	Etiology
Stasis	Arrhythmias
	Heart failure
	Immobilization
	Obesity
	Varicose veins
	Dehydration
Blood vessel injury	Trauma
	Fracture
Increased coagulability	Neoplasm
	Oral contraceptives
	Pregnancy
	Surgery
	Polycythemia
Previous thromboembolism	

The physician must be sure of the diagnosis of deep venous thrombosis before embarking on anticoagulation therapy because this form of treatment may result in complications. Warfarin products especially have the highest frequency of outpatient complications of any pharmaceutical agent.

Therapy for deep venous thrombosis includes acute anticoagulation with intravenous heparin followed by conversion to oral warfarin on an outpatient basis. The usual regimen for anticoagulation is a bolus of 5000 U of heparin intravenously, followed by hourly dosage of around 1000 U/hour adjusted to the partial thromboplastin time at 2 times normal. Heparin therapy is continued for approximately 1 week. Oral anticoagulation therapy with Coumadin is begun early on in the hospital course and is continued on an outpatient basis after the heparin therapy is discontinued. Once a prolonged prothrombin time of 1.5 to 2 times control value is achieved, warfarin is continued on an outpatient basis for 3 to 6 months. In addition to anticoagulation, compression hose may be prescribed to provide external compression and reduce venous stasis. Thrombolytic therapy, with urokinase and streptokinase, has been used for deep venous thrombosis with success. Usually the thrombolytic agents are used for a 24-hour period followed by systemic heparinization. Some studies have shown that the therapeutic benefit of thrombolytic agents over standard anticoagulation with heparin is the preservation of the venous valves. However, thrombolytic therapy carries a significant risk of bleeding and must be administered in an intensive-care setting. The major complications of untreated deep venous thrombosis include pulmonary embolus and postphlebitic syndrome.

Superficial Thrombophlebitis

Superficial thrombophlebitis refers to a thrombotic process in the superficial veins of the lower extremity, namely the long and short saphenous veins. The clinical presentation includes erythema, pain, swelling, and a tender edematous segment of the involved superficial vein. In fact, this condition may well be associated with an infectious process in the superficial vein and is often confused with lymphangitic streaks or cellulitis. Because superficial thrombophlebitis is associated with thrombosis in the vein, there is no flow detected when Doppler ultrasonography examination is carried out in that vein.

The most common cause of superficial thrombophlebitis is the presence of an intravenous catheter in a superficial vein, but intravenous catheters are not used commonly in the lower extremity. A special instance of superficial thrombophlebitis is called migratory thrombophlebitis, which refers to bouts of inflammation of the superficial veins in various parts of the body and may be associated with an underlying intra-abdominal malignancy or collagen vascular disorder. Treatment includes elevation of the affected extremity, moist heat application, and antibiotic therapy. In the case of a persistent thrombophlebitis at an old intravenous catheter site, it may become necessary to remove the segment of vein involved.

Iliofemoral thrombosis, which has already been referred to as phlegmasia cerulea dolens, refers to massive thrombosis of the venous system of the lower extremity, including the iliac veins. As already stated, this condition is a rare but striking complication. The picture of a cyanotic, swollen, moderately painful lower extremity is not easily forgotten. The predominant risk factors are the same as those for deep venous thrombosis. Therapy is moist heat to the affected area, bed rest, and elevation. Thrombolytic therapy may also be considered for this problem.

Chronic Venous Insufficiency

Chronic venous insufficiency states include varicose veins and postphlebitic syndrome. Varicose veins are tortuous, elongated, and enlarged veins. Superficial as well as deep and communicating veins may be involved. Deep venous thrombosis may or may not be involved. There is a strong family history in patients who have this problem. Varicose veins are usually associated with venous hypertension, which is an increased venous pressure that occurs in the upright position and with ambulation. Normally there is a pressure of 100 mm Hg in the veins of the foot on standing still. This pressure drops dramatically to 20 to 30 mm Hg with ambulation. This drop is due to the venous pump mechanisms provided by the lower extremity musculature and competent venous valves in returning blood in the veins toward the heart. When venous valves are malfunctioning or absent, most commonly owing to prior deep venous thrombosis, the pressure in the venous system is significantly higher with ambulation (i.e., 40 to 50 mm Hg or more). Instead of flowing toward the heart, blood in the veins demonstrates a retrograde flow under increased pressure, causing dilatation, and results in varicose veins. As already stated, the deep superficial system of veins in the lower extremity as well as the communicating veins may be involved with the inability to handle venous flow in the usual fashion. This inability results in a pooling of blood in the lower extremity in the upright position under increased pressure. This pooling ultimately explains all the clinical manifestations seen with varicose veins in postphlebitic syndrome.

On examination, a varicosed vein easily observed in the superficial system of the veins in the lower extremity is tortuous, dilated, and engorged with blood. Trendelenburg's test has been used in the past to delineate involvement of the deep communicating and superficial system of veins. Pain often accompanies distended engorged veins, and this results from stretching of the vein wall, impinging on surrounding nerve fibers in the subcutaneous tissue. Swelling of the lower extremity may result most commonly from involvement of the deep venous system. Stasis dermatitis and ulceration, along with pigmentation of the skin from rupture of capillary plexus under undue venous pressure, may be observed. The examining physician must search for concomitant arterial insufficiency, especially with indolent venous stasis ulcers.

Venography was the mainstay in the diagnosis of venous disorders of the lower extremities until the advent of noninvasive modalities. The common noninvasive methods used today are ultrasonography techniques, phleborheography, impedance plethysmography, segmental plethysmography, and photoplethysmography (see Noninvasive Evaluation of the Venous System).

Therapeutic Approaches to Venous Diseases

Therapy is directed at eliminating the varicosities by surgical excision or stripping. In addition, injection sclerotherapy is employed. A majority of these patients should wear compression stockings for life. An exception to this rule may be those patients who have arterial insufficiency as well as venous insufficiency. In the past, stripping of the long saphenous vein was a common procedure. However, because of the use of this vein as a bypass conduit, this procedure is carried out less commonly at present. Localized excision of tributaries of the long and short saphenous veins, which may be carried out under local anesthesia, is undertaken with regularity. The surgical technique involves cutting down in the skin and subcutaneous tissue over the varicosed segment locally, tying off the varicosed vein, and removing it. Multiple incisions may need to be undertaken with this technique. Patients who seem to benefit the most by surgical removal of varicose veins are those who are the most symptomatic, that is, those with pain and swelling. Although many patients undergo this procedure for cosmetic ends, many note that one problem is replaced by another, that is, the presence of multiple surgical scars postoperatively.

Injection sclerotherapy, using morrhuate sodium and other sclerosing agents, can be successful in drying up varicose veins. This technique involves injecting a sclerosing agent perhaps many times into a varicosed venous segment and wrapping the involved area with an Ace compression bandage. The sclerosing agent induces an obliteration of the vein lumen by apposition of the vein walls with compression, which is achieved by wrapping the involved area.

The postphlebitic syndrome represents a series of end-stage signs and symptoms resulting from deep vein thrombosis and varicose veins. These symptoms include edema of the lower extremity, stasis dermatitis and ulceration, skin pigmentation, and leg pain. The venous outflow obstruction commonly present with this syndrome causes symptoms of leg pain that are exacerbated with exercise. Such pain is referred to as venous claudication. The patient must stop exercising and elevate the leg to achieve relief from pain. Venous ulceration and hyperpigmentation characteristically occur around the ankle area. This location is very infrequently involved with pure arterial insufficiency states, which usually cause ulcerations in the foot and toe areas. That is not to say that there may not be concomitant arterial insufficiency with a venous ulcer in the area of the ankle. The natural course of a venous ulcer is eventual formation of granulation tissue and epithelialization. Of course, formation of granulation tissue and epithelialization do not occur if there is concomitant arterial insufficiency. Stasis dermatitis occurs with drying and malnutrition of the skin due to chronic edema and inability of the skin and subcutaneous tissue to resist the ever-present microbes that reside in the skin. The pigmentation that is commonly present is brown and results from chronic deposition of heme in the skin and subcutaneous tissue from burst capillaries caused by venous hypertension. This finding can be striking and quite prominent in and around the area of the ankle and lower calf. All these findings may co-exist in a patient with advanced disease as well as an element of cellulitis, which is the principal differential diagnosis. The diagnostic modalities with this syndrome are those already described for the other venous disorders, including venography, Doppler ultrasonography, and other noninvasive modalities. The important objectives of the diagnostic techniques are to identify valvular incompetence and deep venous obstruction.

Therapy is designed to counteract the chronic venous hypertension that inevitably is present. This hypertension is most easily treated by compression hose. Most patients do not need hose that extend above the knee. Patients need to be encouraged to use the hose because they are often difficult to put on, especially for elderly patients. The hose need not be worn in bed at nighttime. Patients should be encouraged to keep their legs elevated when seated and to avoid the dependent position of the lower extremities for prolonged periods of time. Antibiotic therapy may be indicated to control temporary infections associated with venous stasis ulcerations. A medicated absorbent bandage wrapped around the ankle area (Unna's boot) can be very effective in treating chronic venous stasis ulcerations.

Surgical therapy aimed at minimizing the effect of the incompetent venous communicating veins in and around the area of the most commonly involved tissue, that is, at the ankle level and lower calf, includes Linton's procedure, which ligates the subcutaneous perforating veins between the superficial and deep venous system in the lower calf. This procedure and those similar to it are not commonly performed because they are not usually effective in controlling the signs and symptoms of these disorders. Superficial vein stripping also does not control the advanced sequelae of the postphlebitic syndrome. A number of innovative venous reconstructive procedures, including venous bypass around obstructed femoral or iliac veins and venous valve repairs or transposition, most commonly from the brachial vein to the femoral vein, have been devised. Improvements in the patient's condition have been noted with many of these procedures. However, these procedures are still being evaluated for efficacy.

Common Lymphatic Disorders

Lymphedema

Swelling of the lower extremity may be produced by arterial and venous processes, such as arterial ischemia and deep venous thrombosis, but uncommonly may be produced by a disorder of the lymphatic system. Lymphedema may be due to obstruction of the lymphatic system, trauma, or infection. Lymphedema may occur congenitally or idiopathically, which is termed primary lymphedema. In primary lymphedema, most commonly there is a deficiency in the number of lymphatic chains emanating from the lower extremity. In 25% of patients, there appears to be varicosities in the lymphatic vessels. Functional abnormalities appear to limit the effectiveness of the lymphatics to remove protein from the interstitial fluid in these patients. Secondary lymphedema from obstruction, trauma, or infection eliminates functioning lymphatic vessels. The most common causes of obstruction are parasitic infection, as in filariasis, and blockage by tumor cells. Iatrogenic removal of lymphatic tissue either via operation or radiation therapy causes the same result.

Symptoms may be slight or severe and not necessarily dependent on the degree of leg edema. Characteristically swelling diminishes overnight but never disappears. The most common symptom is fatigue. Physical examination reveals firm, nonpitting edema. The firm nature of the skin and subcutaneous tissue is from fibrosis, which occurs in long-standing diseases. The process may be hastened with frequent bouts of cellulitis. Differential diagnosis must include edematous states, such as congestive heart failure, chronic renal failure, and hypoalbuminemic conditions. The aforementioned conditions all normally have bilateral involvement, whereas lymphedema in not uncommonly unilateral. Thrombophlebitis is commonly confused with cellulitis of lymphedema. In fact, insufficiency of the venous system and lymphedema may co-exist. Diagnosis of lymphedema is confirmed via lymphangiography and analysis of protein in edema fluid, which is elevated.

Conservative therapy consists of leg elevation, wearing of elastic hose, diuretics, and control of infection when present. Operations for this condition are varied, indicating there is no single effective procedure. Charles's procedure is the classic operation. This operation removes skin, subcutaneous fat, and fascia from the limb and is followed by split-thickness skin grafts. Microsurgical reconstruction of lymphatic-venous anastomosis may produce some improvement in lymphedema.

Lymphangitis

Lymphangitis is usually bacterial in origin and is an inflammation of the lymphatic vessels. In most cases, the responsible organism is hemolytic streptococcus or coagulase-positive *Staphylococcus aureus*. The bacteria gain access via local trauma or ulcerations. No identifiable portal of entry can be found in many instances. Infection spreads from the lymphatics to the regional lymph nodes. Various stages of inflammation are found in the subcutaneous tissue and regional lymph nodes. The local manifestation of lymphangitis consists of a red streak that appears at the site of initial entry of the infective organism and extends to the regional lymph

nodes. The lymph nodes are swollen and tender. There may be a surrounding area of cellulitis. Systemic accompaniments of infection may constitute the presenting manifestations.

The local manifestations of lymphangitis and the systemic reactions are usually sufficient to make the diagnosis. Leukocytosis with predominance of polymorphonuclear leukocytes may be present. Confirmation is obtained by culturing the organism from the portal or entry or from the subcutaneous tissues. Acute lymphangitis may be difficult to distinguish from generalized cellulitis or thrombophlebitis.

With treatment, the prognosis is good when one is dealing with an initial attack in an otherwise normal limb. In the case of recurrent attacks, lymphedema may develop and residual increase in the girth of the limb may occur. The treatment consists of systemic administration of the appropriate antibiotics. In addition, surgical drainage of the focus of infection is important. Supportive measures, including rest and elevation of the infected limb and local warm, wet dressings, are also helpful. The use of elastic support hose may be necessary for a period of several weeks to prevent lymphedema. In recurrent cases, causes of secondary lymphedema should be sought.

Bibliography

Abramson D: Vascular Disorders of the Extremities, 2nd ed. New York: Harper & Row Publishers, 1974.

Allen EV, et al.: Peripheral Vascular Diseases, 2nd ed. Philadelphia: WB Saunders Co, 1955.

Baker WH, Strong ST, Hayes AC, et al.: Diagnosis of peripheral occlusive disease: Comparison of clinical evaluation and noninvasive laboratory. Arch Surg 113:1308, 1978.

Barnes RW: Noninvasive diagnostic techniques in peripheral vascular disease. Am Heart J 97:241, 1979.

DeLaurentis DA: Do you know the treatment of choice in peripheral arterial occlusive disease? Geriatrics 34(10):33, 1979.

Janson L: Smoking cessation and peripheral circulation: A population study in 59-year-old men with plethysmography and segmental measurements of systolic blood pressure. Vasa 4:282, 1975.

Mannick JA, Coffman JD: Ischemic Limbs: Surgical Approach and Physiological Principles. New York: Grune & Stratton, 1973.

Prineas RJ, Harland WR, Janson L, et al.: Recommendations for use of non-invasive methods to detect atherosclerotic peripheral arterial disease in population studies. Circulation, 65:1561A, 1982.

Schroll M, Munck O: Estimation of peripheral arteriosclerotic disease by ankle blood pressure measurement in a population study of 60-year-old men and women. J Chronic Dis 34:261, 1981.

Spittell JA, Jr: Office diagnosis of occlusive arterial disease. J Cardiovasc Med, Feb, p 107, 1984.

Strandness DE, Jr: The use of ultrasound in the evaluation of peripheral vascular disease. Prog Cardiovasc Dis 20:403, 1978

Sumner DS: Evaluation of venous circulation using the ultrasonic Doppler velocity detector. In Rutherford RB (ed): Vascular Surgery. Philadelphia, WB Saunders Co, 1977.

Yao JST, William RF, Bergan JJ: Noninvasive vascular diagnotic testing: Techniques and clinical applications. Prog Cardiovasc Dis 26:459, 1984.

Wolf PA, Kannel WB, Sorlie P, et al.: Asymptomatic carotid bruit and risk of stroke. JAMA 245:1442, 1981.

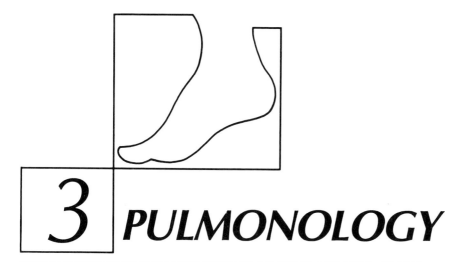

3 PULMONOLOGY

ROBERT A. SANDHAUS

OVERVIEW

The study of pulmonary disease has both obvious and subtle links to surgery in general and podiatry in particular. The preoperative evaluation of the surgical candidate often centers on the individual's pulmonary function. Some diseases of the lower extremities, such as thrombophlebitis, have prominent pulmonary manifestations.

An evaluation of the lower extremities may tell much about the state of the lungs. A patient wearing worn running shoes probably has normal pulmonary function (although the fortuitous finding of a localized pulmonary lesion should not be ruled out). Peripheral edema or the wearing of support hose may indicate right-sided heart failure, often caused by chronic lung disease. An infected joint may be secondary to pneumococcal pneumonia. Peripheral cyanosis may be the first clue to a worsened oxygen transport in chronic obstructive lung disease. Clubbing of the toes may lead one to suspect a primary pulmonary problem.

PATHOPHYSIOLOGY

The architecture of the lungs (Fig. 3–1) is designed to provide a vast area of intimate contact between the blood and the external environment. In fact, the lungs, with a surface area larger than that of a tennis court, offer our largest and most vulnerable contact with the outside world. This vulnerability is due to the gas exchange function of the lungs; the blood

99

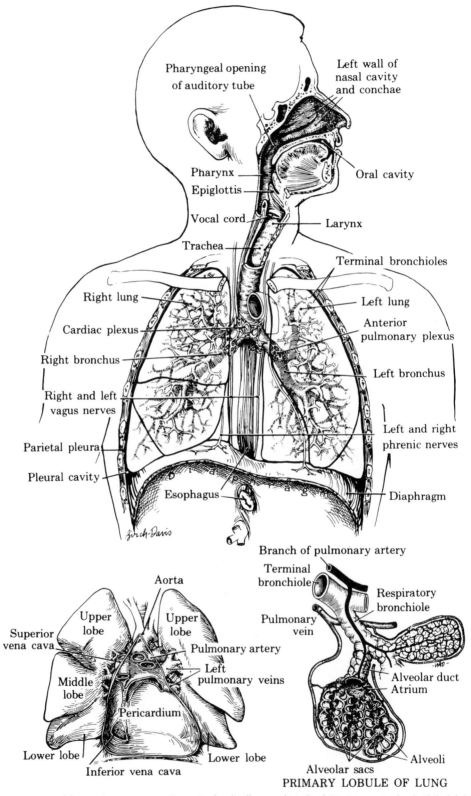

Pharyngeal opening
of auditory tube

Left wall of
nasal cavity
and conchae

Pharynx

Epiglottis

Vocal cord

Trachea

Oral cavity

Larynx

Terminal bronchioles

Right lung

Cardiac plexus

Right bronchus

Right and left
vagus nerves

Parietal pleura

Pleural cavity

Esophagus

Left lung

Anterior
pulmonary plexus

Left bronchus

Left and right
phrenic nerves

Diaphragm

Birch-Davis

Branch of pulmonary artery

Terminal
bronchiole

Respiratory
bronchiole

Pulmonary
vein

Aorta

Upper
lobe

Upper
lobe

Superior
vena cava

Pulmonary artery

Left
pulmonary veins

Middle
lobe

Pericardium

Alveolar duct

Atrium

Lower lobe

Inferior vena cava

Lower lobe

Alveoli

Alveolar sacs

PRIMARY LOBULE OF LUNG

Figure 3–1. Organs of the respiratory system. (From Dorland's Illustrated Medical Dictionary, 27th ed. Philadelphia: WB Saunders Co, 1988.)

supply is often less than a micron away from the air that continually bathes the lungs' internal surface.

In order to fulfill the gas exchange function (i.e., providing oxygen to the tissues via the blood and removing toxic products of metabolism such as carbon dioxide), the lungs utilize a bellows-like arrangement of the chest wall, which actively fills the lungs with air during inhalation and passively allows the exhalation of carbon dioxide–enriched air. This passive exhalation is driven by the elastic tissues of the lungs and chest wall.

There are two primary physiologic abnormalities that can be identified by classic pulmonary function testing, obstructive and restrictive defects. In their simplest forms, obstructive defects are abnormalities of exhalation, and restrictive defects are abnormalities of inhalation.

Commonly we think of obstructive defects as physical blockage of an airway such that, during exhalation, the flow of air out of the lungs meets an increased resistance, as in asthma, in which the muscular bundles around the airways contract, and there is increased mucus production and delivery of mucus to the airways. The facts may be more complex, however. In emphysema a loss of the elastic tissue of the lungs occurs. These elastic fibers normally tether the small airways so that they remain open during the act of exhalation. Loss of these fibers means that these airways close prematurely, which prevents the normal airflow out of the lungs and traps air at the end of exhalation. Thus an individual suffering from an obstructive lung disease often demonstrates a reduced flow of exhaled air and trapped air within the lungs.

A restrictive process, usually characterized by scarring and fibrosis (the laying down of fibrous tissue) within the lungs, makes the lungs stiffer, increasing the elastic recoil that drives exhalation. Inhalation becomes increasingly more difficult against this increased force, which tends to keep the lungs from expanding. Thus, reduced maximum lung volumes are seen in individuals suffering from a restrictive lung disease.

Smoking. A discussion of the pathophysiology of lung disease would be incomplete if there were no mention of the role of the products of tobacco combustion in lung pathology (Fig. 3–2). The two most

Carcinogenic Effects
Lung Cancer
The death rate from cancer of the lung is 60 times greater in the heavy smoker than in the nonsmoker and 15 times greater in the one half to one pack per day male smoker.

Airflow Obstruction
Bronchitis
Emphysema

Potentially Reversible Effects
Chronic bronchitis/Airflow obstruction
Cessation of smoking reduces rate of deterioration.

Synergistic Effects
Cigarette smoke may act jointly with air pollution or occupational irritants to produce greater morbidity and mortality.

Infections
Respiratory infections are more common and more serious among smokers.

Figure 3–2. Harmful effects of cigarette smoking. (Data from Luckman, J, Sorenson, KC: Medical-Surgical Nursing: A Psychophysiological Approach, 2nd ed. Philadelphia, WB Saunders Co, 1980.)

common causes of pulmonary morbidity and mortality, lung neoplasms and pulmonary emphysema, are directly associated with the chronic inhalation of cigarette smoke. The postoperative morbidity of patients who smoke cigarettes is more than twice that of patients who do not smoke. This morbidity can be greatly reduced by cessation of smoking in the week prior to surgery. By aiding a patient in an effort to quit smoking, the health professional can help reverse the effects of this greatest preventable cause of death in today's society.

Environmental Risk Factors. An important aspect of the evaluation of a pulmonary process is the identification of other environmental risk factors that can lead to lung disease. These include occupational exposures to inhaled agents, such as asbestos, oxides of nitrogen, and allergens as well as exposures in the home that are not immediately apparent, such as agents released from pets (bird droppings and dog dander), fungal contamination of a humidifer, and the side-stream tobacco smoke of a family member.

PRESENTING FEATURES

Subjective Symptoms

A pulmonary history elicits subjective symptoms of pulmonary disease (Table 3–1).

Cough. The act of coughing is one of the major protective mechanisms of the lung, providing clearance of foreign material and mucus via a violent exhalation. The cough produces maximal flows in the large airways, driving the offending material up into the nasopharynx where it is swallowed or expectorated. An impairment of the cough reflex, caused by a neurologic abnormality or the inability of a diseased lung to generate the flows necessary to produce an effective cough, can lead to the accumulation of mucus and foreign material and can produce increased airflow obstruction, pulmonary infection, or both.

Similarly, the suppression of physiologic cough by medications can lead to impaired clearance from the lung and can result in lung disease. Some coughs, however, are not generated by the need to clear secretions from the large airways. Such coughs may be due to the stimulation of receptors in the airways by lung problems such as asthma or viral infections in the nasopharynx or large airways. Extrapulmonary mass lesions, including aortic aneurysms, can lead to mechanical distention of nerves and airways and can lead to cough as a primary or secondary symptom. The cough may be severe and debilitating but serves no useful purpose to the lungs.

Dyspnea. Dyspnea, or the subjective sensation of being breathless, is one of the most common symptoms of lung disease. It can be due to an abnormality of gas transport in the lung, leading to hypoxia, the build-up of carbon dioxide in the blood, or both (Table 3–2). Dyspnea can also be due to the inability to move air well, as in an acute asthma attack. We have all experienced a temporary sensation of dyspnea after a hard workout or long run. The individual suffering from pulmonary disease may not be able to recover from this sense

---

Table 3–1. PULMONARY HISTORY

General State of Health
  Family health history; e.g., is asthma, emphysema, tuberculosis, or lung cancer present in the family?
  Medications. Is the patient taking bronchodilators, diuretics, antibiotics, heart medications, or any other drugs for a chronic or acute medical condition?
Specific Respiratory History
  Chest pain. Is it associated with breathing, exercise, etc.?
  Shortness of breath. When does it occur; is it painful; what causes it to improve?
  Cough. When does it occur; is sputum produced; is it associated with pain; how often does it occur; is blood observed in the sputum?
  Sputum production. How much; what color; what time of day is the most productive; does position affect the acount of production; is there any odor to the sputum?
  Hemoptysis (blood in the sputum). How often; when does it occur; is pain associated with the raising of blood?
  Exercise Tolerance. How much activity can the patient usually perform; what limits the degree of activity; when did a change in the amount of exercise tolerated start?
  Wheezing. What causes the wheeze (exercise, emotions, exposure to allergens or other external factors)?
  Allergies that produce respiratory distress, e.g., pollens, molds, etc. When did the allergic symptoms begin; when were they diagnosed?
  Occupational History. Length of time exposed to occupational irritants, e.g., welding, coal mining, sandblasting, etc.
  Personal Pollution History—this includes smoking history. Smoking history is reported in number of "pack years." To determine this figure, multiply the number of years cigarettes have been smoked by the average number of packs of cigarettes smoked per day. Two packs per day × 40 years of smoking = 80 pack years.

Table 3–2. HYPOXEMIA AND HYPERCAPNIA: SIGNS AND SYMPTOMS

Hypoxemia	Hypercapnia
Tachycardia	Impaired ventilation
Tachypnea	Lethargy
Loss of consciousness	Cerebral vasodilation
Bradycardia	Papilledema
Bradypnea	Twitching, tremor
Coma	Somnolence
Apnea	Coma
Confusion	Restlessness
Agitation	Hypertension
Progressive irritability	Headache
Progressive muscle weakness	
Cyanosis	
Diplopia	
Difficulty with coordination	
Impaired judgment	
Somnolence	

of breathlessness once it begins, as can the healthy jogger.

Sputum Production. Sputum production is any noticeable expectoration of pulmonary secretions (Table 3–3). This sputum may represent an overproduction of normal secretions or the generation of abnormal material, as in the purulent secretions of pneumonia, consisting of exudated fluid, white blood cells, and bacteria. The yellow-green color of purulent sputum is due to the presence of myeloperoxidase, an enzyme with a characteristic green color, packaged in the granules of the neutrophilic granulocyte.

Hemoptysis. Bloody sputum, or the coughing up of whole blood, is never a normal symptom or sign. It can represent simple bronchial inflammation, however. In fact, the most common cause of hemoptysis is bacterial bronchitis. In contrast, massive hemoptysis is a life-threatening condition. Life-threatening hemoptysis requires rupture or erosion of a blood vessel functioning at systemic arterial pressures (e.g., bronchial artery). In contrast, pulmonary arterial pressures are usually much lower than systemic arterial pressures except in pulmonary hypertension, in which pulmonary pressures are elevated, leading to rare instances of massive hemoptysis.

The causes of massive hemoptysis include pulmonary neoplasms (both benign and malignant), cavitary disease of the lung with formation of a bronchial artery aneurysm (Rasmussen's aneurysm), mitral stenosis, and primary pulmonary hypertension. Pulmonary infection and pulmonary embolism or thrombosis are less likely to lead to life-threatening bleeding from the lungs.

Wheezing. The sensation of whistling or musical sounds within the chest is often the cardinal sign, to both patient and physician, of asthma. However, any obstruction in a relatively large bronchiole or bronchus or the trachea itself can lead to wheezing. There must be sufficient flow of air past the airway obstruction or no sound will be produced. Thus, when an asthmatic patient reports that his or her wheezing has stopped, this may imply that the airflow obstruction has lessened and the patient is improving, *or* that the airflow obstruction has worsened to the point that the wheezing sound cannot be generated.

Chest Pain of Pulmonary Origin. Chest pain is a relatively common complaint, and a pulmonary source may often exist. Naturally, chest pain of cardiac origin must always be ruled out, even when the primary manifestation of pain is chest wall tenderness. Once a cardiac origin is ruled out, the multitude of pulmonary and chest wall processes must be considered.

Classically, pulmonary hypertension produces a vague central chest pain. A patient with pulmonary infection can present with localized chest pain. Most pulmonary processes produce chest pain when they lead to inflammation or pressure on the pleural surfaces. The pleurae are endowed with a wealth of sensory nerve endings. The result of stimulation of these nerves is classic pleuritic chest pain, which is related to the respiratory excursions of the lungs and chest wall.

Objective Signs

Physical Examination

A physical examination of the lungs reveals objective signs (Table 3–4). The lungs require evaluation using the classic fourfold approach: inspection, palpation, percussion, and auscultation.

Inspection. Inspection should first concentrate on the general appearance of the patient. Is the patient breathing comfortably, or is the breathing labored? Are there scars of previous thoracic surgery? Does the patient have a plethoric appearance, or is there generalized cyanosis? Does the pa-

Table 3–3. SPUTUM CHARACTERISTICS IN SPECIFIC DISORDERS

Abscess—large quantities, foul odor
Asthma—mucoid
Bronchiectasis—periodic large quantities; separates into three layers upon standing
Bronchitis (chronic) or emphysema—tenacious; thick
Carcinoma (bronchogenic) or tuberculosis (advanced)—contains frank blood
Edema—large quantities; pink and frothy
Pneumonia (pneumococcus)—sticky, small amounts, rusty or pink
Suppuration—large quantities; purulent; yellow or green
Tracheobronchitis—mucoid

Table 3–4. PHYSICAL SIGNS OF CHRONIC
RESPIRATORY DYSFUNCTION

Overdeveloped sternomastoid muscles
Elevated sternum
Increased anteroposterior diameter of chest
Barrel-shaped chest
Pursed-lip breathing pattern or a prolonged expiratory
  phase
Posture that elevates the ribs and increases the size of the
  thorax (shoulders usually elevated)
Clubbing of the fingers and toes
Signs of heart failure, e.g., swelling of the feet and ankles;
  noisy respirations
Cough and noisy respiration
Nicotine stains on fingers
Retraction of the spaces between the ribs during inspira-
  tion

(Data from Luckmann J, Sorensen KC: Medical-Surgical
Nursing: A Psychophysiological Approach, 2nd ed. Philadelphia: WB Saunders Co, 1980.)

tient aid his or her exhalation by pursing
the lips? Are there cigarette stains on the
hands or teeth? Does the patient have signs
of clubbing or arthritis? These can be assessed during the initial handshake.

After a general assessment, the breathing pattern should be observed. Is it regular? If not, is there a pattern to the irregularity? The regular, extremely deep
breathing pattern of Kussmaul's respiration is a sign of metabolic acidemia, as in
diabetic ketoacidosis. The pattern of
Cheyne-Stokes respiration (gradually increasing depth of breath followed by gradually more shallow breathing followed
with an apneic period) is a nonspecific
indicator of metabolic or neurologic derangement. Disorders of the breathing
mechanism can occur, especially when
respiratory muscle weakness is present,
and these can lead to paradoxical respiration, a breathing pattern in which the abdomen moves inward during exhalation
and outward during inhalation.

It is also important to observe the position of the chest wall and its musculature
during breathing. Severe chronic obstructive diseases of the lungs lead to an increase in the anteroposterior diameter of
the chest wall, the so-called barrel-chested
appearance. The chest is at near-maximum
expansion even at the end of expiration. In
order to move the chest wall at all, accessory muscles of respiration, especially
those in the neck such as the sternoclei-
domastoids, are called into play.

The diaphragm is usually flat in these

individuals. The contraction of this muscle, tethered to the lower ribs, simply flat-
tens the dome of the diaphragm in the normal individual. In patients with chronic
obstructive pulmonary disease (COPD),
one often sees the paradoxical inward
movement of the lower ribs during inspiration, as the already flattened diaphragm
contracts.

Inspection should also include a look at
the spine. Kyphoscoliosis and other skeletal deformities can lead to restriction of
airflow and pulmonary abnormalities.

Palpation and Percussion. Palpation of
the chest can detect poor respiratory movements, areas of tenderness along the chest
wall, lymph nodes that signal a pulmonary
neoplasm, or the transmission of lung
sounds or vocalization that suggests a localized parenchymal process. *Percussion*
of the chest can yield a great deal of information about the underlying contents of
the chest cavity. An advantage one has in
this type of evaluation is the symmetry of
the chest cavity. The left side can be repeatedly compared with the right, always
accounting for incidental organs such as
the heart.

Poor excursion of the diaphragm can be
identified by percussion of the location of
the dullness that represents the location of
this muscle before and after a full inspiration. Dullness to percussion indicates a
space-occupying process, such as fluid in
the parenchyma or outside the lung (as in
a pleural effusion). Resonance to percussion suggests an abundance of air is underlying the point of percussion, as in
pneumothorax or advanced emphysema
with bullae.

Auscultation. Auscultation of the lung
usually employs the diaphragm of the
stethoscope, since most respiratory sounds
are predominantly high-pitched. During
auscultation, all areas of the lung should
be assessed. To avoid overlooking any one
area, evaluate all lobes. The upper and
lower lobes appear superiorly and inferi-
orly on the back. Left and right should be
compared during auscultation. The major
surfaces of the right middle lobe and the
lingula on the left are along the lower anterior chest wall.

Specific names that describe the various
auscultatory findings communicate physical findings. This communication may be
from the examiner to him- or herself, as

when one wants to place an accurate description of current findings in the record for later comparison, or the communication may be to another health care provider. Therefore, it is appropriate to explain in detail some of the auscultatory findings that have been named (Fig. 3–3).

Air Movement. Listen for air movement. The normal respiratory sounds, if not auscultating close to a central airway, transmit loudest during midinspiration and midexpiration. There should be a silent period between inspiration and expiration. As the stethoscope is moved toward the location of the central airways, this silent period grows shorter. No silence between inspiration and expiration is called

bronchial breath sounds. Pulmonary consolidation, as caused by bacterial pneumonia, will transmit these bronchial breath sounds out to the parenchyma, and thus this sign can be a valuable diagnostic tool. The inspiratory and expiratory times should be roughly equivalent. When this ratio is exceeded, and expiratory time becomes greater than twice the inspiratory time, an obstruction of airflow should be suspected such as asthma, emphysema, chronic bronchitis, or lesion of major airways.

Rales. Pulmonary adventitial sounds are called crackles. Wet crackles, called rales, are a soft crackling sound, usually heard during end-inspiration but some-

Bronchial breath sounds over peripheral lung

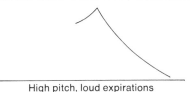

High pitch, loud expirations

Medium rales: lower, more moist sound, heard about halfway through inspiration
Found in clients with pneumonia or pulmonary edema (not cleared by cough)

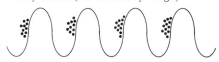

Rhonchi: small airway noise
Sibilant rhonchi (wheeze): musical noise like squeak
May occur during inspiration or expiration, but usually louder during expiration

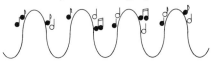

Pleural friction rub: dry, rubbing or grating sound usually due to inflammation of pleural surfaces; heard throughout inspiration and expiration; loudest over lower anterior lateral surface

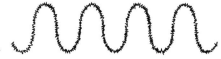

Adventitious sounds, including rales and fine rales, high-pitched crackling sound, heard toward end of inspiration; indicates inflammation or congestion

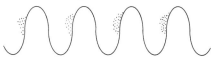

Coarse rales: loud, bubbly noise, heard during inspiration
Found in clients with pneumonia (not cleared by coughing)

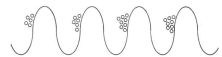

Sonorous rhonchi (wheeze): low, loud, coarse sound like snore; may occur at any point of inspiration or expiration; usually means obstruction of trachea or large bronchi (coughing may clear sound)

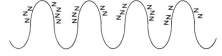

Figure 3–3. *A,* Deviations from normal auscultatory findings. (From Thompson JM, Bower AC: Clinical Manual of Health Assessment. St Louis: CV Mosby Co, 1980.)

Illustration continued on following page

Rales (Crackles)

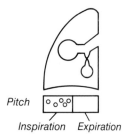

Pitch

Inspiration   Expiration

Rhonchi or Wheezes

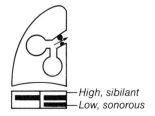

High, sibilant
Low, sonorous

Pleural Friction Rub

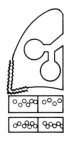

Rales are discrete, noncontinuous crackling sounds that may be imagined as dots in time in contrast to dashes. They are represented here by open circles. They are usually inspiratory. Inspiratory rales are probably secondary to delayed reopening of previously deflated airways. Conditions in which they are heard include congestive heart failure, bronchitis, pneumonia, and pulmonary fibrosis. Rales may or may not change with coughing.

Rhonchi or wheezes last longer than rales and are shown here as dashes. They may be inspiratory, expiratory, or both. These sounds indicate partial obstruction to air flow in passages narrowed by secretions, mucosal swelling, tumors, and so on. They often change with coughing. Texts disagree in their definitions of wheezes versus rhonchi. The terms may be used interchangeably. Differences in pitch depend primarily on differences in velocity of air flow across the obstruction. Some sounds are high-pitched, sibilant, and musical; others are lower and sonorous.

A pleural friction rub is a crackling, grating sound produced when two roughened or inflamed pleural surfaces rub across each other during respiration. Friction rubs are usually heard in both inspiration and expiration but may be limited to inspiration. They are not affected by cough. Recordings have shown that rubs comprise a series of discrete crackles and may be difficult to differentiate from rales, especially when confined to inspiration. The crackles may be so frequent that they coalesce into a continuous sound.

B

Figure 3–3 *Continued B,* Adventitious sounds in the chest examination.

times present throughout the respiratory cycle. The sound of rales can be approximated by holding some hair near the ear and rubbing the hair between two fingers. Empirically, rales are caused by inflammation or edema of the interstitium of the alveoli. Thus rales are a characteristic finding of left ventricular congestive heart failure with pulmonary edema and the various interstitial lung diseases. The interstitial lung diseases are said to have dry rales or "Velcro rales," but these may be due to the fact that these rales are often loud and occur throughout the respiratory cycle. Rales due to the failing left ventricle are first heard at the base of the lung posteriorly, often on the right before the left, but as frank pulmonary edema occurs, the rales can extend up and eventually be heard throughout both lung fields (Table 3–5).

Rhonchi. Dry crackles, or rhonchi, are coarser, more central sounds often caused by mucus or sputum in the airways. Rhonchi may clear, move, or change character after a voluntary or spontaneous cough. The implications of rhonchi are nonspecific. Rhonchi often occur in the presence of wheezing or rales and may be an indi-

cation that whatever process caused the accompanying sound has affected the larger airways. Isolated rhonchi, especially when localized, can be an indication of disease in the bronchi or trachea.

Wheezes. Wheezes, as previously discussed, are more musical, whistling sounds that classically occur during expiration but often obscure the entire respiratory cycle. It is important, but often difficult, to distinguish true lower respiratory wheezing from sounds high in the respiratory tract. Everyone can make wheezing sounds by closing the glottis, larynx, or both during a forced expiration. Some individuals do this unconsciously, either in an effort to keep end-expiratory pressures high and reduce air trapping or because of a dysfunction of the vocal cords. Every effort should be made, therefore, to relax the oropharynx during the inspiratory and expiratory efforts of a physical examination.

Rubs. Rubs differ from the sounds previously described in that they are not intrapulmonary in origin but rather are generated by the movement of inflamed visceral and parietal pleurae across each other during respiration. This movement

Table 3–5. PHYSICAL SIGNS IN SELECTED ABNORMALITIES OF BRONCHI AND LUNGS

Condition	Description	Percussion Note	Tactile Fremitus, Voice Sounds, Whispered Voice Sounds	Breath Sounds	Adventitious Sounds
Normal	The tracheobronchial tree and alveoli are clear; the pleurae are thin and close together; the mobility of the chest wall is unimpaired	Resonant	Normal	Vesicular except perhaps for bronchovesicular sounds near the large bronchi	None except perhaps for a few transient inspiratory rales at the bases after recumbency or sleep
Left-Sided Heart Failure	Some airways in the dependent portions of the lungs are deflated abnormally during expiration; the bronchial mucosa may be swollen	Resonant	Normal	Normal or sometimes prolonged expiration	Rales at lung bases; sometimes wheezes
Pleural Fluid or Thickening	Pleural fluid or fibrotic thickening muffles all sound	Dull to flat	Decreased to absent; however, when fluid compresses the underlying lung, bronchophony, egophony, and whispered pectoriloquy may appear	Decreased vesicular or absent; however, when fluid compresses the lung, a bronchial quality may appear	None unless there is underlying disease
Pulmonary Consolidation (e.g., Lobar Pneumonia)	A consolidated lung is dull to percussion but so long as the large airways are clear, fremitus, breath, and voice sounds are transmitted as if they came directly from the larynx and trachea; abnormally deflated portions of the lungs produce rales	Dull	Increased, with bronchophony, egophony, whispered pectoriloquy	Bronchial	Rales

Labels on diagrams (left column): Normal — Bronchus, Pleura, Alveoli. Left-Sided Heart Failure — Swollen mucosa (sometimes), Deflated airway. Pleural Fluid or Thickening — Pleural fluid or thickening. Pulmonary Consolidation — Deflated airway, Alveoli filled with fluid, red and white cells.

Table continued on following page

Table 3–5. PHYSICAL SIGNS IN SELECTED ABNORMALITIES OF BRONCHI AND LUNGS *Continued*

Condition	Description	Percussion Note	Tactile Fremitus, Voice Sounds, Whispered Voice Sounds	Breath Sounds	Adventitious Sounds
Bronchitis Bronchial constriction / Deflated airway	There may be partial bronchial obstruction from secretions or constrictions; abnormally deflated portions of lung may produce rales	Resonant	Normal	Normal or prolonged expiration	Wheezes or rales
Emphysema Overinflated alveoli with destruction of walls	A hyperinflated lung of emphysema is hyper-resonant; the overfilled air spaces muffle the voice and breath sounds	Hyper-resonant	Decreased	Decreased vesicular, often with prolonged expiration	None or signs of bronchitis

(From Bates B: A Guide to Physical Examination, 2nd ed. Philadelphia: JB Lippincott Co, 1974.)

results in a localized, coarse rubbing sound, often described as "leathery," that is always synchronized with the chest movements during respiration. Pleuritic chest pain may be localized by the patient to the exact area where the rub is appreciated.

Clubbing. Clubbing (Fig. 3–4) is an abnormality of the nail and nail bed of the fingers, toes, or both of individuals who suffer from any of several apparently unrelated pulmonary conditions. Its etiology is not clear at this time. Clubbing is characterized in its earliest stages by a reddening, swelling, and "sponginess" of the nail bed. The nail seems to be floating at its base when finger pressure is applied to the nail bed. In later stages, the nail itself changes. First, the nail, which usually arises from the nail bed at an acute angle to the axis of the digit when viewed from the side, loses this angle and arises parallel to the axis of the finger. Eventually the whole nail assumes a rounded appearance similar to the convex side of a spoon, and in its extreme, the entire distal phalanx of the hand or foot can become enlarged and bulbous.

Clubbing is often due to an intrathoracic problem such as a chronic suppurative pulmonary lesion (bronchiectasis, chronic lung abscess, tuberculosis); an intrathoracic neoplasm (most prominently bronchogenic carcinomas and pleural malignancies); or any lung disease that leads to chronic hypoxemia, although the association between this category of lung disease and clubbing is far from constant. There are several other causes of clubbing. Hereditary clubbing, a condition that is merely an interesting incidental finding of little clinical significance, is one of the most dramatic forms of clubbing. The individual has had hereditary clubbing all his or her life and can usually report that one or both parents had nails with the same characteristics. Among individuals with acquired clubbing, nonpulmonary causes may become apparent, such as cyanotic congenital heart defects and extrapulmonary neoplasms. The extreme of clubbing occurs in the symptom complex known as hypertrophic osteoarthropathy. This condition, which can be idiopathic, hereditary, related to malignancy (often intrathoracic neoplasms), or related to pulmonary inflammatory processes, leads to severe clubbing and periosteal changes in the distal long bones.

Cyanosis. Cyanosis is the observation of poorly oxygenated hemoglobin as manifested by a bluish appearance of the skin or

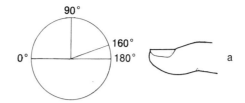

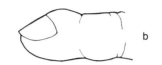

Figure 3–4. Clubbing: *a,* normal base angle; *b,* clubbed finger; *c,* normal finger; *d,* curved nail; *e,* early clubbing (loss of base angle); *f,* advanced clubbing. (From Groer ME, et al.: Basic Pathophysiology: A Conceptual Approach. St Louis: CV Mosby Co, 1979.)

mucous membranes. Often this appearance is first noted in the extremities, presumably because the extremities are subject to vasoconstriction when cold, and thus there is more complete stripping of oxygen from hemoglobin in these areas. But the lips, face, or another, more central location can be involved. The observation of cyanosis requires only that at least 5 g of hemoglobin be unoxygenated. Thus cyanosis can occur in an individual with polycythemia of any cause, even with normal pulmonary and cardiac function, when the normal amount of hemoglobin is saturated with oxygen but the excess hemoglobin is not. There can be many other nonpulmonary causes of cyanosis, including low cardiac output states, arteriovenous malformations and intracardiac shunts, and hypothermia.

Laboratory and Physiologic Data

Arterial Blood Gas Values. The measurement of the partial pressure of oxygen and carbon dioxide, of pH, and of oxygen saturation in arterial blood reflects the current state of the body's gas exchange and oxygen transport systems (Table 3–6). The normal values for arterial blood gases can be affected by body temperature, the altitude, and the instantaneous respiratory history at the time the blood was obtained. Oxygenation is assessed by evaluating the partial pressure of oxygen in the arterial

blood (pO_2) and the oxygen saturation of hemoglobin. Because of the sigmoid shape of the oxyhemoglobin saturation curve, the pO_2 can drop substantially before there is a significant change in the oxygen saturation of the blood. Thus, the oxygen saturation measurement, if it is directly measured instead of calculated, as in some laboratories, can be a more accurate indication of tissue oxygen delivery, whereas the pO_2 can be a more sensitive measure of oxygen delivery from the lungs to blood.

Table 3–6. ACID-BASE DISORDERS

Terminology	Typical Values		
	pH	pCO₂	HCO₃
Respiratory acidosis	7.10	80.0	24.0
Compensated respiratory acidosis	7.40	80.0	48.0
Respiratory alkalosis	7.70	20.0	24.0
Compensated respiratory alkalosis	7.40	20.0	12.0
Metabolic acidosis	7.10	40.0	12.0
Compensated metabolic acidosis	7.40	20.0	12.0
Metabolic alkalosis	7.70	40.0	48.0
Compensated metabolic alkalosis	7.40	80.0	48.0
Mixed respiratory and metabolic acidosis	↓	↑	↓
Mixed respiratory and metabolic alkalosis	↑	↓	↑
Normal	7.40	40.0	24.0

(From Groer ME, et al.: Basic Pathophysiology: A Conceptual Approach. St Louis: CV Mosby Co, 1979.)

An examination of the partial pressure of carbon dioxide (pCO_2) and the pH can reveal a great deal about the acid-base status of a patient (Fig. 3–5). This is a very complex subject; therefore, only the basics will be mentioned. The pH of the blood is normally maintained within very narrow limits. When it is below approximately 7.4, the patient is acidemic; when the pH is above approximately 7.5, the patient is alkalemic. If one examines only the pH, one can be misled as to the actual severity of an individual's metabolic derangement because the body has several effective compensatory mechanisms that attempt to maintain the pH of the blood within the normal range. Acutely, the body changes the respiratory cycle of the lungs to either hyperventilate, thereby blowing off CO_2 and raising the pH, or hypoventilate, thereby lowering the pH, although this latter mechanism is often not as dramatic as hyperventilation.

Thus if a patient has a pH of 7.35 with a pCO_2 of 10 mmHg (normally 35 to 45 mmHg), although the actual acidemia appears mild according to the pH, it is actually quite severe but can be corrected *toward* normal by marked hyperventilation. This patient is described as having a marked metabolic acidosis with respiratory compensation. Any compensatory mechanism, be it respiratory or metabolic, can only correct *toward* normal, not all the way to normal or beyond, unless a second process is at work. If the aforementioned patient were to continue to be severely acidotic over the course of hours, the kidneys would begin to excrete hydrogen ions and to retain bicarbonate in an attempt to compensate for the acidosis on a more long-term basis. Thus over hours or days, if the acidosis were not corrected by treating the underlying cause, the serum bicarbonate level would rise, the pCO_2 would return toward normal, and the pH might remain unchanged. After these had occurred, the patient would have metabolic acidosis with metabolic compensation. The patient would have to be followed in order to reach this conclusion; a single arterial blood gas determination after a metabolic compensation for a metabolic process might appear quite normal.

If one evaluates only the pCO_2, the actual acid-base status of the patient remains unknown, which is similar to the previous example, in which an examination of pH alone would have been misleading. If one sees a pCO_2 of 10 mmHg, this might be the result of hyperventilation as a compensation for a metabolic problem or a primary hyperventilation, leading to alkalemia. The combined evaluation of both pH and pCO_2 leads to a more correct diagnosis of the metabolic situation.

The immediate circumstances at the time of arterial puncture must be evaluated in conjunction with the numbers obtained. A patient may acutely hyperventilate at the time of arterial puncture or may be receiving supplemental oxygen. The patient may have normal or near normal oxygenation when sitting in a chair, but minimal exer-

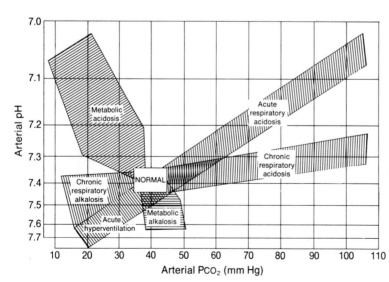

Figure 3–5. Blood gas interpretation. Acid-base graph that allows diagnosis of acid-base abnormalities from PCO_2 and pH. (From Groer ME, et al.: Basic Pathophysiology: A Conceptual Approach. St Louis: CV Mosby Co, 1979.)

tion may lead to marked arterial oxygen desaturation.

Pulmonary Function Testing. The evaluation of lung function on the basis of physiologic measurements can provide remarkable insight into pulmonary disease processes (Table 3–7). Simple spirometry, in which the patient is evaluated on the basis of the volume of air exhaled during

Table 3–7. RESPIRATORY PARAMETERS

Lung Volumes

Tidal volume (V_T)	Volume of air inspired and expired with a normal breath (400–500 ml or 5 ml/kg body weight)
Inspiratory reserve volume (IRV)	Maximal volume that can be inspired from the end of a normal inspiration
Expiratory reserve volume (ERV)	Maximal volume that can be exhaled by a forced expiration after a normal expiration
Residual volume (RV)	Volume of gas left in lung after maximal expiration
Minute volume (MV)	Amount of air inspired per minute

Lung Capacities

Vital capacity (VC)	Maximal amount of air that can be expired after a maximal inspiratory effort (70 ml/kg body weight)
Inspiratory capacity (IC)	Maximal volume that can be inspired after a normal expiration (V_T + IRV)
Functional residual capacity (FRC)	Volume of air left in lungs after a normal expiration (ERV + RV)
Total lung capacity (TLC)	Total volume of gas in lungs after maximal inspiration (IRV + V_T + ERV + RV) (Men: 3.6–9.4 L; women: 2.5–6.9 L)

Flow Rates

Forced expiratory volume (FEV, FEV_1, FEV_2, FEV_3)	Volume of air forcibly exhaled after a maximal inspiration in 1-, 2-, and 3-second intervals
Maximal expiratory flow (MEF)	Total amount of air expired per minute, breathing as rapidly as possible (approx. 400 L/min)
Maximal inspiratory flow (MIF)	Total amount of air inspired per minute, breathing as rapidly as possible (approx. 300 L/min)
Peak expiratory flow rate (PEFR)	Highest rate of flow sustained for 10 msec or more at which air can be expelled from the lungs

(From Groer ME, et al.: Basic Pathophysiology: A Conceptual Approach. St Louis: CV Mosby Co, 1979.)

a forced maneuver, can provide a great deal of information about both the nature and severity of the pulmonary problem.

In order to understand pulmonary function testing, it is necessary to understand the compartmentalization of gases in the lungs. This division of inhaled and exhaled gas into compartments is more functional than actual.

The vital capacity is the volume of gas exhaled from full inspiration to the end of a forced expiration (Fig. 3–6). The residual volume is the gas remaining in the lung at the end of a complete exhalation. Normal values for these volumes are dependent on an individual's height, weight, age, and sex. There is also some ethnic variation.

Simple spirometry measures the forced vital capacity (FVC) and the volume of this FVC exhaled during the first second (FEV_1). Together these values can often suggest the predominant physiologic defect in the individual being studied. The diagrams in Figure 3–6 indicate that the FVC will be decreased in both airway obstruction and restrictive disease, and in general this is the case. Because there is increased resistance to the flow of air in obstructive processes, the FEV_1 will often be the differentiating factor. In airways obstruction, the FEV_1 will be low; less of the FVC will be exhaled during the first second than in the normal individual. In restrictive lung disease, the FEV_1 is often increased; in severe restriction, the FEV_1 may actually approach the value of the FVC.

Spirometry can also be used to detect the response to bronchodilators. If spirometry performed after administration of a bronchodilator reveals an improvement in FVC, FEV_1, or both compared with the preadministration values, there is an element of reversible airway obstruction (e.g., asthma). One must be cautious in interpretation of negative results or in quantification of a responsive patient. The administration of a single dose of a bronchodilator can produce highly variable responses even in individuals with well-documented asthma. Thus a lack of response to a bronchodilator does not necessarily exclude the diagnosis of asthma, and an incomplete response does not necessarily imply an element of irreversible airway obstruction.

Although spirometry can be an ex-

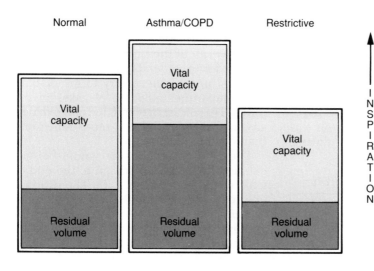

Figure 3–6. Total lung capacity. Each box represents the amount of gas in the lungs at the end of a maximum inspiration. Subdivisions of vital capacity and residual volume are shown.

tremely sensitive and reliable screening technique, there are situations in which additional physiologic measurements are useful. Spirometry cannot measure the total lung capacity or residual volume, and it tells nothing about the gas exchange function of the lungs. More sophisticated methods of pulmonary function measurement are therefore required in situations in which several lung processes may be coexistent (e.g., both a restrictive and an obstructive defect) or in which a more definitive diagnosis is desired (e.g., asthma versus emphysema). In these situations, a variety of physiologic measures is available to the pulmonary specialist, including body plethysmography, gas dilution detection techniques, and diffusing capacity measurements. In addition, the measurement of pulmonary function and gas exchange during exercise is often helpful.

Sputum Examination. The examination of expectorated sputum can provide a virtually instantaneous window on the pathologic processes at work in the lungs. Sputum should be examined for its gross appearance, odor, and volume. Greenish or yellowish sputum or frank pus indicates the presence of white blood cells and often a pulmonary infection or abscess. Frank blood is hemoptysis by definition. Bloody or "rusty"-appearing sputum may suggest pneumococcal pneumonia. Reddish gelatinous-looking sputum is often associated with *Klebsiella pneumoniae.* Voluminous sputum that settles into several layers is associated with bronchiectasis.

After the gross examination of sputum, and depending on the clinical situation,

microscopic examination is often helpful. In the evaluation, it is often sufficient to examine sputum directly, without staining. This examination can reveal the prominent eosinophilia often associated with the sputum of asthmatics. In suspected pulmonary infections, further evaluation using Gram's stain and an acid-fast stain can help in an initial determination of the organisms involved. Thereafter, more definitive diagnosis can be determined by sputum culture and assessment of the sensitivity of the pathogenic organisms to representative antimicrobial agents.

Chest Roentgenogram, Computed Tomography, and Magnetic Resonance Imaging. Radiologic evaluation of the chest has been the mainstay of pulmonary medicine for about a century. The chest roentgenogram (Fig. 3–7), or chest x-ray, can reveal the presence of any lesion that absorbs x-rays more than the surrounding lung, such as pulmonary infiltration with fluid (Fig. 3–8) or scar tissue, a pleural effusion, or a tumor mass, and it can reveal processes that absorb x-rays less than normal lung tissue, such as a pneumothorax or bullous emphysema. Because the mechanics of respiration depend on the integrity of the chest wall, a preliminary evaluation of the ribs and spine can be made with a routine chest roentgenogram. The diaphragm should be examined. The diaphragm is flattened in diseases that lead to airway obstruction and air trapping. Similarly the anteroposterior dimensions of the chest are increased on the lateral view of the chest when the total lung capacity is increased. An abnormally elevated diaphragm sug-

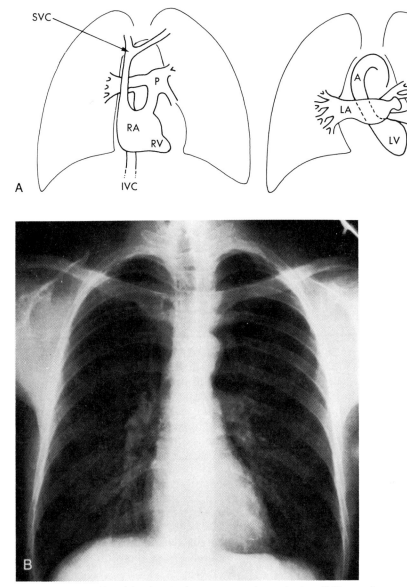

Figure 3–7. *A*, The x-ray film of the chest in the posteroanterior projection. SVC, superior vena cava; IVC, inferior vena cava; RA, right atrium; RV, right ventricle; P, pulmonary artery; LA, left atrium; LV, left ventricle; *A*, aorta. (From Tilkian SM, Conover MB, Tilkian AG: Clinical Implications of Laboratory Tests. St Louis: CV Mosby Co, 1979.) *B*, Normal chest radiograph. (From Fraser RG, Paré JAP: Diagnosis of Diseases of the Chest, Vol 1, 2nd ed. Philadelphia: WB Saunders Co, 1977.)

gests a loss of volume of the lung on that side, a diaphragmatic paralysis, or an abdominal process forcing the diaphragm to elevate.

Further advances in the use of radiographs and the computerized processing of their images have led to the widespread use of computed tomography (CT) in the evaluation of the chest. Computed tomography has proved especially important in the localization of lesions of the lungs or along the chest wall. In many medical centers, CT has become a standard method of evaluating pulmonary neoplasms, tracheal obstructions, and pleural diseases. Several reports have suggested that the relative malignancy of a given lung lesion suspected of being an aggressive tumor can be assessed with chest CT. In an individual patient, however, this technique can rarely, if ever, be used in place of obtaining a tissue specimen, at least with the current state of the art.

Magnetic resonance imaging (MRI [for-

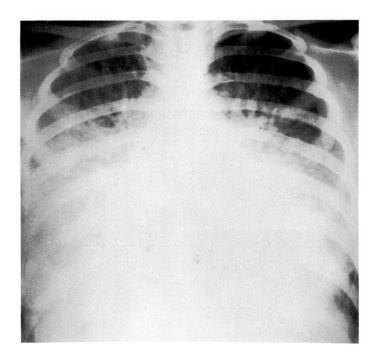

Figure 3–8. Acute pulmonary edema secondary to left ventricular failure. A posteroanterior radiograph reveals extensive consolidation of both lungs extending out to the visceral pleural surfaces. Much of the consolidation is homogeneous, but individual acinar shadows can be identified in the upper lung zones. The heart is moderately enlarged. (From Fraser RG, Paré JAP: Diagnosis of Diseases of the Chest, 2nd ed. Vol II. Philadelphia: WB Saunders Co, 1978.)

merly nuclear magnetic resonance]) produces images of sufficient resolution to be used diagnostically. An important advantage of this imaging technique is that it does not require that the patient be exposed to ionizing radiation. The image is obtained by placing the patient within the field of an extremely powerful magnet, and the perturbations of individual atomic magnetic fields in response to a radio frequency stimulus are measured. Computerized evaluation of these measurements produces an image that appears very similar to a CT image.

In addition to the presumed safety of this technique compared with those that require exposure to x-rays, MRI provides different information, since the changes in image intensity are not related to x-ray absorption. Magnetic resonance imaging has been used with great success in the evaluation of mediastinal processes because the elements of the mediastinum are much more clearly delineated with MRI compared with x-ray techniques. Future research will reveal the relative importance of MRI in the evaluation of lung disease.

Ventilation/Perfusion Scan. The mainstay of noninvasive evaluation of the pulmonary circulation is the ventilation/perfusion scan. This technique uses two radioisotopically labeled agents, one to evaluate the pulmonary circulation and

one to evaluate the ventilation of the lungs. The circulation is evaluated by intravenous injection of a radioactive aggregated substance, such as albumin, and the imaging of the radioactive substance trapped in the pulmonary circulation by an external detection system. Areas of the lung that are poorly perfused or where circulation has been interrupted do not trap the radioactive aggregates and appear as "cold" areas. The most common indication for such a study is the suspicion of pulmonary embolic disease. Pulmonary embolism causes regional loss of blood flow, often in several areas of the lung.

The ventilation study is a necessary addition because loss of the ventilation to an area of the lung is often accompanied by disruption of the circulation to that area. Thus COPD often produces an abnormal perfusion scan, but the areas of poor perfusion are matched by areas of poor ventilation on the accompanying ventilation scan.

Pulmonary Angiography. When the lung scan is inconclusive and it is necessary to determine definitively whether pulmonary embolic disease is present, the "gold standard" is the pulmonary angiogram. The angiogram is indicated whenever the pulmonary artery circulation must be clearly visualized. In contrast, the angiogram is relatively contraindicated in the presence of severe pulmonary hypertension because of the significantly increased mortality of this procedure when elevated pulmonary artery pressures are present.

Bronchoscopy and Lung Biopsy. The introduction of the flexible fiberoptic bronchoscope has led to an era of safe diagnostic procedures in lung disease. Through the bronchoscope, with direct visualization or with the aid of fluoroscopy, biopsy forceps, needles, and brushes can be directed to pulmonary lesions, often allowing a tissue diagnosis without major surgery. The limitations of this procedure are related to the anatomy of the lung. Because the biopsy instrument must be directed to the lesion via the airways, the closer a lesion is to a central airway and the larger the lesion is, the more likely one is to be able to obtain a tissue specimen. A related consideration is that a negative result rarely settles a diagnostic question. One must repeat the bronchoscopic procedure or use another method to obtain the diagnosis.

The use of a "skinny needle" biopsy technique has proved quite successful with lesions too small or too peripheral to be reached using bronchoscopic techniques. This method involves the percutaneous introduction of a small needle through the chest wall and placement in the lesion under radiographic direction (fluoroscope or CT scan). Saline is then introduced into the lesion through the needle, and the suspension of cells in saline is then withdrawn for cytologic evaluation. In the right hands, this technique can be highly successful.

ASSESSMENT OF COMMONLY ENCOUNTERED PROBLEMS

Preoperative Pulmonary Evaluation

The preoperative pulmonary evaluation of the podiatric patient should include, as with other organ systems, a detailed history and physical examination (Fig. 3–9). The functional status of the lungs requires direct evaluation. The importance of this is often overlooked in individuals who are undergoing procedures that require only local anesthesia. In fact, postoperative

morbidity and mortality are increased significantly in an individual with pulmonary disease whether anesthesia is local or general.

In a young, otherwise healthy individual, the history may replace detailed pulmonary function testing (Table 3–8). If the individual reports that he or she runs 5 miles a day and has no significant history of pulmonary diseases such as asthma or of previous thoracic surgery, clinical judgment suggests that it is unlikely that an increased surgical risk exists owing to underlying lung disease. The question becomes less academic as an individual's lung function becomes worse. Any underlying lung disease increases surgical and postoperative morbidity. Often these risks can be minimized with good preoperative management. This may involve the preadmission of a surgical candidate for the express purpose of improving pulmonary toilet, beginning an aggressive regimen of bronchodilators, if indicated, and in severe asthmatic patients or those with COPD and a bronchodilator response, beginning a course of corticosteroids.

There are inevitably those individuals whose surgical risk is so great because of their pulmonary disease that one must ask whether anesthesia and surgery can be tolerated at all. In these individuals, the risk of surgery must be weighed against its ben-

Table 3–8. PULMONARY HISTORY AND PHYSICAL EXAMINATION

Important Points to Consider When Taking a History

Previous episodes of hemoptysis
History of chest disease
Exercise tolerance
Medication history
Bleeding tendencies
Careful investigation of current episode (duration, quantity, and rate of bleeding)

Physical Examination

State of consciousness
Changes in pulse and blood pressure
Evidence of chest trauma
Splinting of chest wall
Breath sounds (may help localize area of bleeding)
Clubbing, adenopathy, wasting in cancer patients, increased AP diameter, and low diaphragm in severe emphysema are all signs that may suggest the underlying process

(Data from Luckmann J, Sorensen KC: Medical-Surgical Nursing: A Psychophysiological Approach, 2nd ed. Philadelphia: WB Saunders Co, 1980.)

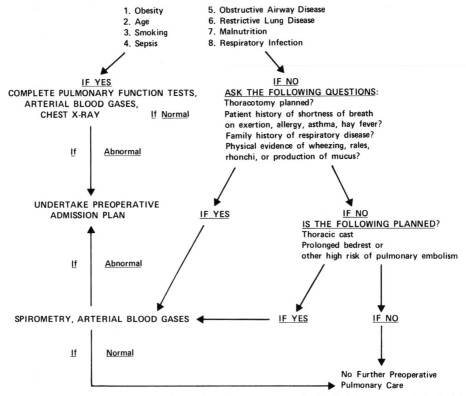

ARE RISK FACTORS PRESENT?

1. Obesity
2. Age
3. Smoking
4. Sepsis

5. Obstructive Airway Disease
6. Restrictive Lung Disease
7. Malnutrition
8. Respiratory Infection

IF YES
COMPLETE PULMONARY FUNCTION TESTS,
ARTERIAL BLOOD GASES,
CHEST X-RAY   If Normal

IF NO
ASK THE FOLLOWING QUESTIONS:
Thoracotomy planned?
Patient history of shortness of breath
on exertion, allergy, asthma, hay fever?
Family history of respiratory disease?
Physical evidence of wheezing, rales,
rhonchi, or production of mucus?

If   Abnormal

UNDERTAKE PREOPERATIVE
ADMISSION PLAN   IF YES

IF NO
IS THE FOLLOWING PLANNED?
Thoracic cast
Prolonged bedrest or
other high risk of pulmonary embolism

If   Abnormal

SPIROMETRY, ARTERIAL BLOOD GASES   ◄——— IF YES   IF NO

If   Normal

No Further Preoperative
Pulmonary Care

Figure 3–9. Flow chart for preoperative care plan and evaluation. (From Molitch ME: Management of Medical Problems in Surgical Patients. Philadelphia: FA Davis Co, 1982.)

efits and a decision made based on the best available evidence.

Postoperative Management of Patient with Pulmonary Disease

In the postoperative period, the individual with pulmonary disease is at great risk of an exacerbation of the underlying disease as well as at increased risk of a superimposed problem such as infection or pulmonary embolic disease. Postoperatively these patients are recovering from anesthesia; receiving sedatives, analgesic medications, or both; and restricting their activities. This combination of events leads to poor clearance of secretions and organisms from the lung, especially in patients whose pulmonary status has been previously compromised by underlying lung disease. This is most dramatically demonstrated following general anesthesia, especially in individuals requiring prolonged intubation and ventilatory support or in those with known pulmonary disease prior to surgery.

All patients require attention to their pulmonary status in the postoperative period, but this is especially true for patients with pulmonary disease (Table 3–9). Intravenous bronchodilator therapy, when appropriate; chest physical therapy; mechanical lower extremity venous stimulation, such as simple support hose or more exotic external pumps; and often subcutaneous heparin injections can minimize postoperative morbidity in these patients.

Chronic Obstructive Pulmonary Disease

Chronic obstructive pulmonary disease classically describes the spectrum of lung disease bounded by pulmonary emphysema and chronic bronchitis. The majority of individuals affected by COPD have a

Table 3–9. ACUTE RESPIRATORY DISEASES

Disease	Description	Recognition	Laboratory Tests	Treatment
Bronchial asthma	Acute airway obstruction owing to allergic/ nervous response; little or no hypoxemia	Respiratory distress; wheezing	CO_2 usually normal; O_2 decreased	Medication (adrenalin); IPPB*; expectorants; bronchodilators
Bronchitis	Airway obstruction owing to edema secondary to inflammation	Fever; chest pain; dyspnea; cough	White blood cell count (WBC) increased	Antibiotics; IPPB; expectorants; humidification
Pneumonia	Pneumococci; bacterial pathogens; gram-negative bacilli; *Staphylococcus aureus*	Fever; productive cough; pulmonary infiltration	WBC increased; pO_2 decreased; pCO_2 may be increased	Antibiotics; IPPB; expectorants; humidification; hydration to thin secretions
Pulmonary edema	Acute heart failure; hypernatremia and fluid retention	Edema; weight gain; hypertension; dyspnea	Urine Cl decreased; serum sodium normal; hemoglobin normal or decreased	Diuretics; salt and fluid restriction
Pulmonary emboli	Capillaries plugged with clots	Chest pain; increased blood pressure	Lactate dehydrogenase (LDH) increased	Anticoagulants
Respiratory depression	Insensitive respiratory center; sometimes accompanies obesity	CO_2 narcosis	pO_2 decreased; pCO_2 increased	Endotracheal tube; supportive breathing; respiratory stimulants
Spontaneous pneumothorax	Ruptured lung	Blood pressure and pulse decreased; movement of chest wall decreased; cyanosis	X-ray	Release air by inserting catheter into intrapleural space through second intercostal space anteriorly; prophylactic antibiotics

* IPPB, Intermittent positive-pressure breathing.

mixture of these two disorders with one predominant. In addition, there is often a component of reversible obstructive disease (e.g., asthma). There are pathologic, physiologic, and historical details that distinguish between emphysema and chronic bronchitis (Table 3–10).

Emphysema is characterized pathologically by lung parenchymal destruction. This results in dilatation of the alveoli and

Table 3–10. DIFFERENTIATING BETWEEN CHRONIC BRONCHITIS AND EMPHYSEMA

	Chronic Bronchitis	Emphysema
Exposure to airway irritants	Almost invariably a history of cigarette smoking	Usually a history of cigarette smoking
Presenting symptom	Persistent cough and sputum production	Gradually progressive exertional dyspnea
Dyspnea	Variable	Persistent
Respiratory infections	Frequent episodes of wheezing, dyspnea, and purulent sputum	Infrequent respiratory infections
Physical examination	Tendency to overweight	Tendency to thinness
	Expiratory wheezes	Expiratory wheezes may not be prominent
		Diminished basilar breath sounds that do not increase in intensity with deep breathing
Chest film	May be normal	Overinflation
	"Dirty chest" with increased bronchovascular markings	Flattened hemidiaphragms
		Increased retrosternal air space
		Increased lucency of lower third of lung fields
Pulmonary function tests	Reduction in FEF (forced expiratory flow) 25–75% (early)	Reduction in FEF 25 to 75%
	Reduction in FEV_1 (later)	Reduction in FEV_1
	Normal diffusing capacity	Reduction in diffusing capacity

(From Speir WA, Jr: How to improve management of chronic obstructive lung disease. Consultant 17:168, 1977.)

a loss of the elastic properties of the lungs' connective tissue. In extreme cases, the decreased surface area available for gas exchange leads to abnormalities in oxygen uptake and in carbon dioxide elimination from blood.

Chronic bronchitis is characterized by chronic sputum production and airflow limitation. Pathologically, there is hypertrophy of the bronchial mucous glands and increased mucus delivery to the airways. Both emphysema and chronic bronchitis are, except in rare instances, diseases of the middle-aged and elderly.

Pathogenesis. The majority of COPD is caused by the long-term inhalation of products of tobacco combustion (i.e., cigarette addiction). The mechanisms by which cigarette smoke leads to lung damage are just beginning to be understood. In order to understand the role of cigarettes in these processes, it is helpful to understand a less common cause of emphysema, the hereditary form. Hereditary, or familial, emphysema is associated with a genetic deficiency of a particular serum protein, alpha$_1$-antitrypsin (also known as alpha$_1$-proteinase inhibitor). Individuals with this deficiency often develop emphysema before age 40 even in the absence of a significant smoking history.

Research indicates that the lung destruction of emphysema is due to the action of white blood cell enzymes. These white blood cells, the polymorphonuclear leukocytes and, perhaps, the alveolar macrophages, produce potent elastases, enzymes capable of degrading the lung connective tissue elastin. The primary protection of the lungs against the action of elastase is serum alpha$_1$-antitrypsin, which constantly bathes the lungs. Deficiency of this important protein leaves the lungs unprotected so that these elastases can destroy the lungs' connective tissue, producing emphysema.

Tobacco combustion releases a multitude of reactive chemical species, including several that are potent oxidizing agents. It has been shown that exposure of alpha$_1$-antitrypsin to chemical oxidants destroys this protein's ability to inhibit elastase. Thus it appears that all emphysema is due to alpha$_1$-antitrypsin deficiency. In the rare individuals with hereditary emphysema, the deficiency of alpha$_1$-antitrypsin is genetic. In the vast majority who

develop emphysema as a result of cigarette smoke inhalation, the deficiency is functional. The result of each form of deficiency is lung destruction.

The obstruction to expiratory airflow seen in emphysema is the direct result of elastin degradation. The elastin fibers in the lung parenchyma act as tethers, holding open the small airways as the lungs deflate during exhalation. When these fibers are destroyed by the action of white blood cell elastases, these airways collapse during exhalation, trapping air in the lungs and increasing the expiratory resistance in the airways.

The pathophysiology of chronic bronchitis is not fully understood. It has been demonstrated that, as in emphysema, products derived from white blood cells are capable of causing some or all of the changes noted in human chronic bronchitis. The association with cigarette smoke inhalation is a statistical one.

Clinical Presentation. The presenting symptoms in individuals with COPD are usually of insidious onset. Symptoms include exertional dyspnea, cough, sputum production, and shortness of breath. Often a patient will notice an increasing inability to keep up with peers in daily physical activities. This inability will be gradually progressive until, after months or years, the shortness of breath occurs with minimal exertion and, finally, at rest.

A common clinical setting in which symptoms are noted is immediately following a respiratory infection. An individual may feel entirely well or have minimal symptoms of COPD but after a respiratory infection note a dramatic worsening of pulmonary reserve and exercise tolerance. In patients with COPD, many of whom appear to have an increased susceptibility to respiratory infections, the clinical picture may be one of frequent, precipitous decrements in lung function accompanying each infection.

Diagnosis. The diagnosis of COPD is based on the clinical picture of irreversible airway obstruction combined with physical findings and laboratory confirmation. The history almost invariably includes heavy cigarette use. In addition to the history of exertional dyspnea, shortness of breath, and cough, patients with COPD may describe an inability to sleep in the fully recumbent position because of shortness of breath (orthopnea). This must be distinguished from orthopnea seen with left-sided congestive heart failure. Individuals with chronic bronchitis will expectorate significant amounts of sputum each day for many months.

The physical appearance of the patient with emphysema has been described as the "pink puffer." The complexion is described as pink because the emphysema sufferer maintains fairly good oxygenation until the very end stages of the disease. The habitus is generally thin but with a barrel-shaped chest and hypertrophy of the accessory muscles of respiration, especially in the neck.

The patient with chronic bronchitis is described as a "blue bloater" because the oxygenation is often poor for prolonged periods, leading to cyanosis. This poor oxygenation can lead to pulmonary vascular hypertension and eventually to right-sided congestive heart failure, called cor pulmonale in this setting. Cor pulmonale leads to liver congestion and peripheral edema. The clinical course of the patient with chronic bronchitis is often marked by exacerbations and improvements.

Physical examination of the chest usually reveals decreased breath sounds, sometimes accompanied by wheeze, and a prolonged expiratory phase. Rarely clubbing of the extremities occurs, although this is not characteristic of COPD.

The laboratory evaluation of the COPD patient reveals polycythemia if the patient has been hypoxemic for a prolonged period. Arterial blood gas values can be quite informative in these patients. Patients with emphysema maintain relatively normal blood gas values, except for mild hypoxemia, until the disease is quite severe. Respiratory acidosis in a patient with emphysema with elevated pCO_2 and decreased pH indicates either end-stage disease or an acute episode of respiratory failure. In contrast, the arterial blood gas values of patients with chronic bronchitis can be extremely deranged, with chronic respiratory acidosis continuing for years. Also, the values can change dramatically in a given patient over the course of the disease, first worsening and then improving.

Pulmonary function testing is the primary mechanism for the determination of the disease process in an individual with airway obstruction. Simple spirometry may not be sufficient, however. Spirometry in individuals with COPD, asthma, or both will reveal a decreased FEV_1 and FEV_1/FVC ratio. Classically, reversibility of these abnormalities following bronchodilator administration suggests the diagnosis of asthma, whereas lack of reversibility suggests COPD. Unfortunately, many times asthma does not completely reverse following a single inhalation of a bronchodilator, and individuals with COPD frequently have a component of their disease that is reversible.

Beyond simple spirometry, a patient with COPD often has an increase in total lung capacity primarily caused by a marked increase in residual volume. This represents the air trapping mentioned previously. In emphysema, a decrease in the diffusing capacity is a very sensitive marker of this disease. Furthermore, the relationship between pleural pressure (as detected by changes in esophageal pressure readings) and lung volume (the pressure/volume curve of the lungs) can indicate a loss of elastic recoil in emphysema. No specific testing for chronic bronchitis is currently available, but the presence of irreversible airflow obstruction in the correct clinical setting is usually used to make the diagnosis.

Exercise testing with oximetry can help determine the etiology of exertional dyspnea. Patients with COPD can demonstrate marked hypoxemia with minimal exercise even if resting arterial blood gas values are near normal.

The chest roentgenogram in COPD shows hyperlucent lung fields, flat diaphragm, increased anteroposterior diameter, and increased retrosternal air space, all representative of air trapping. In some forms of emphysema, large, thin-walled spaces can develop, called bullae, which may appear on the roentgenogram as circular areas devoid of lung markings. Such a patient has an increased risk of pneumothorax, and so a careful evaluation of the roentgenogram is necessary to rule out this serious complication of bullous COPD.

The definitive diagnosis of COPD is made by lung biopsy. This diagnostic measure is rarely necessary, however, and carries an extremely high morbidity if undertaken.

Treatment. The lung destruction of emphysema and, probably, the pathologic changes of chronic bronchitis are irreversible by current medical science. Treatment is concentrated in three main areas: halting the progression of disease, treating any reversible (asthmatic) component, and improving hypoxemia when present. The progression of the disease can be slowed or halted by removing the etiologic agent of COPD, that is, by cessation of smoking. In addition, aggressive therapy of pulmonary infections is indicated as well as yearly influenza immunization and pneumococcal antigen immunization.

As mentioned, most patients with COPD have a component of their airway obstruction that is reversed by bronchodilators. A patient with COPD may benefit from a trial of the regimen outlined subsequently for the patient with asthma. Often a corticosteroid trial is effective, especially when sputum production is a prominent symptom. Vigorous pulmonary toilet is also effective in such an individual.

The administration of supplemental oxygen can be extremely effective in selected individuals with COPD. The presence of cor pulmonale is an indication for nocturnal supplemental oxygen. It has been shown that oxygen administration, for at least 8 hours of every 24, can lead to a reduction in the pulmonary hypertension associated with hypoxemia, and an improvement in the right-sided congestive heart failure and can result in a marked diuresis. Exertional dyspnea caused by hypoxemia with exercise can often be substantially improved by administration of supplemental oxygen during exercise. In the most severe stages of COPD, it is often necessary to administer continuous supplemental oxygen.

The use of supplemental oxygen is not without risk. There are local effects of oxygen administration such as drying of mucous membranes and sinusitis when the nasal cannula is used for delivery. More serious is the observation that many patients with COPD severe enough to require supplemental oxygen use a "hypoxemia drive" mechanism to control respiration. In normal individuals, the level of CO_2 in the blood is the primary message that the respiratory center uses for determining respiratory rate and depth. In patients with severe COPD, in whom the pCO_2 may vary widely, the respiratory center relies instead on the blood oxygen content for control of respiration. Thus if the pO_2 rises sufficiently, the respiratory center may cause the patient to hypoventilate or even shut off respiration entirely. This can be seen when a patient with COPD with hypoxic drive is given high-flow supplemental oxygen. It is advised that supplemental oxygen flow rates for patients with COPD rarely exceed 2 to 3 L/minute unless the patient is under close supervision.

Patients with COPD represent one of the major perioperative high-risk groups. They have a significantly increased morbidity following anesthesia whether general or regional. General anesthesia carries a likelihood of prolonged ventilatory support in the postoperative period. These risks can be reduced by preoperative therapy, which includes enforced smoking cessation; bronchodilator therapy including corticosteroids, if indicated; and a vigorous pulmonary toilet.

Asthma

Asthma, or reversible obstructive airway disease, can affect all age groups. It is characterized by paroxysmal episodes of bronchoconstriction, which can be quite severe, even life-threatening. Asthma is distinguished from COPD by the reversible nature of the airflow obstruction. Classic asthma is divided into extrinsic and intrinsic forms (Table 3–11). *Extrinsic asthma*, usually seen in children, is thought to be chiefly related to sensitivity to environmental agents and primarily an allergic process. *Intrinsic asthma*, seen in adults, describes the disease when no external allergic agents can be identified.

Pathogenesis. The biochemical mechanisms that cause an individual to develop asthma are not fully understood. Much is known about the mediators that can produce bronchoconstriction, but the question of why one individual has asthma and another does not has not been answered. It is clear that all individuals have an element of bronchial reactivity; that is, given sufficient, appropriate stimulation, any individual, asthmatic or nonasthmatic, will respond with detectable bronchoconstriction. The asthmatic patient is often described as having bronchial hyper-reactiv-

Table 3–11. CLINICAL CHARACTERISTICS OF EXTRINSIC (ATOPIC) AND INTRINSIC (NONATOPIC) ASTHMA

	Extrinsic (Atopic) (Allergic)	Intrinsic (Nonatopic) (Infective/Idiopathic)
Onset of symptoms	Usually during childhood	Usually in adults over age 35
Family history of atopy	Positive	Usually negative
History of infantile eczema	Positive	Negative
Identifiable allergy to inhaled and ingested substances	Positive	Negative
Passive transfer of IgE (skin-sensitizing) antibody	Positive	Negative
Reactions to skin test with inhalant allergens	Positive	Negative
Association with Type I, IgE reaction	Positive	Negative
Eosinophilia	Positive	Positive
In vitro release of histamine from washed leukocytes	Positive	Negative
Hyposensitization therapy	Favorable response	Equivocal
Typical attack	Acute and usually self-limiting	Often fulminant and severe
Relationship of acute attack to infection	May be present	Often present
Symptoms and physical findings	Identical for both types of asthma	
Aspirin sensitivity	Negative	Positive
Prognosis	Generally favorable	Less favorable
Death during acute attack	Rare	May occur

ity. This can be defined as an altered sensitivity to stimulatory agents such that levels of stimulatory agents found in the environment are sufficient to produce a bronchoconstricting effect. For up to 2 months following a viral upper respiratory infection, all individuals, whether asthmatic or not, will demonstrate a marked increase in sensitivity to stimuli that can cause bronchoconstriction, such as histamine and methacholine.

The pathologic findings associated with asthma include hypertrophy of the bronchial and bronchiolar smooth muscles; copious, tenacious sputum in all airways; and pulmonary hyperinflation. These findings were noted in pathologic specimens of individuals who died with asthma. Therefore, the pathology of mild asthma is assumed to be less dramatic.

Clinical Presentation. The asthmatic patient complains of recurrent episodes of shortness of breath often accompanied by wheeze. Frequently there will be a triggering event such as a lung infection or cold, but there are a variety of other triggers that certain asthmatics can identify. These include exercise, inhalation of cold air, certain foods or drinks, certain odors or scents, certain seasons or pollens, certain medications, and emotional stresses.

There are other specific triggers that deserve further mention. Exercise-induced bronchospasm is a well-described entity that affects many patients with asthma. Its identification is important because prophylaxis with agents such as cromolyn sodium (see under Treatment) can be very effective in preventing such attacks.

The triad of aspirin sensitivity, asthma, and nasal polyps was one of the first examples of drug-related asthma described. It is sufficiently common that many physicians recommend that all their asthmatic patients abstain from aspirin.

Two food additives have been associated with the triggering of asthma, metabisulfite and tartrazine. Metabisulfite and other sulfiting agents are used as preservatives. They are added in large amounts to dried fruits and vegetables; to wine and beer; and to exposed foods, such as in a restaurant salad bar, to prevent discoloration. Tartrazine is a common yellow food dye.

Some asthmatics have bronchoconstriction that is induced by fungi or bacteria living within their airways. The classic example is that of bronchopulmonary aspergillosis. This disease is characterized by shortness of breath with wheeze, eosinophilia, pulmonary infiltrates, bronchiectasis, *Aspergillus* in the sputum, and precipitating antibodies to *Aspergillus* antigens in the blood. The identification of this disease is important because permanent lung damage can occur if not properly treated with corticosteroids.

Many asthmatic patients have symptoms that are most prominent at night or in the very early morning. There are several possible mechanisms that can lead to this nocturnal asthma pattern. Probably the most common problem relates to drug dosage schedules. Most medications used to treat asthma do not have a duration of action that spans an entire night, and it is difficult to have asthmatic patients arise from sleep to take medications. Fortunately, newer agents are being introduced with prolonged actions that can prevent this cause of nocturnal asthma. Additional causes exist that can be treated, however. Chronic sinusitis with postnasal drip can exacerbate asthma, and the sinuses often drain into the lungs at night. Gastroesophageal reflux can exacerbate asthma during sleep as well.

Diagnosis. The diagnosis of asthma is made on the bases of a history of paroxysmal episodes of shortness of breath, often with wheeze; confirmatory pulmonary function testing; and response to appropriate therapy. Wheezing is neither necessary for diagnosis of asthma nor pathognomonic. As mentioned earlier, individuals with COPD may present with wheezing. Asthmatic patients will have wheeze only when there is sufficient airflow through a confined air space to produce the whistling sound. Thus when asthma is mild or quiescent, there is often no wheeze. In contrast, when asthma is so severe that sufficient airflow cannot be generated, there will be no wheeze (Table 3–12).

Additional physical findings during an attack include intercostal retractions caused by the high negative intrathoracic pressures generated during the inspiratory effort. Similar pressures can lead to the finding of pulsus paradoxus, the observation that arterial blood pressure varies with respiratory excursion, dropping during inspiration.

Pulmonary function testing reveals evidence of airway obstruction with a decreased FEV_1 and FEV_1/FVC ratio. As in COPD, there can be air trapping with resultant increased total lung capacity and residual volume. In contrast to COPD, there is often marked improvement in these pulmonary function abnormalities after initiation of bronchodilator therapy.

Arterial blood gas values are often normal during the quiescent period of an asthmatic patient. During an attack, depending on the severity of the episode, there can be marked abnormalities. Mild to moderate hypoxemia can be found. Early in the course of an attack the pCO_2, usually normal in mild asthma, may fall as compensatory hyperventilation is stimulated by the increased obstruction to airflow. If the attack becomes more severe and the pa-

Table 3–12. STAGING OF THE SEVERITY OF AN ACUTE ASTHMA ATTACK

Stage	Symptoms and Signs	FEV₁ or FVC	pH	PaO₂	PaCO₂
I (mild)	Mild dyspnea; diffuse wheezes; adequate air exchange	50–80% of normal	N* or ↑	occasionally N or most often ↓	N or ↓
II (moderate)	Respiratory distress at rest; hyperpnea; marked wheezes; air exchange N or ↓	50% of normal	generally ↑	↓	generally ↓
III (severe)	Marked respiratory distress; marked wheezes or absent breath sounds; check for pulsus paradoxus >10 mm; sternocleidomastoid retraction	25% of normal	N or ↓	↓	N or ↑
IV (respiratory failure)	Severe respiratory distress; lethargic; confused; prominent pulsus paradoxus; sternocleidomastoid retraction	10% of normal	↓ ↓	↓	↑ ↑

* N, Normal.

(Reproduced from The Merck Manual, 13th ed. Copyright under the Universal Copyright Convention and the International Copyright Convention 1977 by Merck & Co, Inc, Rahway, NJ, USA.)

tient begins to tire, the pCO_2 may rise, leading to a respiratory acidosis, the immediate precursor of respiratory failure. Thus a single blood gas determination showing a normal pCO_2 may indicate that the patient is doing well or that the patient is going into respiratory failure. The clinical picture and repeat blood gas determination answer this question. The chest roentgenogram can be normal or show evidence of air trapping.

Treatment. The treatment of asthma relies on removal of inciting agents (e.g., aspirin, metabisulfite, allergens) as appropriate and administration of bronchodilators. In some asthmatic patients, the removal of an inciting agent or the administration of a single bronchodilator agent is sufficient to control the disease. However, most asthmatics require the administration of multiple bronchodilator agents. The advantage of using multiple agents is that the side effects of giving a single agent at a high dosage can be minimized by giving several agents with additive effects, each at a lower dosage. The disadvantage of using multiple agents is the complexity of the dosage schedule with resultant loss of patient compliance.

There are several categories of bronchodilator medications. The theophylline compounds are the mainstay of most long-term asthma therapies. The development of effective sustained-release preparations has aided in the administration of this class of medications. It is important to adjust the dosage of theophylline based on determinations of blood level because individuals may vary considerably in their absorption and clearance of this medication. Additionally, several drugs affect the clearance of theophylline, notably cimetidine and erythromycin, which prolong the circulatory life of theophyllines and thus can increase the blood level of these drugs. Theophyllines are available for both oral and intravenous administration.

The use of a sympathomimetic agent is often the first line in asthma therapy. Epinephrine (Adrenaline) given subcutaneously is the usual first step in the treatment of an acute asthmatic exacerbation. Medications with more beta$_2$-receptor specificity and longer duration of action have become available for oral, subcutaneous, intravenous, and inhalational administration. These include isoetharine, metapro-

terenol, terbutaline, albuterol, and fenoterol. Their beta$_2$-receptor specificity reduces most of the systemic side effects associated with sympathomimetic agents.

Anticholinergic agents such as atropine have joined our armamentarium. They are given by inhalation and are commonly used in asthmatic patients in whom cough is a prominent symptom. Cromolyn sodium and ketotifin are provided for prophylaxis of asthma. Ketotifen, given orally, or cromolyn, given by inhalation, can prevent asthmatic exacerbations in certain individuals. Their mechanism of action is not known, but they do appear to have the ability to block the influx of calcium into respiratory smooth muscle and thus prevent bronchoconstriction. Cromolyn has found wide acceptance in the prophylaxis of exercise-induced asthma.

The most potent bronchodilators are the corticosteroids. Unfortunately, when administered over the long term, they produce serious side effects, such as adrenal suppression, exacerbation of diabetes, bone demineralization, cataracts, metabolic alkalosis, skin atrophy, capillary fragility, and all the stigmata of iatrogenic Cushing's disease. Short-term therapy, however, is quite safe and effective. Inhaled preparations can greatly reduce the systemic effects of steroid administration. Still, a severe exacerbation may require the administration of an oral or parenteral corticosteroid preparation.

As with COPD, patients with asthma have an increased risk of morbidity in the perioperative period. Prior vigorous bronchodilator therapy, including corticosteroid administration if indicated, can reduce this risk. It is important to obtain a detailed history of corticosteroid usage in patients underoing surgery. Adrenal suppression can be present up to a year following cessation of long-term corticosteroid administration. Such individuals, if not given supplementary steroids during the perioperative period, reveal adrenal suppression by developing total circulatory collapse during the stress of surgery.

Hyperventilation Syndrome

Hyperventilation syndrome describes an episode of acute, sometimes profound respiratory alkalosis without a specific organic cause.

Pathogenesis. The signs and symptoms of hyperventilation syndrome all relate to an acute respiratory alkalosis with a low pCO_2 and an elevated pH. The primary etiologic event is often believed to be related to stress or emotional tension. The sensations provoked by this alkalosis often lead to further stress and panic, exacerbating the problem.

Clinical Presentation. The patient presents with acute shortness of breath and "air hunger." The distal extremities and lips develop paresthesias or numbness. In extreme cases, there can be altered mentation and carpopedal spasm.

Diagnosis. Arterial blood gas determination is usually not required. The success of treatment and the reproduction of the symptom complex by voluntary hyperventilation more commonly confirm the diagnosis.

Treatment. A rebreathing apparatus, such as a paper bag held over the mouth, is commonly successful in treating this syndrome. If the patient is cooperative, breath holding can be equally effective. The prevention of recurrent attacks requires that the patient have a thorough understanding of the syndrome. This explanation should be given once the current attack is well controlled. Voluntary hyperventilation will usually recreate the symptoms and can be instructive to the patient.

The understanding of this syndrome will aid in the differentiation from more serious pulmonary diseases.

Aspiration

Pulmonary aspiration and aspiration pneumonia are serious complications of derangements in the protective mechanisms of the hypopharynx. There is the immediate danger of asphyxiation after an aspiration event. Soon thereafter, the danger of a chemical pneumonitis emerges. Several days after this, the danger of a serious aerobic or anaerobic pulmonary infection occurs.

Pathogenesis. Pulmonary aspiration occurs with the loss of the glottic and laryngeal defenses of the upper airways at a time when material is being delivered to the esophagus from the mouth or when gas-tric contents are being regurgitated. The regurgitation of gastric contents is particularly dangerous because the low pH of this material can be directly damaging to lung tissue. This loss of the normal defenses can occur if the patient has a reduced level of consciousness; if there is a lesion of the central or peripheral nervous system; if there is musculoskeletal disease of the hypopharynx; if there is an anatomic abnormality; or if there has been an iatrogenic breakdown in the laryngeal mechanism, as occurs during an endotracheal intubation or topical anesthesia.

One of the common scenarios leading to increased risk of aspiration is the reduced level of consciousness associated with ingestion of drugs such as ethanol, sedatives, or opiates. These agents cause a patient to be particularly prone to aspiration because such agents may induce vomiting as well as depress the level of consciousness.

The events that occur after an aspiration follow a logical progression. The initial danger involves the obstruction of airways by the aspirated foreign material. Small particles may block minor airways, leading to obstructive pneumonia or atelectasis. Larger material may obstruct major airways and even lead to immediate death by asphyxiation.

The character of the aspirated material determines the next phase. If the material is caustic or injurious, such as gastric acid, a chemical pneumonitis ensues. Bland substances, such as blood, will often produce no such damage.

Within 3 to 5 days a secondary bacterial infection may emerge. Secondary infections are more likely if there has been a chemical pneumonitis or if the aspirated substance contained large numbers of organisms, as when material is aspirated from the mouth of a patient with severe oral disease.

Clinical Presentation. An aspiration event may be observed, or the clinical setting and the progression and location of a pulmonary lesion may suggest an unobserved aspiration.

Diagnosis. The diagnosis of aspiration may be quite simple if the aspiration was observed. If not, an appropriate clinical setting, with a patient who is possibly losing the hypopharyngeal defenses of the upper airways, and an appropriate clinical course determine the diagnosis. Immediately after an aspiration, unless there is obstruction due to a foreign body, there is often no change in any physical or laboratory parameters. There may be a slight, unexplained hypoxemia when arterial blood gas values are analyzed.

Within the first several hours to 24 hours, if the conditions are correct for a chemical pneumonitis, the first signs of a pulmonary process appear. There are often roentgenographic abnormalities (Fig. 3–10) and more severe hypoxemia associated with this chemical pneumonitis. Thereafter, at 3 to 5 days, if a secondary bacterial infection appears, the abnormalities can become much more severe, and signs of sepsis can emerge. An aspiration need not lead to any of the abnormalities noted.

A distinct entity known as chronic aspiration pneumonia should be mentioned. This is seen in patients with recurrent aspiration events over the course of months or years. The clinical picture is one of scarring and infiltration of dependent lung field with no other explanation.

Treatment. The primary treatment for aspiration is prevention. In individuals at risk of aspiration, a simple precaution such as positioning so that pharyngeal contents are more likely to be expectorated than aspirated can be extremely helpful. When more protection is required, as in a stuporous patient with a suspected overdose in which gastric lavage is necessary, elective endotracheal intubation may be required. An additional prophylactic measure in patients at risk of aspiration of gastric contents is the administration of antacids or H_2-receptor antagonists to reduce gastric acidity and thus lessen the likelihood of an aspiration-induced chemical pneumonitis.

Once an aspiration has occurred, the therapy becomes more controversial. The use of corticosteroids has been advocated in aspiration pneumonia. Studies have demonstrated a beneficial effect for corticosteroids only if administered prior to or simultaneous with an aspiration event. Thus corticosteroids should probably be limited to administration immediately after an observed aspiration.

The second area of controversy is use of prophylactic antibiotics after an observed or suspected aspiration. Because there are a wide range of organisms that may develop into a secondary pulmonary infection after an aspiration, and since, in many instances, no secondary infection develops at all, it would seem reasonable to closely monitor the Gram's stain and culture of the

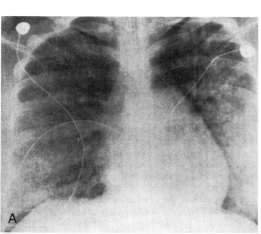
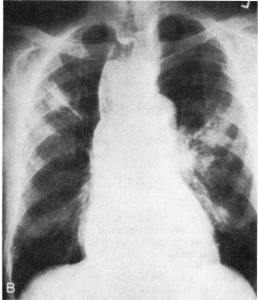

Figure 3–10. *A,* Diffuse pulmonary edema appearing after gastric aspiration, which occurred during obstetric anesthesia. Air bronchograms characteristic of any form of alveolar filling are clearly seen, especially in the upper lobes. *B,* Patchy fibrosis and pneumonia after aspiration in a patient with achalasia of the esophagus. The barium-filled esophagus is also visible. (From Stein JH [ed]: Internal Medicine. Boston: Little, Brown & Co, 1983.)

sputum as well as the patient's clinical course before choosing an antimicrobial regimen.

Prevention of aspiration is the best therapy. The perioperative period following general anesthesia or regional anesthesia accompanied by sedation is a high risk time for aspiration.

Pulmonary Thromboembolism

Pulmonary embolic disease is one of the major causes of death in the United States. Estimates have placed the death rate from pulmonary embolism at about 200,000 per year, with the majority of these deaths occurring without a premortem diagnosis of pulmonary embolism.

Pathogenesis. Pulmonary thromboembolism is the obstruction of elements of the pulmonary artery circulation by blood clots orginating at a site distant from the lung. The most common site of origin of these clots is the deep venous system of the lower extremities, although various other sites have been reported, in particular the great veins of the abdomen, the uterine and ovarian venous system, and the axillary veins of the upper extremities.

In addition to the death rate mentioned earlier, it is likely that there are many times that number of nonlethal and even subclinical episodes of pulmonary thromboembolism. The most common predisposing factor for the development of deep vein thrombosis large enough to cause hemodynamically significant pulmonary thromboembolism is immobilization (Table 3–13). Most commonly this immobilization is due to a medical or surgical illness, although sitting for long periods during travel has been implicated in the development of deep vein thrombosis. There are more rare causes of thrombosis, such as abnormalities of the coagulation or fibrinolytic cascades.

Once a clot has formed and propagated, the development of pulmonary signs and symptoms is a function of the patient's underlying pulmonary status and the percentage of the pulmonary vascular cross section that has been obstructed.

Clinical Presentation. The clinical manifestations can be quite protean in pulmonary embolic disease (Table 3–14). The classic picture of acute pulmonary embo-

Table 3–13. RISK FACTORS FOR VENOUS THROMBOSIS

Stasis: Congestive heart failure (CHF)
      Chronic venous insufficiency
Previous venous disease
Advanced age
Immobilization: Orthopedic
             Paralysis
             Bed rest
Surgery: Pelvic (gynecologic, urologic)
       Orthopedic (hip surgery, lower extremity)
Trauma: Lower extremity fractures
       Other lower extremity trauma
Obesity
Malignant disease
Sickle hemoglobin
Parturition (pregnancy)
Hormonal contraception (estrogen)

lism is described, followed by mention of the many exceptions.

The patient with pulmonary embolic disease may complain of sudden onset of dyspnea, pleuritic chest pain, and profound sense of apprehension. Hemoptysis and cough may be present. Examination of the patient reveals tachypnea, tachycardia, and increased pulmonary second heart sound. Arterial blood gas values show fairly marked hypoxemia accompanied by a respiratory alkalosis (decreased pCO_2, increased pH). The ECG may show signs of right-sided heart strain. The chest roentgenogram reveals pulmonary infiltrates, an elevated diaphragm, and a pleural effusion.

Unfortunately, it is rare that this picture emerges with the clarity of that just de-

Table 3–14. THROMBOEMBOLISM—SIGNS AND SYMPTOMS

	Per cent
PO₂	
<90 mmHg	95
<80 mmHg	80
ECG	
Nonspecific abnormality	65
Acute right ventricular strain	10
Dyspnea	81
Pleural pain	71
Apprehension	59
Cough	54
Hemoptysis	34
Sweats	26
Syncope	14

(Data from Luckmann J, Sorensen KC: Medical-Surgical Nursing: A Psychophysiological Approach, 2nd ed. Philadelphia: WB Saunders Co, 1980.)

scribed. The clinical setting proves most important. Another tenet of medicine is extremely important in the evaluation for pulmonary embolic disease: You must think of the diagnosis before you can make it.

Diagnosis. The diagnosis of pulmonary embolism depends on the clinical setting, the presentation as outlined previously, and the examination of the pulmonary vasculature with the pulmonary ventilation/perfusion scan, the pulmonary angiogram, or both. These latter two procedures have been discussed previously in this chapter.

An alternate approach to diagnosis can be undertaken in an individual in whom the lung scan is inconclusive but the pulmonary angiogram is contraindicated. This approach seeks documentation of deep venous disease of the lower extremities. There are several invasive and noninvasive methods for evaluation of the deep venous system, including contrast venograms, ^{125}I-labeled fibrinogen, and impedance plethysmography. The venogram is the most direct and accurate method of deep venous observation, but it carries the risk of postvenogram phlebitis. The other methods are more indirect and less accurate.

Treatment. The treatment of choice for pulmonary embolic disease is anticoagulation. Supportive therapy with supplemental oxygen and pressor agents may be required, but the prime goal is often the prevention of new clot formation during the time when the patient's own thrombolytic defenses are working to dissolve the obstructing clots. Therapy with intravenous heparin is the initial choice. Once the patient is stable (5 to 10 days) an oral warfarin compound is begun; this oral therapy is continued for 1 to 6 months.

In patients with dire hemodynamic compromise following massive pulmonary embolization, the administration of thrombolytic agents during the first 12 to 24 hours should be considered as an adjunct to heparin therapy. In life-threatening disease, surgical embolectomy should be considered as a last resort.

Patients with recurrent emboli from lower extremities who are not candidates for chronic anticoagulation are sometimes considered for surgical inferior vena cava interruption. This procedure is plagued by considerable surgical morbidity and even

if successful is often only a temporary solution. Large venous collaterals form quite quickly after an interruptive procedure.

The use of "mini-dose heparin" has been advocated as a prophylactic measure for patients at risk of deep vein thrombosis. This procedure involves the subcutaneous injection of small doses of heparin every 8 to 12 hours. The related literature contains conflicting reports regarding the efficacy of such treatment, but its safety has led to widespread acceptance. Lower extremity venous pumps and stockings, while a patient must remain immobile, are other safe and reportedly effective means of deep vein thrombosis prophylaxis.

The podiatric patient is at high risk for pulmonary thromboembolic disease. Often such a patient must remain in bed during the perioperative period. Surgical procedures to the lower extremities are considered by some to place any patient at risk of developing deep vein thrombosis. These high-risk individuals should be considered for prophylactic treatment with "mini-dose heparin" and/or mechanical lower extremity devices and should be evaluated frequently for signs and symptoms of both deep vein thrombosis and pulmonary embolism.

Fat Embolism

The fat emboli syndrome, seen in patients with fractures of the long bones, pelvis, or both, is a dramatic, severe systemic illness.

Pathogenesis. The pathogenesis of the fat emboli syndrome is not fully understood. It is known that fat escaping from the marrow of fractured bones embolizes to distant organs such as the lungs, and that this fat is then broken down to toxic free fatty acids, which can damage lung tissues as well as other tissues to which they are exposed. The aspect of this illness that has thus far escaped explanation is why only a subpopulation of individuals with long bone fractures and venous fat embolization develop the full syndrome.

Clinical Presentation. Individuals who develop the fat emboli syndrome begin to show signs about 24 to 48 hours following trauma to a long bone, the pelvis, or both. The syndrome begins with cough; shortness of breath; apprehension; confusion;

and development of a characteristic pete-chial rash, especially over the anterior chest. This progresses rapidly to severe hy-poxemia, altered mental status, and circu-latory collapse.

Diagnosis. The diagnosis is made on the basis of the clinical setting and the clin-ical course. The chest roentgenogram re-veals a diffuse consolidation throughout all lung fields. The laboratory picture is often consistent with that of diffuse intravascular coagulation.

Treatment. There is some evidence that the anti-inflammatory effects of corti-costeroids may be beneficial in patients who suffer from the fat emboli syndrome. Other than supportive measures, no defin-itive therapy is known for these individu-als. The prognosis is often grave.

During evaluation and care of patients with massive trauma, the fat emboli syn-drome is one of the sometimes unexpected causes of unexplained deterioration in those who appear to be doing well.

Pulmonary Neoplasms

The topic of pulmonary neoplasms is a broad one and is discussed in three parts: benign neoplasms, malignant neoplasms, and metastatic neoplasms.

Benign Neoplasms. Benign neoplasms include hamartomas, fibromas, heman-giomas, lipomas, papillomas, bronchial ad-enomas, and leiomyomas. These tumors, although benign to the extent that they do not cause metastatic disease, can cause morbidity and sometimes death. The mechanisms that account for this morbidity include airway obstruction that can result in pneumonia or suffocation, hemoptysis that can be severe, or transformation that can result in malignant tumors. Those le-sions that have the potential to transform into malignancy include fibroma and leio-myoma.

Malignant Neoplasms. Malignant neo-plasms of the lungs are classified according to the suspected cell of origin and include epidermoid carcinomas (squamous cell carcinomas), small-cell undifferentiated carcinomas (oat-cell carcinomas), large-cell undifferentiated carcinomas, adeno-carcinomas, carcinoid tumors, sarcomas, mesotheliomas, and melanomas. These le-sions result in morbidity and mortality be-cause of their rapid growth, spread to other organs, or compromise of pulmonary func-tion.

Metastatic Neoplasms. Metastatic ma-lignancies, those tumors that arrive in the lung by spread from a site outside the lung, can pose significant diagnostic dilemmas if the primary tumor site is unknown. Meta-static disease to the lungs can be multiple or diffuse. It can arrive at the lungs via the blood vessels, the lymphatics, or the air-ways. Tumors distant from the lungs can result in morbidity and mortality because of metastatic lung disease.

Pathogenesis. The evolution (or de-ev-olution) of normal cells into cancer cells is the topic of intense investigation. Among the primary bronchogenic carcinomas, ap-proximately 80% are attributable to the in-halation of cigarette smoke. The combi-nation of cigarette smoke and asbestos exposure is an extremely potent pulmo-nary carcinogen. Asbestos exposure is uni-versally seen in patients with mesothe-lioma. Although the specific molecular mechanisms of the transformation of nor-mal cells into cancer is not fully under-stood, the result is that cells that were pre-viously normal in appearance, function, and growth acquire defects in the control of these characteristics and proliferate, change their morphology, and sometimes develop aberrant control of their metabo-lism such that they secrete agents that can have systemic effects.

Clinical Presentation. Most commonly the diagnosis of pulmonary neoplasm is made in an asymptomatic individual on the basis of a routine chest roentgenogram. When symptoms are present, they can in-clude hemoptysis, weight loss, cough, re-current pneumonia, and pain. There can be pleural involvement or involvement of the vessels or nerves of the chest. Hor-monal imbalances can be characteristic of certain tumors.

The chest roentgenogram can reveal a single mass, or a tumor may appear with more unusual findings, such as signs of a pneumonia, cavitary lesion, diffuse in-volvement, or multiple masses. Occasion-ally the chest roentgenogram may be en-tirely normal.

Diagnosis. The diagnosis of neoplasm relies entirely on pathologic identification of the tumor cells. A cytologic evaluation of expectorated cells can be performed, or the cells can be obtained by any number of biopsy techniques that range from bronchoscopic to open surgical procedures.

Treatment. Treatment of a pulmonary neoplasm depends entirely on the type of tumor identified. Benign lesions as well as certain malignant tumors require simple resection. In the case of malignant tumors, resection may be accompanied by radiation therapy, chemotherapy, or immunotherapy or some combination of these. Certain malignant tumors of the lung such as the undifferentiated carcinoma are treated with one or more of these modalities in the absence of resection. It is extremely rare to treat metastactic lesions in the lung except by the systemic management of the primary tumor. Several tumors have no effective therapy at this time, notably mesotheliomas.

Tumors of the lower extremities, especially osteogenic tumors, can metastasize to lung. Routine preoperative pulmonary evaluation may detect unsuspected lung neoplasms.

Pulmonary Infections

Pulmonary infections fall into many categories, depending on the causative organism and the patient's response to that organism. Infections can be caused by viruses, bacteria, *Chlamydia*, *Rickettsia*, *Mycoplasma*, mycobacteria, fungi, and parasites. The emergence of the acquired immunodeficiency syndrome (AIDS) has brought many previously rare agents to the fore.

The lung, if it is able, responds to all infectious agents with manifestations of the acute and chronic inflammatory response, which includes activation of complement, influx of inflammatory cells, and generation of various locally acting and systemic agents. The organism responsible for the infection may succumb to these defenses or may overwhelm them, leading to worsening infection of the lungs, and eventually may spread to other parts of the body.

Pathogenesis. All the aforementioned organisms use the lungs as a breeding ground. Some organisms live quite comfortably in the pulmonary tree without ill effects, but when an organism increases in number or when an organism with more damaging effects becomes established, the body's response is pneumonia. Access to the lungs can be obtained from either the airways or the blood supply. The result can be overwhelming infection or localization of the process as occurs in lung abscess or cavity formation.

Viruses, *Chlamydia*, *Rickettsia*, and *Mycoplasma* are rarely, if ever, free-growing organisms and require living cells as their life support. Mycobacteria, a group of organisms that includes the agent responsible for tuberculosis can cause gradually progressive disease. Bacterial infections can be fulminant or indolent, life-threatening or a mere nuisance. The fungi and parasitic agents often are found in patients with an underlying disease condition such as diabetes mellitus or AIDS. However, there are vast areas of the United States in which *Histoplasma* and *Coccidioides*, two common fungi that cause histoplasmosis and coccidioidomycosis, respectively, are endemic.

Clinical Presentation. The patient with a pulmonary infection often has the systemic symptoms and signs that accompany inflammation, release of toxins by the infecting organism, or both. Fever is often present, and the patient feels generally ill. Specifics depend on the etiologic organism. The classic case of pneumococcal pneumonia is a patient who presents with cough, sputum production, high fevers, shaking chills, and pleuritic chest pain. Tuberculosis, in contrast, presents with an indolent course with chronic weight loss, low-grade fevers, night sweats, and sputum.

Diagnosis. The diagnosis of pulmonary infection relies on the history, physical signs, and the setting. A history consistent with pulmonary infection may be present. Travel history can be important. A patient who has recently traveled in the Ohio River valley causes one to consider histoplasmosis, and California's central valley is the endemic area for coccidioidomycosis. Several of the parasitic organisms that can infect lungs have suggestive geographic distributions.

Infections of the lung that result in pneumonia produce physical findings of consolidation, including bronchial breath sounds transmitted to the lung periphery and crackles.

The chest roentgenogram is often quite suggestive of the agent involved. Consolidation suggests bacteria, viruses, and other of the more rapidly damaging organisms. Cavitary disease and disease of the apices of the lungs suggest pulmonary tuberculosis (Fig. 3–11). A diffuse, vague pattern is often seen in early *Pneumocystis carinii* infection. However, none of these patterns is exclusive to the diseases mentioned.

The final diagnosis of pulmonary infections depends on the isolation and identification of the organism itself. A sputum Gram's stain examination may be sufficient, in the proper clinical setting, to make

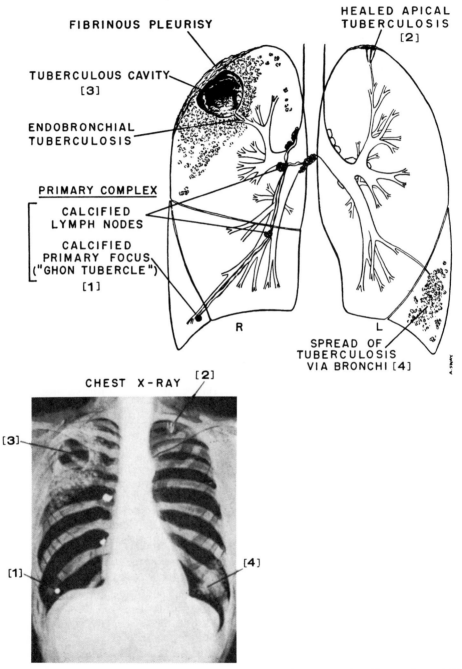

Figure 3–11. Chronic pulmonary tuberculosis. The drawing identifies lesions (correlated by numbers) visible on the radiograph below. (From Introduction to Respiratory Diseases, 4th ed. Copyright American Lung Association. Reprinted with permission of American Lung Association.)

the diagnosis. More often, the organism must be isolated, usually by culturing the infective agent, before identification can be made. In the case of slow-growing organisms such as *Mycobacterium tuberculosis*, this culturing can take several weeks. Fortunately, there are special stains, some employing specific antibody/antigen detection techniques, that have made the identification of such organisms as *Pneumocystis carinii*, mycobacteria, and fungi more rapid. In certain infections, a tissue specimen must be obtained before identification of the infecting organism can be made.

Treatment. The treatment of pulmonary infections is wholly dependent on the causative organism. Most viral infections have no specific treatment, although prevention by immunization and certain drugs with antiviral potential is effective. Bacterial infections are treated with antibiotics. The emergence of bacterial strains resistant to many antibiotics has led to a proliferation of these drugs. Sensitivity testing, to determine the best agent in a given infection, is routine. The treatment of mycobacterial diseases is plagued by the emergence of resistant organisms as well. Routine pulmonary tuberculosis should be treated with at least two drugs to which the organism is known to be sensitive. Atypical tuberculosis, caused by mycobacteria other than *M. tuberculosis,* and drug-resistant tuberculosis are often treated with six or more drugs.

Pulmonary infections are the most common cause of postoperative morbidity. Sepsis of the joints in the foot may have had their source in the lung.

Interstitial Lung Disease

The interstitial lung diseases (ILD) are characterized by diffuse inflammation, fibrosis of the pulmonary interstitium, or both. Many of these diseases have no known etiologic agent. Even when the trigger is known, the biochemical mechanisms leading to the processes of inflammation and fibrosis are not understood. These diseases usually lead to a restrictive pulmonary physiology with decreased lung volumes and decreased pulmonary compliance (small, stiff lungs). For many of

these diseases, treatment is palliative or nonexistent.

The diseases that fall into the ILD category include idiopathic pulmonary fibrosis, the collagen vascular diseases, lymphoid interstitial pneumonia, sarcoidosis, and certain occupational lung diseases. This list is more inclusive than most but leaves out some of the rarer interstitial processes, such as lymphangiomyomatosis, which are more appropriate for a pulmonary text. The nomenclature of ILD is currently in a state of flux. Idiopathic pulmonary fibrosis has been named usual interstitial pneumonitis by some workers, whereas others prefer chronic fibrosing alveolitis. Until there is some mutually agreed upon nomenclature, these diseases will remain obscure both in name and pathogenesis.

Pathogenesis. The pathogenesis of many of these diseases is not known. In certain occupationally related forms of ILD, the inciting agent, such as beryllium, is known. This information has not yet led to an understanding of the cellular mechanisms that connect an exposure to beryllium with the development of pulmonary granulomas.

Many of these diseases lead to pulmonary inflammation. This inflammation can be acute (neutrophil infiltration), chronic (predominance of lymphocytes, monocytes, and macrophages), or granulomatous (chronic inflammation with characteristic architecture, giant cells, or necrosis, or caseation or their combination). An additional sequela is often fibrosis, although there are those workers who dispute whether inflammation necessarily precedes fibrosis.

Clinical Presentation. Patients suffering from ILD often complain of dyspnea on exertion. Asymptomatic patients may be discovered on routine chest roentgenograms. There may be nondescript chest discomfort.

Progression of symptoms is almost universal; however, the rate of progression varies widely. The disease can be fulminant, as in the Hamman-Rich syndrome, or the disease can progress slowly over many years.

Diagnosis. The diagnosis of ILD depends on the symptom complex, the proper setting in the case of occupational and environmental causes, the chest roentgeno-gram revealing a diffuse interstitial increase in density, the pulmonary function testing showing a restrictive defect and a diminished diffusing capacity, and the tissue biopsy findings. The most reliable method of obtaining a tissue diagnosis is the open lung biopsy. In many cases a fiberoptic bronchoscopic transbronchial lung biopsy is sufficient, especially when the pathology is unique, such as sarcoidosis. Asbestosis can often be diagnosed in the absence of a tissue specimen if the history of a significant asbestos exposure is obtained and if an interstitial pattern on chest roentgenogram combined with the pleural or diaphragmatic plaques is obtained that is characteristic of this process.

Treatment. Interstitial lung diseases have been treated with corticosteroids or a combination of corticosteroids and immunosuppressive agents. The use of these agents is largely empiric; they work in some patients but not in others with similar pathology. Corticosteroids are often extremely effective in sarcoidosis, but often sarcoidosis will regress spontaneously without any treatment. It appears unlikely that pulmonary fibrosis itself will respond to any current therapy, but those processes that include an inflammatory reaction have the potential to respond to these medica-tions. The use of supplemental oxygen is indicated when the ILD has progressed to the point where hemoglobin desaturation has occurred.

As with other chronic lung diseases that impair oxygenation, individuals with ILD are at increased operative risk.

Adult Respiratory Distress Syndrome

The adult respiratory distress syndrome (ARDS) is presented as a paradigm of acute respiratory failure. Adult respiratory distress syndrome is a catchall term used to describe the end result of any of a number of pulmonary insults (Table 3–15). This end result is the development of generalized, noncardiogenic pulmonary edema. This leads to profound hypoxemia, tremendous loss of pulmonary compliance, and ventilatory failure. Adult respiratory distress syndrome carries a mortality rate of approximately 70%, and this rate has changed little since it was first described in 1971.

Pathogenesis. The alveolar air spaces are protected from the influx of fluid from blood and the surrounding tissues by the tightly arranged lining cells of the capillaries and the alveolar epithelium. The in-

Table 3–15. DISORDERS ASSOCIATED WITH ADULT RESPIRATORY DISTRESS SYNDROME

Shock of any cause	*Inhaled toxins*
Infection	Oxygen
Gram-negative sepsis	Smoke
Pneumonia	Corrosive chemicals
Viral	Nitrous oxide, chlorine, ammonia,
Bacterial	phosgene, cadmium
Fungal (rare)	*Hematologic disorders*
Pneumocystis carinii (rare)	Intravascular coagulation
Trauma	Massive blood transfusion
Fat emboli	Postcardiopulmonary bypass (?)
Lung contusion	*Metabolic and toxic disorders*
Nonthoracic trauma	Pancreatitis
Head injury	Uremia
Liquid aspiration	Paraquat ingestion
Gastric juice	*Miscellaneous*
Fresh or salt water	Lymphangitic carcinomatosis
Hydrocarbon fluids	Increased intracranial pressure
Drug overdose	Eclampsia
Heroin	Postcardioversion
Methadone	Radiation pneumonitis
Propoxyphene (Darvon)	
Barbiturates	

(From Brown M, Andrews JL, Jr: How to manage adult respiratory distress syndrome. Geriatrics 34:39, 1979.)

flux of protein-rich fluid during the development of ARDS, often in the absence of any increase in pulmonary vascular pressure, has been shown to represent the breakdown of these barriers to fluid movement. This breakdown appears to be the result of direct injury to the cells that constitute these barriers.

There are many underlying abnormalities that can lead to the development of ARDS. The classic examples include sepsis, massive trauma, hemorrhagic shock, pancreatitis, gastric aspiration, drug reactions, viral pneumonias, oxygen toxicity, disseminated intravascular coagulation, and cardiopulmonary bypass. That all of these processes should lead to a final common pathway of lung cell injury would seem surprising. Although all the biochemical events leading to the picture of ARDS are not yet known, animal models have provided some insight into this enigma.

Currently there is evidence that two classes of injurious agents play a cooperative role in provoking the barrier derangement characteristic of ARDS. These are oxidants and proteases. Either alone is capable of mimicking the damage seen in ARDS when given in large doses, but given together, minute quantities of each are able to produce tremendous fluid movement into the alveoli. The proteases and oxidants studied are products derived from the human polymorphonuclear leukocyte, and this is consistent with the observation that virtually all the predisposing conditions that are known to lead to ARDS can result in polymorphonuclear leukocyte sequestration and activation in the lungs.

Adult respiratory distress syndrome usually develops in the absence of underlying lung disease. Individuals with an identical clinical course of underlying systemic disease may diverge for no obvious reason as one develops ARDS while the other recovers. Although predisposing risk factors can be identified and a primitive understanding of cellular events leading to ARDS exists, there is currently no way of making a prospective judgment as to the likelihood of a given patient developing the syndrome.

Clinical Presentation. Adult respiratory distress syndrome usually appears hours to days after a predisposing insult (Table 3–16). Initially the patient develops

Table 3–16. ADULT RESPIRATORY DISTRESS SYNDROME

Stages of ARDS
Stage 1
Interstitial pulmonary edema
Pulmonary capillary congestion
Electron microscopy findings:
widening of junction of endothelial cells and swelling of endothelial cells
Stage 2
Intra-alveolar pulmonary edema
Eosinophilic proteinaceous fluid in alveoli
Stage 3
Cellular response
Hyaline membrane formation
Type II pneumocyte hyperplasia
Capillary endothelial regeneration
Fibrogenesis, then fibrosis

(From Brown M, Andrews JL, Jr: How to manage adult respiratory distress syndrome. Geriatrics 34:39, 1979.)

dyspnea, anxiety, and hypoxemia with little if any changes on the chest roentgenogram. Over the next 12 to 48 hours, the roentgenogram begins to evolve, first showing patchy areas of consolidation that eventually coalesce into massive air-space consolidation in all lung fields. The hypoxemia worsens during this time, and if the patient is not given mechanical ventilatory support, profound respiratory acidosis ensues.

The patient almost always requires endotracheal intubation and mechanical ventilatory support. High inspired-oxygen concentrations are required to maintain adequate tissue oxygenation, and frequently positive end-expiratory pressures (PEEP) are required as well.

Diagnosis. The clinical setting and course determine the diagnosis of ARDS. A predisposing, usually systemic disease is invariably present. The clinical presentation previously outlined should be seen. It is important to rule out other causes of pulmonary edema. Cardiogenic pulmonary edema due to congestive heart failure, fluid overload, or both can appear in a similar fashion, although the heart size is usually enlarged and left atrial pressures, as assessed by pulmonary capillary wedge pressure measurement, are elevated when a primarily cardiac etiology exists. Massive pulmonary thromboembolic disease can present with a clinical course similar to ARDS, although elevated pulmonary artery pressures, profound shock, and ab-

Table 3–17. THERAPEUTIC MODALITIES FOR ADULT RESPIRATORY DISTRESS SYNDROME

Oxygen (controlled dose)
Mechanical ventilation with positive end-expiratory pressure (PEEP)
Fluid restriction
Diuretics
Cardiotonic/vasopressor agents
Hypothermia
Antibiotics
Steroids (?)
Heparin (?)
Extracorporeal membrane oxygenation (?)

(Adapted from Brown M, Andrews JL, Jr: How to manage adult respiratory distress syndrome. Geriatrics 34:39, 1979.)

normal pulmonary angiogram findings confirm emboli as the cause.

If a pulmonary artery pressure catheter is placed during the development of ARDS, one should note normal or low pulmonary capillary wedge pressures and normal pulmonary artery pressures. The chest roentgenogram should reveal a normal heart size.

Treatment. The treatment of ARDS is supportive (Table 3–17). Maintenance of adequate oxygenation, support of vascular pressures without raising the left atrial pressure to a level that might cause greater fluid movement into the lungs, and maintenance of appropriate acid-base status are paramount. Corticosteroids and lately certain prostaglandins have been advocated, but neither has shown any objective benefit.

A major goal of any treatment regimen for ARDS, or for any disease that requires prolonged intubation and mechanical ventilation, is the prevention of complications of therapy and the prompt identification and resolution of such complications should they occur. These complications include superinfection of the lungs with a hospital-acquired organism; sepsis; pneumothorax/pneumomediastinum; trauma to the trachea and vocal cords; occult bacterial otitis, sinusitis, or both; aspiration; and pulmonary thromboembolic disease. Surveillance is the key to rapid identification and treatment of such common complications.

The surgical patient often falls into one of the groups at risk for this rare complication of systemic processes. Recognition of the early stages of acute respiratory failure can improve chances of survival.

References

Brown M, Andrews JL, Jr: How to Manage Adult Respiratory Distress Syndrome. Geriatrics 34:39, 1979.

Fontana RS, Sanderson DR, Taylor WF, et al.: Early lung cancer detection. Am Rev Respir Dis 130:561, 1984.

Fraser RG, Paré JAP: Diagnosis of Disease of the Chest, 2nd ed, Vol II. Philadelphia: WB Saunders Co, 1978.

Goldmann DR, et al. (eds): Medical Care of the Surgical Patient: A Problem-Oriented Approach to Management. Philadelphia: JB Lippincott Co, 1982.

Hurst JW (ed): Medicine for the Practicing Physician. Boston: Butterworth Publishers, 1983.

Molitch ME: Management of Medical Problems in the Surgical Patient. Philadelphia: FA Davis Co, 1982.

Raffin TA: Indications for aterial blood gas analysis. Ann Intern Med 105:390, 1986.

Rubenstein E, Federman DD (eds): Scientific American Medicine. New York: Scientific American, Inc, 1987.

Stulberg M: Evaluating and treating intractable cough. West J Med 143:223, 1985.

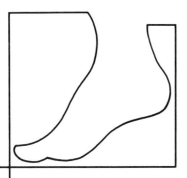

4 RHEUMATOLOGY

JAMES A. DAVIS

OVERVIEW

There is no other medical specialty that interfaces as closely with podiatry as rheumatology. Many areas of podiatric medicine and biomechanics are intimate parts of clinical rheumatology. Crystal and septic arthritides are seen quite frequently in busy podiatric practices. Podiatric clinics in large university centers see many patients with pedal manifestations of systemic diseases such as rheumatoid arthritis, Reiter's syndrome, and systemic lupus erythematosus (SLE). The podiatric physician must have a thorough clinical understanding of rheumatologic disease.

PATHOPHYSIOLOGY

Arthritis is defined as a swelling of one or more joints. In order to determine whether someone is indeed suffering from arthritis, the normal anatomy of a joint must be understood (Fig. 4–1). In a normal synovial joint, the periarticular bone is abutted by hyaline articular cartilage. Inserting into the periarticular bone adjacent to the hyaline cartilage is a synovial lining membrane. Over this is the joint capsule; inserting into the joint capsule are tendons, and adjacent to this is the periosteum.

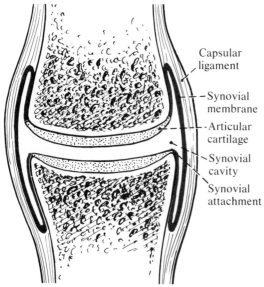

Figure 4–1. Schematic diagram of a diathrodial joint. (From Polley HF, Hunder GG: Rheumatologic Interviewing and Physical Examination of the Joints. Philadelphia, WB Saunders Co, 1978.)

Capsular ligament

Synovial membrane

Articular cartilage

Synovial cavity

Synovial attachment

Each of these is the target of specific arthritic syndromes. For example, the articular cartilage is the primary target of degenerative arthritis, the synovium the primary target of rheumatoid arthritis, the tendinous insertions the primary target of the seronegative spondyloarthropathies, and the bursae the primary target of bursitis.

PRESENTING FEATURES

The history and physical examination enable the clinician to determine whether the patient is suffering from arthritis as opposed to another condition that may cause pain in an extremity or around a joint, such as peripheral neuritis or peripheral vascular disease. Once it is decided a patient has arthritis, it is important to determine whether one is dealing with inflammatory arthritis, degenerative arthritis, or periarticular disease such as tendonitis or bursitis. The patient's signs, symptoms, and distribution of arthritis enable one to make this differentiation. The subjective symptoms and objective signs of arthritis are explored subsequently.

Subjective Symptoms

Pain and Stiffness

The pain associated with degenerative arthritis is predominantly present during use and absent during rest. This is in contrast to pain in conjunction with inflammatory arthritis, which occurs predominantly at rest and seems to improve as the joint is used. Degenerative arthritis is associated with minimal morning stiffness, typically lasting less than half an hour. In contrast, patients with inflammatory arthritis have several hours of morning stiffness. They also experience a "gel" phenomenon after sitting for prolonged periods of time; that is, the joint stiffens up after prolonged sitting.

Onset

The type of onset of the various arthropathies also helps one to differentiate between them. The degenerative arthropathies generally have an insidious onset over several weeks to months. The onset of the inflammatory arthropathies is quite variable. Rheumatoid arthritis, systemic lupus erythematosus (SLE), and the seronegative spondyloarthropathies generally have an insidious onset over several days to weeks. However, these disorders can also have acute presentations. Gout classically has an acute presentation, frequently having its onset in the late evening or awakening the patient in the morning. Whenever one encounters an acute onset of arthropathy, especially if it involves only one joint, septic arthritis must be considered.

Systemic Features

Degenerative arthritis is not associated with systemic symptomatology. Inflammatory arthropathies are often associated with systemic illness because of the inflammation seen in conjunction with these diseases. Often these patients experience malaise, fever, weight loss, and anorexia. The type of systemic symptoms seen in conjunction with arthritis is helpful in differentiating between the various types of arthropathies. For example, patients with SLE, in addition to suffering from arthritis, frequently also experience fever, marked malaise, alopecia, an erythematous rash on the face, and symptoms suggestive of renal or cardiorespiratory disease. The arthritis of rheumatoid arthritis in the early stages is identical to that of SLE. However, the patient with rheumatoid arthritis frequently experiences malaise but not the other systemic symptoms seen in SLE. These features can help to differentiate between these two arthropathies.

Loss of Function

Both inflammatory and noninflammatory arthropathies lead to loss of function. The loss of function in both emanates from pain. With time, both degenerative and inflammatory arthritis lead to destruction of the joint with deformity, loss of range of motion, and as a result loss of function.

Objective Signs

Swelling, Heat, and Redness

As previously defined, arthritis is swelling of a joint. Both inflammatory and non-inflammatory arthritis result in joint swelling. In both conditions, this can result from soft tissue swelling and the accumulation of fluid within the joint. However, in degenerative arthritis, there can also be a bony swelling as a result of osteophyte formation.

Degenerative arthritis is not associated with heat or redness of the joint because it is a noninflammatory arthritis. Occasionally, there can be a mild inflammatory component to osteoarthritis, which can result in some heat and redness, usually seen in the small joints of the hand. In contrast, the inflammatory arthropathies can be associated with heat and redness. The extent of this heat and redness can often aid the clinician in differentiating between various types of inflammatory arthritis. For example, rheumatoid arthritis is associated with heat and occasionally redness localized to the joint itself. The heat, redness, and swelling frequently correspond to the extent of subjective symptoms the patient is experiencing. In contrast, patients with inflammatory arthritis of SLE usually have less heat, redness, and swelling than those with rheumatoid arthritis. The heat, redness, and swelling are frequently much less than one would anticipate from the severity of the patient's subjective complaints. Also, distribution of the heat and swelling can aid one in differentiating between the various types of inflammatory arthritis. The heat, swelling, and tenderness of the seronegative spondyloarthropathies are localized both to the joint and to the tendinous insertions around the joint. Thus in this disease, one sees not only arthritis but often a diffusely swollen digit (sausage digit), which results from this tendinous inflammation. The heat, redness, and swelling of gout often involves both the joint and the soft tissue around the joint, appearing somewhat like cellulitis. This feature would not be seen in rheumatoid arthritis or SLE.

Joints of the Foot and Arthritis

Distribution of arthritis is paramount in determining the type. An examination of each of the joints of the foot shows how the various arthritides involve them.

Metatarsophalangeal Joints. Diffuse swelling of a toe is pathognomonic of the seronegative spondyloarthropathies, most commonly psoriatic arthritis and Reiter's syndrome. When this is seen, it is called a sausage digit. The metatarsophalangeal joints can be quickly screened on physical examination by squeezing all of the joints between the thumb and index finger. If pain is elicited, each of the joints should be examined independently. This can be done by pressing the metatarsophalangeal joint between the thumb and forefinger while moving the toe. Swelling and bony deformity can also be appreciated. The first metatarsophalangeal joint is the major target of osteoarthritis because it is the major weight-bearing surface in the foot. It is also the major target of gout. Diffuse involvement of the metatarsophalangeal joints occurs in conjunction with rheumatoid arthritis. Radiographically, rheumatoid arthritis commonly involves the fifth metatarsophalangeal joint prior to involving the others. The seronegative spondyloarthropathies can also involve the metatarsophalangeal joints but more commonly involve the other joints of the foot and toes.

Ankle Joint. The true ankle joint is landmarked by both of the malleoli and is responsible for flexion and extension of the foot. Involvement of the ankle is not seen in conjunction with osteoarthritis unless there is an unusual mechanical stress on the ankle. This might result from previous trauma to the leg causing abnormal stresses across the joint or from an unusual occupational stress to the ankle, for example, in ballet dancers. Swelling of the ankle can be observed in conjunction with all the inflammatory arthropathies. However, when in conjunction with rheumatoid arthritis, SLE, or a seronegative spondyloarthropathy, usually other joints are involved in addition to the ankle. Monoarticular involvement of the ankle suggests a septic process or gout.

Talonavicular Joint. The talonavicular joint or midfoot is responsible for rotation of the foot and is examined by using one hand to support the ankle and subtalar joint while rotating the foot with the other hand. This joint can be involved in osteoarthritis. However, if one sees marked degenerative changes in the talonavicular joint, one should consider a Charcot or neuropathic joint. This would occur in the clinical setting of a peripheral neuropathy, most commonly in conjunction with diabetes mellitus. The talonavicular joint is also involved with rheumatoid arthritis, but less commonly with the seronegative spondyloarthropathies. Soft tissue swelling of the midfoot is the second most common target for acute gout.

Subtalar Joint. The subtalar joint is halfway between the calcaneus and medial malleolus and is responsible for inversion of the foot. This joint is examined by supporting the ankle with one hand and inverting the calcaneus with the other hand. The subtalar joint is rarely involved in degenerative arthritis, but it can be seen in conjunction with all the inflammatory arthritides. It would be unusual for this joint to be involved in an isolated fashion, and if tenderness is elicited one should rule out a fracture of the calcaneus.

Achilles Tendon. The Achilles tendon is best examined by palpating the insertion of the tendon into the calcaneus. It is best visualized with the patient in the kneeling position and the clinician looking down onto the Achilles tendon. By doing this, subtle swelling can be appreciated. Achilles tendonitis is not found in conjunction with osteoarthritis. All the inflammatory arthropathies can involve this tendon. However, isolated Achilles tendonitis is seen most commonly in conjunction with the seronegative spondyloarthropathies, especially Reiter's syndrome and psoriatic arthritis. When one treats an acute Achilles tendonitis in conjunction with one or two other swollen joints, especially in a younger, sexually active individual, the diagnosis of disseminated gonococcal arthritis must be considered. It is frequently very difficult to differentiate gonococcal arthritis from a seronegative spondyloarthropathy. Achilles tendonitis can be associated with rheumatoid arthritis but is always associated with other joint involvement.

Plantar Fascia. Plantar fasciitis is best appreciated by palpating the insertion of the plantar fascia into the calcaneus on the sole of the foot. Plantar fasciitis is seen most commonly in conjunction with a mechanical spur. It can also be a target of the inflammatory arthropathies in a fashion similar to that discussed under Achilles tendonitis.

Laboratory Evaluation

After the clinician has obtained a history and has examined the patient, laboratory studies help to corroborate impressions about the arthritis. Laboratory tests are not helpful without clinical correlation and can often be misleading, as no laboratory test is diagnostic of a clinical disease. This point cannot be overemphasized.

Laboratory tests can be useful both in diagnosing a specific rheumatic disease and in monitoring the activity of the patient's rheumatic disease. Laboratory tests can be viewed in three categories: nonspecific indicators of inflammation, specific indicators of rheumatic disease, and synovial fluid analysis.

Nonspecific Indicators of Inflammation

The tests that are nonspecific measures of inflammation include the erythrocyte sedimentation rate (ESR) and a complete blood count (CBC).

Erythrocyte Sedimentation Rate. ESR is one of the best measures of inflammation available. It is a simple test and relatively inexpensive. In degenerative arthritis, this test is normal because there is no inflammation present. In the inflammatory arthropathies—rheumatoid arthritis, SLE, the seronegative spondyloarthropathies, and gout—the ESR is elevated. This test can also be useful in the monitoring of these diseases, as with adequate control of these diseases, the ESR normalizes.

Complete Blood Count. The CBC is also a nonspecific indicator of inflammation. In rheumatoid arthritis, the seronegative spondyloarthropathies, and gout, the white blood cell count is frequently elevated. In SLE, because of antibodies against lymphocytes, often in the presence of a markedly elevated ESR, one sees a lowered white blood cell count. The hematocrit and hemoglobin are also indicators of inflammation. Chronic inflammation usually causes the hematocrit and hemoglobin to decline. If the hemoglobin is less than 10 g or the hematocrit is less than 30, one must consider another source for the anemia in addition to the chronic inflammatory arthropathy. This source may include hemolytic anemia, especially if one is dealing with SLE, or anemia of

iron deficiency, which might occur secondary to gastrointestinal blood loss, especially if the arthritis is being treated with a nonsteroidal anti-inflammatory drug (NSAID).

Specific Indicators of Rheumatic Disease

The blood tests used to identify specific rheumatic diseases include uric acid; rheumatoid factor; antinuclear antibody (ANA); anti-DNA antibody; complement studies including C_3, C_4, and total hemolytic complement (CH_{50}); and HLA-B27.

Uric Acid. The uric acid level is an important test if one suspects gout. However, a normal uric acid level does not exclude the diagnosis of gout, just as an elevated uric acid level does not establish the diagnosis.

Rheumatoid Factor. If one suspects rheumatoid arthritis, a rheumatoid factor should be obtained. This is a measure of IgM antibody directed against IgG immunoglobulin. The most common laboratory tests used to measure IgM rheumatoid factor are the latex agglutination test, in which human IgG is attached to a latex particle, and the sheep cell agglutination test, in which rabbit IgG is attached to sheep red blood cells. In both, if the patient's serum contains IgM rheumatoid factor, there is agglutination of the latex particles or the sheep red blood cells on the slide. The rheumatoid factor test is not specific for rheumatoid arthritis. The result is positive in approximately 80% of patients with rheumatoid arthritis but is negative in a significant percentage of patients with early rheumatoid arthritis. In addition, rheumatoid factor is present in a number of other conditions, such as any chronic infection, especially subacute bacterial endocarditis, and certain cancers, especially multiple myelomas. Rheumatoid factor is also present in 25% of patients over the age of 55 who never develop rheumatoid arthritis.

Antinuclear Antibody. If one suspects the diagnosis of SLE, an ANA can be obtained. In this test, the patient's serum is exposed to a source of nuclei. If the patient's serum contains antibodies to these nuclei, the antibodies attach to the nuclei. The antibodies are then stained with a fluorescent dye and examined under a fluorescent microscope. If the patient's serum contains antibodies to these nuclei, the antibodies are then visualized under the fluorescent microscope. The ANA is positive in 98% of patients with SLE. The ANA is also positive in a number of other rheumatic diseases, including scleroderma. Sjögren's syndrome, and 10% of rheumatoid arthritis cases.

Anti-DNA Antibody and Complement Studies. If the ANA is positive, to further assess the patient's SLE or related disease, an antibody against native DNA can be requested as well as a C_3, C_4, and total hemolytic complement, to assess the activation of the complement cascade. Antibody to DNA antibody and activation of the complement cascade are frequent in active severe SLE, especially with renal involvement.

HLA-B27. The HLA-B27 is a measure of one of the specific determinants in the human leukocyte antigen system. Although the test results are positive in most patients with ankylosing spondylitis and Reiter's syndrome, it is a test that is rarely indicated. See Reiter's Syndrome for further discussion.

Synovial Fluid Analysis

The examination of the synovial fluid can be extremely helpful. This is especially important if one is dealing with an arthritis of unknown etiology. The synovial fluid analysis is mandatory if one is dealing with a monoarticular arthritis, in which case a septic joint is possible. The only contraindication to arthrocentesis is cellulitis. One should not enter the joint through a cellulitis because the infection could be introduced into the joint. A joint should always be aspirated using sterile technique with topical anesthesia in the form of either lidocaine (Xylocaine) or local freezing.

The ankle is the most common joint that requires arthrocentesis in the foot. The ankle should be at a 90°-angle, and an 18- to 20-gauge needle should be used. The ankle should be entered just medial to the tibialis anterior tendon and lateral to the medial malleolus. The other joints of the foot are more difficult to aspirate. The subtalar joint can be aspirated by entering just inferior to the tip of the lateral malleolus.

The talonavicular joint is extremely difficult to aspirate without radiologic assistance. The first metatarsophalangeal joint is aspirated posteriorly by palpating the joint space with the toe flexed and entering directly into the joint.

Even if a very small amount of fluid is removed, it can be examined microscopically and should not be discarded. Analyzing the synovial fluid can give one an accurate determination of the type of arthritis (Table 4–1). In addition to looking at the joint fluid grossly, the fluid should be sent to the laboratory for a cell count, microscopic evaluation for crystals, Gram's stain, and culture. A protein determination can also be helpful but generally correlates with the cell count. Early in rheumatoid arthritis, a rheumatoid factor can be positive prior to the serum being positive, so this can be a helpful test. The glucose and lactic acid tests add little besides cost to these determinations.

Types of Synovial Fluid. As shown in Table 4–1, synovial fluid can be broken down into three types or classes. Class I, or noninflammatory joint fluid, is seen with osteoarthritis, traumatic arthritis, and SLE. Class II joint fluid is observed in the inflammatory arthropathies, including rheumatoid arthritis, the seronegative spondyloarthropathies, and the crystal-induced arthritides gout and tuberculosis. A class III joint fluid occurs in conjunction with an acute septic arthritis. Exceptions to this are gonococcal arthritis and tuberculous arthritis. Gonococcal arthritis can result in a class I, class II, or class III fluid, and tuberculous arthritis generally results in a class II joint fluid.

Gross Appearance. On gross appearance, class I joint fluid is clear or bloody if one is dealing with a traumatic arthritis. Class II joint fluid is cloudy, but light can still be transmitted through it. Class III joint fluid is very cloudy, and no light can be transmitted through it.

The mucin clot test and string sign are measures of the viscosity of the joint fluid. Normal joint fluid, when dropped into 1% acetic acid, holds together like oil dropped into water. This represents a good mucin clot. Normal knee or ankle joint fluid can be stretched between 1 and 2 cm between the thumb and first finger before it breaks, which is the string sign. In class II and class III joint fluid, the inflammation

Table 4–1. CLASSIFICATION OF SYNOVIAL EFFUSIONS

Gross Examination	Normal	Noninflammatory (Class 1)	Inflammatory (Class II)	Septic (Class III)
Volume (ml) (knee)	<3.5	Often >3.5	Often >3.5	Often >3.5
Viscosity	High	High	Low	Variable
Color	Colorless–straw	Straw–yellow	Yellow	Variable
Clarity	Transparent	Transparent	Translucent	Opaque
Routine laboratory tests:				
WBC	<200	200–2000	2000–75,000	Often >100,000
PMN (%)	<25	<25	>50 often	>75
Culture	Negative	Negative	Negative	Often positive
Mucin clot	Firm	Firm	Friable	Friable
FBS	Nearly = to blood	Nearly = to blood	<50 mg/dl lower than blood	>50 mg/dl lower than blood
Crystals	None	None	*Gout* negative birefringence *Pseudogout:* positive birefringence	None
Differential diagnosis	—	DJD Trauma Osteochondritis dissecans Neuropathic arthropathy Pigmented villonodular synovitis SLE Scleroderma	Rheumatoid arthritis Scleroderma Gout Pseudogout Reiter's syndrome Ankylosis spondylitis SLE Psoriatic arthritis Arthritis associated with ulcerative colitis, regional enteritis	Bacterial infection

DJD, Degenerative joint disease; FBS, fasting blood sugar; PMN, polymorphonuclear neutrophils; SLE, systemic lupus erythematosus; WBC, white blood count.

leads to a breakdown of the hyaluronic acid and results in a loss of the synovial fluid's viscosity. With this, one develops a poor mucin clot test. Instead of holding together like a drop of oil in the 1% acetic acid, the synovial fluid breaks up into many small droplets. Inflammatory joint fluid can be stretched only a few millimeters before breaking, which represents a poor string sign.

Cell Count. The cell count in a class I joint fluid is less than 1000, almost all of which are lymphocytes. In SLE, the cell count in joint fluid is generally less than 1000 but can be up to 5000. Rarely, one may encounter a class II joint fluid in a patient with SLE. The cell count in a class II joint fluid ranges from 5000 to 30,000 with a mean of approximately 10,000. The cells are predominantly polymorphonuclear. Cell counts in class III joint fluids are greater than 100,000 white blood cells and are almost completely polymorphonuclear.

Microscopic Evaluation. The microscopic evaluation of the joint fluid is obtained by taking one drop of joint fluid and placing it on a slide with a coverslip. In a class I joint fluid, one sees rare white and red blood cells with no crystals. In a class II joint fluid, one observes abundant white blood cells. In rheumatoid arthritis, one can see abundant cytoplasmic inclusions within the polymorphonuclear cells, but no crystals are apparent. The crystal of gout is a needlelike crystal that bisects the white blood cell (Fig. 4–2) and is negatively birefringent under a polarizing microscope with a color compensator. The calcium pyrophosphate crystal that is in pseudogout is more difficult to see. It is a rhomboid-shaped crystal, which is weakly positively birefringent under a polarizing microscope (Fig. 4–3). This crystal is often quite difficult to observe because it refracts the light poorly under a polarizing microscope.

Gram's Stain and Culture. If one sees an abundance of white blood cells microscopically, a Gram's stain and culture should be obtained. A note of caution in evaluating the Gram's stain is that patients

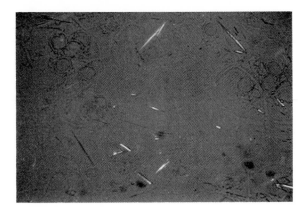

Figure 4–2. Monosodium urate crystals from a gouty synovial fluid, as viewed with compensated polarized light. The crystals are yellow parallel to the axis of slow vibration marked on the compensator (negative birefringence). (From Kelley WN, et al.: Textbook of Rheumatology, 2nd ed. Philadelphia: WB Saunders Co, 1985.)

with inflammatory arthropathies have a great deal of protein in their synovial fluid, which makes the Gram's stain difficult to interpret.

ASSESSMENT

Osteoarthritis

Osteoarthritis is the most common type of arthritis. Of the population over 65 years of age, 75 to 80% suffer from at least mild osteoarthritis.

There are two types of osteoarthritis: primary and secondary. *Primary osteoarthritis* is more common in women. Of women, 60% who suffer from this have a positive family history of osteoarthritis. Primary osteoarthritis has a propensity to involve the proximal and distal interphalangeal joints of the hands (Fig. 4–4).

Secondary osteoarthritis is mainly due to mechanical factors and is the more commonly type of osteoarthritis. It is most commonly due to recurrent microtrauma of the joint and therefore follows the distribution of the weight-bearing joints of the body. The most common joint involved in the foot is the first metatarsophalangeal, which is the major weight-bearing joint of the foot. Secondary osteoarthritis can also involve the other metatarsophalangeal joints but tends to spare the ankle. Its other major targets are the knees, hips, lower back, lower cervical spine, and first carpometacarpal joint of the hand.

There are several factors that place abnormal stresses on a joint and predispose a person to the development of osteoarthritis. These factors consist of the hypermobile joint syndrome, previous damage that disrupts the normal architecture of the joint, a congenital anomaly such as an aplastic hip that causes abnormal alignment of the leg, and work-related activities that put unusual stresses on the joints. For example, ballet dancers can experience osteoarthritis in the ankle because of the abnormal stresses placed on it, whereas other individuals tend not to experience osteoarthritis in this joint.

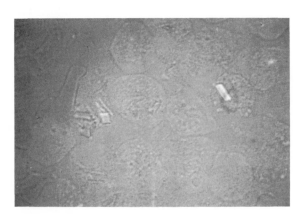

Figure 4–3. Calcium pyrophosphate dihydrate (CPPD) crystals can be needle-shaped, rod-shaped, or rhomboid-shaped but usually have blunt ends. (From Kelley WN, et al.: Textbook of Rheumatology, 2nd ed. Philadelphia: WB Saunders Co, 1985.)

Subjective Symptoms

The symptoms of osteoarthritis are pain and stiffness predominantly with activity. Osteoarthritis is frequently asymptomatic when a patient is at rest. Initially, patients may have symptoms only with the extremes of activity, but as the arthritis progresses, symptoms occur with just minimal use. These patients have mild morning stiffness that generally lasts only a few minutes. Patients can also experience crepitation as they walk because of the disrupted articular cartilage.

Objective Signs

Swelling of the joint usually occurs, but this is not associated with heat or erythema. The swelling can be soft but is generally bony secondary to osteophyte formation. This osteophyte formation and progressive deformity can result in the classic hallux valgus deformity of the foot, which is the combination of an osteophyte forming over the first metatarsal head with a valgus deformity of the first toe (Fig. 4–5). There can also be crepitation on physical examination of the joint, and with time there is a markedly diminished range of motion, resulting in a hallux rigidus. Patients can develop secondary bursitis,

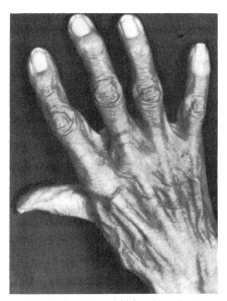

Figure 4–4. *A.* An 85-year-old female with primary osteoarthritis of the right hand. The distal interphalangeal joints are involved, producing the bulbous deformities called Heberden's nodes; the proximal interphalangeal joints are involved to a lesser extent, resulting in milder deformities called Bouchard's nodes; and the carpometacarpal joint of the thumb is involved, making abduction of the thumb difficult and producing the square hand often seen in this form of osteoarthritis. (From Kelley WN, et al.: Textbook of Rheumatology, 2nd ed. Philadelphia: WB Saunders Co, 1985.)

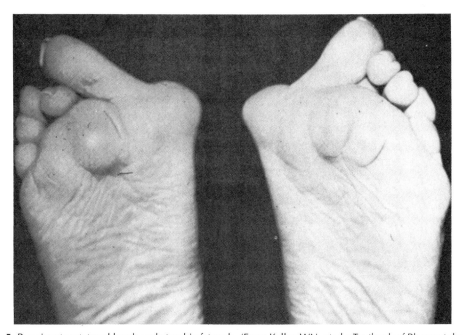

Figure 4–5. Prominent metatarsal heads and atrophic fat pads. (From Kelley WN, et al.: Textbook of Rheumatology, 2nd ed. Philadelphia: WB Saunders Co, 1985.)

which is frequently the case in the first metatarsophalangeal joint.

Laboratory Data

Because this is a noninflammatory arthritis, the laboratory studies in osteoarthritis are normal. A class I joint fluid is seen.

Pathophysiology

In order to understand the pathophysiology of osteoarthritis, one must first have a basic understanding of the articular cartilage. The articular cartilage has no blood vessels within it and is nourished by the synovial fluid. The articular cartilage is made up of proteoglycan subunits. The backbone of the proteoglycan consists of two mucopolysaccharides that are very negatively charged. These are keratin sulfate, which has a molecular weight of 5000 to 10,000, and chondroitin sulfate, which has a molecular weight of 10,000 to 30,000 (Fig. 4–6). These mucopolysaccharides contain abundant sulfide bonds, which result in the negative charge of these mucopolysaccharides. The negative charge causes these macromolecules to repel one another and to stand quite rigidly. These proteoglycan subunits are attached to a core of protein, forming a larger proteoglycan with a molecular weight of 2 million to 3 million.

This macromolecule has the appearance of a large coil. The coil expands and contracts with weight bearing and is responsible for the elastic nature of the articular cartilage and its ability to absorb the trauma of weight bearing. In addition, because of its negative charge, this macromolecule is able to keep larger macromolecules such as degradative enzymes out of the articular cartilage and allows smaller amino acids, glucose, and some water into the articular cartilage for nutrition.

In degenerative arthritis, this proteoglycan subunit breaks down, becoming more fragmented. As a result, larger macromolecules and larger amounts of water are allowed to enter into the articular cartilage. The articular cartilage, as a result, becomes heavier and loses its elastic quality. Degradative enzymes, such as collagenase, are able to enter into the articular cartilage. The earliest pathologic change is a crack-

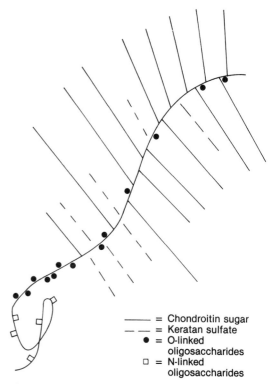

= Chondroitin sugar
= Keratan sulfate
= O-linked oligosaccharides
= N-linked oligosaccharides

Figure 4–6. Proteoglycan molecule, depicting bottlebrush configuration and heterogeneity of the core protein with respect to attachment sites for chondroitin sulfate and keratan sulfate and hyaluronate-binding region. (From Kelley WN, et al.: Textbook of Rheumatology, 2nd ed. Philadelphia: WB Saunders Co, 1985.)

ing or fissuring of the articular cartilage. There is also a proliferation of chondrocytes. With time, the cracking of this articular cartilage becomes more marked, and fissures develop. As this pathologic process progresses, the articular cartilage becomes eroded, resulting in asymmetric loss of the articular surface.

With the loss of the articular cartilage, weight is progressively borne by the subchondral bone. In reaction to this, sclerosis or eburnation of the subchondral bone develops. With the repeated trauma to the subchondral bone, the body makes an effort to repair itself by the formation of new bone. This new bone formation occurs at the margin of the joint, where it results in an osteophyte.

Radiology

The radiology of the osteoarthritic joint stems directly from the pathophysiologic changes that have been described. One sees asymmetric joint space loss, sclerosis or eburnation of the subchondral bone, and osteophyte formation. The radiographic changes are asymmetric both within the joint itself and in terms of its distribution within the body (Fig. 4–7).

Therapy

The therapy of osteoarthritis is largely symptomatic because there is no cure for the disease. Likewise, there is no known prevention of osteoarthritis.

Maintenance of Muscle Tone and Mobility. Maintaining good muscle tone and mobility of the joints can be somewhat protective. Patients with early osteoarthritis can obtain marked symptomatic improvement by working on muscle tone and range of motion. Physical therapists and occupational therapists can instruct the patient in muscle-strengthening exercises and facilitate active range of motion. Occupa-

tional therapists aid the patient in splinting and in providing adaptive devices to take some of the pressure off already damaged joints.

Pharmacologic Therapy. Nonsteroidal anti-inflammatory drugs are the backbone of the pharmacologic therapy of osteoarthritis. Because osteoarthritis is not an inflammatory disease, these can be given in low analgesic doses rather than the larger, more toxic doses necessary to obtain anti-inflammatory effects. In addition, these drugs can be given at the time of activity when the patient is exhibiting the most symptoms. Aspirin remains the NSAID of choice. The half-life of aspirin is approximately 4 hours when given in low doses. Therefore, it can be given with a meal just prior to activity so that the patient can feel the analgesic effects of the medication while he or she is using his or her joints. If the patient is unable to tolerate aspirin,

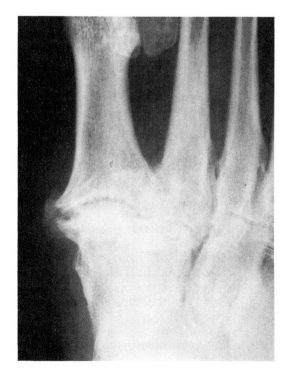

Figure 4–7. Osteoarthritis of the first tarsometatarsal joint. Findings include joint space narrowing, sclerosis, and osteophytes at the first (medial) tarsometatarsal joint and to a lesser extent at the second tarsometatarsal space. (From Resnick D, Niwayama G: Diagnosis of Bone and Joint Disorders, 1st ed. Philadelphia: WB Saunders Co, 1981.)

the physician's discretion determines which other NSAID is used. Acetaminophen, which has analgesic but no anti-inflammatory effect, can be used to treat the pain of osteoarthritis. Its advantage is that it does not result in dyspepsia or tinnitus, which are common complications of aspirin and the other NSAIDs. If a patient has extensive pain from osteoarthritis, occasionally small doses of codeine may be necessary to control the pain. However, this should be done with great caution because osteoarthritis is a chronic disease, and a patient may require long-term analgesic therapy.

Podiatric Implications

The podiatrist has a great deal to offer in terms of local orthotic devices, which take the weight off involved joints. Often a simple metatarsal pad, placed proximal to the first metatarsophalangeal joint, can bring the patient a dramatic degree of symptomatic relief. If this measure is not successful, surgery is often necessary.

Rheumatoid Arthritis

Rheumatoid arthritis is a chronic systemic inflammatory disease involving predominantly the peripheral synovial-lined joints. The major targets of this disease are the small joints of the hands and feet. This is a common disease with a prevalence of approximately 3% and worldwide distribution. Rheumatoid arthritis involves women more commonly than men with a 3 to 1 ratio. The peak age of onset is 25 to 50 years, but it can involve any age group.

Subjective Symptoms

The most common onset is a *polyarticular symmetric arthritis*, which occurs in approximately 75% of patients. The most common initial joints to be involved are the small joints of the hands and feet. This is the characteristic onset in 60% of patients. Typically, patients begin with the insidious onset of pain and swelling symmetrically of the small joints of the hands or feet, in conjunction with a great deal of morning stiffness and malaise. This stiffness can last any time from 1 hour to an entire day. Pa-

tients also notice a gel phenomenon; that is, after sitting or lying for a prolonged period of time, their joints again stiffen.

Twenty-five per cent of patients have a presentation of monoarticular rheumatoid arthritis. When this occurs, the knee is the most common target of the arthritis, accounting for 50% of the monoarticular presentations. The other half have a monoarticular arthritis involving the shoulder, wrist, ankle (Fig. 4–8), or elbow. When rheumatoid arthritis occurs as a monoarticular arthritis, it can mimic a septic joint, an acute gout, or Reiter's syndrome. It is often initially impossible to firmly establish the diagnosis of rheumatoid arthritis. When a patient presents in this fashion, it is mandatory to perform an arthrocentesis. If a class II joint fluid is found with no crystals and culture results are negative, the patient can usually be treated with NSAIDs.

Another presentation of rheumatoid arthritis is *palindromic arthritis*. Patients with this disorder develop episodic attacks of arthritis involving one or two joints. These joints become intensely painful and swollen over a few hours, and the acute attack spontaneously abates over 1 to 3 days. Of these patients, 30% go on to develop rheumatoid arthritis.

Objective Signs

Podiatric Involvement. The most common joints of the foot to be involved in rheumatoid arthritis are the metatarsophalangeal joints, which are involved in 95% of patients with rheumatoid arthritis, followed by the ankle, talonavicular, and subtalar joints. Initially, one may see dif-

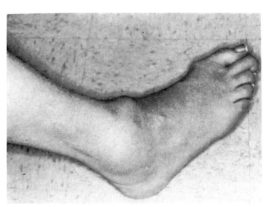

Figure 4–8. Marked synovial proliferation in the ankle joint of a 43-year-old woman with rheumatoid arthritis. (Courtesy of James L McGuire, MD.)

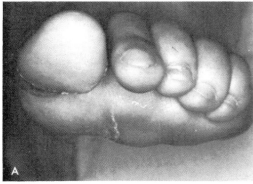

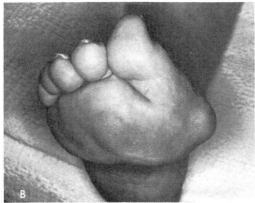

Figure 4–9. Foot problems in rheumatoid arthritis. *A,* Discrete cystic proliferation below subluxed metatarsal heads (2 and 3) in the foot of a patient with rheumatoid arthritis. *B,* Marked hallux valgus with proliferative tissue in the form of a "bunion" at the first metatarsophalangeal joint in a patient with rheumatoid arthritis. There is, in addition, diffuse cystic swelling below the metatarsal heads. (Courtesy of James L McGuire, MD.)

fuse swelling of the metatarsophalangeal joints, which can create widened spaces between the toes. Upon palpation of the joints, one elicits tenderness over the metatarsophalangeal joints and occasionally notes fullness, erythema, and warmth. The involvement of the feet tends to be symmetric. With time, the patient develops widening of the forefoot and a valgus deformity of the toes (Fig. 4–9). The ankle and subtalar joint can likewise develop marked swelling, tenderness, warmth, and occasionally erythema. With time, the ankle (Fig. 4–10) and subtalar joints can sublux.

Other Joint Involvement. Rheumatoid arthritis commonly involves the knees. When it does, there is mild to massive swelling of the knees. A patient can develop the complication of a baker's cyst. This is a swelling in the popliteal space. The cyst can rupture and dissect down into the calf, resulting in pain and swelling that can mimic thrombophlebitis. This is called the pseudothrombophlebitis syndrome. The cyst can also result in an ecchymotic area behind the lateral malleolus. To confirm the diagnosis, one can perform an ultrasonographic or a computed tomography (CT) scan of the knee. Occasionally it is necessary to do an arthrogram, which demonstrates the extension of dye into the calf, confirming the diagnosis of a ruptured Baker's cyst.

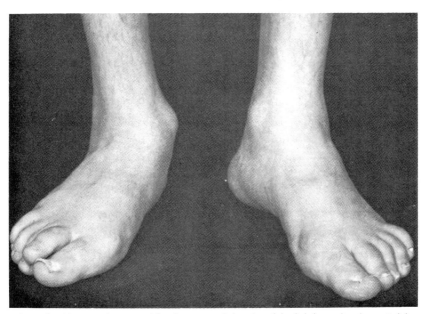

Figure 4–10. Valgus of ankle, pes planus, and forefoot varus deformity of the left foot related to painful synovitis of the ankle, forefoot, and metatarsophalangeal joint in a 24-year-old man with severe rheumatoid arthritis. (From Kelley WN, et al.: Textbook of Rheumatology, 2nd ed. Philadelphia: WB Saunders Co, 1985.)

All the peripheral joints of the body can be involved with rheumatoid arthritis. The other major target of rheumatoid arthritis is the small joints of the hands. Clinically, one sees diffuse swelling of all the small joints of the hands with the exception of the distal interphalangeal joints. Initially, in a similar fashion to that in the foot, there is fusiform swelling of the small joints of the hands with moderate tenderness, erythema, and warmth. Rheumatoid arthritis also involves the tendon sheaths, resulting in tenosynovitis of both the flexor and extensor tendons of the hand. The deformities of rheumatoid arthritis stem from a combination of intrinsic tightness of tendons and weakening of tendons, placing an abnormal stress on already damaged joints.

Rheumatoid arthritis does not involve the low back, sacroiliac joints, or thoracic spine. However, the upper cevical spine or atlantoaxial joint, first cervical vertebra (C-1), and second cervical vertebra (C-2) are involved in 40% of patients with rheumatoid arthritis. This is important to recognize, especially if the patient is undergoing surgery. He or she may have atlantoaxial subluxation, which would warrant the use of a cervical collar during anesthesia to avoid marked flexion of the neck (Fig. 4–11), which can result in damage to the spinal cord and severe neurologic deficit.

Extra-Articular Manifestations

SYSTEMIC SYMPTOMS

Rheumatoid arthritis is systemic inflammatory arthritis. In addition to morning stiffness that patients invariably experience in conjunction with rheumatoid arthritis, patients also experience fatigue, weight loss, malaise, and occasionally a low-grade fever.

RHEUMATOID NODULES

This is the most common extra-articular manifestation of rheumatoid arthritis, occurring in 20% of patients. Nodules occur most commonly over pressure points, especially over the elbow and Achilles tendon (Fig. 4–12). Nodules tend to occur in patients who have more virulent rheumatoid arthritis and in those patients who are

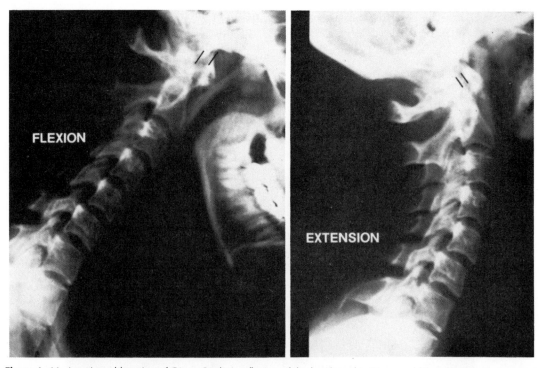

Figure 4–11. Anterior subluxation of C1 on C2 during flexion of the head. In this 21-year-old female, there is a normal 3-mm distance between the atlas and the odontoid process while her head is held in extension (*right*). In flexion radiograph (*left*), subluxation to 7 mm has developed. (Courtesy of Gary S Hoffman, MD.)

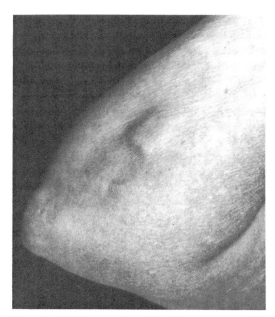

Figure 4–12. Rheumatoid nodule. Subcutaneous nodule over the ulnar aspect of the forearm in a patient with rheumatoid arthritis. (From Kelley WN, et al.: Textbook of Rheumatology, 2nd ed. Philadelphia: WB Saunders Co, 1985.)

rheumatoid-factor positive. Histologically, the nodule is a granulomatous vasculitis. There is a central area of caseous necrosis surrounded by palisading histiocytes, around which are chronic inflammatory cells.

SJÖGREN'S SYNDROME

Sjögren's syndrome is seen in 25 to 30% of patients with rheumatoid arthritis. The major subjective symptoms of Sjögren's syndrome are dry eyes (keratoconjunctivitis sicca), dry mouth (xerostomia), dry vagina resulting in dyspareunia, dry skin, and occasionally involvement of the lungs with an interstitial pneumonitis.

The clinical manifestations of keratoconjunctivitis sicca include a gritty sensation in the eye. Often this is quite severe in the morning, with the accumulation of a thick secretion in the inner aspect of the eye when the patient awakens, which can result in the eyelids being stuck together. These patients are at increased risk for developing conjunctivitis. On physical examination, there is frequently decreased collection of tears in the eye and erythema of the conjunctiva.

The symptoms of xerostomia consist of a dry sensation in the mouth and difficulty in swallowing dry food. This dryness can be so severe that patients need to carry water with them in their purse or car.

Sjögren's syndrome histologically is a lymphocytic infiltration of the secretory glands. Diagnosis can be confirmed by doing a minor salivary gland biopsy of the inner lip. Decreased tear production can be confirmed by Schirmer's test, in which case a piece of litmus paper shows less than 5 mm of wetness after being inserted in the eye for 5 minutes.

PULMONARY INVOLVEMENT

Pulmonary involvement occurs in less than 10% of patients with rheumatoid arthritis. The most common pulmonary manifestation is that of an asymptomatic pleural effusion. The other pulmonary manifestations, in decreasing order of frequency, include interstitial fibrosis; rheumatoid nodules within the lung; and Caplan's syndrome, which is a nodular pneumoconiosis.

FELTY'S SYNDROME

Felty's syndrome is the complex of leukopenia, splenomegalia, and rheumatoid arthritis. Patients can also develop hyperpigmentation, predominantly of the lower extremities, and leg ulcers. The leukopenia can predispose a subset of these patients to severe recurrent infections.

OTHER EXTRA-ARTICULAR MANIFESTATIONS

A small percentage of patients with rheumatoid arthritis develop generalized lymphadenopathy, splenomegaly, and inflammatory myopathy. Patients can also develop a symptom complex similar to polyarteritis nodosa, which is a vasculitis involving the small to medium-sized blood vessels.

Pathophysiology

The earliest lesions of rheumatoid arthritis are hypertrophy of the synovial lining cells and inflammation of the blood vessels within the synovium. The normal synovial lining membrane is one to two cell layers thick. In early rheumatoid arthritis, hyperplasia of the synovial lining cells of 6 to 10 cells deep occurs. The normal stroma of the synovium, which is rich in small blood vessels, becomes infiltrated with lymphocytes and polymorphonuclear cells.

This early stage of rheumatoid arthritis is nonspecific. Identical features can be seen in acute self-limited arthritis of unknown etiology, seronegative spondyloarthropathy, and SLE. A patient with rheumatoid arthritis, however, experiences a transformation of this nonspecific synovitis into an immunoglobulin-producing lymphoreticular-like structure and into a pannus, which also has destructive potential. Each of these aspects of the transformation of the rheumatoid synovium is discussed.

Immunoglobulin Transformation. The rheumatoid synovium undergoes a histologic transformation with the occasional development of small nodules of lymphocytes that in some ways resemble lymph nodes. There is also a massive hypertrophy of the synovium. With this hypertrophy and histologic transformation, the synovium develops the potential to produce tremendous amounts of immunoglobulins. These immunoglobulins include IgM and IgG rheumatoid factors and antinuclear antibodies. The immunoglobulins are secreted into the synovial fluid and produce an inflammatory reaction. The IgG and IgM rheumatoid factors and ANAs form immune complexes that activate the complement system, which further fosters an inflammatory reaction. The synovial fluid is thereby transformed into a class II inflammatory joint fluid with a cloudy yellow appearance, a poor mucin clot test, a poor string sign, 5000 to 30,000 white blood cells that are predominantly polymorphonuclear, and greater than 2.5 mg/dl of protein. The immune complexes and other immunoglobulins are phagocytized by these polymorphonuclear cells. Lysosomal enzymes, including collagenases, elastases, and proteases, are released into the synovial fluid. Oxidative products of metabolism, superoxide ions, are released by the phagocytosis of these immune complexes. In addition, prostaglandins and leukotrienes are released into the synovial fluid. As a result, the synovial fluid has the ability to destroy the articular cartilage and subchondral bone.

Pannus Transformation. The other process that occurs is the transformation of the rheumatoid synovium into a pannus. This is a markedly vascular granulation tissue that is composed of proliferating fibroblasts, numerous small blood vessels, and inflammatory cells. The pannus invades the articular cartilage and also releases products that are able to turn on the chondrocytes, which facilitates the absorption of the articular cartilage and subchondral bone adjacent to the pannus. Thus the inflammatory synovial fluid and pannus together have the ability to destroy the rheumatoid joint.

Etiology

The etiology of rheumatoid arthritis is not known. It is most likely the combination of an unidentified underlying immunologic predisposition combined with an environmental trigger.

Of patients with rheumatoid arthritis, 60 to 70% are HLA-DR4 positive. This is a marker on the surface of most nucleated cells that identifies a particular immune response. Normal individuals who are HLA-DR4 positive without rheumatoid arthritis have been shown in at least one laboratory to have an abnormal immune response to collagen.

Sixty-five percent of patients with rheumatoid arthritis have been shown to have a precipitin within their serum that reacts with nuclear antigen extracted from cells infected with the Epstein-Barr virus. In addition, several investigators have shown that the lymphocytes from patients with rheumatoid arthritis have abnormal immune responses when infected with the Epstein-Barr virus. Normal lymphocytes from patients without rheumatoid arthritis, when stimulated by the Epstein-Barr virus, produce immunoglobulin, including rheumatoid factor. However, they then develop an appropriate suppressor response that turns off this immunoglobulin production. Patients with rheumatoid arthritis lack this suppressor response.

Other infectious agents have also been implicated as possible precipitating factors in rheumatoid arthritis. The earliest agent was *Mycoplasma*. However, later studies have not confirmed *Mycoplasma* as an etiologic factor. Other investigators have shown evidence that a bacterial cell wall fragment, peptidoglycan, may lodge itself within the synovium and possibly incite an inflammatory response.

In summary, some as yet unidentified factor such as the Epstein-Barr virus may become lodged within the synovium. This may initially elicit a nonspecific self-limiting inflammatory response. However, in a patient destined to the development of rheumatoid arthritis, there may be an abnormal immune response to this infection. Possibly HLA-DR4 in a patient is a marker of such an abnormal immune response. The patient then develops chronic synovitis and rheumatoid arthritis.

Laboratory Data

Most patients with rheumatoid arthritis have elevations of the nonspecific indicators of inflammation. Thus the ESR is frequently elevated. Patients also frequently develop mild normochromic, normocytic anemia. If the hemoglobin is less than 10 g or the hematocrit is less than 30, other causes for anemia should be sought, especially iron deficiency anemia that is secondary to gastrointestinal blood loss due to an NSAID.

Of patients with rheumatoid arthritis, 80% become rheumatoid-factor positive. Frequently, early in the course of rheumatoid arthritis, the rheumatoid factor analysis is negative and may become positive later in the disease. The techniques for measurement of rheumatoid factor are discussed under Laboratory Evaluation, under Presenting Features. High titers of rheumatoid factor are seen in patients with more aggressive erosive rheumatoid arthritis and in patients with rheumatoid nodules.

Radiology

The earliest change seen radiographically in rheumatoid arthritis is soft tissue swelling. Next periarticular osteoporosis occurs. With time, there can be mild joint space narrowing and a pannus, and the patient develops a small marginal erosion. Marginal erosions occur from the invading pannus attacking the periarticular bone where there is no articular cartilage to protect it. As the disease progresses, there are marked joint space losses and large periarticular erosions. Subsequently there can be tremendous damage to the joint and de-

formities, as discussed previously in the clinical presentation (Fig. 4–13).

Therapy

The therapeutic approach to rheumatoid arthritis is outlined in Figure 4–14. The basic program for treatment consists of aspirin, rest, therapeutic exercises, and education.

Aspirin

Aspirin remains the drug of choice in the treatment of rheumatoid arthritis. In order to achieve the anti-inflammatory effects of aspirin necessary for treatment, often large amounts may be given, up to $4\frac{1}{2}$ g/day. A serum salicylate level should be obtained after the patient has started taking the aspirin, aiming for a therapeutic level of 20 to 25 mg/dl. When this amount is given, the half-life of aspirin increases. The half-life of one or two aspirin is 4 hours, whereas the half-life of 3 g of aspirin is 15 to 20 hours. Thus aspirin can be given two to three times a day. This increases the convenience of dosage and also enables the patient to take aspirin with meals and thereby diminish any gastrointestinal toxicity. Buffered aspirin has not been shown

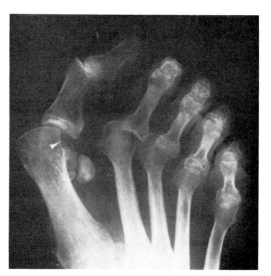

Figure 4–13. Rheumatoid arthritis. The classical forefoot deformities are well illustrated in this patient. Note the subluxation and fibular deviation at the metatarsophalangeal joints and the prominent marginal erosions of the first metatarsal head (arrowhead). (From Resnick D, Niwayama G: Diagnosis of Bone and Joint Disorders, Philadelphia, WB Saunders Co, 1981.)

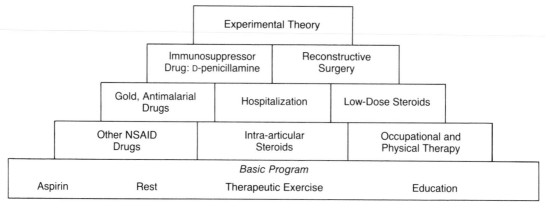

Figure 4–14. Therapeutic approach to rheumatoid arthritis.

in endoscopy studies and in gastrointestinal blood loss studies to be significantly better than plain aspirin. However, enteric-coated aspirin has been demonstrated to be less toxic to the stomach when given in large doses. Enteric-coated aspirin is probably preferable to plain aspirin in long-term treatment of rheumatoid arthritis.

The major mechanism of action of aspirin is the inhibition of prostaglandin synthesis. However, aspirin also interferes with other inflammatory processes such as granulocyte migration and phagocytosis. The major toxicities of aspirin and other NSAIDs stem from their inhibition of prostaglandin synthesis. Aspirin and other NSAIDs interfere with the enzyme cyclooxygenase, which converts arachidonic acid into endoperoxidases, which are then converted into prostaglandins, thromboxane, and prostacyclins. Thromboxanes and prostacyclins control clotting. In addition, the inhibition of the cyclooxygenase on the platelet cell wall plays a role in platelet function. Interfering with prostaglandins, thromboxane, and prostacyclins is the mechanism by which aspirin and other NSAIDs impede clotting. In addition, prostaglandins increase cellular and humoral immunity, are potent vasodilators, sensitize pain receptors, and cause fever. Interfering with these functions of prostaglandins is the major mechanism by which aspirin impedes the inflammatory response. However, prostaglandins also inhibit gastric acid secretion, help maintain the gastric mucosal barrier, and increase blood flow to the stomach. Interference with this function is the major

mechanism by which aspirin results in gastric toxicity.

Prostaglandins also play a role in regulating renal blood flow in patients with underlying renal disease. Therefore, in patients with congestive heart failure or underlying renal disease, aspirin and other NSAIDs, with the possible exception of sulindac, should be given with caution because they can precipitate renal failure. Prostaglandins cause smooth muscle relaxation within the lungs, so aspirin can result in smooth muscle contraction and thereby precipitate asthma. In the uterus, prostaglandins cause muscle contraction. Interference with this function is the most likely cause for the beneficial effect of NSAIDs on menstrual cramps. However, by a similar mechanism, aspirin given at the time of labor can cause its prolongation.

REST, EXERCISE, AND EDUCATION

The other aspect of the basic program in the treatment of rheumatoid arthritis consists of rest. Total body rest to conserve energy is recommended with rest of the involved joints, which includes splinting and joint protection. Patients should also be instructed in a set of therapeutic exercises to maintain strength and range of motion in the affected joints. Education is a critical part of this regimen. Patients must be educated as to the natural history of the disease and the potential toxicities of the drugs for its therapy. The better educated patients are about the nature of their disease, the better they are able to cope with it. There are many forms of quackery available to patients with arthritis; education helps to avoid these potentially dangerous and costly therapies.

There have been several controlled studies regarding the benefit of diet on rheumatoid arthritis. There is some suggestion, though statistically not proven, that a diet low in saturated fats and high in fish oil may be beneficial. Patients should, however, eat a well-balanced diet with adequate amounts of calcium.

OTHER NONSTEROIDAL ANTI-INFLAMMATORY DRUGS

If this program is not sufficient in controlling the activity of rheumatoid arthritis, one should then use an alternative treatment regimen. If the patient is unable to tolerate aspirin, or it is not efficacious, another NSAID should be instituted. It is arbitrary which NSAID is chosen. None of the newer NSAIDs are more effective than aspirin in terms of their anti-inflammatory effects. In addition, they all have similar toxicities, though there seems to be less gastrointestinal toxicity with some and less tinnitus, which can be a problem in the treatment of elderly patients. All the newer NSAIDs are significantly more expensive than aspirin. This is an important point when one considers that this is a chronic disease and patients take these medications for years.

Phenylbutazone. There is no indication for the use of phenylbutazone in the treatment of rheumatoid arthritis.

Aspirin Congeners. Choline magnesium trisalicylate and salicylate are excellent aspirin substitutes. These agents seem to have less gastrointestinal toxicity than regular aspirin, and there are indications in vitro that they have no significant effect on platelet function. Thus they offer an alternative for individuals being treated with sodium warfarin (Coumadin). They are given twice per day generally with an initial dose of 3 g. This can be slowly increased while monitoring the patient's serum salicylate level.

Propionic Acid Derivatives. The propionic acid derivatives, ibuprofen, naproxen, and fenoprofen, are excellent substitutes for the treatment of rheumatoid arthritis. Ibuprofen, the first propionic acid derivative available, should be given in three to four doses per day, generally starting with a dose of 600 mg four times/day. The gastrointestinal toxicity of ibuprofen is similar to that of aspirin. Naproxen, an excellent anti-inflammatory drug, has the advantage of being given only twice per day. Fenoprofen is generally given in a dosage of 600 mg four times/day.

Indole Acetic Acids. The indole acetic acids include indomethacin, tolmetin sodium, and sulindac. Sulindac is an indine derivative of indomethacin. Indomethacin is effective in treatment of rheumatoid arthritis, but its gastrointestinal toxicity is similar to that of aspirin. Patients who take this drug can develop headaches and some clouding of their sensorium. Tolmetin sodium is an effective anti-inflammatory drug given in a dosage of 400 mg four times/day. Sulindac is given in a dosage of 200 mg twice/day. It is suggested that in patients with underlying renal disease, sulindac may be a safer drug than other NSAIDs. However, it can cause the patient to retain sodium.

Diclofenac sodium is a new NSAID with toxicity similiar to that of the other NSAIDs that is given in doses of 50 to 75 mg twice a day.

Intra-Articular Steroids. Intra-articular steroids can be very effective in the control of a joint that is somewhat more inflamed than the others. In addition, there is some systemic absorption of cortisone, which frequently gives the patient temporary relief while other therapeutic modalities are being instituted. A dose of 20 mg of methylprednisolone or triamcinolone can be used in an ankle joint. Approximately 10 mg should be used in other joints of the foot. Caution should be taken in injecting a joint; if one joint is more inflamed than other joints, a superimposed septic arthritis may be the cause.

OCCUPATIONAL THERAPY AND PHYSICAL THERAPY

Occupational therapy and physical therapy play tremendous roles in the treatment of rheumatoid arthritis. The occupational therapist can assist the patient with activities of daily living, joint protection, and splinting. Physical therapists are useful in maintaining the patient's full ranges of motion and muscle tone.

DISEASE-REMITTIVE DRUGS, HOSPITALIZATION, AND LOW-DOSE STEROIDS

If the aforementioned modalities are ineffective or if the patient has erosive disease, the next alternative approach includes disease-remittive drugs, frequently a short course of hospitalization, and occasionally low-dose steroids.

Chrysotherapy. Chrysotherapy remains the major treatment when using disease-remittive drugs. There are three gold preparations available: gold sodium thiomalate, aurothioglucose, and auranofin. The injectable preparations and oral preparations of gold (auranofin) will be looked at separately.

Injectable Preparations. Gold sodium thiomalate and aurothioglucose if tolerated are effective in placing rheumatoid arthritis into remission in approximately 70% of patients. However, it takes 2 to 3 months for gold to begin to work. The major mechanisms of action of gold are the inhibition of lysosomal-enzyme release and the modification of immune response at the level of the macrophage. A gold preparation is given as a weekly intramuscular injection, beginning with a test dose of 10 mg followed the next week by 25 mg and then 50 mg each week until the patient goes into remission. The dosage is then slowly tapered to every other week and eventually to once a month.

Side effects occur in 25 to 40% of patients. The most common side effect is a nonspecific pruritic dermatitis. Patients can also develop stomatitis. Leukopenia and thrombocytopenia can occur; therefore, a platelet count and a blood count prior to each injection of gold should be done. Membranous glomerulonephritis is a late complication of gold therapy as a result of immune complex deposition in the kidney. Patients should be screened for membranous glomerulonephritis with a ureal dipstick testing for urinary protein prior to each gold shot. Gold sodium thiomalate can result in a nitritoid-type reaction in which the patient experiences tachycardia, flushing, and hypotension. This side effect can be avoided by the use of aurothioglucose.

Oral Preparations. Auranofin, an oral gold preparation, is given in a dosage of 3 mg twice/day and takes approximately 4 months to be effective. Auranofin also modifies the immune response, but it appears to have a somewhat different mechanism of action than injectable gold. Preliminary studies have suggested that auranofin is not quite as effective as injectable gold but is safer. The incidence of leukopenia, thrombocytopenia, and glomerulonephritis is minimal. Patients should be screened once per month with a CBC and urinalysis.

Antimalarials. Antimalarials, hydroxychloroquine and chloroquine, are almost as effective as injectable gold in the treatment of rheumatoid arthritis. Their mechanism of action is not clearly understood, but antimalarials appear to work by binding to nucleic acids and suppressing lymphocyte responsiveness. These drugs also take 2 to 3 months to be effective. They are given in a dosage of 400 mg/day, which can be slowly tapered after the patient achieves remission.

The major side effects of antimalarials are nausea, headache, and occasionally skin rash. The most feared reaction is that of retinopathy, which is very unusual. Hydroxychloroquine and chloroquine can build up in the macula and result in blindness. Because hydroxychloroquine has less retinal toxicity, it is the drug of choice. Even though blindness is a rare side effect, patients should be initially screened by an ophthalmologist, then re-evaluated every 4 to 6 months while receiving the drug. If such build-up is present, the drug must be discontinued.

Sulfasalazine. There have been several studies suggesting that sulfasalazine, a sulfanamide, is an effective disease-remittive drug in the treatment of rheumatoid arthritis.

Hospitalization. Hospitalization is effective in patients with extremely active rheumatoid arthritis. A 1- to 2-week stay in the hospital, with physical and occupational therapy, has been shown in several studies to significantly quiet the activity of rheumatoid arthritis.

Prednisone. In patients with extremely active rheumatoid arthritis, low doses of prednisone (5 to 10 mg) are often necessary. This is not a disease-remittive agent and has significant toxicity when given over a long period of time. Prednisone is very rarely given without the concurrent use of a disease-remittive drug. Unfortunately, once started, it is extremely difficult to wean a patient from prednisone because rheumatoid arthritis is exquisitely sensitive to small changes in dosage. Long-term side effects, especially osteoporosis, can become more devastating than the disease itself.

D-PENICILLAMINE, IMMUNOSUPPRESSIVE DRUGS, AND RECONSTRUCTIVE SURGERY

If the aforementioned modalities are ineffective, one should use D-penicillamine or an immunosuppressive drug. Often, reconstructive surgery is also necessary.

D-Penicillamine. D-Penicillamine has been widely used in the past for treatment of rheumatoid arthritis. However, studies have shown that its efficacy diminishes with time. Other studies have suggested that it is no better than placebo in treatment. The mechanism of action of D-penicillamine appears to interfere with leukocyte proliferation, especially with T-helper cell function. Side effects occur in 35% of patients and are identical to those of gold. Occasionally a patient may develop an autoimmune disease such as myasthenia gravis or an SLE–like syndrome.

Immunosuppressive Drugs. The immunosuppressive drugs methotrexate, azathioprine, and cyclophosphamide have been effective in the treatment of rheumatoid arthritis. In addition to their bone marrow–suppressive effects, there has been some question that these drugs may potentiate the development of malignancy. However, all have been shown to be effective in patients with recalcitrant rheumatoid arthritis. Cyclophosphamide, because of its potentially more serious side effects, is reserved for the patient with fulminant life-threatening rheumatoid arthritis.

Reconstructive Surgery. Reconstructive surgery, consisting of joint replacement and metatarsal head resection, is important in the treatment of rheumatoid arthritis. Synovectomy has a limited role in treatment because the synovium always grows back. A disease-remittive drug should be instituted at the time of synovectomy so that the synovium that grows back is less virulent. In controlled studies, the only joint with which synovectomy has been shown to be of benefit is the knee. Tenosynovectomies of the extensor tendon of the hand are indicated when a tendon rupture is threatened.

OHER MODES OF THERAPY

Several experimental modes of therapy have been investigated, most notably lymphoplasmapheresis and total lymph node irradiation. Plasmapheresis has been ineffective in the treatment of rheumatoid arthritis. Lymphoplasmapheresis appears to put the patient into remission while a disease-remittive drug is being instituted. However, they are very expensive and probably no better than a short-term large dose of prednisone or hospitalization. Total lymph node irradiation has been an effective treatment, but is extremely toxic with a high rate of mortality in two of the preliminary studies. These therapeutic modalities should be reserved for the patient who has been refractory to all treatment and should be done only at a medical center conducting controlled studies.

Systemic Lupus Erythematosus

The spectrum of disease in SLE involves almost every organ of the body (Table 4–2). Systemic lupus erythematosus is caused by an immunologically mediated tissue injury. Systemic lupus erythematosus predominantly affects young black women. It is a relatively rare disease with an incidence of 7.5 per 100,000.

Table 4–2. SYSTEMIC LUPUS ERYTHEMATOSUS: SPECTRUM OF DISEASE

Involvement	Percentage (%)
Arthritis	90
Fever	85
Fatigue	80
Dermatitis:	80
Butterfly rash	50
Photosensitivity	35
Discoid rash	20
Alopecia	60
Raynaud's phenomena	20
Myalgia-Myositis	45
Gastrointestinal	50
Adenopathy	40
Pulmonary	50
Cardiac	50
Renal	50
Central nervous system	35

Manifestations of Systemic Lupus Erythematosus

The criteria for classification of SLE are listed in Table 4–3. *Arthritis* is the most common finding. Subjectively, patients complain of a great deal of pain and stiffness. The stiffness can last several hours. Objectively, when one examines a patient with SLE, one usually finds mild swelling and occasionally some deformity. This deformity is not fixed because the joints can be moved back into their proper positions. Often, the objective findings are much less than the severity of the patient's subjective symptoms. Systemic lupus erythematosus can involve all the joints of the body, but its major targets are identical to those of rheumatoid arthritis, predominantly the small joints of the hands and feet.

Fever is present in 85% of patients at some time in the course of the disease. The fever results from inflammation, emanating from the immunologically mediated tissue injury. In conjunction with this fever, patients often experience a great deal of malaise. Systemic lupus erythematosus results in *dermatitis* in 80% of patients, which is discussed in Chapter 12. The most characteristic rash is in a butterfly pattern occurring in a malar distribution on the sun-exposed areas of the face. Patients with SLE develop a photosensitivity rash. This rash often precipitates generalized flares of SLE. *Alopecia* occurs in 50% of patients. This can be a nonscarring

Table 4–3. CRITERIA FOR CLASSIFICATION OF SYSTEMIC LUPUS ERYTHEMATOSUS

Criterion	Definition
Malar Rash	Fixed erythema, flat or raised, over the malar eminences; tends to spare nasolabial folds
Discoid Rash	Erythematous raised patches with adherent keratotic scaling and follicular plugging; atrophic scarring may occur in older lesions
Photosensitivity	Skin rash as a result of unusual reaction to sunlight; by patient history or physician observation
Oral Ulcers	Oral or nasopharyngeal ulceration, usually painless; observed by a physician
Arthritis	Nonerosive arthritis involving 2 or more peripheral joints, characterized by tenderness, swelling, or effusion
Serositis	Pericarditis, documented by ECG, rub, or evidence of pericardial effusion *or* Pleuritis, convincing history of pleuritic pain or rub heard by a physician or evidence of pleural effusion
Renal Disorder	Persistent proteinuria greater than 0.5 g/day or greater than 3 + if quantitation not performed *or* Cellular casts, may be red cell, hemoglobulin, granular, tubular, or mixed
Neurologic Disorder	Seizures, in the absence of offending drugs or known metabolic derangements (uremia, ketoacidosis, or electrolyte imbalance) *or* Psychosis, in the absence of offending drugs or known metabolic derangements (uremia, ketoacidosis, or electrolyte imbalance)
Hematologic Disorders	Hemolytic anemia, with reticulocytosis *or* Leukopenia, less than 4000/mm total on 2 or more occasions *or* Lymphopenia, less than 1500/mm total on 2 or more occasions *or* Thrombocytopenia, less than 100,000/mm in the absence of offending drugs
Immunologic Disorders	Positive lupus erythematosus cell preparation *or* Anti-DNA antibody to native DNA in abnormal titer *or* Anti-Sm, presence of antibody to Sm nuclear antigen *or* False positive serologic test for syphilis known to be positive for at least 6 months and confirmed by *Treponema pallidum* immobilization or fluorescent treponemal antibody absorption test
Antinuclear Antibody	An abnormal titer of antinuclear antibody by immunofluoresence or an equivalent assay of any point in time and in the absence of drugs known to be associated with "drug-induced lupus syndrome"

(From Kelley WN, et al.: Textbook of Rheumatology, 2nd ed. Phildelphia: WB Saunders Co, 1985.)

or scarring type of alopecia with permanent hair loss. Raynaud's phenomenon is present in 20% of patients, myalgia and myositis in 45%, and nausea or vomiting from pancreatitis or serositis of the abdominal viscera in approximately 40%.

Of patients, 40% have *pulmonary involvement*, which is most commonly pleuritis but can be a patchy interstitial pneumonitis, which can develop into interstitial pneumofibrosis. Fifty per cent of patients have *cardiac involvement*, with the most common manifestation being pericarditis and a less common manifestation being myocarditis. Patients treated with long-term corticosteroids can develop premature arteriosclerotic cardiovascular disease.

The most dreaded complication is *glomerulonephritis*. Almost 100% of patients with SLE have some degree of renal involvement. The spectrum of this involvement includes mesangial deposition of immune complexes, which occurs in almost all patients and can be asymptomatic, to a rapidly proliferative glomerulonephritis, which can result in renal failure.

One third of patients have *central nervous system involvement*. The most common type is depression. However, these patients can also experience seizure disorders, peripheral neuropathies, migraine headaches, and aseptic meningitis.

Laboratory Data

Routine laboratory tests for inflammation usually reveal an ESR and mild anemia. This is most commonly anemia of chronic disease but may also be secondary to an immunologically mediated hemolytic anemia. Leukopenia commonly occurs secondary to the presence of antibodies against leukocytes. Patients can also have thrombocytopenia. The urinalysis, if the patient has glomerulonephritis, reveals proteinuria, red blood cells, and often red blood cell casts. If the patient does have glomerulonephritis, there can be an elevation of the blood urea nitrogen (BUN) and creatinine levels. Analysis of joint fluid reveals a class I fluid with less than 5000 white blood cells, which are predominantly mononuclear cells.

The hallmark of SLE is a positive ANA finding. There are four patterns of a positive ANA analysis. The homogeneous pattern is nonspecific and is seen in patients

with SLE, in approximately 30% of individuals over 65 years old, in patients with drug-induced lupus, and in 20% of patients with rheumatoid arthritis. The rim pattern is thought to be more suggestive of antibodies to DNA and is found in patients with SLE, especially in those with glomerulonephritis. The nucleolar pattern is seen most commonly in patients with scleroderma. A speckled pattern of ANA can be observed in patients with SLE and those with mixed connective tissue disease as well as a number of other rheumatic diseases associated with non–DNA-containing antigens (Table 4–4).

Therapy

Therapy for SLE depends on the manifestations of the disease. Just as there is a spectrum of disease manifestations, there is a spectrum of treatments. If a patient has arthritis, fever, and fatigue, the treatment is predominantly rest and administration of NSAIDs. If a patient has dermatitis or alopecia, topical steroids and antimalarials can be used. With more serious manifestations of renal or central nervous system involvement, steroids and occasionally immunosuppressive drugs may be necessary.

Reiter's Syndrome

Reiter's syndrome is the most common of the seronegative spondyloarthropathies. The seronegative spondyloarthropathies consist of Reiter's syndrome, psoriatic arthritis, arthritis in conjunction with inflammatory bowel disease, ankylosing spondylitis, and juvenile ankylosing spondylitis.

Table 4–4. SYSTEMIC LUPUS ERYTHEMATOSUS LABORATORY TESTS

Test	Percentage (%)
Anemia	80
Leukopenia	50
Thrombocytopenia	20
Positive VDRL	20
Positive ANA	99
Hypocomplementemia	50

ANA, Antinuclear antibody; VDRL, Venereal Disease Research Laboratory.

Reiter's syndrome is probably the most common inflammatory arthritis afflicting young men. The average age of onset is 30. The male to female ratio is 9 to 1. Reiter's syndrome consists of four symptoms: arthritis, urethritis, conjunctivitis, and dermatologic lesions. Arthritis occurs in virtually all patients. There are three predominant targets of arthritis of Reiter's syndrome: larger joints of the lower extremity, sacroiliac joints, and tendinous insertions.

Arthritis

The most common sites of involvement of arthritis are the knee and ankle, with involvement of the metatarsophalangeal joints being less common. Pauciarticular arthritis usually involves three to four joints in an asymmetric distribution. These patients can often have an explosive onset of arthritis with large, very painful swelling of one or two joints. The onset can also be more insidious over several weeks. Objective signs include massive, warm effusions, especially of the knees and to a lesser degree of the ankles. One of the characteristics of arthritis is the rapid reaccumulation of fluid after arthrocentesis and initiation of steroids. For this reason, Reiter's syndrome can often mimic a septic joint.

Sacroiliitis

Approximately 30% of patients with Reiter's syndrome develop sacroiliitis. Subjectively, these patients, most of whom are young men, generally present with morning stiffness and pain of the lower back, which gradually improves during the course of the day. This is in contrast with the back pain seen in conjunction with osteoarthritis or with a mechanical low back syndrome, in which patients generally feel better in the morning with the pain becoming more severe in the course of the day and with use. With repeated attacks of Reiter's syndrome, an increased number of patients experience back pain.

Objectively, it is often difficult to distinguish on physical examination between a mechanical low back syndrome and an inflammatory sacroiliitis. In inflammatory sacroiliitis, there is often pain with direct palpation of the sacroiliac joints and pain referred to the area of the sacroiliac joint when the hip is taken to any full range of its motion and then stressed.

Ankylosing Spondylitis

Approximately 30% of patients with Reiter's syndrome develop ankylosing spondylitis. If this develops, patients complain of more diffuse back pain. On physical examination, there is evidence of decreased mobility of the lumbosacral spine. This can be evaluated by performing a Schoeber's test. With the patient erect, 10 cm are measured with a tape measure over the lower lumbar spine. The patient is then asked to bend forward; this area should open up by at least 4 cm. In the patient with ankylosing spondylitis, this opening is much diminished, and the patient does not reverse his or her normal lordotic curve with bending.

Enthesopathy

One of the major signs of Reiter's syndrome and the seronegative spondyloarthropathies is inflammation of tendinous insertions. Clinically a patient presents in two ways, with a sausage digit or tendonitis (Fig. 4–15).

A sausage digit is pathognomonic for seronegative spondyloarthropathies. Subjectively, patients note diffuse swelling and frequently pain of one or more of their toes. On physical examination, there is diffuse swelling of the digit that is often quite painful but can be asymptomatic. This dif-

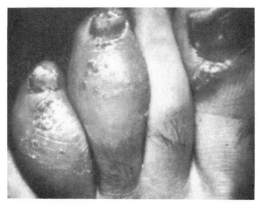

Figure 4–15. Reiter's syndrome. Note two "sausage" digits (dactylitis) and typical nail change. (From Kelley WN, et al.: Textbook of Rheumatology, 2nd ed. Philadelphia: WB Saunders Co, 1985.)

fuse swelling is precipitated by inflammation of the tendinous insertions along the entire margin of the toe. Similarly, there can be inflammation of tendinous insertions, with the Achilles tendon and insertion of the plantar fascia into the calcaneus being the most common targets. Subjectively patients note swelling of the Achilles tendon, which is painful, or a painful heel on ambulation. The pain can be quite severe when the patient first gets out of bed in the morning, which is why this problem is referred to as a "lover's heel". This can be a chronic problem and a source of great disability.

Extra-Articular Manifestations

CONJUNCTIVITIS AND IRITIS

A mild conjunctivitis is seen in up to 50% of patients with Reiter's syndrome. This is usually nonpurulent and minimally asymptomatic. Iritis, a painful inflammation of the eye, can occur in 25% of patients with Reiter's syndrome.

DERMATOLOGIC LESIONS

Dermatologic lesions of Reiter's syndrome consist of keratoderma blennorrhagicum, balanitis circinata, superficial erosions of the tongue,and periungual hyperkeratotic changes.

Keratoderma blennorhagicum is a pustular lesion occurring predominantly on the sole of the foot, which can progress to a very scaly hyperkeratotic lesion (Fig. 4–16). Histologically, the lesion is identical to pustular psoriasis. A patient can also develop a similar hyperkeratotic lesion in the umbilicus. *Balanitis circinata* is a hyperkeratotic scaly lesion seen most commonly on the glans penis. Of all the dermal manifestations of Reiter's syndrome, this can be the most chronic. A patient can also develop *superficial erosions* on the tongue and palate. These are usually asymptomatic and are not usually found unless there is an index of suspicion for them. The *nail changes* of Reiter's syndrome are identical to those seen in psoriasis (Fig. 4–17). The similarity of the skin lesions of Reiter's syndrome to those in psoriasis illustrates one of the difficulties that occurs in differentiating Reiter's syndrome from psoriatic arthritis.

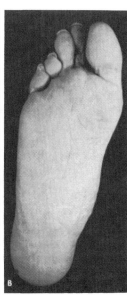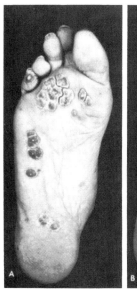

Figure 4–16. Reiter's syndrome. *A,* Keratodermia blennorrhagica on sole of foot. Note hyperkeratotic lesions. *B,* Same foot as shown in *A,* 6 weeks later. Note total healing of lesions. (From Kelley WN, et al.: Textbook of Rheumatology, 2nd ed. Philadelphia: WB Saunders Co, 1985.)

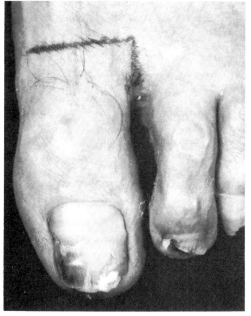

Figure 4–17. Reiter's syndrome. Nail lesions. Note typical destructive nature of change with subungual hyperkeratotic accumulation of material. (From Kelley WN, et al.: Textbook of Rheumatology, 2nd ed. Philadelphia: WB Saunders Co, 1985.)

URETHRITIS

Urethritis is the fourth component of the symptom complex in Reiter's syndrome. This was previously believed to be a sterile urethritis. However, evidence of a *Chlamydia* infection is present in 50% of patients with Reiter's syndrome who suffer from urethritis. In addition, 85% of patients with acute Reiter's syndrome give a history of a recent new sexual contact.

The finding of *Chlamydia* infection in up to 50% of patients with Reiter's syndrome illustrates that this syndrome is a reactive arthritis found in conjunction with bacterial infection. In the United States, Reiter's syndrome most commonly follows urethritis, whereas in Europe it frequently occurs in conjunction with infectious diarrheas. Reiter's syndrome has been seen in conjunction with *Salmonella, Shigella, Campylobacter,* and *Yersinia* dysentery. In Scandinavia, about 33% of patients infected with certain serotypes of *Yersinia enterocolitica* develop Reiter's syndrome. Frequently, arthritis following infectious diarrhea consists only of the arthritis of Reiter's syndrome without extra-articular manifestations.

Laboratory Data

The nonspecific measures of inflammation are generally abnormal in patients with Reiter's syndrome, with ESR and commonly a mild normochromic normocytic anemia. Of patients with Reiter's syndrome, 95% are HLA-B27 positive. The joint fluid is a class II fluid.

Radiology

The radiographic findings of Reiter's syndrome are similar to those of rheumatoid arthritis. Reiter's syndrome tends not to result in periarticular osteoporosis, but can result in bony ankylosis of joints that have been affected for a long time. A patient can also develop a very destructive arthritis that results in a severe "pencil and cup" deformity because of the resorption of the end of the phalanx (Fig. 4–18).

The radiographic findings of the enthesopathy reveal periosteal new bone formation around the periarticular area and the area of tendinous insertions. This bone formation is most commonly seen at the in-

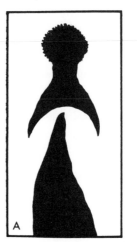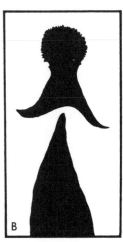

Figure 4–18. Negatives of radiographs showing (*A*) osteolysis resulting in "pencil-in-cup" appearance, and (*B*) osteolysis resulting in "fishtail" deformity of the proximal end of the distal phalanx. (From Kelley WN: Textbook of Rheumatology, 2nd ed. Philadelphia: WB Saunders Co, 1985. After Wright and Moll.)

sertion of the plantar fascia into the calcaneus (Fig. 4–19). Initially one may observe soft tissue swelling in the area, but with time a fluffy, poorly defined periosteal new bone formation develops. This formation is in contrast with the sharply demarcated spurs of a mechanical osteophyte in this area. Similar changes can occur at the insertion of the Achilles ten-

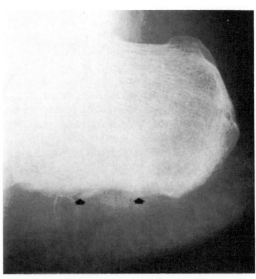

Figure 4–19. Psoriatic arthritis. The inferior surface of the calcaneus reveals the characteristic combination of erosive and proliferative changes (arrows) that form the hallmark of the seronegative spondyloarthropathies. (From Kelley WN, et al.: Textbook of Rheumatology, 2nd ed. Philadelphia: WB Saunders Co, 1985.)

don. A small erosion can develop at both areas.

The earliest radiographic finding of sacroiliitis is that of pseudowidening of the joint. Initially there are small erosions that tend to occur in the lower third of the sacroiliac joint, most commonly on the iliac side. In conjunction with these erosions, there can be some sclerosis of the surrounding bone (Fig. 4–20). With time and healing, bony ankylosis of the sacroiliac joints develops, which results in obliteration of the joint space. These changes can be unilateral in Reiter's syndrome, as contrasted with ankylosing spondylitis in which the changes tend to be bilateral.

Etiology and Pathophysiology

The etiology of Reiter's syndrome is not clear. There are several speculations about how the HLA-B27 haplotype predisposes patients to the development of seronegative spondyloarthropathy. Up to 15% of HLA-B27–positive individuals develop seronegative spondyloarthropathy. The polymorphonuclear cells of HLA-B27–positive individuals tend to migrate more actively toward a source of inflammation. However, the predominant inflammatory infiltrate in Reiter's syndrome and ankylosing spondylitis is a lymphocyte rather than a polymorphonuclear cell. The other possible cause is molecular mimicry. The HLA-B27 haplotype may be similar to a

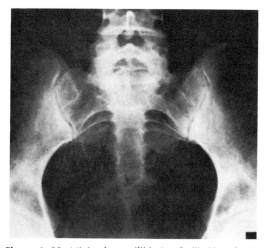

Figure 4–20. Minimal sacroiliitis (grade II). Note juxta-articular sclerosis, blurring of joint margin, minimal erosions, and some joint-space narrowing in this 35-year-old woman. (From Kelley WN, et al: Textbook of Rheumatology, 2nd ed. Philadelphia: WB Saunders Co, 1985.)

bacterial cell wall product, especially Y. enterocolitica. Patients with Reiter's syndrome who live in Los Angeles, with no known exposure to Y. enterocolitica, have leukocytes that cross-react with this organism. There is also evidence to suggest that the HLA-B27 cell surface marker can be altered by an environmental agent. This modification could then alter an immune response and predispose the individual to the development of arthritis.

Pathologically, the synovitis of Reiter's syndrome is identical to that of rheumatoid arthritis with the exception of a tendency toward less synovial lining cell hypertrophy. Also, it is very unusual to develop lymphoid follicles within the synovium. The earliest lesion of the enthesopathy is lymphocytic infiltrate. With time, there is a fibrous transformation of the inflammatory lesion. With healing of this scar, there tends to be ossification that results in a bony periosteal new bone formation or, as is the case in the sacroiliac joint and occasionally in the peripheral joints, bony ankylosis.

Therapy

In order to understand the therapeutic approach to Reiter's syndrome, one must understand its natural history. The duration of the initial attack of Reiter's syndrome is approximately 4 months. Ninety per cent of patients have complete resolution of their initial attack within 6 months. Fifty per cent of patients relapse. Many patients with Reiter's syndrome develop chronic arthritis. Heel pain is one of the poor prognostic signs. In one series, 45% of patients who presented with heel pain had chronic symptoms. Five years after the development of Reiter's syndrome, approximately 70% of patients have persistent symptoms. Of these, 20% have annoying symptoms. Of patients with Reiter's syndrome who are HLA-B27 positive, 40% develop chronic back pain in contrast to those who are HLA-B27 negative, in which case only 15% develop back pain. Aside from this feature, patients who are HLA-B27 positive and those who are HLA-B27 negative have identical diseases.

The therapy of acute Reiter's syndrome consists of administration of NSAIDs, rest, joint protection, and education. The NSAID of choice for Reiter's syndrome is indomethacin. This should be started in an initial dose of 25 mg three to four times/ day and slowly raised to a maximum of 150 mg and rarely 200 mg/day. If this is not effective or if the patient is unable to tolerate indomethacin, all other NSAIDs have been shown to be effective. Some clinicians have noted that aspirin is less effective than other NSAIDs in the seronegative spondyloarthropathies. Phenylbutazone should be reserved for those patients who have been refractory to all other NSAIDs. Great caution should be used if a patient is given long-term treatment with phenylbutazone; the dosage should never exceed 400 mg/day. Patients should be followed with frequent CBCs if treated with phenylbutazone for any period of time. If these modalities are ineffective in controlling arthritis, patients have been shown in uncontrolled studies to respond to hydroxychloroquine (Plaquenil), gold, and methotrexate.

Rest is important. Both total body rest to conserve the patient's energy and rest of the involved joints with splinting, padded shoes, and proper orthotics are important.

Education is paramount. Reiter's syndrome was initially believed to be a self-limiting disease, but as discussed previously, it is now recognized to be chronic arthritis. Patients must understand this in order to comply with the trials of different medications often necessary to bring the arthritis into remission.

Psoriatic Arthritis

Of patients with psoriasis, 6% develop arthritis. There is no distinguishing pattern of the skin lesion that predisposes the patient to psoriatic arthritis. The onset of arthritis can precede the psoriasis by months to years, but it occurs most commonly after or concomitant with the development of psoriasis. The peak age of onset of psoriatic arthritis is 40 years, and the sex ratio is approximately equal.

There are several different patterns of psoriatic arthritis. This disorder was initially categorized as distinct types of arthritis, but it is now appreciated that because of the wide overlap among these various types of arthritis, they cannot be specifically distinguished.

Psoriatic arthritis is similar in many ways to Reiter's syndrome. As discussed under Reiter's Syndrome, it is often extremely difficult to distinguish between these diseases.

Presentation

The most common lesion of psoriatic arthritis is the sausage digit similar to that in a patient with Reiter's syndrome. A patient can also have involvement of the distal interphalangeal joints, commonly in conjunction with a psoriatic nail (Fig. 4–21). Subjectively, patients complain of pain and swelling of this joint with significant morning stiffness and pain with use. Patients can also develop pauciarticular arthritis, predominantly involving large joints. In contrast to Reiter's syndrome, this can involve joints of both the upper and lower extremities. Patients can also develop polyarticular, somewhat symmetric arthritis similar in many ways to rheumatoid arthritis with the exception that there tends to be more distal interphalangeal joint involvement in psoriatic arthritis than there is in rheumatoid arthritis. Patients can develop sacroiliitis with ankylosing spondylitis as well. Ankylosing spondylitis in conjunction with psoriatic arthritis is identical to that in Reiter's syndrome. In contrast to ankylosing spondylitis, there is an asymmetric spondylitis that tends to be associated with large syndesmophytes (Fig. 4–22).

The onset of psoriatic arthritis tends to be insidious as opposed to the frequently acute onset of Reiter's syndrome.

Laboratory Data

The nonspecific measures of inflammation, an ESR and normochromic normocytic anemia, are frequently seen in patients with psoriatic arthritis. The incidence of HLA-B27 positivity in patients with psoriatic arthritis is approximately 30%. The distribution of arthritis predicts the frequency of HLA-B27 positivity. Those with predominantly peripheral joint involvement have no greater incidence of HLA-B27 positivity than the general population. However, those patients with sacroiliitis and spondylitis have a 60% incidence of HLA-B27 positivity. This illustrates the lack of usefulness of this test. Initially, the HLA-B27 haplotype enabled

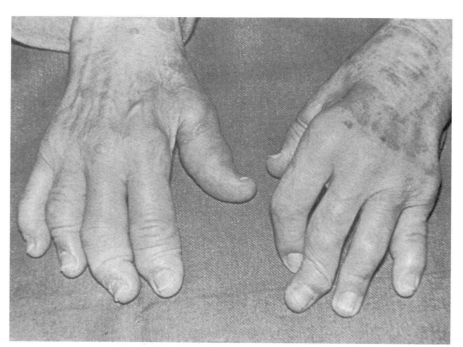

Figure 4–21. Hands of a patient with psoriatic arthritis showing pronounced distal joint involvement. (From Kelley WN, et al.: Textbook of Rheumatology, 2nd ed. Philadelphia: WB Saunders Co, 1985.)

rheumatologists to identify this whole group of arthropathies. However, this test was so successful in delineating this group of diseases that it is now rarely necessary to obtain the test to establish a diagnosis.

Hyperuricemia is occasionally seen in

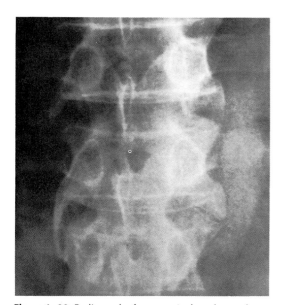

Figure 4–22. Radiograph of nonmarginal syndesmophytes of the lumbar spine in psoriatic arthritis. (From Kelley WN, et al.: Textbook of Rheumatology, 2nd ed. Philadelphia: WB Saunders Co, 1985.)

patients with psoriasis because of the increased skin turnover. However, gout is not commonly seen in this population.

Radiology

The radiographic changes of psoriatic arthritis are similar to those of Reiter's syndrome but show more destruction (Fig. 4–23). There is a tendency for these changes to occur especially in the distal joints.

Pathophysiology

The histologic changes of psoriatic arthritis are identical to those of Reiter's syndrome. It is not understood why some patients with psoriasis develop arthritis.

Natural History. Psoriatic arthritis can have a quite variable course. It can be a self-limited arthritis, however, most patients develop a chronic arthritis that is often quite difficult to control. A small percentage of patients develop arthritis mutilans. Over the course of a few months, marked destruction of joints can occur, which can be refractory to all medications.

Therapy

The therapeutic approach to psoriatic arthritis is similar to that of Reiter's syn-

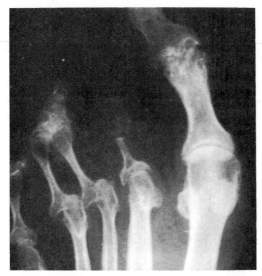

Figure 4–23. Radiograph of dissolution of phalanges of second toe in psoriatic arthritis. (From Kelley WN, et al.: Textbook of Rheumatology, 2nd ed. Philadelphia: WB Saunders Co, 1985.)

drome. An effort should be made to control the skin lesions. However, only 50% of patients have a correlation between the activity of the skin disease and the activity of the arthritis.

The NSAID of choice for psoriatic arthritis is indomethacin. If this is not effective, all other NSAIDs, with the possible exception of aspirin, have been effective. If the patient's arthritis cannot be controlled with an NSAID and rest, hydroxychloroquine, gold, and methotrexate have been effective. However, there is an incidence of severe exfoliative dermatitis in patients treated with hydroxychloroquine.

Arthritis in Inflammatory Bowel Disease

There are two types of arthritis seen in conjunction with inflammatory bowel disease (e.g., Crohn's disease and ulcerative colitis). Patients can develop a *pauciarticular arthritis* of the lower extremities identical to that seen in conjunction with Reiter's syndrome. Interestingly, there is not an increased incidence of HLA-B27 positivity in this group. The activity of this arthritis tends to correlate with the activity of the bowel disease. Occasionally, patients also have erythema nodosum, which is a warm, painful raised erythematous skin

lesion that tends to occur over the tibia (Fig. 4–24). The therapeutic approach to this group of patients is to first control the activity of the bowel disease. Nonsteroidal anti-inflammatory drugs, especially indomethacin, can be useful in the control of arthritis.

The other type of arthritis found in conjunction with inflammatory bowel disease is *ankylosing spondylitis*. The course of this arthritis is independent of the activity of the inflammatory bowel disease. Sixty per cent of patients are HLA-B27 positive.

Crystal-Induced Arthritis

There are three types of crystal-induced arthritis: gout, which is secondary to the uric acid crystal; chondrocalcinosis, which is secondary to the calcium pyrophosphate dihydrate crystal; and hydroxyapatite-deposition disease, which is secondary to the hydroxyapatite crystal. This group of arthropathies shares many similarities, which are discussed subsequently.

Gout

Gout is the most common of the crystal-induced arthropathies, affecting approximately 3% of the population. This is predominantly a male disease, with only 5% of cases involving females, and is extremely rare prior to menopause. Gout is

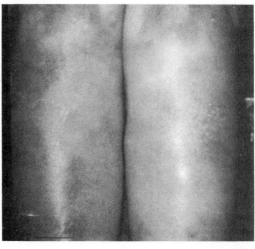

Figure 4–24. Erythema nodosum. Healing subcutaneous nodules on the anterior tibial surfaces resembling multiple contusions. (From Kelley WN, et al.: Textbook of Rheumatology, 2nd ed. Philadelphia: WB Saunders Co, 1985.)

commonly associated with hyperuricemia. Every patient with hyperuricemia does not have gout, and an acute attack of gout is possible in a patient with a normal uric acid level (Table 4–5).

Podiatric Involvement. Of all the crystal-induced arthropathies, gout is the only arthropathy to commonly involve the foot. The patient complains of the acute onset of erythematous, painful swelling of the foot. Gout classically begins in the evening or early morning. It can occur with local trauma, with an acute medical illness, following a surgical procedure, or following a high-purine diet or alcohol binge.

The major target of gout is the first metatarsophalangeal joint. Ninety per cent of patients have involvement of their first metatarsophalangeal joint (podagra) at some time, and 50% of patients have an initial attack that involves the first metatarsophalangeal joint. The next most common target of gout is the soft tissue of the midfoot followed by the ankle. All the peripheral joints have been involved with acute gout.

Gout is not only an arthritis, but also a soft tissue inflammation. Thus a characteristic physical finding is not only acute swelling of the joint but inflammation of the surrounding tissue. For this reason, gout can be confused with acute cellulitis.

Other Involvement. Of acute attacks of gout, 15% involve more than one foci. Because this is an inflammatory reaction, in addition to severe pain, patients occasionally experience low-grade fever and malaise.

ETIOLOGY

Gout tends to occur in previously damaged joints. The first metatarsophalangeal joint has the highest incidence of degenerative arthritis of any of the joints in the body. During the course of the day, because of microtrauma to this joint, a small effusion often develops. At night, this effusion is resorbed approximately 50% faster than the uric acid within it. As a result, the uric acid crystals can precipitate gout, causing an acute attack of podagra,

Table 4–5. CLASSIFICATION OF HYPERURICEMIA AND GOUT

Type	Metabolic Disturbance	Inheritance
Primary		
1. Molecular defects undefined		
Underexcretion (90% of primary gout)	Not established	Polygenic
Overproduction (10% primary gout)	Not established	Polygenic
2. Associated with specific enzyme defects		
PP-ribose-P synthetase variants: increased activity	Overproduction of PP-ribose-P and uric acid	X-linked
Hypoxanthine-guanine phosphoribosyltransferase deficiency, partial	Overproduction of uric acid; increased purine biosynthesis de novo driven by surplus PP-ribose-P	X-linked
Secondary		
1. Associated with increased purine biosynthesis de novo		
Glucose 6-phosphatase deficiency or absence	Overproduction plus underexcretion of uric acid; glycogen storage disease, Type I (von Gierke)	Autosomal recessive
Hypoxanthine-guanine phosphoribosyltransferase deficiency, complete	Overproduction of uric acid; increased purine biosynthesis de novo driven by surplus PP-ribose-P, Lesch-Nyhan syndrome	X-linked
2. Associated with increased nucleic acid turnover	Overproduction of uric acid	Most not familial
3. Associated with decreased renal excretion of uric acid	Decreased filtration of uric acid, inhibited tubular secretion of uric acid, or enhanced tubular reabsorption of uric acid	Some autosomal dominant, some not familial, most unknown
Unknown		Unknown

(From Kelley WN, et al.: Textbook of Rheumatology, 2nd ed. Philadelphia: WB Saunders Co, 1985.)

which explains why acute attacks tend to occur more commonly in the late evening or early morning. Another reason that gout involves the foot is that uric acid is less soluble at cooler temperatures. At normal body temperature, 37° C (98.6° F), the solubility of uric acid is 6.8 mg/dl. At 30° C (86° F), the solubility of uric acid is 4.5 mg/dl. The temperature of the normal ankle joint is 29° C (84.2° F). Therefore, uric acid is less soluble in the cooler environment of the foot. This explains why acute gout can occur with a normal uric acid level and why gout tends to involve the foot. Uric acid is more soluble in proteoglycans, a major constituent of articular cartilage and joint fluid, which is the reason why gout does not occur more commonly in patients with normal uric acid levels.

There are several clinical settings in which acute gout can occur. These are most commonly associated with fluctuations of uric acid. Common settings include those involving acute medical illness and following surgery in the postoperative period. These situations involve mild dehydration, lactic acidosis, and discontinuation of medications that lower uric acid levels. All these can result in an acute elevation of the uric acid level. Dehydration results in a decrease in glomerular filtration of uric acid and thereby an increase in serum uric acid. Lactic acidosis diminishes uric acid secretion by the kidney. Postoperatively, patients often cannot take anything by mouth; as a result their uric acid drugs are discontinued, which further contributes to the acute elevations of uric acid.

Malignancies, especially lymphoproliferative malignancies, can result in increased uric acid levels because of increased cellular turnover. When these malignancies are treated and a great number of cells are killed, there can be a large elevation of serum uric acid level and consequently acute gout; often renal disease can occur as well.

Any change in the body's uric acid level may result in an acute attack of gout. Thus lowering of uric acid level with the institution of a uric acid–lowering drug can also precipitate acute attacks of gout. During this period of time, urate is being mobilized from the body's tissues and joints, resulting in local fluctuations in uric acid concentrations. It is for this reason that it is necessary to administer a prophylactic NSAID or colchicine to the patient while the uric acid level is being lowered medically.

DIAGNOSTIC TESTS

The diagnosis of acute gout is made by obtaining the characteristic uric acid crystal from an aspirate of the soft tissue or joint. It is mandatory to perform an aspiration on any undiagnosed patient suspected of having acute gout unless the patient has an acute attack of podagra that responds promptly to an NSAID or to colchicine. When the aspirated fluid is examined microscopically, needlelike crystals bisecting white cells are seen. The needlelike morphology of this crystal is as important in establishing the diagnosis as the negative birefringent nature of the crystal when it is placed under a polarizing microscope. Beause the uric acid crystal is negatively birefringent, when the crystal is parallel to the lane of the polarizer, it appears yellow, and when it is perpendicular to the plane of the polarizer, it appears blue.

Once gout is suspected, a serum uric acid determination should be obtained. As previously mentioned, an elevated uric acid level helps confirm that one is dealing with gout. However, an elevated uric acid level does not establish the diagnosis of gout, just as a normal uric acid level does not exclude it.

If one suspects an acute attack of gout, it is also important to examine the patient for evidence of tophi. These are collections of urate that tend to occur in areas of decreased temperature such as the helix of the ear, over the olecranon bursa of the elbow, over the Achilles tendon (Fig. 4–25), and occasionally on the hand. One should also seek a history of kidney stones, type IV hyperlipidemia, and hypertension, which occurs with increased frequency in patients with hyperuricemia. In addition, one should ask if there is a positive family history for gout.

Gout can be conceptualized as two disease processes. One is acute gout, and the other is the deposition phase of the disease. Acute precipitation of the uric acid crystal results in an acute attack of gout. However, it is the chronic tophaceous

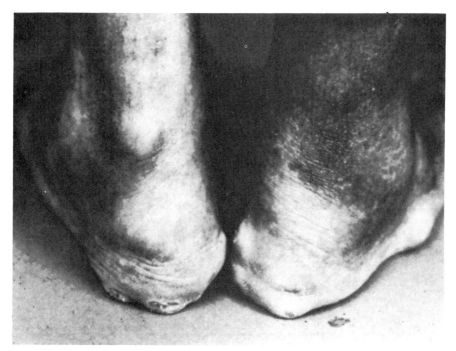

Figure 4–25. Tophi of Achilles tendons and their insertions in a black patient with gout. (From Kelley WN, et al.: Textbook of Rheumatology, 2nd ed. Philadelphia: WB Saunders Co, 1985.)

deposition of urate that results in the destructive changes one sees within joints.

If one aspirates a tophus, one sees abundant uric acid crystals but few white blood cells. If one were to biopsy a chronic tophaceous joint, one would see large collections of uric acid crystals at the margins of the joint with often a migration of this urate into the joint. Within the articular cartilage, collections of uric acid can also occur (Fig. 4–26). Within these collections, there is little evidence of inflammation. These local collections of uric acid destroy the local area of cartilage, whereas the remainder of the cartilage is well preserved. It is this local infiltration of uric acid that results in the damage to the joint rather than the inflammation of the acute attack of gout.

RADIOLOGY

In an acute attack of gout, generally there are no radiographic findings aside from soft tissue swelling. Because gout has a propensity to involve previously damaged joints, there can be some changes of degenerative arthritis in the joint involved with gout.

The radiologic findings stem directly from the pathologic process described earlier. One sees a local "rat-bite" type erosion commonly at the margin of the joint (Fig. 4–27). As the tophus wedges into the joint, there can often be an overhanging edge of normal bone over the tophus. There can also be localized areas of destruction within the joint with the remainder of the joint being well preserved. There is no periarticular osteoporosis. The soft tissue swelling adjacent to a chronic gouty joint frequently calcifies with time.

THERAPY

The therapy for gout is twofold. First, treatment is given for the acute attack, and secondly, once the acute attack has resolved for at least 2 weeks, treatment is given for the hyperuricemia. The drugs of choice for treatment of acute gout include NSAIDs, colchicine, and local cortisone injections.

Acute Attack of Gout
Nonsteroidal Anti-Inflammatory Drugs.
Indomethacin is the NSAID of choice. Indomethacin (Indocin) should be used in large doses. One should begin with an initial dose of 50 mg, with 150 mg being given within the first 24 hours. The med-

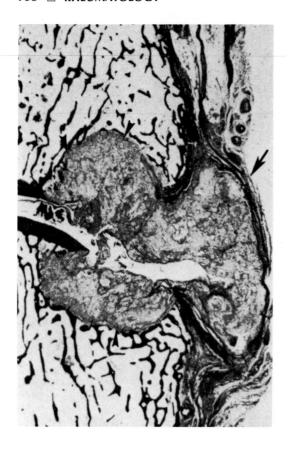

Figure 4–26. Osseous alterations (5 ×). At a metatarso-phalangeal joint, urate deposition has resulted in capsular distention (*arrow*) and invasion of articular cartilage and subchondral bone (*arrowheads*). (From Jaffe HL: Metabolic Degenerative and Inflammatory Diseases of Bone. Philadelphia: Lea & Febiger, 1972.)

ication should then be continued at 100 to 150 mg/day until the acute attack has resolved. Unfortunately, at these dosages there is a high incidence of central nervous system changes, especially headache, clouded sensorium, and gastrointestinal intolerance. An excellent alternative to indomethacin is phenylbutazone (Butazolidin), especially if the patient is a young person. One should begin with an initial dose of 200 mg, with 600 mg being given within the first 24 hours, followed by 100 mg four times/day for the next few days. All the NSAIDs can be used in treatment of acute gout with the exception of aspirin and aspirin congeners. Aspirin increases uric acid levels at low doses and is uricosuric at higher doses. The resultant fluctuation in the serum uric acid level makes it more difficult to control the acute attack.

Colchicine. Colchicine is an extremely toxic drug. There are two settings in which it can be recommended for treatment of an acute attack of gout. In the postoperative period, when a patient can take nothing by mouth, 2 mg of colchicine can be given intravenously through a rapidly running intravenous line, followed by 1 mg in 4 to 6 hours. A patient should never receive more than 4 mg of colchicine intravenously in a 24 hour period because of the risk of aplastic anemia. Colchicine should be given in a rapidly running intravenous line because any extravasation of colchicine into the surrounding soft tissue can result in marked tissue necrosis. The clinical setting in which colchicine can be given orally is when the clinician is not sure if he or she is dealing with gout. Gout promptly responds to colchicine, which is almost diagnostic of acute gout. Occasionally, pseudogout responds to colchicine, but none of

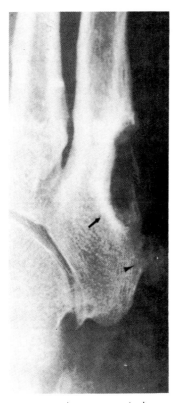

Figure 4–27. Gout. A large extra-articular erosion of the lateral aspect of the fifth metatarsal shaft is bordered by reactive bony sclerosis (arrow). A smaller erosion is present more proximally (arrowhead) with an adjacent calcified soft tissue tophus. (From Resnick D, Niwayama G: Diagnosis of Bone and Joint Disorders. Philadelphia, WB Saunders Co, 1981.)

the other inflammatory arthropathies or infections respond to it. Thus colchicine can be given as a diagnostic/therapeutic drug, helping in both relieving the patient's acute gout attack and in confirming the diagnosis. Colchicine is given in a 1-mg loading dose, and then 0.5 mg/hour is given until the patient gets marked gastrointestinal symptoms or the gout responds.

Cortisone. An alternative mode of therapy for the acute attack of gout is to inject the inflamed area with cortisone.

Hyperuricemia. Treatment of hyperuricemia should not commence until the acute attack has completely resolved for 2 weeks. During the period of time that the uric acid is being lowered, the patient should be prophylactically treated with a low dose of NSAIDs or colchicine in a dose of 0.5 mg two to three times/day.

If a patient has only one attack of gout and has mild hyperuricemia (i.e., a uric acid level of less than 10 mg/dl) and no evidence of tophi or renal disease, it is often not necessary to treat the hyperuricemia but rather to follow the patient closely and institute therapy only if he or she has frequent attacks of gout.

Etiology. Before a patient's hyperuricemia is treated, the etiology of the hyperuricemia should be determined. There are two primary mechanisms of hyperuricemia. The first and most common is a primary renal mechanism in which one sees an underexcretion of uric acid by the kidneys. The second is an overproduction of uric acid, in which case one sees a normal excretion of uric acid by the kidney in the presence of hyperuricemia. This determination can be made by collecting a 24-hour urine sample for analysis of uric acid. A patient with less than 600 mg of uric acid in a 24-hour urine sample is considered to be an underexcreter and to have a renal mechanism for the hyperuricemia. A patient with over 600 mg in a 24-hour sample is considered to be an overproducer of uric acid with a normal renal clearance of uric acid.

Eighty per cent of patients have a renal mechanism of hyperuricemia and thus are found to be underexcreters of uric acid. The most common cause of this is diuretic therapy. Other associated disorders that can cause an underexcretion of uric acid are hypertension, aspirin ingestion, decreased renal function, lead intoxication, and lactic acidosis. Overproduction of uric acid is associated with two enzymatic defects: an underactivity of hypoxanthine guanine phosphoribosyltransferase and an overactivity of the enzyme phosphoribosylpyrophosphate synthetase. Overproduction of uric acid can be seen in conjunction with certain cancers, especially lymphomas and leukemias, and in conjunction with hemolytic anemias, psoriasis, obesity, and alcohol ingestion. In addition, hyperuricemia is associated with type IV hyperlipidemia and obesity. If one of these conditions is present, efforts should be made to treat it.

Drug Therapy. If the patient's mechanism of hyperuricemia is an underexcretion of uric acid by the kidney, the drugs of choice are probenecid and sulfinpyrazone, which increase the renal excretion of uric acid. With both of these drugs, one should start with a low dosage and slowly increase it. The initial dosage of probenecid is 250 mg/day, which can slowly be increased to 1 to 2 g/day. The initial dose of sulfinpyrazone is 50 mg twice/day, which can slowly be increased to 200 mg twice/day.

Allopurinol is the drug of choice for patients who are primarily overproducers of uric acid, have evidence of tophaceous deposits, have a history of renal disease, are receiving chemotherapy for cancer, or have allergies to probenecid or sulfinpyrazone. The dose of allopurinol is 300 mg/day. This should be lowered in elderly patients and in patients with azotemia.

Diet. A purine-free diet can lower uric acid by 1 mg/dl. Patients should be instructed in regard to a relatively low-purine or purine-free diet and should abstain from organ meats, such as sweetbread, liver, and kidney; anchovies; sardines; rich gravies; and alcohol.

Chondrocalcinosis

Chondrocalcinosis is secondary to the calcium pyrophosphate dihydrate crystal. This is a quite common disease in the elderly, with an incidence of up to 27% on radiographs of the knees in patients over the age of 80. In younger individuals, chondrocalcinosis is associated with certain metabolic diseases. Gout is most commonly associated with chondrocalcinosis, and it is not unusual to see gout and pseudogout in the same joint. Other metabolic diseases associated with chondrocalcinosis include hyperparathyroidism, hemochromatosis, hemosiderosis, hypothyroidism, hypomagnesemia, hypophosphatemia. Steroid therapy has been potentially linked with chondrocalcinosis as well. These are thought to possibly alter cartilage metabolism and predispose the patient to the deposition of calcium pyrophosphate within the articular cartilage.

PRESENTATION

The clinical presentation of chondrocalcinosis is quite variable and can mimic many of the more common arthropathies. The joint most frequently involved in chondrocalcinosis is the knee. It is often said that the knee is to pseudogout what the big toe is to gout. Other commonly involved joints include the wrists, elbows, shoulders, metacarpophalangeal joints, and occasionally ankles.

The most common presentation of chondrocalcinosis is that of pseudogout. Subjectively, the patient complains of acute painful swelling, most commonly of the knee. In conjunction with this, patients often experience marked systemic symptoms, with a high-grade fever and a toxic-appearing condition with occasionally mental obtundation. Objectively, on physical examination there is warm, painful swelling of the joint with a limited motion secondary to the pain. Another presentation is pseudo-osteoarthritis with the subjective complaints predominantly of osteoarthritis. On physical examination, there is a component of mild inflammation with moderate joint swelling and often involvement of atypical joints for osteoarthritis. For example, the patient may have the appearance of osteoarthritis but have involvement of the ankle or the wrist, joints that are not commonly involved in osteoarthritis. In this case, chondrocalcinosis should be considered.

Patients with chondrocalcinosis can also present with symptoms of pseudorheumatoid arthritis. In these cases, there are symptoms similar to those of rheumatoid arthritis with a symmetric polyarticular arthritis. However, larger joints tend to be involved, with sparing of the smaller joints of the hands and feet. Rarely, chondrocalcinosis can be a very destructive arthritis similar to that of Charcot's joint.

Of patients with chondrocalcinosis, 25% are asymptomatic; radiographic findings of chondrocalcinosis are the only evidence of disease.

DIAGNOSIS

The diagnosis of chondrocalcinosis is established by the typical radiographic finding of calcification of the articular cartilage or meniscus (Fig. 4–28). If one has a patient with an acute inflammatory arthritis and one aspirates the joint and finds the classic calcium pyrophosphate crystal, pseudogout is diagnosed. Pseudogout cannot be determined by radiographic diagnosis. The crystal of chondrocalcinosis is rhomboid-shaped and weakly refracts light. This makes the crystal often difficult to find, and thus one must have a high index of suspicion for this disease in order

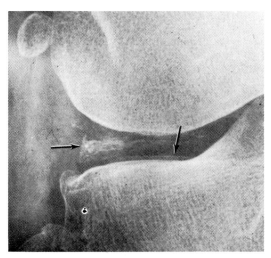

Figure 4–28. Punctate and linear mineral deposition in the fibrocartilage of the lateral meniscus as well as in hyaline articular cartilage, demonstrated by the magnification technique of Genant. (From Genant HK: In McCarty DJ [ed]: Proceedings of the Conference on Pseudogout and Pyrophosphate Metabolism. Arthritis Rheum 19:Suppl 3. May–June, 1976.)

to identify the crystal. The crystal is positively birefringent so that when it is parallel to the plane of the polarizer, it appears blue, and when it is perpendicular to the plane of the polarizer, it appears yellow. However, the calcium pyrophosphate crystal is only weakly birefringent, so this color change is not as dramatic as with the uric acid crystal.

LABORATORY DATA

There is no characteristically abnormal laboratory data in pseudogout. The nonspecific indicators of inflammation are abnormal, with an ESR and rarely a lowered hemoglobin. Once the diagnosis of chondrocalcinosis is established, one should screen for underlying metabolic diseases associated with gout, as described earlier. This should always include uric acid, calcium phosphorus, magnesium, and thyroxine (T_4) analyses.

THERAPY

The therapy for inflammation of chondrocalcinosis is administration of NSAIDs, with indomethacin being the drug of choice. If the patient is unable to tolerate indomethacin, often a short course of phenylbutazone may be necessary to control the acute inflammation. However, any of the NSAIDs in full therapeutic doses can be used to treat acute pseudogout. Colchicine is inconsistently effective; intra-articular steroids can be extremely effective. Unfortunately, there is no therapy for the underlying chondrocalcinosis.

Hydroxyapatite-Deposition Disease

Hydroxyapatite-deposition disease is caused by the hydroxyapatite crystal. This crystal is now recognized as being responsible for calcific tendonitis and possibly contributing to advanced osteoarthritis. It is also responsible for the calcinosis seen in conjunction with scleroderma, polymyositis, neuropathic disorders, chronic renal failure, hypercalcemia, hyperphosphatemia, and myositis ossificans.

THERAPY

The therapy for the inflammation in conjunction with hydroxyapatite-deposition disease is administration of NSAIDs and local steroid injection. Colchicine has been of limited success in this disease. Medical treatment for calcinosis has been uniformly ineffective. Occasionally surgical removal of the calcinosis is necessary.

Septic Arthritis

There are three predominant types of septic arthritis: gonococcal arthritis, nongonococcal bacterial arthritis, and tuberculous arthritis. Fungal arthritis is quite rare and usually occurs secondary to an underlying osteomyelitis.

Gonococcal Arthritis

The target of this infection is the young, sexually active population, but it can be seen in any age group. The typical presentation is that of prodromal fever, malaise, and migratory polyarticular arthritis. Initially, this arthritis frequently involves several joints in rapid succession over a 24- to 72-hour period and then settles into one or two joints, predominantly the smaller peripheral joints of the body. In addition, there is frequently an acute tenosynovitis. In a clinical setting in which a young woman or man presented with an acute tenosynovitis or arthritis of the foot, gonococcal arthritis would have to be actively excluded because this presentation is identical to that in Reiter's syndrome (Table 4–6). To help distinguish gonococcal arthritis, an additional objective sign of a typical skin rash might be found (Fig. 4–29). Generally, this rash is a small pustule on an erythematous base that is slightly painful and can occur singularly or in masses; more than 20 of these lesions can occur predominantly on the extremities. Occasionally these lesions can be atypical can occur as small blisters. In the healing stage, the pustule often develops a central necrotic ulcerative lesion.

Most commonly, patients with disseminated gonococcemia have no pelvic inflammatory disease or urethritis. The gonococcal organism tends to disseminate during menses and in early pregnancy. The organism that causes disseminated gonococcemia may be of a different strain than that which causes pelvic inflammatory disease. There are much data to suggest this. First, the organism that causes disseminated gonococcemia has different nutritional requirements in culture than the organism that causes pelvic inflammatory disease. Second, normal human serum is bactericidal against the gonococcal organism. The organism that causes disseminated gonococcemia is relatively resistant to this bactericidal action.

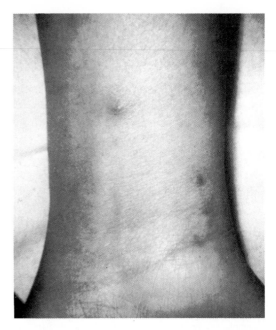

Figure 4–29. Skin lesions of disseminated gonococcal infection. The major lesion is vesicopustular, surmounting a hemorrhagic base. The other two smaller lesions appear more necrotic and probably represent older lesions. (From Kelley WN, et al.: Textbook of Rheumatology, 2nd ed. Philadelphia: WB Saunders Co, 1985.)

LABORATORY DATA

Once disseminated gonococcemia is suspected, the urethra, oropharynx, vagina, and rectum should be cultured for gonococcus even if the patient is asymptomatic.

Table 4–6. DIFFERENCES BETWEEN REITER'S SYNDROME AND GONOCOCCAL ARTHRITIS

	Reiter's Syndrome	Gonococcal Arthritis
Sex	Males > females	Males < females
Personal or family history of arthritis	+	−
Uveitis	+	−
Gonococcus culture:		
Joint	−	? +
Skin	−	? +
Pharynx	−	? +
Rectum	−	? +
Back pain	+	−
Migratory arthralgia	−	+
Joint distribution	Lower > upper	Lower < upper
Achilles tendonitis	+	−
Plantar fascitis	+	−
Massive recurrent knee effusion	+	−
Stomatitis	+	−
Balanitis	+	−
Keratoderma blennorrhagicum	+	−
Response to penicillin	−	+
HLA-B27 (%)	80	5
Course	Recurrent/chronic	Acute

The organism is infrequently isolated from joint fluid or skin lesions.

THERAPY

The therapy of choice for disseminated gonococcemia is 10,000 U of aqueous penicillin given intravenously each day until the skin lesions and arthritis subside, followed by 2 g of ampicillin in divided doses to complete a 10-day course. Because of several reports of penicillin-resistant disseminated gonnorrhea, some clinicians suggest ceftriaxone sodium or another third-generation cehalosporin as the initial therapy. Regimens of tetracycline and ampicillin administered orally have been effective. It is usually not necessary to repeatedly drain joints infected by gonococcemia because they resolve with adequate antibiotic therapy.

Nongonococcal Bacterial Arthritis

As contrasted with gonococcal arthritis, nongonococcal bacterial arthritis appears as an acute, exquisitely tender monoarticular arthritis. The patient generally is clinically ill, complaining of a high fever and marked malaise. Nongonococcal bacterial arthritis can involve any age group, from young children to the elderly. The most common joint involved in the foot is the ankle, and the most common joint involved in the body is the knee. However, any peripheral joint can be involved. A patient with a septic joint always has a source for the infection. The risk factors for development of a septic joint include evidence of an extra-articular infection. The most common source of extra-articular infection occurs in intravenous drug abusers who inject bacteria into their bodies by using contaminated needles. Other individuals at risk are elderly patients with underlying acute infection such as pyelonephritis or cholecystitis. Joints that have been previously affected by an arthritic process are at greatest risk for developing infection. This factor can present problems in making the diagnosis. For example, a patient with rheumatoid arthritis may have one joint that is inflamed out of proportion to the others. This can often be misdiagnosed as a flare of the underlying rheumatoid arthritis, and the bacterial infection can go undiagnosed for a period of time. Thus any time a patient presents with an acute monoarticular arthritis or with one joint inflamed out of proportion to the others, this joint must be aspirated, and the aspirate must be cultured. Other patients who are at increased risk for developing septic joint include those who are experiencing underlying chronic illnesses and who are immunocompromised because of the nature of their illness or medications.

DIAGNOSTIC TESTS

The nonspecific indicators of inflammation are almost always elevated, with an ESR and an elevated white blood cell count. Because of the acute nature of this problem, anemia is infrequent.

The diagnosis of a septic joint is established with an arthrocentesis. The joint fluid is a class III joint fluid, appearing grossly purulent with a count of greater than 100,000 white blood cells that are predominantly polymorphonuclear. The Gram's stain can be difficult to interpret because of large amounts of protein within the synovial fluid.

The culture results are invariably positive. The most common organism responsible for a septic joint is *Staphylococcus aureus*; the second most common organisms are *Streptococcus pneumoniae* and *Streptococcus viridans*. In the elderly, gram-negative infections, especially secondary to *Escherichia coli*, can be seen. In the pediatric population, septic joints secondary to *Haemophilus influenzae* can be seen. *Salmonella* infections occur in patients with sickle cell anemia. In heroin addicts, many unusual gram-negative organisms, especially *Pseudomonas*, have been isolated.

RADIOLOGY

The radiographic findings of a septic joint are initially periarticular osteoporosis with rapid development of destruction of the articular surfaces (Fig. 4–30). With a long-standing infection, periarticular new bone formation can occur. A distinctive radiographic finding is the asymmetry of the destruction. Often the changes in a septic joint could be confused with the changes in rheumatoid arthritis. However, the destructive changes occur quite rapidly, and the involved joint shows radiographic

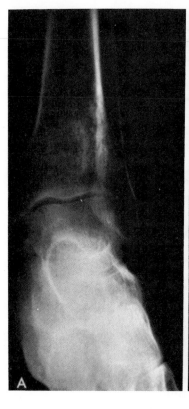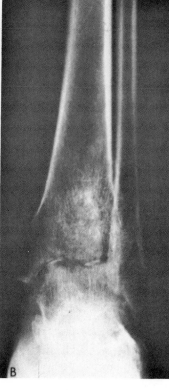

Figure 4–30. Progressive destructive radiographic changes in an ankle secondary to staphylococcal arthritis. *A*, Baseline radiograph of involved ankle space. Incidental bone infarct is noted. *B*, Ankle radiograph 2 months later detailing marked destruction of articular surfaces and obliteration of joint space. (Generously provided from the Philadelphia General Hospital X ray Teaching File at the Mütter Museum of the College of Physicians of Philadlephia.)

changes out of proportion to the contralateral joint.

THERAPY

If a class III joint fluid is obtained on arthrocentesis, therapy must be instituted even before the return of the joint fluid culture results. A septic joint should be treated as if it were an abscess. Thus drainage is necessary. Closed drainage with a large-bore needle is the preferred method. Initially this is necessary at least once and occasionally twice per day. Cell counts can be followed to monitor the adequacy of therapy. If inadequate drainage is obtained using closed drainage, surgical drainage is necessary. Often this also includes débridement of the area to facilitate adequate drainage of the entire joint surface.

The patient should be treated with large doses of intravenous antibiotics to which the organism is sensitive. It is not necessary to instill antibiotics directly into the joint because they avidly enter into infected joints when administered intravenously, with good levels of antibiotics being achieved within the joint.

The degree of morbidity in a septic joint is related to the length of time that it takes to establish the diagnosis. If diagnosed within the first 4 days, the prognosis is excellent. If diagnosed after a week, the prognosis for preservation of the normal architecture of the joint is poor.

Tuberculous Arthritis

The patient with tuberculous arthritis presents with a chronic, slowly destructive arthritis and few if any systemic symptoms. Tuberculous arthritis is the rarest form of septic arthritis. The distribution of this arthritis has changed in the postantibiotic era, with an older age group being involved and predominantly peripheral joints being infected. Prior to the advent of tuberculosis therapy, the major target of this arthritis was the axial skeleton and large weight-bearing joints. In addition, this disease was predominantly a pediatric one. All the small joints of the feet have been reported to be involved with tuberculous arthritis. As mentioned, these patients have few systemic symptoms but rather present with a slowly destructive, chronically inflamed joint.

Diagnosis

One should have a high index of suspicion for tuberculous arthritis if one observes a joint that has become slowly destroyed over a long period of time. Radiographs of the involved joint show nonspecific destructive changes. There are generally periarticular osteoporosis and occasionally sequestered bone around the area of destruction. In addition, there can be periosteal new bone formation in the vicinity of the joint. Laboratory studies generally show a mildly ESR. The purified protein derivative (PPD) is positive in approximately 95% of patients with tuberculosis. The chest radiograph findings are positive in only 50% of patients with tuberculous arthritis. These patients rarely have active tuberculosis but rather have evidence of old, inactive tuberculosis. The joint fluid in tuberculosis is generally a class II joint fluid. The Ziehl-Neelsen stain of the joint fluid is positive in less than 20% of patients and is positive on culture in approximately 80% of patients. The diagnosis of tuberculous arthritis is established by synovial biopsy. The biopsy is positive histologically for tuberculosis 95% of the time and yields the organism on culture in 95% of patients. The classic histologic picture of tuberculosis includes caseating granuloma and Langhans' giant cells.

Therapy

Tuberculous arthritis is managed with isoniazid and either rifampin or ethambutol given for a period from 1 year to 18 months. Usually it is not necessary to surgically débride the infected joint.

Viral Arthritis

Patients with viral arthritis have a much different clinical presentation than that of patients with bacterial arthropathies or tuberculous arthritis. The clinical presentation is similar to early rheumatoid arthritis or SLE, with a patient presenting with a symmetric small joint arthritis with a great deal of morning stiffness and swelling. The most common viral arthritis is the prodrome of hepatitis B. This disease is analogous to a serum sickness model of arthritis. Prior to the clinical onset of hepatitis, the patient develops a symmetric small joint arthritis. With the development of frank hepatitis, the patient's arthritis generally resolves. The diagnosis is confirmed in the laboratory by finding a positive hepatitis surface antigen and generally a mild increase in the liver transaminase concentrations. A similar clinical presentation can be seen in conjunction with hepatitis A, rubella, rubella vaccination, and adenovirus infection.

Lyme Disease

This arthritis is caused by the spirochete *Borrelia burgdorferi* transmitted by the *Ixodes dammini* tick. The disease classically begins as an expanding skin rash, erythema chronicum migrans (Fig. 4–31). This can often begin as a red macule or papule that gradually expands to form a large annular lesion with a flat erythematous border. Shortly after the development of the rash, patients can experience a migratory polyarthritis and tendonitis. Usually these patients have minimal morning stiffness. Later in the course, patients can develop a persistent arthritis involving predominantly the knees and to a lesser degree the ankles.

Specific IgM and IgG antibody titers can be obtained for diagnosis. These patients can have a positive fluorescent treponemal antibody absorption (FTA-ABS) test result.

Oral penicillin or tetracycline can eradicate the early manifestations of Lyme disease. Approximately 40% of patients with the late arthritis respond to large doses of penicillin or ceftriaxone.

Perioperative Considerations in Rheumatic Diseases

When considering perioperative management of rheumatic diseases, one must look at each of the rheumatic diseases individually.

Osteoarthritis. There are no specific perioperative considerations for the management of osteoarthritis. However, the elderly seem to be predisposed to the development of this disease, and these patients generally have a number of other medical problems that must be considered.

Rheumatoid Arthritis. Many patients

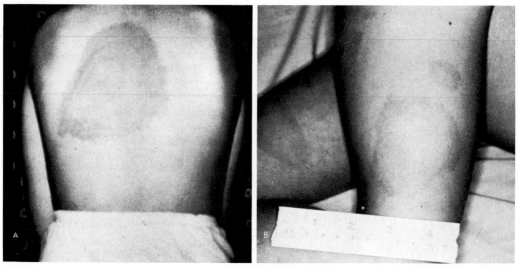

Figure 4–31. Two patients are seen, one with erythema chronicum migrans (*A*), the other with secondary annular lesions (*B*). The lesions began as red macules that expanded to form large rings. In *A*, the outer border is an intense red, the middle shows partial clearing, and the center is indurated. In *B*, the outer rims are red, and centers show nearly complete clearing. The lesions were hot to touch. (Reproduced, with permission, from Steere AC, et al.: Ann Intern Med 86:685, 1977.)

coming to surgery for the treatment of rheumatoid arthritis have been on long-term steroids. These suppress the pituitary adrenal axis, and these patients require corticosteroid coverage during their perioperative period. This should be given even if it has been a year since the patient has received cortisone for rheumatoid arthritis. It is not necessary to treat a patient with adrenocorticosteroids if they have received only intra-articular injections of cortisone. The appropriate dosage of adrenocorticosteroids is discussed in Chapter 5.

The one articular consideration in the operative patient is the atlantoaxial joint of the neck. Even if a patient has not had neck symptoms, a lateral view of the neck in flexion should be done. If there is greater than a 4-mm distance between the anterior arch of C-1 and the odontoid process, the patient should be sent to surgery with a cervical collar in place. The collar prevents marked flexion of the neck during the induction of anesthesia, which could possibly result in damage to the spinal cord and neurologic impairment.

Nonsteroidal anti-inflammatory drugs and disease-remittive drugs can safely be stopped for several days during the perioperative period.

Systemic Lupus Erythematosus. If the patient has received corticosteroids within the last year prior to surgery, he or she, similar to the patient with rheumatoid arthritis, should receive stress-coverage levels of replacement corticosteroids during the perioperative period (see Chapter 5). Because SLE is a multisystem disease, a careful history should be taken and the patient should be given a physical examination prior to surgery to make sure there is no significant organ impairment that would interfere with the induction of anesthesia.

Reiter's Syndrome, Psoriatic Arthritis, and Colitic Arthritis. There are no specific perioperative considerations for these diseases.

Crystal-Induced Arthritis

Gout. Patients with gout are at increased risk for developing an acute attack during the perioperative period, as discussed previously. The reasons for this are discussed in the section on gout but emanate from an acute rise in the uric acid, which can occur in the perioperative period for several reasons. It is not necessary for the patient to receive prophylactic colchicine during the perioperative period, but if the patient should develop an acute attack of gout postoperatively, intravenous colchicine or a local injection of cortisone directly into the inflamed area or joint is the treatment of choice. Either one of these agents generally promptly ameliorates an acute attack of gout, especially if given early. The patient's uric acid–lowering drugs should be reinstituted as soon as possible postoperatively.

Chondrocalcinosis. There are no specific perioperative considerations for this disease.

Septic Arthritis. A patient should never undergo surgery if there is any chance that the joint is infected. If there is a past history of infection, specimens should be taken at the time of surgery for histologic evidence of infection and for cultures.

Bibliography

Kelley WN, Harris ED, Ruddy S, Sledge CB (eds): Textbook of Rheumatology, 3rd ed. Philadelphia: WB Saunders Co, 1989.

Moskowitz RW: Clinical Rheumatology: A Problem-Oriented Approach to Diagnosis and Management, 2nd ed. Philadelphia: Lea & Febiger, 1982.

Resnick D, Niwayama G: Diagnosis of Bone and Joint Disorders, 2nd ed. Philadelphia: WB Saunders Co, 1988.

Rodnan GP, Schumacher R, Zaifler NJ (eds): Primer of the Rheumatic Diseases. Atlanta: Arthritis Foundation, 1983.

Snyderman R (ed): Advances in Rheumatology. Med Clin North Am 70:215, 1986.

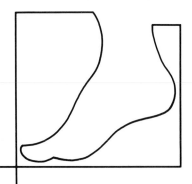

5 ENDOCRINOLOGY

BENNETT G. ZIER

OVERVIEW

Endocrinology is the study of the normal and disordered function of the hormone-secreting cells of the endocrine organs and their metabolic consequences. The endocrine glands are responsible for homeostasis in health and disease (Fig. 5–1). They synthesize, store, and secrete hormones from specific organ tissues that affect the functioning of other organs. The endocrine glands have an extremely important role in maintaining stability of the internal environment of the organism in the face of stress such as trauma, surgery, and infection.

PATHOPHYSIOLOGY

The principal organs involved in the endocrine system are the pituitary, thyroid,

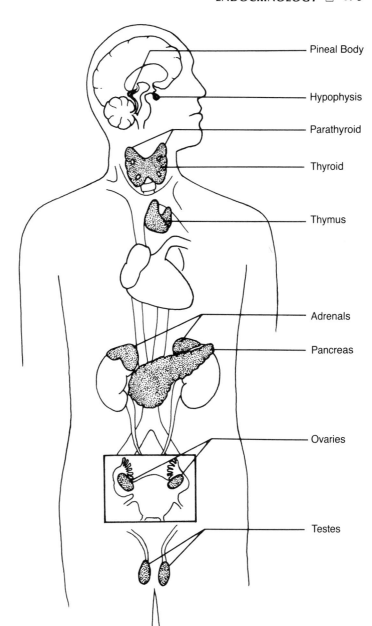

Pineal Body

Hypophysis

Parathyroid

Thyroid

Thymus

Adrenals

Pancreas

Ovaries

Testes

Figure 5–1. The glands of the endocrine system.

parathyroid, adrenal, pancreatic islet cells, testes, and ovaries. Each of these glands secretes particular hormones with specific actions on target tissues (Table 5–1). In order for the endocrine system to maintain stability of the internal environment, it must perceive and react to stimuli. Before endocrine hormones can be secreted, there must be recognition of the stimuli by the nervous system. Therefore, the nervous and endocrine systems are intimately integrated. The stimuli must first be appreciated by the nervous system, which then sends neural impulses to specific endo-

crine organs. The endocrine organs may then send hormones to other endocrine organs. A specific example is the appreciation of stress by the nervous system, whereupon hypothalamic factors and catecholamines are secreted. These hypothalamic factors and catecholamines stimulate the anterior pituitary and its target organs. Every cell in the body is activated by this reaction until a new steady state is achieved in response to the stimulus.

The clinical approach to endocrinologic problems begins with identifying patients with true endocrinologic disorders from

Table 5–1. HORMONES: TARGET TISSUES AND ACTIONS

Gland	Hormones	Target Tissue	Action
Anterior pituitary	ACTH	Adrenal cortex	Stimulates synthesis, release of corticosteroids and adrenocorticotropics
	TSH	Thyroid gland	Stimulates synthesis, release of thyroxine and triiodothyronine
	GH	Generalized effect	Promotes growth through protein anabolism, insulin antagonism, and lipolysis
	Prolactin	Mammary glands	Stimulates production of breast milk
	LH	Follicle (female)	Stimulates ovulation, progesterone secretion, luteinization of ovarian follicle
	FSH	Follicle (female)	Stimulates follicle maturation; estrogen secretion
		Testes (male)	Stimulates spermatogenesis
	ICSH	Testes (male)	Stimulates secretion of testosterone
	αMSH, βMSH	Melanocytes	Promote pigmentation
Posterior pituitary	Vasopressin (ADH)	Kidney collecting ducts, distal tubules, blood vessel walls	Promotes water retention, decreases urinary output, smooth muscle contraction
	Oxytocin	Mammary alveoli, uterus	Stimulates milk ejection into duct, uterine contraction
Thyroid	Thyroxine, triiodothyronine	Generalized effect	Stimulates catabolic metabolism, organ growth, and differentiation; affects nervous system function
Parathyroid	PTH	Generalized effect	Regulates calcium and phosphorus metabolism
Adrenal cortex	Glucocorticoids	Generalized effect	Regulates intermediate carbohydrate, protein metabolism, increases blood sugar
	Mineralocorticoids	Generalized effect	Regulates sodium and fluid balance, affects serum sodium and potassium levels
	Androgens	Generalized effect	Governs certain secondary sex characteristics
Adrenal medulla	Epinephrine	Generalized effect	Elevates blood pressure, increases heart rate, dilates bronchioles, elevates blood sugar
	Norepinephrine	Generalized effect	Elevates blood pressure owing to peripheral resistance
Pancreas (islets of Langerhans)	Insulin	Generalized effect	Promotes metabolism of carbohydrates, proteins, and fat
	Glucagon	Generalized effect	Raises blood glucose via mobilized glycogen stores
Ovaries	Estrogen, progesterone	Generalized effect	Secondary sex development, endometrial repair after menses
Testes	Testosterone	Reproductive organs	Secondary sex development, normal reproductive function

among patients with nonspecific complaints that can mimic symptoms associated with these disorders. Many endocrine diseases begin subtly and progress very slowly. It is one thing to make the diagnosis of hypothyroidism in someone who has a huge goiter, but quite another to diagnose the same disease in someone who has a common complaint such as fatigue. When an endocrine disorder is suspected, the next step is to identify more specific signs in physical findings and then to carry out laboratory studies that support the diagnosis. The last step is laboratory confirmation of endocrine dysfunction. Fortunately, there is increased sophistication in measuring hormone concentrations in body fluids. Radioimmunoassay (RIA) of specific hormones can be done for many endocrine organs. However, there must be careful correlation of hormonal assay values with clinical signs and symptoms.

When the diagnosis of an endocrine disease is established, it is important to determine its etiology. In the first half of the 20th century, infectious diseases were a common cause of endocrine gland destruction. However, in the last 30 years or so, the phenomenon of autoimmune destruction has assumed more of this etiologic role.

Endocrinologic problems usually do not create serious complications for patients who need surgery if the diagnosis is known. Complications arise in the patient who has unsuspected hypothyroidism, diabetes, or adrenal insufficiency that is found either intraoperatively or postoperatively. The podiatric practitioner must be aware of signs and symptoms consistent with endocrine dysfunction as well as understand the management of endocrine problems during clinical podiatric situations, whether they be medical or surgical.

PRESENTING FEATURES

Subjective Symptoms

Weight Change. Probably the most important factor in determining weight change is to document that the weight change has indeed occurred. Weight loss is a very nonspecific symptom that is associated not only with endocrine dysfunction, but with many other systemic problems such as neoplasms and gastrointestinal dysfunction. Endocrinologically, weight loss may indicate adrenal insufficiency, hyperthyroidism, or uncontrolled diabetes mellitus. Weight gain is most commonly due to overeating. However, certain endocrinologic problems such as Cushing's syndrome (i.e., glucocorticoid hyperfunction) are marked by a specific type of weight gain. In Cushing's syndrome, the fat is redistributed centrally; that is, the face is full and rounded, and there are supraclavicular pads of fat and a "buffalo hump" (an accumulation of fat in the back between the shoulders). However, the arms and legs are thin owing to loss of muscle mass. Hypothyroidism is also associated with weight gain; the patient presents with increased puffiness of the face and other subcutaneous tissues throughout the body.

Mass in Neck. When a patient complains of a mass in the neck and it involves an enlargement of the thyroid gland, this is called goiter. A goiter can refer to either a diffuse or a localized enlargement of the thyroid gland. It may be due to either hypothyroidism or hyperthyroidism.

Anxiety, Irritability, and Palpations. The aforementioned symptoms point out how subtle certain endocrine diseases may appear. Anxiety, irritability, and palpations as well as insomnia are cardinal symptoms of hyperthyroidism. These symptoms are also consistent with pheochromocytoma, which is an adrenal medullary tumor that produces excessive amounts of catecholamines. Of course, these symptoms may also be consistent with depression. It is impor-

tant to separate these symptoms and correlate them with a careful laboratory diagnosis.

Weakness, Fatigue, and Lethargy. These symptoms are not very specific and may also indicate an underlying psychologic problem. Disorders in other systems that can produce these symptoms include arthritis, disease of the central nervous system, heart disease, and respiratory disease as well as neoplasms and infections. Endocrinologically, patients with hypothyroidism present with weakness, fatigue, and lethargy. Adrenal insufficiency, hyperparathyroidism, and uncontrolled diabetes mellitus may also be associated with these symptoms.

Polyuria and Polydipsia. These symptoms are classic findings for poorly controlled or new-onset diabetes mellitus. Uncommonly, patients with hypercalcemia and hyperaldosteronism may also present with these symptoms.

Hyperhidrosis. Hyperhidrosis is a very common podiatric complaint. Patients with hyperthyroidism, pheochromocytoma, and hypoglycemia may all present with hyperhidrosis.

Pruritus. This is one of the classic symptoms of diabetes mellitus and hyperthyroidism.

Bone Pain. Bone pain is a podiatric complaint that may relate to hyperparathyroidism and osteomalacia.

Edema of the Extremities. This may reflect cardiovascular system pathology, namely, congestive heart failure. Edema of the extremities may also be a sign of Cushing's syndrome.

Objective Signs

Physical Examination

Striae. Striae are streaks or bands on the epidermis that are distinguished by color, texture, and depression or elevation from surrounding skin. Striae are found in pregnancy and obesity. In endocrine disease, striae are characteristically found in conditions of glucocorticoid excess. These striae are characteristically broad and purple and usually appear on the anterior abdominal wall. They are much broader and deeper than the striae in pregnancy or obesity, and they have an intense color. The intense color is due to heightened outpouring of adrenocorticotropic hormone

(ACTH), which causes hyperpigmentation.

Hyperpigmentation. Adrenocorticotropic hormone and melanocyte-stimulating hormone (MSH), both of which are produced by the pituitary gland, can directly increase pigmentation of the skin. These pigmentary changes occur when there is hypersecretion of endogenous ACTH, as in adrenal insufficiency. Also in adrenal insufficiency, hypersecretion of MSH occurs. Usually there is a diffuse tan over the nonexposed as well as the exposed parts of the body. The skin looks dirty, particularly over the knees, elbows, and other pressure points.

Onycholysis. Onycholysis is separation of the nail plate at its free edge from the nail bed. Onycholysis can be seen in psoriasis and fungal infections of the nails. In endocrine disease, it is often observed in diabetes mellitus and thyrotoxicosis.

Ecchymoses. Ecchymoses occur most often in an exccessive glucocorticoid state, in which there is increased protein metabolism and thus increased skin fragility.

Diaphoresis. Diaphoresis refers to sweating, which occurs in hypermetabolic states such as fever and, of course, in exercise. One of the classic signs of acute hypoglycemia is acute diaphoresis. This is due to an outpouring of epinephrine, which raises blood glucose and causes increased sweating. Patients with thyrotoxicosis or hyperthyroidism may also present with diaphoresis as a prominent feature.

Skin Ulcers. One of the most common ischemic and neuropathic complications of diabetes mellitus is skin ulcers over the tips of the toes, the heels, the metatarsal heads, and the dorsal arches.

Seizures. Although seizures may indicate an underlying idiopathic disorder, they may also be a consequence of hypoglycemia as well as other metabolic abnormalities such as hypocalcemia and hyponatremia.

Laboratory and Physiologic Data

Electrolyte Abnormalities. Patients with endocrine disorders can present commonly with electrolyte abnormalities. Hypernatremia may be indicative of adrenal insufficiency. Low potassium, or hypokalemia, may be a sign of hyperaldosteronism.

Calcium. Hypocalcemia is a very important finding in hypoparathyroidism, and hypercalcemia is a classic sign of hyperparathyroidism.

Glucose. Hyperglycemia is a cardinal manifestation of diabetes mellitus. Hypoglycemia indicates any one of a number of underlying conditions and is commonly encountered as a consequence of excessive insulin administration.

Serum Ketones. Serum ketones are mainly found in two conditions, diabetic ketoacidosis and starvation.

Anemia. Anemia is a nonspecific finding that may indicate underlying hypothyroidism as well as adrenal insufficiency.

Abnormalities in Urinalysis. Glycosuria is found in diabetes mellitus and in gestational diabetes; urinary ketones are found in diabetic ketoacidosis as well as in starvation.

Electrocardiogram Abnormalities. The electrocardiogram (ECG) is an important tool in diagnosing acute electrolyte abnormalities. Patients with *hyperkalemia* may present with *elevated T waves*. Patients with *hypokalemia* often exhibit *low-amplitude T waves*. Patients with *hypercalcemia* may present with a *short QT* interval, and patients with *hypocalcemia* may present with a *prolonged QT* interval. The ECG is particularly helpful in situations that are medical emergencies in which immediate information regarding suspected electrolyte imbalances must be rapidly confirmed.

Thyroid Function Tests. Thyroid function tests are discussed under Thyroid Disorders.

Adrenal Function Tests. Adrenal function tests are discussed under Adrenal Disorders.

Glycosolated Hemoglobin. Glycosolated hemogloben is discussed under Diabetes Mellitus.

ASSESSMENT OF CLINICAL SYNDROMES AND DISEASE STATES

Diabetes Mellitus

Pathogenesis

Diabetes mellitus refers to a group of diseases that share glucose intolerance as a

Table 5–2. CLASSIFICATIONS OF DIABETES MELLITUS

1. Insulin-dependent (IDDM), type I, juvenile-onset, or ketosis-prone diabetes
2. Non–insulin-dependent (NIDDM), type II, adult-onset, maturity-onset, or nonketotic diabetes
3. Secondary:
    a. Pancreatic disease: hemochromatosis, pancreatic deficiency, pancreatectomy
    b. Hormonal: Cushing's syndrome, acromegaly, pheochromocytoma
    c. Drug-induced: thiazides, diuretics, steroids, phenytoin
    d. Genetic syndromes: lipodystrophy, myotonic dystrophy, ataxia, telangiectasia
4. Impaired glucose tolerance (IGT), also known as chemical, latent, borderline, or subclinical
5. Gestational: glucose intolerance with onset during pregnancy

cardinal feature. Insulin produced by beta cells in the pancreas decreases blood glucose by inhibiting glycogen breakdown and facilitates entry of glucose into tissue cells. When tissues fail to use glucose, this results in hyperglycemia and glycosuria. If tissues cannot use glucose fats are broken down at an increased rate, and this causes ketosis, as found in the serum and in the urine.

Diabetes affects approximately 2 to 5% of the population in the United States. There are a number of subtypes of diabetes mellitus (Table 5–2).

Clinical Features

Type I (IDDM). Insulin-dependent diabetes mellitus was formerly called juvenile-onset diabetes mellitus but is now referred to as type I because it is not restricted to the juvenile age group. It is characterized by abrupt onset, polyuria, polydipsia, polyphagia, and often rapid weight loss.

Type II (NIDDM). Non–insulin-dependent diabetes mellitus was formerly called adult-onset diabetes mellitus. The symptoms are less pronounced than in type I. Patients with NIDDM present classically with thirst, pruritus, and fatigue. Obesity is present in 60 to 90% of these patients (Table 5–3).

Diagnosis

The diagnosis of diabetes mellitus has serious medical, psychologic, and financial (eligibility for health and disability insurance) implications. There must be objective data to support the diagnosis. The most objective laboratory measurement is elevation of blood glucose concentration, or hyperglycemia. In the absence of stress or glucose-raising drugs, diabetes mellitus may be diagnosed in patients with classic symptoms (polyuria, polydipsia, and polyphagia) and definite hyperglycemia (fasting plasma glucose level greater than 140 mg/dl on more than one occasion).

When diabetes mellitus is suspected and fasting plasma glucose level is greater than 140 mg/dl, a standardized oral glucose tolerance test (OGTT) may be done. The Na-

Table 5–3. DISTINGUISHING FEATURES OF DIABETES MELLITUS

Features	IDDM*	NIDDM†
Age of onset	< 30 yrs	> 40 yrs
Prevalence	0.2–0.3%	2–4%
Ketosis	Common	Rare
Weight	Normal	Obese (80%)
Complications	Frequent	Frequent
Genetics: HLA‡	Yes	No
Monozygotic twins	40–50%	Concordance near 100%
Islet cell antibodies	Yes	No
Insulin secretion	Severe deficiency	Variable: Moderate to hyperinsulinism
Insulin treatment	Always	Usually not required
Insulin resistance	Occasional: Poor control, excessive antibodies	Usual: Receptor, postreceptor defects

* IDDM, Insulin-dependent diabetes mellitus; also called juvenile-onset diabetes mellitus and type I diabetes mellitus.
† NIDDM, Non–insulin-dependent diabetes mellitus; also called adult-onset diabetes mellitus and type II diabetes mellitus.
‡ HLA, Human leukocyte antigen.

tional Diabetes Data Group recommends giving a 75-g glucose dose dissolved in 300 ml of water for adults after an overnight fast in subjects who have been receiving at least 150 to 200 g of carbohydrate daily for 3 days before the test. A diagnosis of diabetes mellitus requires plasma glucose levels to be above 200 mg/dl at both 2 hours and at least one other time between zero and 2 hours.

Carbohydrate intolerance can be caused by special situations, and the resultant hyperglycemia should not be classified as diabetes mellitus. Such situations include pregnancy; advanced age; use of drugs such as glucocorticoids, thiazide diuretics, oral contraceptives, or diphenylhydantoin; and stress.

The hemoglobin A_{1C} (glycosylated hemoglobin) blood test is utilized in diagnosis of diabetes mellitus. Diabetics have a two- to threefold elevation in this minor hemoglobin, which is present in normal individuals at a concentration of 3 to 6%. Its concentration is a rough reflection of the mean level of circulating glucose for the previous 2 to 3 months. It is a useful index of 2- to 3-month hyperglycemic control, whereas blood glucose levels are subject to instantaneous fluctuations related to many variables. Hemoglobin A_{1C} is a helpful supplement to blood glucose values.

Treatment

Data suggest that persistent hyperglycemia may be the trigger that sets off the development of micro- and macrovascular changes associated with complications of diabetes mellitus. A normal fasting blood glucose value and a 2-hour postprandial blood glucose value of 150 mg/dl or less are considered good control, meaning that there is infrequent hyperglycemia.

DIET

Diet is the cornerstone of diabetic treatment (Table 5–4). The objectives are to provide nutrition with balance of protein, carbohydrates, and fats and to normalize weight. The importance of weight reduction for the obese diabetic cannot be overstated. Most diabetes mellitus is manifested by obesity. Thus most overt diabetes mellitus in obese patients is potentially "curable" by weight reduction, provided that the disease has not been present for more than a few years.

ORAL HYPOGLYCEMICS

In the past, many NIDDM patients with symptomatic disease have been treated with oral hypoglycemic drugs (Table 5–5). Such treatment may improve glucose tolerance, although no evidence exists to support this. A controversial study of long-term use of tolbutamide suggests that the drug itself may increase the frequency of cardiovascular problems. This study has been criticized by many observers; however, the result of this study is that oral hypoglycemics have been less in favor as antidiabetic agents than in the past.

Oral hypoglycemic therapy for modest elevations of fasting plasma glucose level is not warranted. The official recommendation of the American Medical Association Council on Drugs as well as the American Diabetic Association is that sulfonylureas should be limited to patients with symptomatic NIDDM who cannot be controlled by diet and in whom an addition of insulin is impractical or unacceptable (such as the blind diabetic who lives alone). Sulfonylureas can cause hypoglycemic reactions that can be quite severe and can last for several days. These drugs are contraindicated in patients with he-

Table 5–4. ELEMENTS OF DIET TREATMENT REGIMENS FOR DIABETES MELLITUS

1. Fundamental element of therapy: well-balanced, nutritional
2. Obese, mild hyperglycemia: weight reduction, caloric restriction
3. Insulin-dependent, nonobese: timing of meals, periodic snacks, exchange list
4. Caloric restriction for obtaining and maintaining ideal weight
5. With weight reduction no greater than 1–1.5 kg/week (1500–2000 calories) and even slower weight reduction in the older patient
6. Distribution of caloric intake: widest timing possible of meals during day
7. Avoidance of rapidly absorbed carbohydrate loads
8. Exchange lists caloric distribution: breakfast 20%, lunch 30%, dinner 40%, bedtime snack 10%
9. Exchange list content: protein 15–20%, fat 30–35%, carbohydrate 45–50%

Table 5-5. ORAL HYPOGLYCEMIC AGENTS

	Generic Name	Trade Name	Duration (hrs)	Dosage (mg)
First Generation	Tolbutamide	Orinase	6–12	500–3000
	Tolazamide	Tolinase	10–18	100–1000
	Chlorpropamide	Diabinese	36+	100–500
	Acetohexamide	Dymelor	12–24	250–500
Second Generation	Glyburide	DiaBeta	24	1.25–5.0
	Glipizide	Glucotrol	24	5–40
	Glyburide	Micronase	24	2.5–3.0

patic and renal insufficiency. Special attention must be given to drug interactions. Acetylsalicylic acid, phenytoin, propranolol, barbiturates, ethanol, clofibrate, phenylbutazone, and acetaminophen all can affect the hypoglycemic activity of sulfonylureas.

Oral Hypoglycemic Management During Surgery. For a discussion of oral hypoglycemic management during surgery, see under Podiatric Implications.

INSULIN THERAPY

Insulin is used primarily for the type I (IDDM) diabetic who is hypoinsulinemic and prone to ketosis. It can also be provided for the overweight type II diabetic who is not compliant with diet. Insulin therapy may be given on a short-term basis in pregnant patients with severe gestational diabetes or in other patients with severe infctions, stress (i.e. surgery), or both.

Types of Insulin. There are several different types of insulin (bovine, bovine-porcine, and human) with varying lengths of activity (short, intermediate, and long) (Table 5–6). When animal insulin is introduced into the human body, it acts as a foreign substance, causing formation of anti-bodies that results in a form of insulin resistance. Use of human insulin eradicates this problem. Human insulin may be semisynthetic or may be produced by recombinant DNA technology. Both types of human insulin are structurally identical to the insulin produced naturally in the body and therefore cause no antibody formation. Many patients with a single morning dose of intermediate-acting insulin (insulin zinc suspension [Lente] or NPH) can achieve near normal blood glucose levels. Other patients require mixtures of various forms of insulin (usually regular and intermediate-acting) and may require more than a single dose per day, usually before breakfast and before dinner. Insulin therapy together with proper diet can prevent diabetic ketoacidosis and other diabetic complications (see under Complications of Diabetes). Insulin is the most physiologic hypoglycemic medication. The axiom "You can always give insulin, but never neurons" is an extremely useful reminder that insulin-induced hypoglycemia should be carefully avoided. If a patient has "brittle" diabetes (type I diabetes mellitus that is poorly controlled owing to wide, unpredictable fluctuation of blood glucose levels) the patient's glucose level should al-

Table 5-6. COMMERCIALLY AVAILABLE INSULINS

Type	Onset (hrs)	Peak of Action (hrs)	Duration (hrs)
Rapid-acting			
Regular	½–1	2–4	5–7
Semilente	½–1	2–4	12–16
Intermediate-acting			
NPH	1–2	6–12	24–48
Lente	1–4	6–12	24–28
Long-acting			
Ultralente	4–8	18–24	36+
Protamine zinc	4–8	20–30	36+

ways be on the side of hyperglycemia—not hypoglycemia. See Table 5–6 for commercially available insulins.

Insulin Management in Surgery. For discussion of insulin management in surgery, see under Podiatric Implications.

Complications of Diabetes

ACUTE

Diabetic ketoacidosis accounts for approximately 10% of diabetic deaths. The mortality from diabetic ketoacidosis ranges from 1 to 20%. Precipitating factors are usually infection, omission of insulin, new onset of diabetes, or stress. Diabetic ketoacidosis is characterized by hyperglycemia and ketosis both in the blood and urine. In diabetic ketoacidosis, there is

relatively absolute insulin deficiency, which causes increased lipolysis, resulting in a rise in fatty acids in the blood, leading to ketosis. Hyperglycemia leads to an osmotic diuresis and depletion of water and then dehydration. The ketosis leads to acidosis and potential cardiac arrhythmias. Treatment is administration of fluids and electrolyte therapy as well as insulin therapy. If the underlying cause is infection, it obviously must be treated (Fig. 5–2, Table 5–7).

HYPEROSMOLAR NONKETOTIC HYPERGLYCEMIC COMA

Hyperosmolar nonketotic hyperglycemic coma is defined as significant hyperglycemia (blood glucose value greater

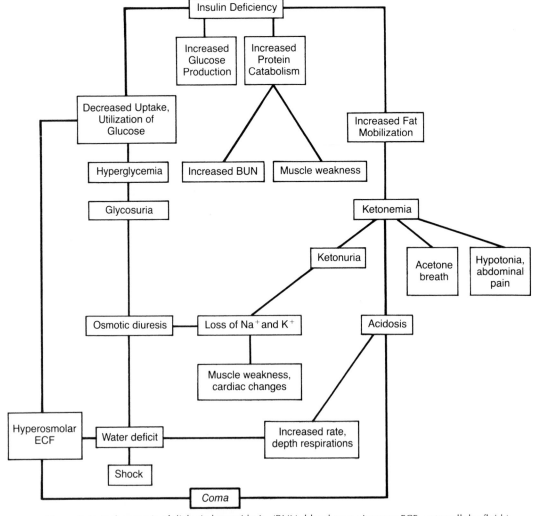

Figure 5–2. Pathogenesis of diabetic ketoacidosis. (BUN, blood urea nitrogen; ECF, extracellular fluid.)

Table 5–7. TREATMENT FOR DIABETIC KETOACIDOSIS

Prevention

Recognition of early symptoms and signs
Supplemental regular insulin for persistent ketonuria, glycosuria
Replenish fluids and electrolytes; broth, lightly salted tomato juice
Contact physician if ketonuria persists, if vomiting occurs, or if insulin pump adjustment does not correct ketonuria or hyperglycemia

Emergency Measures
Therapeutics

Hospitalize for correction of hyperosmolarity, ketoacidemia
Monitor vital signs, diagnostic laboratory values as related to therapy (urine glucose and ketones, arterial pH, plasma glucose, acetone, bicarbonate, electrolytes)
Indwelling catheter if comatose, nasogastric tube with sodium bicarbonate lavage
No sedatives or narcotics

Insulin Replacement

Regular insulin initially in all cases of severe ketoacidosis
Loading dose 0.3 U/kg IV bolus followed by 0.1 U/kg/hr continuous IV drip or IM
Repeat loading dose if glucose level falls < 10% in first hour
Insulin resistance requires doubling dose q 2–4 h with no improvement in hyperglycemia after first 2 doses (anaphylaxis may occur in resistant patients requiring high IV doses)
Continue insulin q 2–4 h until ketonemia has cleared

Fluid and Electrolyte Replacement

4–5 Fluid deficit, *solution of choice—normal saline* 1000 ml in first hour, then 0.45% Saline 300–500 ml/hr if glucose > 500 mg/dl
5% Glucose solution if glucose falls to 250 mg/dl or less (maintain between 200–300 mg/dl)
1–2 Ampules of sodium bicarbonate (44 mEq) added to hypotonic saline solution if pH = 7 or less or bicarbonate < 9 mEq/l
Monitor potassium carefully, normal or high until after first few hours of treatment; replace as necessary
Replace phosphate that develops during insulin therapy in small amounts and slowly to prevent tetany (3 mmol/h)
Potassium and phosphate should be replaced separately

Treatment of Associated Infection

Often a precipitating cause
Appropriate antibiotics

---

than 600 mg/dl) and without significant ketosis or acidosis. This complication carries an excessive mortality rate of 40 to 70%. The clinical presentation is usually in an elderly, mildly diabetic patient with neurologic signs, (lethargy, confusion, seizure, and coma), hypertension, polyuria, and polydipsia. There is a frequent association with infection (usually gram-negative sepsis). The treatment is administration of fluids and very low-dose insulin (Table 5–8).

Table 5–8. TREATMENT FOR HYPEROSMOLAR NONKETOTIC HYPERGLYCEMIC COMA

Fluid Replacement

Initiate with 0.45% saline or isotonic saline in circulatory collapse
4–6 l may be required in the first 8–10 hrs
Monitor blood pressure and urine output to determine IV solution
Hypotonic if maintained; after insulin therapy may need isotonic to avoid hypotension
Blood glucose reaches 250 mg/dl, may use D5W, D5/0.45 saline or 0.9% saline solution
Urine output of 50 ml/hr or more is end point of fluid therapy

Insulin

Initial dose—Regular 15 U subcutaneously
Monitor blood glucose during initial fluid replacement, which reduced hyperglycemia
Continue subsequent doses not greater than 10–25 U subcutaneously q 4 h

Potassium

Initiate early because of rapid decline with insulin therapy
Potassium chloride 10 mEq in initial bottle if serum potassium is not elevated
No initial hyperkalemia with the absence of acidosis and during initial stages of glycosuria

Phosphate

Replace phosphate that develops during insulin therapy in small amounts and slowly to prevent tetany (3 mmol/hr)
Potassium and phosphate should be replaced separately

D5W, 5% Dextrose in water; D5, 5% dextrose.

INFECTION

An impairment of host defenses occurs with diabetes. This may in part be due to granulocyte dysfunction as well as defective phagocyte ingestion. Specific infections seen in diabetes include vulvovaginal candidiasis, epidermophytosis, and ascending urinary tract infection*; pyelonephritis; septicemia; and gas infections.

Many of the infections mentioned can be prevented. Foot care can prevent or minimize infection in patients with poor vascular supply. Great caution must be taken before placing urinary catheters in diabetic patients. Influenza immunization is routinely indicated in all diabetic patients to reduce the risk of severe influenza infection. It is of utmost importance to remember that diabetics who are most prone to developing infection have some impairment of renal function. Renal function is the most important factor for determining antimicrobial selection in the diabetic. Penicillin or a cephalosporin is much more preferable than an aminoglycoside in terms of avoiding drug-induced nephrotoxicity. If one must use an aminoglycoside the patient's renal function must be closely watched. Peak and trough levels of the aminoglycoside must be monitored to be sure the patient is achieving a therapeutic level and is excreting the drug appropriately.

CHRONIC COMPLICATIONS

With the administration of insulin and improved diet, patients with diabetes mellitus are living longer. With increased longevity, the occurrence of chronic complications is a major problem. The complications correlate with the duration of the disease. Whether they correlate with the degree of control of the diabetic state is debatable. The common bias is that the worse the control, the worse the complication and the earlier it appears in the course of the disease.

Atherosclerosis. This occurs twice as frequently in the diabetic as in the nondiabetic. Diabetes mellitus seems to accelerate the arteriosclerotic process. How it does this is unknown. The incidence of coronary artery disease is greater in dia-

betics, and survival after myocardial infarction is shorter. Although most diabetics experience classic symptoms, approximately 10% experience little or no pain during a myocardial infarction. This is probably due to decreased pain appreciation in the diabetic as a result of autonomic neuropathic disease.

Cerebral Vascular Disease. Strokes frequently occur in diabetic patients owing to arteriosclerotic involvement of the cerebral vascular system.

Peripheral Vascular Disease. Of all nontraumatic amputations in the United States, 70% are a result of diabetes mellitus. Peripheral pulses are usually absent when large arterial involvement is present. However, in 20% of diabetics, the pulses are present, and signs of peripheral vascular disease are seen as a result of involvement of smaller arteries without significant involvement of large arteries. Small as well as large arteries are affected in diabetics; thus it is common to first see small distal areas involved before larger areas.

Diabetic Foot. This is a complex result of several processes that include (1) peripheral vascular disease; (2) thickening in the basement of the microscopic vessels, the arterioles; (3) peripheral neuropathy (Table 5–9); and (4) infection. The end result can be ulceration, leading to infection, gangrene, tissue loss, and amputation. It is important clinically to make the judgment as to whether the foot lesion has resulted from ischemia or neuropathy (Table 5–10). This differentiation has significance in that neuropathic disease has a better prognosis than ischemic disease. The objective of therapy for the diabetic foot is to preserve tissue, that is, to heal the foot lesion without amputation. Unfortunately, if this is not

Table 5–9. SUMMARY OF SIGNS AND SYMPTOMS OF DIABETIC NEUROPATHIC FOOT

Hyperesthesia	Loss of vibratory and position sense
Hypoesthesia	Heavy callus formation over pressure points
Pressure points	Infection complicating trophic ulcers
Radicular pain	Changes in foot shape
Anhydrosis	Muscle atrophy
Charcot's joint	Changes in bone and joints
Demineralization	Osteolysis

---

* Do not catheterize diabetics unnecessarily.

Table 5–10. SUMMARY OF UPPER AND LOWER EXTREMITY DIABETIC NEUROPATHY

Features	Symmetric	Asymmetric
Frequency	Common	Less common
Pathogenesis	Metabolic	Vascular
Onset	Usually slow	Usually rapid
Course	Poor prognosis	Variable
Sensory:		
Numbness	Feet, hands, stocking-glove	Spotty
Dysesthesia	Common	Common
Lightning pain	Common	Common
Cranial	Unusual	Frequent
Autonomic	Common	Common
CSF*	Protein elevated usually	Protein elevated usually
Nerve conduction	Generalized slowing: Sensory and motor	Focal slowing: Involved nerve

* CSF, Cerebrospinal fluid.

possible, amputation must be used as the final therapeutic option.

Ophthalmic Complications. The leading cause of blindness in the United States is diabetes mellitus. There are two types of eye lesions:

1. *Cataracts.* This begins with swelling of the lens due to increased osmolarity (from increased glucose in the lens). The lens protein then denatures, and cataracts form.

2. *Diabetic retinopathy.* This is usually observed 10 to 15 years after onset of diabetes mellitus. Diabetic retinopathy is thought to be related to ischemia of the retina due to diabetes mellitus.

Neuropathy. Clinical neuropathy usually begins about 10 years after the onset of diabetes mellitus. Different elements of the nervous system are involved (Table 5–11). *Peripheral neuropathy* occurs as a bilateral "stocking and glove" distribution (symmetric distal extremity location) with motor and sensory functions affected. This can lead to Charcot's joint and incapacitating pain syndrome. *Mononeuropathy* is a disorder of a single peripheral nerve, either mixed, spinal, or cranial. Onset is rapid and is accompanied by loss of motor and sensory function of the involved nerve. *Radiculopathy* is caused by an infarction of the nerve root. This causes a sensory syndrome in which symptoms and signs are present in the distribution of the nerve route. *Amyotrophy* is an asymmetric wasting and weakness of the muscles of the pelvic girdle. In *autonomic neuropathy*, any autonomic function can be affected by diabetes mellitus. This includes cardiovascular function (tachycardia, hypertension, or silent ischemic heart disease), gastrointestinal function (diarrhea), and genitourinary function (impotence).

Dermopathy. Two types of *dermopathy* are seen in the diabetic. One type is known as "shin spots" and appears as pig-

Table 5–11. ANATOMIC CLASSIFICATION OF DIABETIC NEUROPATHIES

Structure	Disorder	Etiology	Signs and Symptoms
Nerve root	Radiculopathy	Probably vascular	Pain, dermatome sensory loss
Mixed nerve (spinal or cranial)	Mononeuropathy	Probably vascular	Pain, weakness, sensory loss, reflex change
Nerve terminals	Polyneuropathy	Metabolic	Sensory loss: stocking-glove, mild weakness, absent reflex
Nerve terminal (muscle)	Amyotrophy	Unknown	Anterior thigh pain with weakness
Sympathetic ganglion	Autonomic neuropathy	Unknown	Postural hypotension, impotence, gastrophy, vesical atony, anhydrosis, Charcot-type arthropathy

mented atrophic lesions over the shin. The second type is also found in the anterior shin area and appears as a waxy-looking patch in which telangiectatic vessels may be seen centrally. This is called necrobiosis lipoidica diabeticorum (see Chapter 12).

Podiatric Implications

Medical Approach to the Ambulatory Diabetic

Patients with diabetes are commonly seen by internists and podiatrists alike. Just as an internist must be aware of podiatric complications of diabetes mellitus, so too should the podiatrist have a sense of the patient's overall health in regard to the diabetic disease. There should be frequent communication between the podiatrist and the primary physician regarding these matters. If the diabetic patient has no primary health provider, the podiatrist should refer the patient appropriately. The podiatric physician should keep a record of the patient's diabetic status (e.g., 6-month review of medications, recent blood glucose status) in the patient's chart. Preventive care for the diabetic patient is the responsibility of all health care providers, with special emphasis on foot health care rendered by the podiatrist.

Care of the Diabetic Foot

Foot problems are of vital clinical concern when rendering comprehensive care to the diabetic patient (Table 5–12). Diabetics are 17 times more likely to develop gangrene of the foot than are nondiabetics. Diabetes mellitus is a major factor involved in greater than 50% of amputations performed in the United States every year. Diabetic foot problems create significant difficulties in terms of utilization of hospital and economic resources.

Diabetic foot disease may be due to infection alone, may have a neuropathic factor (Table 5–13), or may be caused by ischemia. The patient with neuropathic foot with ischemic changes poses the most difficult therapeutic challenge. Such patients are vulnerable to trauma, which, if is-

Table 5–12. CHRONIC AND PROGRESSIVE COMPLICATIONS OF DIABETIC FOOT

Peripheral Neuropathy
Cranial-truncal-limb
Multiple mononeuropathies
Amyotrophy
Distal symmetric primary sensory polyneuropathy
Sensory and sensorimotor neuropathy
Acute distal motor neuropathy
Autonomic Neuropathy
Cardiovascular, GU, GI
Decreased sweating
Hypoglycemia symptoms response
Vasculopathy
Macrovascular disease—hypertension, MI, CVA
Microvascular disease—neuropathy, nephropathy, retinopathy
Osteoarthropathies
Radiographic signs: demineralization, osteolysis, Charcot's joint, bony deformity, calluses, blisters, "rockersole" callus infection, ulcerations
Dermopathies
Necrobiosis lipoidica diabeticorum, bullous diabeticorum, pruritus, vitiligo, glucagonoma (necrolytic migratory erythema).

CVA, Cardiovascular accident; GI, gastrointestinal; GU, genitourinary; MI, myocardial infarction.

chemia is present, may provide a poor environment for proper healing.

Common foot problems, all of which can be exacerbated by poorly fitting shoes, include the following:

- corns
- calluses
- fungus infections
- ingrown toenails
- blisters
- plantar warts
- fissures
- paronychia
- trauma

Table 5–13. DIAGNOSIS OF DIABETIC FOOT NEUROARTHROPATHIES

Duration
Diabetes 15 yrs or more
History
Peripheral neuropathy, lower extremity
Clinical Features
Early
Soft tissue swelling
Bony foot deformity
Lisfranc's joint involvement
Sequela to "Burnt-out" Process
Arrested: difficulty with shoe gear
Infection
Local complications of bony deformity

Any of these problems may resolve or, depending on the degree of ischemia, neuropathy, or both, may lead to serious infection with abscess, cellulitis, or gangrene.

Neuropathic Disease. Patients with neuropathic disease may complain of anesthesia to pain and temperature, and paresthesias may be present. The neuropathic foot may appear healthy. However, on physical examination, early signs of neuropathy may include absent or diminished ankle reflexes, vibratory sensation, or both. In advanced cases, a footdrop or Charcot-type lesion may be present. The pressure points are the areas that are potentially problematic. Pressure points on the soles and toes can lead to calluses and can cause bruising of the subcutaneous tissues. These localized areas of inflammation can serve as a medium for local bacteria to grow and cause an abscess. Because of neuropathic anesthesia, the patient may be unaware of the presence of an abscess, with the problem finally progressing to the stage of obvious infection. Often the callus is so hard that infection more easily invades the underlying joint capsule and bone, resulting in osteomyelitis.

For diagnosis, radiographic tests and nerve conduction studies are most helpful. Radiographs help to differentiate osteomyelitis, and nerve conduction studies can confirm a clinical diagnosis of neuropathy. Bone scanning is another procedure that may be helpful in differentiating bone resorption caused by either osteomyelitis or neuropathy. A positive technetium bone scan means that an active lesion is present, owing to osteomyelitis or neuropathy. A gallium bone scan is then done, which is positive if a focus of infection is present.

Ischemic Disease. A patient with an ischemic foot often has a history of intermittent claudication, nocturnal leg cramps, and ischemic paresthesias. Physical examination reveals absent or diminished hair growth. The peripheral pulses are diminished or absent, and the foot may be cool to the touch. Blanching with elevation and cyanosis with dependency may be found, with a venous refilling time of more than 15 to 20 seconds.

Diagnostic aids are utilized to find and localize any area of block that may be correlated with symptoms and signs of is-chemia. Noninvasive studies such as oscillometry and Doppler's ultrasonography are helpful. Arterial angiography, which outlines the aorta and iliac, femoral, and distal leg arteries, is the most direct approach and shows the exact condition of the blood vessels when surgery is contemplated.

Prognosis. The major concern is whether therapy is medical, surgical, or both. An estimate of the prognosis of the lesion can be made by evaluating whether there is a neuropathic or ischemic cause or a combination of the two and whether infection is present. All patients with significant foot lesions must be hospitalized and a team approach utilized by the podiatrist and internist.

Diabetes and Surgery

There are many successful regimens that can be used to treat the diabetic patient who is undergoing surgery. There are no data demonstrating the superiority of one approach over another. It is important that the practitioner use a consistent approach, one with which he or she is familiar. Regardless of approach, several principles must be adhered to, including the following:

1. A diabetic patient should be in good metabolic balance prior to surgery. This balance includes normal vital signs, normal electrolytes, and blood glucose level between 100 and 200 mg/dl. Knowledge of the patient's current renal and hepatic function is necessary. A preoperative electrocardiogram is essential in a diabetic patient because of the increased prevalence of atherosclerosis in diabetes.

2. In order to achieve normal metabolism before surgery, it is preferable to admit a diabetic patient to the hospital the day before surgery so as to adjust the patient's insulin or oral antidiabetic agent regimen.

3. Because capillary blood glucose monitoring is so readily available and inexpensive, the patient's blood glucose concentration should be measured frequently before, during, and after surgery. A reasonable approach would be a minimum of once per hour for several hours prior to and several hours after surgery. If the patient has "brittle" diabetes, blood glucose con-

centration measurement may be increased to every 30 minutes.

Management of Diabetes During Minor Surgical Procedures

In a diabetic in whom the anesthesia of choice is a local one and who will immediately be given oral nutrition postoperatively, there should be no change in diet, oral hypoglycemic medication, or insulin regimen. Blood glucose values should be obtained 1 hour before surgery as well as 1 hour after surgery to monitor the level of glycemia.

Management of Diabetes During Major Surgical Procedures

PREOPERATIVE EVALUATION

The following considerations are relevant in preoperative evaluation:

1. The patient's status as a type I (ketosis-prone) or type II diabetic should be determined.

2. The type of diabetic therapy being utilized, that is, diet, hypoglycemics, insulin, or some combination, should be determined.

3. How well controlled the patient's diabetes has been should be evaluated. This is determined by assessing symptoms and utilizing blood glucose determinations as well as glycosylated hemoglobin.

4. The patient should be examined for any chronic diabetic complications, such as arteriosclerosis, nephropathy, retinopathy, and autonomic neuropathy.

5. The patient should be admitted to the hospital a day prior to surgery. If the patient's diabetes mellitus is not well controlled, he or she may require hospitalization 2 to 3 days before surgery to stabilize his or her diabetic state. A fasting blood glucose value and at 4:00 P.M. a random blood glucose value should be obtained while the patient is still on his or her usual antidiabetic regimen. Blood glucose monitoring before each meal and at bedtime should be done to get a gross appreciation of plasma glucose level.

6. Preoperative laboratory and physiologic data should include an ECG, a urinalysis, electrolyte tests and renal function tests (e.g., blood urea nitrogen [BUN] and creatinine), and a glycosylated hemoglobin determination.

7. Surgery should be scheduled early in the day to provide the best equilibrium between morning insulin dose and caloric intake. Insulin should never be given until the intravenous line is in position, because insulin dosing in a fasting diabetic without an intravenous line to provide glucose will clearly lead to hypoglycemia.

8. One can assume that the diabetic treated by diet alone is fairly stable and not prone to ketosis. Such a patient requires no immediate special preoperative therapy other than a fasting blood glucose determination on the morning of surgery.

9. It is assumed that the diabetic treated with oral hypoglycemics is under reasonable control (preoperative blood glucose value is less than 250 mg/dl). The oral agent should be discontinued the morning before the day of surgery. Fasting blood glucose and 4:00 P.M. blood glucose values should be obtained the day before surgery. If control is poor, the patient may be given small doses (5 U) of regular insulin no more frequently than every 4 hours. Type II diabetics are often sensitive to small doses of insulin.

10. It is assumed that the diabetic treated with insulin is usually prone to ketosis. If the patient is under reasonable control (preoperative blood glucose value is less than 250 mg/dl), he or she should be given approximately one half the usual dose of insulin on the morning of surgery at the time the intravenous line is started.

INTRAOPERATIVE AND POSTOPERATIVE MANAGEMENT

The two most important considerations during this period are as follows:

1. Blood glucose should ideally be between 100 to 200 mg/dl. Healing and host defense against infection function best at this level.

2. The axiom that "you can always give insulin but never neurons" reinforces the importance of avoiding iatrogenic hypoglycemia. This may require frequent (every hour) intraoperative blood glucose testing. It is not good practice to use urine glucose as a monitor of blood glucose activity. There are too many variables (e.g., renal glucose threshold, state of hydration, difficulty in voiding) present to consider

this an accurate representation of intraoperative blood glucose.

With major procedures, there are two primary methods of management.

Method 1.   Preoperatively, start intravenous line with 1000 ml of 5% dextrose in water (D5W) with 40 mEq/L of potassium chloride to run at approximately 100 ml/hour.

Administer one half of usual morning insulin. Run a blood glucose test immediately after surgery is completed. Give regular insulin as per this value. Continue the intravenous fluids at a rate of 80 ml/hour, and monitor blood every 4 to 6 hours with appropriate regular insulin coverage.

Method 2.   Use low-dose continuous regular insulin. The intravenous solution consists of 100 U of regular insulin added to 500 ml of 0.5% normal saline solution. A continuous drip of 2 to 3 U of regular insulin is given every hour. Blood glucose is monitored every 30 minutes, and the rate of regular insulin infusion is determined by the blood glucose value.

Blood Glucose Level.   After surgery is completed, the most important information is the state of hydration of the patient as well as the level of blood glucose. In the diet-controlled diabetic, if the blood glucose level remains less than 300 mg/dl postoperatively, the patient can be managed on diet therapy alone, which usually begins 12 to 24 hours after surgery. In the diabetic taking oral hypoglycemics, if the blood glucose level is under control and the patient is eating, the oral agent can be started the day following surgery. These patients usually have blood glucose values in the range of 250 mg/dl or greater in spite of oral hypoglycemic dosing. If this occurs very small amounts of insulin should be used because certain types of diabetics may be very sensitive to insulin. The diabetic who is taking insulin requires frequent (every 4 hours for the first 12 postoperative hours) blood glucose testing. Insulin is to be given only if the patient's blood glucose values are greater than 300 mg/dl. Only regular (rapid-acting) insulin is to be used at intervals of 4 to 6 hours. Avoid giving insulin based on urinary glucose values (the so-called urinary glucose sliding scale).

Nutrition.   Nutrition must be carefully monitored in all postoperative patients, especially in diabetics. Patients may be fed by mouth within 1 to 2 days following surgery. If this is not possible intravenous fluids should be continued with careful attention to proper metabolic balance. Prolonged use of intravenous fluids as the sole source of nutrition should alert the practitioner to obtain a nutrition consultation. The use of nasogastric-tube feeding or total parenteral nutrition is a decision that requires careful deliberation, with consultation by an internal medicine specialist.

Hypoglycemia

Pathogenesis

Symptomatic hypoglycemia occurs when the central nervous system is deprived of sufficient glucose. Chemical hypoglycemia is defined as a plasma glucose level of less than 50 mg/dl, but this may not always be symptomatic. Levels less than 30 mg/dl are almost always associated with symptoms. The symptoms produced by hypoglycemia are caused by catecholamine release ("adrenergic discharge") and tend to manifest initially in lack of glucose in the central nervous system.

The causes of hypoglycemia are numerous. The most common and classic type of hypoglycemia is seen in insulin-dependent diabetics who have an imbalance between too much insulin and too little glucose. The next most common type is reactive hypoglycemia, which is a mismatch in timing between insulin secretion and absorption of food from the gastrointestinal tract.

A few conditions are associated with insulin overproduction. Insulin-producing tumors of the pancreas (insulinoma) can produce hypoglycemia. Fasting hypoglycemia occurs following alcohol ingestion. In this situation, glucose production by the liver can be blocked by alcohol. If a patient needs this source of glucose, which usually occurs after fasting, the ingestion of alcohol can cause profound hypoglycemia. Fortunately, adequate food intake during alcohol ingestion prevents this type of hypoglycemia.

Clinical Features

Regardless of the cause, hypoglycemia is characterized by Whipple's triad, which is a history of hypoglycemic symptoms associated with a blood glucose level of 40 mg/dl or less and immediate recovery following administration of glucose.

Although hypoglycemic symptoms can be nonspecific, they generally fall into two categories:

1. *Epinephrine mediated* (the adrenergic response): sweating, palpations, anxiety, and tremors.

2. *Central nervous system mediated:* blurred vision, headache, weakness, syncope, and seizures.

Diagnosis

Most of the tests designed to diagnose hypoglycemia are directed toward uncovering an insulinoma and involve comparing serum insulin titers to serum glucose levels at prescribed time intervals. The combination of hypoglycemia and increased insulin titers during a fasting state is a classic finding for insulinoma. Interestingly, one must be sure there is no surreptitious administration of hypoglycemic agents (insulin or sulfonylureas) that could simulate this type of hypoglycemia. These patients are usually associated with the health professions. The OGTT is used as a diagnostic tool in hypoglycemia specifically to support the diagnosis of reactive hypoglycemia (the imbalance between the time of insulin secretion and the time food is completely absorbed in the gastrointestinal tract).

Permanent and irreversible brain damage can occur if hypoglycemia becomes a chronic condition. This is usually seen in patients with insulinomas. Delayed diagnosis has often resulted in patients being treated for psychiatric disorders or seizures.

Treatment

The treatment of hypoglycemia is, of course, related to the underlying cause. Insulinomas, when diagnosed early, are treated surgically. Insulin-induced hypoglycemia in diabetics necessitates careful adjustment of insulin dosage and extensive patient education. Reactive hypoglycemia is treated by weight reduction in obese patients as well as dietary regulation. Alcohol-induced hypoglycemia is treated by restricting alcohol or by providing supplementary food intake if the patient continues to drink.

Podiatric Implications

The podiatrist must realize that any of his or her patients who are taking oral hypoglycemics or insulin may present with hypoglycemic symptoms. Usually these symptoms are of the central nervous system–mediated type, namely, headache and blurred vision. The podiatrist needs to be aware of these possibilities when caring for the ambulatory diabetic patient. Hypoglycemia may also occur in the insulin-requiring diabetic during the perioperative period when exogenous insulin requirement varies markedly. Frequent blood glucose monitoring at regular intervals should forewarn of this problem.

Postoperatively, hypoglycemia may occur in patients with severe liver disease who have poor caloric intake. In this situation, glycogen stores become depleted within 48 hours, and hepatic gluconeogenesis may be blocked by the underlying liver dysfunction. Preoperative liver function tests uncover this dysfunction.

Thyroid Disorders

Pathogenesis

The thyroid gland produces hormones in quantities sufficient to meet the needs of the whole organism. Disturbances of thyroid growth and function are among the most common endocrinopathies. Excessive production of thyroid hormones thyroxine (T_4) and triiodothyronine (T_3) results in hyperthyroidism or thyrotoxicosis; decreased hormone production results in hypothyroidism (Table 5–14). Generalized enlargement of the thyroid gland, regardless of cause, is called goiter. A focal enlargement of the thyroid is termed a nodule. Nodules are usually benign but can be malignant. Goiter as well as nodules may be associated with either hyper- or hypothyroidism.

The principal regulatory mechanism of the thyroid is the hypothalamic-pituitary-thyroid negative feedback control system. The hypothalamus secretes thyrotropin-re-

Table 5–14. CLINICAL MANIFESTATIONS OF THYROID DISEASE

Signs and Symptoms	Mechanism
Hyperthyroidism	
Muscle wasting (negative nitrogen balance)	Increased catabolism and heat production
Weight loss	
Increased appetite	
Initially increased physical stamina then fatigue	
Heat intolerance	
Sweating (heat intolerance)	Increased sensitivity to catecholamines
Tachycardia	
Irritability	
Warm hands and feet	
Increased Achilles DTR time	
Increased susceptibility to infection	
Palpations	
Tremors	
Increased nervousness	
Tachycardia	Increased cardiovascular activity
Increased cardiac output	
Increased blood pressure	
Palpations	
CHF	
Diarrhea	Increased gastrointestinal motility and activity
Nausea	
Weight loss	
Vomiting	
Rapid speech	
Emotional instability	
Oligomenorrhea or amenorrhea	
Hoarseness	
Hypothyroidism (Myxedema)	
Weakness	Decreased metabolism with decreased energy production
Easy fatigability	
Lassitude	
Lethargy	
Cold intolerance	Decreased heat production
Decreased cardiac rate and output	
Decreased body temperature	
Decreased blood pressure, dyspnea on exertion	Decreased oxygen requirements
Decreased respiratory effort	
High incidence of atherosclerosis and CAD	Increased blood lipids
	Decreased liver function with increased cholesterol
Capillary fragility with bruising	Decreased tissue synthesis
Xerosis	
Brittle nails	
Dry, sparse hair	
Anemia	
Decreased libido	Decreased reproduction function
Decreased fertility	
Puffy face	Electrolyte imbalance with fluid shifts
Edema	
Weight gain	Decreased gastrointestinal activity
Constipation	
Decreased appetite	
Apathy	
Slow speech	

CAD, Coronary artery disease; CHF, congestive heart failure; DTR, deep tendon reflex.

leasing hormone (TRH), which travels to the pituitary, stimulating release of thyroid-stimulating hormone (TSH). Thyroid-stimulating hormone stimulates many aspects of thyroid activity, including hormone synthesis, thyroid growth, and release of thyroid hormone. Thyroid-stimulating hormone secretion by the pituitary is inhibited by thyroid hormone ("negative feedback").

The thyroid hormones exert their action via a variety of means. A classic effect is on basal metabolic rate (BMR), the oldest laboratory tests for assessment of thyroid status. Other actions include stimulation of oxygen consumption by cells, regulation of protein synthesis, and regulation of membrane physiology. In general terms, thyroid hormone has a stimulatory effect on many metabolic processes. It is essential for optimal growth and development.

Clinical Features

In order to understand the diagnosis of thyroid disorders, it is necessary to first be familiar with thyroid function tests. The diagnosis of thyroid disease rests as much on laboratory tests as on clinical symptoms and signs.

Basal Metabolic Rate. This is a direct measure of metabolic activity. However, the wide range of normal values and changes in BMR caused by nonthyroidal factors makes this test virtually useless and antiquated.

Thyroxine by Radioimmunoassay. Serum T_4 by RIA is commonly used to screen for thyroid dysfunction or to monitor hyperthyroid patients. It is the single most important measurement in clinical evaluation of thyroid disease. However, if thyroid-binding proteins are increased or decreased, there is an increase or decrease in the level of T_4. In these circumstances, T_4 by RIA is not an accurate estimate of thyroid function.

Triiodothyronine Resin Uptake. The triiodothyronine resin uptake (T_3U) is not a thyroid function test but an indirect measurement of plasma thyroxine-binding globulin (TBG). The usefulness of T_3U is in interpreting a given level of T_4. A high or low T_4 can be interpreted as reflecting increased or decreased T_4 secretion only if the plasma-binding T_4 is normal, that is, only if T_3U TBG is normal. For convenience, the T_4 and T_3 uptake tests have been combined to give a so-called free T_4 index (FTI) by simply multiplying one number times another. This calculation compensates for the high or low concentration.

Thyroxine-binding globulin can be affected by many factors. It is increased in pregnancy, in liver disease, and during the use of oral contraceptives. It may be decreased with the use of androgens, steroids, or both and during acute illness or surgical stress.

Thyroid-Stimulating Hormone by Radioimmunoassay. The TSH by RIA is utilized to distinguish hypothyroidism due to primary thyroid failure (TSH is elevated) from hypothyroidism due to pituitary or hypothalamic disease (TSH is not elevated). It is also used as a measure of adequate exogenous thyroid replacement in patients with primary hypothyroidism. In these situations, TSH drops to normal when thyroid replacement is adequate (i.e., patient is euthyroid) and remains elevated when thyroid replacement is inadequate.

Summary. In terms of the aforementioned tests, T_4 by RIA is an excellent screen for thyroid disease. FTI is utilized when there are problems in interpretation of the free T_4 (usually in seriously ill patients). The TSH by RIA is utilized to distinguish between primary and secondary hypothyroidism as well as to check on thyroid replacement therapy.

Other Tests of Thyroid Function

Thyroid Scan. This provides information concerning localization, size, shape, and uniformity of function of the thyroid. It commonly provides information about the function and location of thyroid nodules in the gland.

Thyroid Ultrasonography. This technique is utilized to distinguish between solid nodules and cystic lesions.

Thyroid Antibodies. A relatively high percentage of patients with Graves' disease (i.e., hyperthyroidism, primary hyperthyroidism, and autoimmune thyroiditis [Hashimoto's disease]) have positive test results for thyroid antibodies. These diseases are considered to be autoimmune thyroid diseases. Titers of these antibodies can be quantitated and together with other clinical and laboratory abnormalities can help in diagnosis of these autoimmune diseases.

HYPERTHYROIDISM (THYROTOXICOSIS)

Thyrotoxicosis is a clinical syndrome resulting from excess T_4, T_3, or both. Thyrotoxicosis affects women much more frequently than men. It can occur at any age but usually occurs in early adult life. Symptoms include emotional instability, weight loss, heat intolerance, muscular weakness, and palpations. Signs include hyperkinetic activity, fine tremors, onycholysis, prominent eyes (exophthalmos), tachycardia, and irregular heart rate.

The most common form of thyrotoxicosis is Graves' disease, otherwise known as diffuse toxic goiter, which appears as a palpably large thyroid gland. Although these patients usually have a goiter, they may have a single adenoma, which represents an area of hyperfunctioning thyroid tissue. As excessive thyroid hormone is produced, T_4 by RIA is elevated as well as FTI. Causes of hyperthyroidism other than Graves' disease and a hyperfunctioning adenoma include toxic multinodular goiter (Plummer's disease), acute autoimmune thyroiditis (Hashimoto's disease), and excessive exogenous intake of thyroid hormone given for suppression or replacement therapy. Interestingly, in Graves' disease, an abnormal thyroid-stimulating immunoglobulin is present, which supports the concept of autoimmune etiology.

Management of hyperthyroidism involves different modalities, depending on etiology. Surgery is the treatment of choice only in selected patients. Antithyroid drugs suppress thyroid hormone production, but they do not alter the course of the disease. Radioactive iodine therapy is the most common mode of therapy for Graves' disease in adults. It is contraindicated in children, adolescents, and pregnant women because of possible toxicity from radiation.

Hypothyroidism

Hypothyroidism may be due to failure of the thyroid gland itself (primary) or to failure of TSH production because of pituitary disorders (secondary). Rarely is hypothyroidism due to hypothalamic (tertiary) problems. Hypothyroidism may be a consequence of an inflammatory disorder of the gland (thyroiditis) or of radiation therapy or thyroidectomy done for hyperthyroidism. Symptoms include dry skin, hair loss, weight gain, cold intolerance, constipation, decreased libido, and amenorrhea. Signs include puffiness, slowed speech, hoarseness, decreased activity, and delayed relaxation of the knee or ankle jerk ("hung-up" reflex).

The most common causes of hypothyroidism are idiopathic atrophy of the gland itself, chronic lymphocytic thyroiditis, and loss of tissue due to thyroidectomy or radioactive iodine treatment. The laboratory findings of a low T_4 and FTI are common in all forms of hypothyroidism. The TSH should always be determined, as this distinguishes between primary hypothyroidism (high TSH) and pituitary or hypothalamic causes (normal or low TSH). Thyroid autoantibodies are elevated in a high percentage of patients with idiopathic thyroid atrophy and chronic lymphocytic thyroiditis, indicating the autoimmune basis of these diseases.

Therapy for hypothyroidism rests on replacing thyroid hormone with exogenous preparations.

Goiter

Worldwide, the most common cause of goiter, or thyroid enlargement, is iodine deficiency. This problem has been eliminated in the United States because of dietary iodine supplementation. Goiters can also occur from a variety of mechanisms, including congenital abnormalities in which synthesis of thyroid hormone is impaired, resulting in elevated TSH, which stimulates thyroid tissue growth; hyperthyroidism; and, finally, inflammation of the gland, whether bacterial or autoimmune in nature.

Thyroid Nodule

Thyroid nodules are quite common. They can be detected in up to 4% of the adult population. The incidence increases with age and is seven times greater in women than in men. The important differential diagnosis of the thyroid nodule includes benign adenoma, cyst, and thyroid cancer. The vast majority of nodules are benign; however, a history of x-ray or radiation to the area of the thyroid gland is associated with a definitely increased incidence of thyroid cancer. Thyroid scan, ultrasonography, thyroid biopsy, and aspiration cytology are critical in distinguishing whether the patient has a malignant or benign nodule.

Podiatric Implications

Thyroid disorder should be considered if a patient exhibits clinical symptoms and signs consistent with one of these entities. The patient should then be appropriately referred for further examination. No patient should undergo elective surgery if he or she is either hypothyroid or hyperthyroid. Serious perioperative cardiac and respiratory problems can occur in the form of cardiac arrhythmias or metabolic imbalances. A goiter is a contraindication to elective surgery because it may cause upper airway obstruction and difficulty with intubation.

Parathyroid Disorders

Parathyroid disorders are not commonly encountered in podiatric practice. However, it is important for the podiatric practitioner to be cognizant of these disorders because asymptomatic patients may present with hypercalcemia on routine preoperative laboratory tests that may indicate underlying parathyroid disease. In addition, the distressing bone disease of secondary hyperparathyroidism due to renal failure (renal osteodystrophy) must be recognized by the podiatrist and evaluated within the context of the patient's chronic renal disease.

Hypoparathyroidism

Hypoparathyroidism should be considered when evaluating a laboratory finding of a serum calcium level of < 8.7 mg/dl. True hypoparathyroidism is most commonly seen following thyroidectomy or surgery for parathyroid tumor.

Pseudohypoparathyroidism is a genetic defect associated with short stature, round race, obesity, short metacarpals, hypertension, and ectopic bone formation. The parathyroid glands are present, but the renal tubules do not respond to the hormone because there is a receptor protein defect.

Acute hypoparathyroidism (hypocalcemia) causes tetany, carpopedal spasm, irritability, dyspnea, abdominal cramps, and urinary frequency. *Chvostek's* sign (facial muscle contraction on tapping the facial nerve near the ≤ of the jaw) is positive and Trousseau's phenomenon (carpal spasm with application of a sphygmomanometer) is present. The podiatrist may encounter this entity when evaluating laboratory findings of low serum calcium level, high serum phosphate level, and low to absent urinary calcium level. Parathyroid hormone assay is low or absent in post surgical hypoparathyroidism but normal or elevated in pseudohypoparathyroidism. The emergency treatment of an acute attack of hypoparathyroid tetany requires airway management and infusion of calcium gluconate. The chronic treatment of hypoparathyroidism consists of a high calcium, low-phosphate diet; calcium salts; and calciferol (a vitamin D analog that increases serum calcium concentration).

Hyperparathyroidism

Hyperparathyroidism should be considered when evaluating a laboratory finding of a serum calcium level > 10.7 mg/dl. Hyperparathyroidism is uncommon but should always be suspected in obscure bone or renal disease, especially if renal calculi are present. Most importantly, hyperparathyroidism may be asymptomatic and appear solely as hypercalcemia on routine laboratory screening done preoperatively or as part of a routine health evaluation. About 80% of cases of primary hyperparathyroidism are caused by a single autonomously functioning adenoma. Of cases, 2% are caused by hyperplasia of all four parathyroid carcinoma. Of cases, 2% are caused by parathyroid carcinoma. Multiple neoplasms, often familial, of the pancreas, pituitary gland, thyroid gland, and adrenal gland may be associated with primary hyperparathyroidism due to tumor or hyperplasia of the parathyroids (multiple endocrine adenomatosis).

Secondary hyperparathyroidism is associated with parathyroid gland hyperplasia and is most commonly seen in chronic renal failure.

Hyperparathyroidism causes excessive excretion of calcium and phosphate by the kidney, eventually producing renal stone formation or infiltration of the kidney parenchyma by calcium (nephrocalcinemia). Eventually calcium loss from bones results in diffuse demineralization, pathologic fractures, or cystic bone lesions throughout the skeleton (osteitis fibrosa cystca).

The symptoms of hyperparathyroidism can be classified into skeletal manifestations (back pain, joint pain, and fractures), urinary tract findings (renal stones), and gastrointestinal tract manifestations (nausea, vomiting, and ulcers). Hypertension is not uncommon. Most importantly, hyperparathyroidism is often asymptomatic and is detected when analyzing laboratory data consistent with high serum calcium and normal or low serum phosphate levels. Radioimmunoassay for parathyroid hormone is available to confirm the diagnosis.

The treatment of hyperparathyroidism is primarily surgical excision of either the parathyroid tumor or removal of three of four parathyroid glands in the instance of parathyroid hyperplasia.

Podiatric Implications

Podiatric concerns regarding parathyroid disorders relate in part to asymptomatic hypercalcemia in a preoperative patient. The patient scheduled for surgery who is found to be hypercalemic should be fully evaluated before surgery. Whereas a number of these patients may eventually prove to have hyperparathyroidism, some patients may have underlying malignancies (lung, breast, and multiple myeloma). Thiazide diuretics are a common cause of hypercalcemia, and it is imperative that these drugs be discontinued before a parathyroid hormone assay is done.

The severely hypercalcemic patient (calcium greater than 14 mg/dl) must be treated as an emergency with the first step being adequate hydration. Appropriate consultation should be obtained after beginning parenteral hydration.

Hypocalcemia is rarely encountered in podiatric situations. As previously stated, the most common cause of hypoparathyroidism is surgical excision of the parathyroid glands.

Adrenal Disorders

Pathogenesis

The adrenal gland elaborates hormones from two different sites. The hormones in the adrenal medulla are responsible for blood pressure regulation and for preparing the body for physical activity (i.e., "fight, fright, or flight reaction").

Adrenal Cortex. Although the cortex elaborates more than 25 different types of steroids, the effects of the steroids separate them into three groups:

1. Mineralocorticoids: aldosterone
2. Glucocorticoids: cortisol
3. Sex steroids: testosterone, estrogen, progesterone.

The pathology associated with adrenal cortical dysfunction results from too much or too little of each of these hormones.

Adrenal Medulla. This tissue produces catecholamines (e.g., epinephrine and norepinephrine). Adrenal medullary dysfunction arises from a tumor of the medullary cells (i.e., pheochromocytoma). The tumor may manifest itself as hypertensive disease and is commonly regarded as one of the secondary causes of hypertension. Although such a tumor is uncommon, if discovered surgical excision is usually successful in nonmalignant cases (see Hypertension).

Clinical Features

GLUCOCORTICOID HYPERFUNCTION
HYPERCORTISOLISM

These clinical conditions result from prolonged, excessive exposure to cortisol. The most common cause is iatrogenic, that is, exogenous steroid therapy in large doses for a variety of chronic disorders. Cushing's syndrome may also be brought about by sustained, excessive production of cortisol by the adrenal cortex. This endogenous cause usually indicates a pituitary tumor producing excessive ACTH or, rarely, autonomous cortisol production by a primary adrenal tumor. Very rarely might an extra pituitary malignancy (usually lung cancer) produce ectopic ACTH, a condition called ectopic Cushing's syndrome.

Signs. Regardless of the cause, all patients with chronic hypercortisolism are obese, hypertensive, and plethoric. These signs are directly related to excess cortisol. Cortisol also makes the arterial system hypersensitive to neural stimuli, resulting in hypertension. Protein breakdown is increased, and muscles become weak, which results in thin, weak extremities and osteoporotic bone. Surface capillaries become fragile, and slight traumas cause hematomas. Cortisol also inhibits insulin activity with resultant hyperglycemia. In some, hypercortisolism causes glucose intolerance and often diabetes mellitus. Other signs are central obesity with a "buffalo hump," (as defined previously, an accumulation of fat in the back between the shoulders), a supraclavicular fat pad, a moon facies, muscle weakness, ability to bruise easily, and striae (Fig. 5–3). Hypertension is common. Mental changes, ranging from depression to euphoria, can usually be observed. Osteoporosis is characteristic, and vertebral fractures are commonly seen.

Diagnosis. Endogenous hypercortisolism is diagnosed by demonstrating ele-

vated plasma and urinary cortisol levels. Diagnosis is further reinforced by demonstrating that dexamethasone (a potent steroid) is not able to suppress this response, which should occur if the cortisol were being produced by a gland with a normal negative feedback system. Finally, the assay of ACTH allows differentiation between a pituitary cause (normal ACTH levels) and an adrenal cause (undetectable ACTH). Exogenous hypercortisolism re-

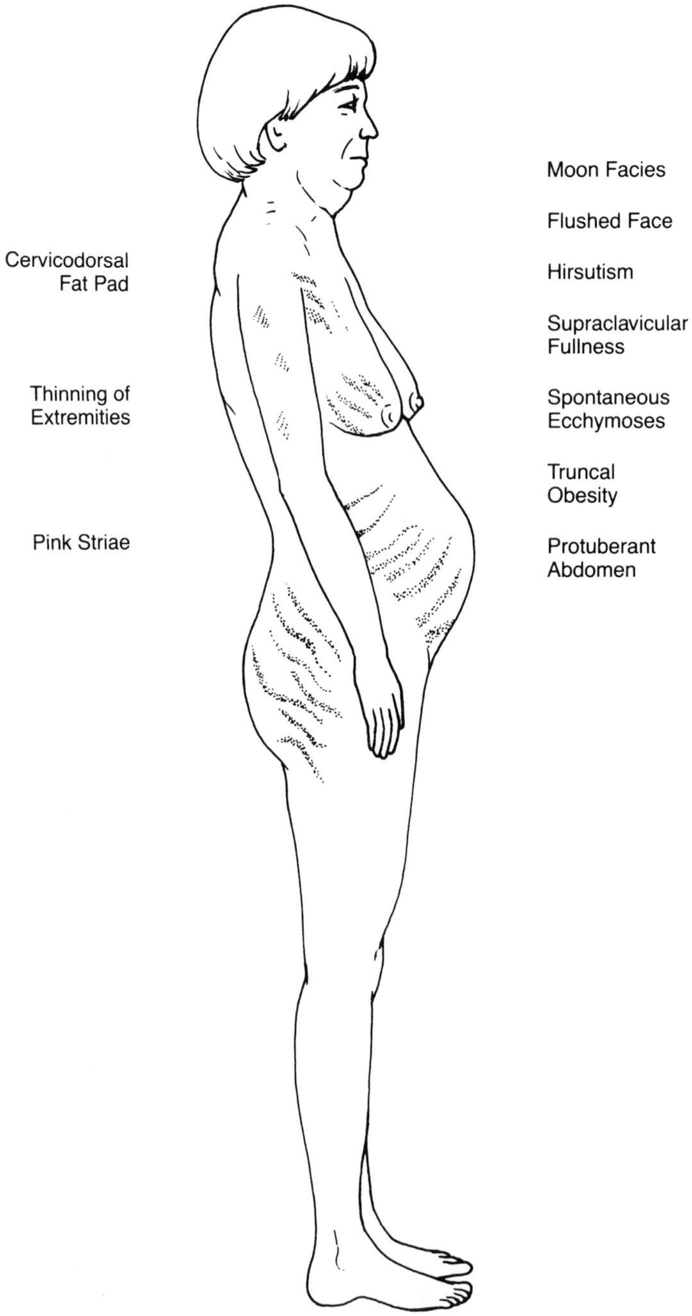

Cervicodorsal Fat Pad

Thinning of Extremities

Pink Striae

Moon Facies

Flushed Face

Hirsutism

Supraclavicular Fullness

Spontaneous Ecchymoses

Truncal Obesity

Protuberant Abdomen

Figure 5–3. Findings in Cushing's syndrome.

quires only a careful history, documenting long-term use of oral or parenteral steroids.

Treatment. Treatment of endogenous hypercortisolism is usually surgically directed to the pituitary gland in the case of a pituitary tumor. Irradiation is sometimes employed as an adjunctive measure. Treatment of Cushing's syndrome, produced by adrenal tumors, is usually surgical excision. Drugs may provide symptomatic relief in this situation. The treatment of exogenous hypercortisolism involves carefully assessing whether the administration of steroids is therapeutically necessary, especially in a patient who is suffering from chronic hypercortisolism. If the use of long-term steroids is therapeutically justified, careful measures must be taken to try to diminish the side effects as much as possible. These measures may include alternate-day steroid treatment and treatment of hypertension and steroid-induced diabetes mellitus.

GLUCOCORTICOID HYPOFUNCTION

This clinical syndrome is due to inadequate production of cortisol. When the cause is a lesion in the adrenal cortex, the disorder is termed *primary adrenal insufficiency* or Addison's disease. If the lesion is due to ACTH deficiency the syndrome is called *secondary adrenal failure*. Although these syndromes are rare, they have enormous importance in terms or surgical morbidity and mortality.

Signs. Addison's disease is characterized by weakness, weight loss, hypotension, electrolyte abnormalities, and nausea and vomiting. The disorder can be chronic or can occur as an acute medical emergency (adrenal crisis) with severe hypotension, fever, electrolyte imbalance, and cardiovascular collapse.

Diagnosis and Treatment. Most cases of Addison's disease have an autoimmune basis. Tuberculosis was the most common offender earlier in the 20th century but is rare now. Diagnosis is made by demonstrating a lack of rise in serum cortisol when synthetic ACTH is administered. The demonstration of high plasma ACTH with low plasma cortisol supports this diagnosis. The treatment of Addison's disease is physiologic steroid replacement.

Secondary adrenal failure can be caused by a variety of pituitary disorders (e.g., tumors and necrosis of ACTH-producing cells), but by far the most common cause is adrenocortical suppression of cortisol due to exogenous long-term steroid use. Supraphysiologic amounts (i.e., greater than 7.5 mg/day of prednisone or its equivalent steroid for 3 weeks or longer) can suppress the pituitary's ability to release ACTH, a condition which may last for up to 1 year. This has significant implications in terms or how such patients are managed in stress situations such as surgery and infection. Absence of plasma ACTH in the presence of low plasma cortisol is an excellent diagnostic test.

Podiatric Implications

The adrenal gland's release of cortisol in response to stress is of great importance. In patients with Addison's disease, adrenal cortical tissue has been destroyed, and thus the patient is unable to produce endogenous cortisol. Daily steroid replacement is given in physiologic doses. However, in periods of stress, the daily steroid dose needs to be supplemented to compensate for the inability of the patient's adrenal gland to respond with increased cortisol.

Steroid Supplementation. In patients with secondary adrenal failure due to supraphysiologic steroid doses given to treat inflammatory, autoimmune, and neoplastic disease and other illnesses, pituitary ACTH production is inhibited and, therefore, so is production of adrenal cortisol. These patients have had their hypothalamic-pituitary-adrenal access suppressed, and they are unable to increase their endogenous cortisol production in response to stress. This suppression, as previously mentioned, can persist up to 1 year following discontinuation of exogenous steroid therapy. It is generally believed that any patient who has received 7.5 mg of prednisone or its equivalent daily for 4 or more weeks should be assumed to have hypothalamic-pituitary-adrenal access suppression lasting 1 year. The podiatrist must be able to identify these patients and to determine if their podiatric therapy will require supplemental steroids. The podiatrist should inquire whether the patient is, or has been in the past year, receiving steroid therapy. A positive response should be followed with specific inquiries regarding the type and dosage of the steroid medication, the length of therapy, the frequency and route of administration, and when the last dose was taken. In response to severe, nonsurgical stress, such as infection, supplemental steroids should be given on a daily basis in two to four times the daily amount of the usual steroid dose. This is given throughout the time the infection is being managed.

·Minor Surgical Procedures. With minor procedures, patients should double their usual steroid dose on the day of treatment. They can then take their normal dose beginning the day after treatment.

Major Surgical Procedures. A major surgical procedure produces maximum stress. Because normal individuals secrete 100 to 300 mg of cortisol in 24 hours in the face of severe stress, the recommended dosage is 300 mg/day of cortisol on the day of surgery. Depending on the duration of postoperative stress, steroid treatment may be tapered over a 4-day period. The usual regimen is to give 50 to 100 mg of hydrocortisone sodium succinate (Solu-Cortef) on the night before surgery to compensate for psychologic preoperative stress. On the day of surgery, 100 mg of hydrocortisone intramuscularly is given on call to the operating room, 100 mg of hydrocortisone intravenously is given during surgery, and 100 mg of hydrocortisone intramuscularly is given in the evening after surgery. On the first postoperative day, 50 mg of hydrocortisone intramuscularly is given every 8 hours; on the second postoperative day, 25 mg of hydrocortisone is given intramuscularly every 8 hours, on the third postoperative day, 25 mg of hydrocortisone is given intramuscularly every 12 hours. Thereafter, the patient's usual maintenance dose is given.

If the postoperative course is stressful or if infection occurs, the rate of tapering is slowed. If there is any question as to whether the patient truly requires steroid coverage, it is far wiser to err on the side of giving steroid coverage. It is always better to administer steroids and taper very slowly, as the benefits of allowing the patient to meet stress adequately outweigh any negative effects of transient high-dose glucocorticoid therapy.

There are certain diseases in which patients receive alternate-day steroid therapy, one of the benefits being that there is no adrenal suppression. It is wise even in these patients to provide glucocorticoid therapy.

Complications. Although it is generally believed that steroid therapy may have a deleterious effect on wound healing, such a complication occurs only if doses are unusually high for long periods of time and protein intake is inadequate. Vitamin A in high doses may help in this regard. This in no way means that steroids should not be withheld if adrenal insufficiency is even suspected. It does, however, call for extra attention to the meticulous care of wounds in patients taking steroids. The incidence of postoperative infection, particularly of the wound, may be increased in steroid-treated patients. The literature, however, does not support the use of prophylactic antibiotics. Again, attention to wound care is of paramount importance. Patients with hyperaldosteronism, as previously mentioned, almost always have hypertension and should be given the usual considerations that any hypertensive patient would receive in undergoing any minor or major surgery. Special emphasis should be placed on correcting the hypokalemia seen in this condition because hypokalemia can predispose the patient to intraoperative and postoperative cardiac arrhythmias.

Hyperlipoproteinemia

The hyperlipoproteinemia diseases have impact on podiatric practice in two areas. One is the presentation of patients with xanthoma tendinosum in the lower extremity, which is a manifestation of familial hyperlipoproteinemia. Secondly, patients who are evaluated preoperatively may have abnormal elevations of cholesterol and triglycerides levels noted on screening. Both these situations require evaluation and referral by the podiatrist. Therefore, it is important for the podiatrist to have a working knowledge of this group of disorders (Table 5–15).

Hyperlipoproteinemia is an abnormal elevation of either or both of the principal blood lipids, cholesterol and triglycerides. This term is more descriptive than hyperlipidemia because it alludes to the important role that proteins play in the patho-

Table 5–15. TYPES OF HYPERLIPOPROTEINEMIA

	Clinical Features	Secondary Causes	Appearance of Blood in Test Tube
Type I (Increased chylomicrons)	Abdominal pain Pancreatitis Eruptive xanthomas Lipemia retinalis	IDDM Dysglobulinemia Lupus erythematosis	Creamy layer present Plasma clear
Type IIa (Increased LDL)	Tendon xanthomas Premature corneal arcus	Nephrotic syndrome Hypothyroidism	Plasma clear
Type IIb (Increased LDL and VLDL)	Xanthelasma Premature CHD	Obstructive liver disease Porphyria Multiple myeloma	Turbid plasma sometimes
Type III (Increased LDL, abnormal lipoproteinemia)	Orange-yellow deposits Palmar creases Tuberoeruptive xanthomas Premature PVD, CHD	Hypothyroidism Dysgammaglobulinemia	Turbid plasma
Type IV (Increased VLDL)	Eruptive xanthoma Hypertension Low HDL cholesterol Abnormal GTT Risk factor for CHD	Diabetes mellitus Nephrotic syndrome Pregnancy GSD Alcoholism Gaucher's disease Niemann-Pick disease	Turbid plasma
Type V (Increased chylomicrons and VLDL)	Pancreatitis Xanthomatosis	IDDM Nephrotic syndrome Alcoholism Myeloma Idiopathic hypercalcemia	Creamy layer present Turbid plasma

CHD, Coronary heart disease; GSD, glycogen storage disease; GTT, glucose tolerance test; HDL, high-density lipoprotein; IDDM, insulin-dependent diabetes mellitus; LDL, low-density lipoprotein; PVD, peripheral vascular disease; VLDL, very low-density lipoprotein.

physiology of these disorders. Elevated plasma levels of lipoproteins predispose the patient to atherosclerosis, peripheral vascular disease, and pancreatitis.

Pathophysiology

The pathophysiology of hyperlipoproteinemia begins with exogenous lipids absorbed from the gastrointestinal tract that are then transported in the circulation in the form of chylomicrons. These contain cholesterol, triglycerides, and phospholipids, which are transported to the liver. Endogenous lipids are synthesized by hepatic cells and are released only when bound to plasma proteins. There are three classes of these lipoproteins: (1) high-density lipoproteins (HDL), (2) low-density lipoproteins (LDL), and (3) very low-density lipoproteins (VLDL) Hyperlipoproteinemias are classified according to the type of lipoprotein and whether or not chylomicrons are present.

Types II and IV hyperlipoproteinemia are the only ones commonly encountered in practice, and both are associated with premature development of coronary heart disease. In type II, the LDL fraction is increased. This type is subdivided into those patients with only increased LDL and those with LDL associated with increased VLDL. In type IV hyperlipoproteinemia, the VLDL, containing about 60% triglycerides and 10 to 15% cholesterol, is elevated. The most common causes of this type of hypertriglyceridemia are obesity, alcoholism, and diabetes.

Although a lipoprotein electrophoresis is the most specific way to classify the type of hyperlipoproteinemia, it is not always necessary. An elevated serum cholesterol level with normal triglycerides suggests type IIA. Increased cholesterol with moderately increased triglycerides suggests type IIB. Normal cholesterol with markedly increased triglycerides suggests type IV.

Diagnosis and Treatment

The diagnosis of hyperlipoproteinemia is somewhat arbitrary. There are no absolute levels of triglycerides or cholesterol that are diagnostic of hyperlipoprotein-emia. In addition to age and sex, there are differences among populations. The mean levels of cholesterol in the United States are higher than those in Japan. The National Institutes of Health (NIH) considers persons with cholesterol levels above the 90th percentile to be at high risk for atherosclerosis and those above the 75th but below the 90th percentile to be at moderate risk.

The NIH has also stated that a person with a normal cholesterol level is at no greater risk for atherosclerosis when the triglyceride level is below 250 mg/dl. The prevalence rate for familial hypercholesterolemia is approximately one individual in 500, whereas the frequency of familial hypertriglyceridemia is approximately one in 1 million.

The treatment of choice for all patients with hyperlipoproteinemias is diet. There are specific diets for the types of hyperlipoproteinemias that have been associated with accelerated atherogenesis. Patients with more severe hyperlipoproteinemia may require drugs as well (Table 5–16). These drugs can be divided into those thought primarily to diminish lipoprotein synthesis (clofibrate, nicotinic acid, and probucol) and those thought to increase cholesterol excretion (cholestyramine, colestipol, and neomycin). Diet and drugs have a synergistic effect in patients.

Acromegaly

The pituitary gland is a complex endocrine organ located in the bony fossa called the "sella turcica" at the base of the brain and consists of two portions, the anterior pituitary and the posterior pituitary. The anterior pituitary gland produces growth hormone, prolactin, ACTH, TSH, follicle stimulating hormone (FSH), and luteinizing hormone. The posterior pituitary gland produces oxytocin as well as antidiuretic hormone (ADH). Adrenocorticotropic hormone is directly involved in production of plasma cortisol, whereas TSH is involved in production of thyroid hormone. Growth hormone has many metabolic and tissue actions, including the promotion of sodium, potassium, chloride, phosphate, and nitrogen retention as well as normal soft tissue and bone growth and gluconeogenesis. It is especially important for normal

Table 5–16. HYPOLIPIDEMIC AGENTS

	Decreased Lipoprotein Synthesis		Increased Lipoprotein Excretion	
	Nicotinic Acid	Clofibrate	Probucol	Colestipol or Cholestyramine
Primary indications	Types III and IV	Type III	Type II	Type II
Other indications	Type II	Type IV		
Initial dose	100 mg tid	1 g bid	250 mg bid	8 g bid
Maintenance dose	1–3 g tid	1 g bid	500 mg bid	8–16 g bid
Major side effects	Flushing, pruritus, nausea, diarrhea	Nausea, diarrhea	Diarrhea, nausea	Constipation, nausea, abdominal distention
Other side effects	Hyperpigmentation, glucose intolerance, hyperuricemia, hepatotoxicity	Leukopenia, myositis, alopecia, abnormal LFTs, cholelithiasis, ventricular ectopy (possible increased), hepatobiliary (possible increased)	? Hyperchloremic acidosis, steatorrhea, biliary tract calcification	
Drug interaction	Increased vasodilation by ganglioplegic antihypertensive agents	Increased hypoprothrombinemic effect of warfarin sodium	?	Decreased absorption of phenylbutazone, thyroid thiazides, tetracycline, phenobarbital, digitalis warfarin sodium
Estimated cost per year	$144	$225	$335	$400 (colestipol) $700 (cholestyramine)

bid, Twice a day; LFTs, liver function tests; tid, three times a day.

growth in childhood. Prolonged exposure to excessive growth hormone levels leads to the clinical features of acromegaly in adults and pituitary gigantism in children.

Clinical Features

Acromegaly is an uncommon disease, but it has special relevance to podiatry in that many of its features are related to complaints that may bring patients to the podiatrist. These complaints include acral enlargement, soft tissue overgrowth, hyperhydrosis, parathesias, and joint pain. Acromegalic patients, male or female, present most often between 30 to 40 years of age, usually with a history of noting changes in their physical features over several years. Patients are aware of enlarging hands and feet and changes in facial appearance, with an increase in jaw, tongue, and nose size. Headaches are present in about 80% of these patients, and heat intolerance, increased sweating, and seborrhea are common. Arthralgias of the peripheral joints, stiffness and pain of the neck and back, and parathesias and weakness of the extremities may all be noted. Many patients are unaware that they may have diabetes mellitus and complain of frequent thirst and urination. On physical examination, generalized enlargement of the body and large spadelike hands and feet with widening of the phalanges and increased soft tissues of the palm and plantar surfaces may be observed. Also noted are prominence of the supraorbital ridge, zygomatic arch, and frontal bosses. A large mandible may be present, often with malocclusion of the mouth and prognathism, and widely spaced teeth and thickened skin with prominent folds as well as hirsutism in women. Hypertension may be present in approximately 30% of patients. Many have bony joint deformities and enlargement of the joints of the hands, feet, elbows, and knees. About 20% of patients may show carpal tunnel syndrome.

Diagnosis and Treatment

The clinical syndrome resulting from excessive growth hormone secretion has been linked to the presence of a pituitary adenoma. Diagnosis is made by the clinical picture as well as the finding of repeated elevation of serum fasting growth hormone levels (greater than 10 mg/ml) that are usually not suppressed after a glucose load. The treatment of acromegaly depends partially on the size of the tumor, particularly whether the mass extends beyond the sella turcica and whether the optic nerves are involved. Surgical ablation as well as external radiation eventually arrest the progress of the disease, but there is a high incidence of hypopituitarism.

One of the most important metabolic consequences of acromegaly is diabetes mellitus. Frank diabetes mellitus is present in approximately 33% of patients. The podiatrist must keep in mind that many acromegalic patients are unaware of their disease and come to learn of it only after other individuals mention to the patients that their physical appearance has undergone a marked change over a short period of time. Therefore, the podiatrist must keep this diagnosis in mind when dealing with patients who appear to have any of the subjective or objective criteria previously listed.

Bibliography

Brown MJ, Asbury AK: Diabetic Neuropathy. Ann Neurol 15:2, 1984.

Fairbairn JF, II, Juergens JL: Principles of medical treatment. In Juergens JL, Spittell JA, Jr, Fairbairn JF, II (eds): Peripheral Vascular Diseases, 5th ed. Philadelphia: WB Saunders Co, 1980.

Gabbe SG: Gestational diabetes. N Engl J Med 315:1025, 1986.

Gerich JE: Sulfonylureas in the treatment of diabetes mellitus—1985. Mayo Clin Proc 60:439, 1985.

Goldmann DR, et al. (eds): Medical Care of the Surgical Patient: A Problem-Oriented Approach to Management. Philadelphia: JB Lippincott Co, 1982.

Hamburger JI: The autonomously functioning thyroid adenoma. N Engl J Med 309:1512, 1983.

Hamburger JI: The various presentations of thyroiditis. Ann Intern Med 104:219, 1986.

Harkless LB, Dennis KJ: You see what you look for and recognize what you know. Clin Podiatr Med Surg 4:331, 1987.

Hurley JR: Thyroid disease in the elderly. Med Clin North Am 67:497, 1983.

Hurst JW (ed): Medicine for the Practicing Physician. Boston: Butterworth Publishers, 1983.

Kahn CR: Insulin resistance: A common feature of diabetes mellitus. N Engl J Med 315:362, 1981.

Kleerekoper M, Sudhaker Rao DS, Frame B: Occult Cushing's syndrome presenting with osteoporosis. Henry Ford Hosp Med J 28:132, 1980.

Kozak GP (ed): Clinical Diabetes Mellitus. Philadelphia: WB Saunders Co, 1982.

Meikle AW, Tyler FH: Potency and duration of action of glucocorticoids: Effects of hydrocortisone, prednisone and dexamethasone on human pituitary-adrenal function. Am J Med 63:200, 1977.

Messer J, Reithman D, Sacks HS, et al.: Association of adrenocorticosteroid therapy and peptic ulcer disease. N Engl J Med 309:21, 1983.

Molitch ME (ed): Management of Medical Problems in Surgical Patients. Philadelphia: FA Davis Co, 1982.

Molnar GD, et al.: Methods of assessing diabetic control. Diabetologia 17:5, 1979.

Nathan DM, Singer DE, Hurxthal K, et al.: The clinical information value of the glycosylated hemoglobin assay. N Engl J Med 310:341, 1984.

Paz-Guevara AT, Hsu T-H, White P: Juvenile diabetes mellitus after 40 years. Diabetes 24:559, 1975.

Raskin P, Rosenstock J: Blood glucose control and diabetic complications. Ann Intern Med 105:254, 1986.

Ross DS: New sensitive immunoradiometric assays for thyrotropin. Ann Intern Med 104:718, 1986.

Rubenstein E, Federman DD (eds): Scientific American Medicine. New York: Scientific American, Inc, 1987.

Schroeder SA, et al. (eds): Medical Diagnosis and Treatment. East Norwalk, CT: Appleton & Lange, 1988.

Wagener D, Sacks JM, LaPorte RE, et al.: The Pittsburgh study of insulin dependent diabetes mellitus: Risk for diabetes among relatives of IDDM. Diabetes 31:136, 1982.

Werner SC: Modalities of medical therapy for nodular goiter. In Werner SC, Ingbar SH (eds): The Thyroid. New York: Harper & Row Publishers, Inc, 1978.

Winegrad AL, Greene DA: The Complications of Diabetes Mellitus. N Engl J Med 298:1250, 1978.

Wyngaarden JB, Smith LH (eds): Cecil Textbook of Medicine. Philadelphia: WB Saunders Co, 1985.

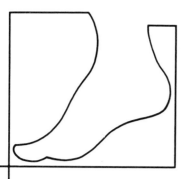

6 GASTROENTEROLOGY

GREG FITZ

OVERVIEW

At first glance, disorders of gastrointestinal function would seem to be of little importance to the practicing podiatrist. The digestive organs, however, are susceptible to a wide variety of toxic, metabolic, and infectious insults. It has been estimated that 15 million people in the United States have acute episodes of digestive disease each year, including such diverse problems as diarrhea, hepatitis, and peptic ulcer disease. Another 20 million have chronic disorders such as cirrhosis, gallstones, and inflammatory bowel disease. These gastrointestinal problems are often exacerbated by the stress associated with podiatric disorders. In addition, podiatric therapeutics rely heavily on a num-

ber of potential gastrointestinal toxins such as aspirin, acetaminophen, other nonsteroidal anti-inflammatory drugs (NSAIDs), and anesthetics (Table 6–1). Consequently, many podiatric patients are likely to have or to develop gastrointestinal disorders that will influence their therapy.

The purpose of this chapter is to provide a framework for the clinical evaluation of common gastrointestinal disorders. Emphasis is placed on the problems that are likely to develop as a consequence of podiatric therapy and on the diseases that, if recognized, should cause an alteration of standard therapy. In addition, special hazards associated with the care of patients with chronic digestive diseases such as cirrhosis are addressed. A more detailed discussion of these and other related issues

Table 6–1. ADVERSE GASTROINTESTINAL EFFECTS OF MEDICATIONS

Adverse Effect	Medication
Diarrhea	Magnesium-containing antacids
	Antibiotics
	Anti-inflammatory drugs
	Quinidine
	Digitalis
Constipation	Aluminum-containing antacids
	Opiate pain medications
	Anesthetic agents
Gastritis	Aspirin
	NSAIDs
	Erythromycin and other antibiotics
	Alcohol
Hepatitis	Alcohol
	Acetaminophen
	Diphenylhydantoin
	Halothane
	Alpha-methyldopa
	Isoniazid
	Phenothiazines

NSAIDs, Nonsteroidal anti-inflammatory drugs.

can be found in *Cecil's Textbook of Medicine* and *The Pathologic Basis of Digestive Disease.*

PATHOPHYSIOLOGY

The diverse organs of the digestive tract can be divided conceptually into two groups, the tubular organs and the accessory organs. The tubular organs consist of the mouth, esophagus, stomach, and small and large intestine (Fig. 6–1). The accessory organs, which empty their products into the lumen of the tubular system, include the salivary glands, pancreas, liver, and biliary tree. This division is obviously artificial because these organs normally work together in a beautifully orchestrated way. Ingested food is propelled down the lumen, where it is digested into its components by mechanical and chemical means. These nutrients are then absorbed across the intestinal mucosa with the aid of pancreatic and biliary secretions. These nutrients are utilized by the liver for a variety of biochemical needs, including protein biosynthesis, carbohydrate metabolism, and drug metabolism.

Tubular Organs. The tubular components of the digestive tract share a common structure comprised of three muscular layers surrounding a central lumen. The mus-cular activity is controlled in part by densely interconnected neural networks between the outer longitudinal and middle circular layers (Meissner's plexus) and between the middle circular and inner longitudinal layers (Auerbach's plexus). Ingested food is propelled away from the mouth by coordinated waves of muscle contraction immediately preceded by relaxation, termed peristaltic waves. This action serves to move intestinal contents down the intestine in a regulated manner, allowing digestion and absorption to take place.

The mucosal cells lining the lumen are highly specialized in each area. In the stomach, parietal and chief cells secrete hydrochloric acid and the potent proteolytic enzyme pepsinogen, respectively. Other cells in the stomach secrete mucus or intestinal hormones. By contrast, small intestine mucosal cells are adapted for absorption of a variety of nutrients. Iron, glucose, most vitamins, and amino acids are absorbed in the proximal small intestine. Mucosal cells in the distal small intestine (ileum) absorb vitamin B_{12} and bile salts. In the colon, little nutrient absorption occurs, but Na^+, Cl^-, and water are reclaimed, and feces is stored for expulsion.

Accessory Organs. The accessory organs of digestion share a common gland-like structure of cells, secreting their products into a central collecting system that then drains into the intestinal lumen to aid digestion. Salivary glands secrete up to a liter of bicarbonate-rich fluid each day to lubricate ingested food and amylase, an enzyme that begins the process of carbohydrate digestion. The breakdown of protein into its amino-acid components occurs mostly in the stomach as a result of acid secretion and breakdown of certain peptide bonds by pepsin. Acidic gastric contents must then be neutralized as they enter the proximal small intestine (duodenum) because most intestinal enzymes do not work at an acidic pH. Pancreatic secretions are rich in bicarbonate and also contain amylase and other potent digestive proenzymes, including trypsinogen and chymotrypsinogen. These are converted into active enzymes in the intestinal lumen to continue the process of carbohydrate and protein digestion. Pancreatic and biliary secretions enter the intestinal lumen via a common duct, the ampulla of Vater (Fig. 6–2). This is located in the duodenum

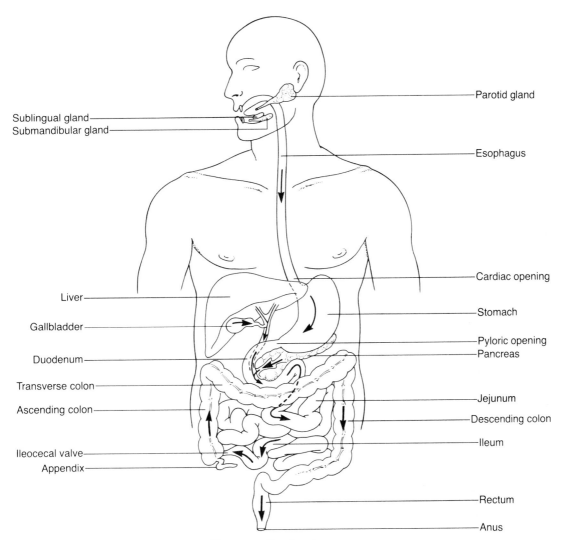

Figure 6–1. The digestive system.

just distal to where acidic gastric contents enter the small intestine.

Bile. Bile is made continuously in the liver and is secreted into the biliary tree. In the fasted state, the ampulla of Vater is closed and bile is stored in the gallbladder. Food entering the duodenum causes the ampulla to relax and the gallbladder to constrict, emptying bile into the lumen. Free fatty acids released from fat digestion are relatively insoluble in water and must be solubilized by bile salts before they can be absorbed. The bile salts, cholic acid, and the chenodeoxycholic acid mix with fats in the lumen, resulting in the formation of aggregates called micelles that are more readily absorbed.

Liver Function. The liver is the largest organ in the body, and it has many complex functions other than bile formation. The liver receives a dual blood supply from the hepatic artery and the portal vein. Following a meal, the portal vein has high concentrations of amino acids, fatty acids, and other basic nutrients. These are transported to the interior of the liver cell for biochemical processing. The principal functions of the liver include protein biosynthesis, lipid and carbohydrate metabolism, drug metabolism, and bile formation. Consequently abnormal liver function has many medically important sequelae. Impaired protein synthesis results in low serum albumin concentrations and a tendency to bleed because of low levels of clotting factors. Similarly the half-life of certain drugs may be prolonged owing to impaired hepatic clearance.

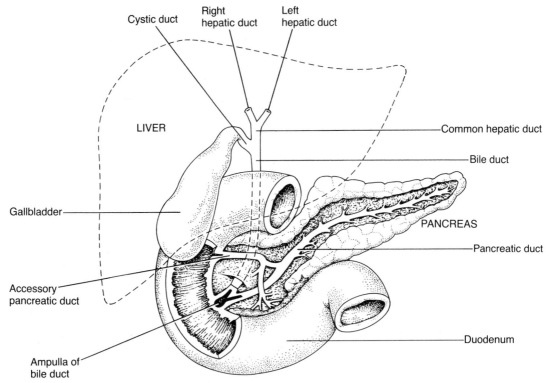

Figure 6–2. Connections of ducts of gallbladder, liver, and pancreas.

Regulating Hormones. A number of important hormones regulate many gastrointestinal processes. The best described are gastrin, secretin, and cholecystokinin-pancreozymin (CCK-PZ). Gastrin is released by G cells in the gastric antrum and is a potent stimulant for gastric acid release. Following a meal, gastrin levels increase and act via a receptor on parietal cells to promote acid secretion. Acid secretion inhibits the release of gastrin, constituting a feedback loop for regulation of acid secretion. In rare patients with Zollinger-Ellison syndrome, a gastrin-secreting tumor is not subject to the same negative feedback, causing abnormally high and sustained acid secretion and resulting in ulcer formation.

Secretin and CCK-PZ are both released from cells in the duodenal mucosa in response to acid and amino acids in the duodenal lumen. Secretin promotes the production of a watery, bicarbonate-rich fluid from the pancreas, and CCK-PZ stimulates the release of pancreatic digestive enzymes and gallbladder contraction. The precise mechanisms and site of action of these and other hormones are currently being defined.

PRESENTING FEATURES

Subjective Symptoms

The structural and functional diversity of the gastrointestinal tract makes the evaluation of gastrointestinal complaints deceptively difficult. Abdominal pain, changes in bowel habits, intestinal bleeding, and jaundice are each symptoms of underlying disease, and a careful history, physical examination, and laboratory evaluation are usually necessary for definitive diagnosis of a specific problem.

Abdominal Pain

Abdominal pain may be somatic, visceral, or referred. Somatic pain is well localized and arises from the abdominal wall or musculature, whereas visceral pain tends to be poorly localized and arises from the intestine, biliary tract, or other tubular structure. Abdominal disease may result in symptoms elsewhere. For example, diaphragmatic or biliary tract inflammation may be associated with pain in the shoulder area. This is known as referred pain

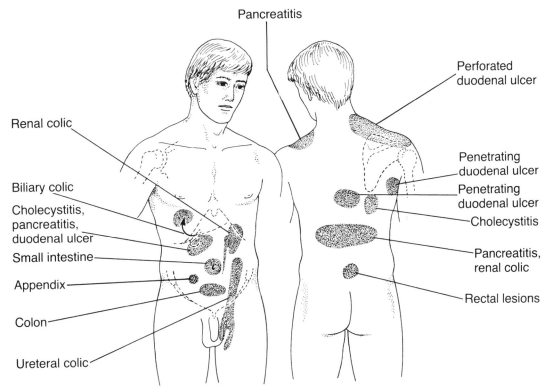

Figure 6–3. Direct and referred pain in intra-abdominal disorders.

and results from innervation by a common nerve root.

The location of pain provides an important clue to its etiology (Fig. 6–3). When combined with other information about the nature and duration of symptoms and about factors that exacerbate or alleviate the pain, an accurate differential diagnosis can generally be made. For example, pain of esophageal origin is generally precipitated by swallowing solids or liquids. It is often described as a sticking or tight sensation in the substernal area and is relieved by passage of the bolus of food.

Pain from peptic ulcer disease or gastritis is often localized in the midepigastrium and is described as a sensation of burning or hunger. It is characteristically relieved by ingestion of food or antacids but is made worse by fasting, ingestion of alcohol, or ingestion of aspirin. It is not unusual for patients with ulcer disease to be awakened by their symptoms 1 or 2 hours after going to bed at night.

In contrast to peptic ulcer disease, pain of biliary tract origin is described as a full or cramping sensation in the right upper quadrant that is often quite severe. It occasionally radiates to the right shoulder or

midepigastrium and tends to wax and wane over a 1- or 2-hour period. The pain is not generally relieved by ingestion of food and may sometimes be exacerbated by fatty food ingestion. Biliary tract disease tends to be chronic, so a history of similar episodes may be helpful.

Pain of small bowel origin tends to be crampy in nature and peaks in intensity every 3 to 10 minutes as a peristaltic wave passes. The pain then recedes as the intestinal wall relaxes. Colonic motility can cause similar pain, but the symptoms are more localized to the left lower quadrant and are often improved by passing of flatus or feces.

Alterations in Bowel Habits

Perhaps the most common gastrointestinal symptoms encountered clinically are diarrhea and constipation. Most individuals have one to three bowel movements per day and a total stool weight of less than 150 g/day, but there is wide variation in these standards. Constipation or diarrhea reflects a change in the frequency, volume, or liquidity of stool, and it is very important to ask specifically what alteration is present, since "normal" bowel function has so much person-to-person variability.

Diarrhea and constipation often result from changing diet and stress associated with hospitalization. Constipation can also be caused by a variety of medications, including aluminum hydroxide–containing antacids and analgesics. Abdominal pain, fever, and failure to pass gas are indications that more worrisome causes may be involved. Diarrhea can also be caused by medications, including antibiotics and magnesium-containing antacids. The irritable bowel syndrome is a common disorder characterized by diarrhea alternating with constipation that recurs over periods of months to years but has no effect on longevity. It is often associated with crampy abdominal pain, and the diarrhea is characteristically exacerbated by stress. Although most episodes of diarrhea are benign and self-limited, there are a number of more worrisome infections and structural causes that require urgent attention. Clues to potentially severe underlying diseases include diarrhea associated with fever, severe pain, or blood or leukocytes in the stool. These patients require a more aggressive evaluation.

Objective Signs

Physical Examination

Examination of the abdomen should always be accompanied by a thorough general medical examination because abdominal complaints are often indicative of major disease elsewhere. The four basic methods of examination—inspection, auscultation, percussion, and palpation—are generally performed in the order listed.

Inspection. With the patient supine in a warm, comfortable location, the abdomen should be inspected for masses, surgical scars, pulsations, and engorged veins. Pulsations from the abdominal aorta are evident in most individuals but may be exaggerated by aneurysmal dilatation of the aorta. A distended, protuberant abdomen may result from an abnormal accumulation of fluid in the peritoneal space. When associated with engorged veins on the abdominal wall, a distended abdomen suggests cirrhosis or portal hypertension. Bluish discoloration around the umbilicus

or flanks may result from blood in the peritoneum, as is seen with severe pancreatitis or abdominal trauma.

Auscultation. Peristaltic waves passing along the intestine can usually be heard in normal individuals as watery or tinkling sounds that peak in intensity every 2 to 3 minutes. Increased bowel sounds often coinciding with episodes of pain may indicate intestinal obstruction. Diminished or absent bowel sounds may occur in adynamic ileus (as in the postoperative patient), severe metabolic disorders, or peritoneal inflammation. Bruits are abnormal vascular sounds caused by turbulent flow in diseased vessels and may be heard over an aortic aneurysm or in a liver scarred by cirrhosis or cancer (Table 6–2).

Percussion and Palpation. Percussion and palpation of the abdomen are used to determine organ size and to localize abdominal tenderness. The liver is located beneath the right rib cage, and so it cannot be directly palpated in most individuals. Its size is usually determined by percussion along the midclavicular line because percussion over the liver produces a dull sound when compared with the resonance of the chest or abdomen. Normal hepatic span is approximately 10 cm. The liver may be shrunken in advanced cirrhosis or enlarged by acute hepatitis, right heart failure, or infiltration. The edge of the liver can often be felt beneath the right costal margin, and it is normally smooth, firm, and not tender. An enlarged, smooth, tender liver is suggestive of hepatitis, whereas a smaller liver with a nodular consistency is suggestive of cirrhosis.

Table 6–2. CLINICAL CONDITIONS THAT MAY CAUSE CHANGES IN PERISTALTIC SOUNDS

Peristalsis Diminished or Absent	Peristalsis Increased
Ileus from peritonitis	Brisk diarrhea
Pneumonia	Early pyloric obstruction
Myxedema	Advanced intestinal
Uremia	obstruction
Spinal cord injury	
Mesenteric thrombosis	
Postoperative adynamic ileus	
Enterocolitic ulceration	
Severe metabolic disorders	
Advanced intestinal obstruction	

The abdomen should also be examined gently in all four quadrants for areas of local tenderness. Gentle palpation to localize tender regions should always precede deeper probing. Deeper palpation for masses or organomegaly should follow, with attention to detection and characterization of specific abnormalities. Splenic enlargement, for example, results in a fullness in the left upper quadrant that is dull on percussion, whereas a gas-filled loop of intestine in the same region is tympanitic. Rectal examination for masses and tenderness and examination of the stool for occult blood are essential parts of any evaluation for intestinal bleeding, diarrhea, or abdominal pain.

PHYSICAL FINDINGS IN PERITONITIS

The possibility of peritonitis, or inflammation of the peritoneal membrane lining the abdominal cavity should be considered during the physical examination of any patient with abdominal pain. Peritonitis has many different causes and often heralds an intra-abdominal catastrophe that requires urgent surgery for correction. Perforation of an ulcer through the duodenal wall, ischemia or gangrene of the intestine, or perforation of an inflamed appendix or gallbladder can cause intestinal contents to spill into the normally sterile abdomen and result in peritonitis. The hallmark of this disorder is severe pain that is exacerbated by any movement, such as walking or coughing, such that most patients lie very still. Bowel sounds are diminished or absent, and the abdominal wall is quite rigid on palpation. The abdomen may feel rigid owing to contraction of the abdominal musculature, which is known as abdominal guarding. Similarly any motion of the abdomen elicits pain. This is detected clinically by rebound tenderness, which is elicited by carefully pressing into the abdominal wall and then rapidly withdrawing. Pain on rapid withdrawal is often indicative of underlying inflammation. When peritonitis is suspected on the basis of these findings, urgent medical and surgical consultation are indicated.

PHYSICAL FINDINGS IN LIVER DISEASE

The cardinal physical features of liver dysfunction are jaundice and ascites.

Table 6–3. CLINICAL MANIFESTATIONS OF PORTAL HYPERTENSION

Caput medusae
Hemorrhoids
Abdominal bruits
Enlarged, palpable spleen
Blood in stool
Ascites with concurrent liver disease

Jaundice. Jaundice is a yellowish discoloration of the skin, mucous membranes, and sclerae that results from the abnormal accumulation of bilirubin. Bilirubin is normally present in the serum in concentrations of 1 mg/dl or less. It is released by the breakdown of hemoglobin and is cleared from the circulation by the liver and excreted in the bile (see later). A variety of hepatic insults interfere with this clearance, and when serum levels exceed 2.5 mg/dl or so, the bilirubin begins to darken the skin and sclerae. Some of the excess bilirubin appears in the urine, and so jaundice is generally associated with darkening of the urine.

Ascites. Ascites is the accumulation of fluid in the peritoneal cavity. The healthy liver is a low-resistance vascular bed that receives essentially all of the nutrient-laden portal venous flow. Fibrosis or swelling of the liver may increase the pressure in the portal venous system (Tables 6–3 and 6–4). Portal hypertension results in a pressure gradient favoring movement of fluid out of the sinusoidal space and into the peritoneal cavity. Ascites formation can also result from other causes of portal hypertension in the absence of liver disease,

Table 6–4. CAUSES OF PORTAL HYPERTENSION

Intrahepatic
 Cirrhosis
 Schistosomiasis
 Tumor
 Fibrosis
 Infiltration
 Polycystic disease
 Sarcoidosis
Portal Vein
 Thrombosis
 Infection
 Tumor
Hepatic Vein
 Veno-occlusive disease
 Thrombosis

including congestive heart failure and hepatic vein thrombosis. It is exacerbated by associated hypoalbuminemia. Ascites is detected in severe cases by the observation of a bulging protuberant abdominal wall. Lesser amounts of fluid can be detected by a fluid wave when one side of the abdominal wall is tapped sharply and the opposite side is felt with the other hand. "Shifting dullness" is another sign of ascites. It is detected by percussing the area of tympany in the abdominal wall, turning the patient to his or her side, and repercussing to determine if the area of tympany changes. Because gas-filled intestine floats in ascitic fluid, the presence of shifting dullness strongly suggests ascites.

There are a variety of other more subtle physical accompaniments of liver disease that might catch the eye of an astute examiner. Palmar erythema, or reddish coloration of the thenar and hypothenar areas, is seen more frequently in patients with cirrhosis. Similarly, spider angiomas are vascular abnormalities on the upper torso, face, and arms that are often seen in these patients. It is important to emphasize, however, that significant liver disease can exist without any overt physical abnormalities.

Laboratory and Physiologic Tests

Laboratory studies provide important corroboration for diseases suspected on clinical grounds. The importance of many of these tests is self-evident and is not discussed in detail. The hematocrit, for example, is essential for evaluation of suspected intestinal bleeding, and the white blood cell count should be obtained whenever an inflammatory process such as cholecystitis, appendicitis, or peritonitis is suspected. Serum electrolyte abnormalities, particularly hypokalemia, occur frequently in patients with bowel obstruction or diarrhea.

Certain tests have greater specificity for gastrointestinal desease. In patients with abdominal pain, an elevated serum amylase level suggests underlying pancreatitis or inflammation of the pancreas. Amylase may also be elevated in other conditions, including parotid gland inflammation, tubo-ovarian abscess, and intestinal ischemia, but the clinical symptoms are distinct. Obstruction of the biliary tract is associated with elevation of alkaline phosphatase and bilirubin levels. Elevation of alkaline phosphatase levels results from increased hepatic synthesis. However, alkaline phosphatase is also found in bone. The hepatic origin can be confirmed by observing elevation of the 5'-nucleotidase. Bilirubin metabolism is more complex. As noted, bilirubin is produced by the metabolism of hemoglobin from senescent red blood cells. Unconjugated bilirubin is released in the circulation, is insoluble in serum, and is carried to the liver bound to albumin. In the liver, bilirubin is made water soluble by conjugation with one or two molecules of glucuronic acid, a reaction catalyzed by the enzyme glucuronyl transferase. By convention, unconjugated bilirubin is referred to as indirect bilirubin, and conjugated bilirubin is referred to as direct bilirubin. Conjugated bilirubin is secreted by the hepatocytes into the biliary tree, where it is stored in the gallbladder and then released into the duodenum by the bile duct. A small amount of this conjugated bilirubin escapes into the blood surrounding the hepatocytes and reaches levels up to 1 mg/dl in the serum. Any disruption of this normal pattern of metabolism results in the accumulation of bilirubin in the serum.

Hepatitis or hepatic injury is associated with elevation of serum aspartate aminotransferase (AST) and alanine aminotransferase (ALT) levels, also known as SGOT and SGPT, respectively. These enzymes found in the hepatocyte are released into the serum whenever there is hepatic damage. In general, the degree of elevation corresponds to the cellular damage. Biliary obstruction from a gallstone, for example, causes large elevations in alkaline phosphatase and bilirubin levels but small increases in AST and ALT levels. By contrast, in hepatitis, the alkaline phosphatase and bilirubin levels are elevated but the AST and ALT levels are much greater owing to the direct hepatocellular necrosis. Other laboratory tests important in assessing liver function include the serum albumin level and prothrombin time. In advanced liver disease, serum albumin concentrations decrease, and the prothrombin time is prolonged. This reflects severely impaired protein synthesis by the liver.

Visualization of Digestive Organs. Radiologic studies using barium to define the intestinal lumen can visualize the upper or lower intestine when structural abnormalities, such as ulcers, polyps, and malignancies, are suspected. Barium studies are widely available, cost less, and are relatively noninvasive. Fiberoptic endoscopy provides direct visualization of the intestinal lumen from the mouth to the second portion of the duodenum (upper tract endoscopy) and the entire colon and rectum (lower tract endoscopy).

Radiographic and endoscopic techniques are complementary, and the choice of techniques depends on local availability and the specific clinical condition. Endoscopy generally provides better mucosal detail and may also allow therapeutic intervention in certain conditions, including variceal hemorrhage, ulcer disease, and intestinal polyps. However, endoscopy is more expensive, and sedation is generally required.

Ultrasonography and computed tomography (CT) provide images of the intra-abdominal structures. Ultrasonography is safe (no radiation) and relatively inexpensive and is the procedure of choice in patients with suspected abdominal aortic aneurysm. Ultrasonography also provides excellent resolution of hepatic lesions, since the sound waves are easily transmitted through the solid organ. Computed tomography is more expensive and utilizes radiation but provides much better spatial resolution (1 cm or less) and better definitions of other intra-abdominal organs and the retoperitoneum. These techniques have been supplemented by magnetic resonance imaging.

ASSESSMENT OF COMMONLY ENCOUNTERED PROBLEMS

In the following sections, specific gastroenterologic problems that are likely to be found in podiatric patients are described in more detail. It is evident that one disease can manifest itself in several ways. Peptic ulcer disease, for example, can occur with abdominal pain, gastrointestinal bleeding, or acute abdomen. Gallstones can cause jaundice or abdominal pain. The evaluation of these clinical problems is usually guided by clinical clues such as guaiac-positive stools or elevated liver function test results.

Gastrointestinal Bleeding

Bleeding from the upper gastrointestinal tract is a serious and distressingly common problem in patients. Approximately 75% are found to have peptic ulcer disease or gastritis. Pain, stress, and use of certain medications increase the risk of hemorrhage in the perioperative period. Because bleeding is associated with significant morbidity and a mortality as high as 10%, an aggressive approach, emphasizing hemodynamic resuscitation and early empiric therapy, is warranted.

Diagnosis. In the patient with suspected upper gastrointestinal bleeding (defined as bleeding proximal to the ligament of Treitz), early attention to the hemodynamic status is far more important than the precise localization of the bleeding site (Fig. 6–4). Clinical assessment of blood loss should include inspection of the patient for signs of weakness, pallor, and mental confusion, all of which imply inadequate circulation; shock or hypotension; and inadequate urine output (less than 30 ml/hr), which implies poor renal perfusion. A nasogastric tube should be placed in order to confirm the upper intestinal origin of the bleeding and to assess its rate. Equivocal results of the nasogastric aspiration should be interpreted with caution for two reasons. A small amount of blood can be produced by tube placement. The absence of blood does not eliminate the possibility of bleeding distal to a competent pylorus. Hematocrit, blood coagulation studies, and blood typing and crossmatching are usually necessary. A normal hematocrit can be misleading in a patient with significant hemorrhage because several hours are necessary for rehydration and hemodilatation to produce a fall in the hematocrit.

Treatment. Patients who are hypotensive or who have evidence of organ hypoperfusion should be resuscitated with blood volume replacement and normal saline before specific diagnostic tests are performed. Early empiric therapy with saline lavage and antacids is appropriate in most patients. There is no clear evidence that early therapy with antacids, cimetidine, or ranitidine helps stop bleeding or prevents rebleeding, but these are safe therapies, and their potential benefit justifies their use.

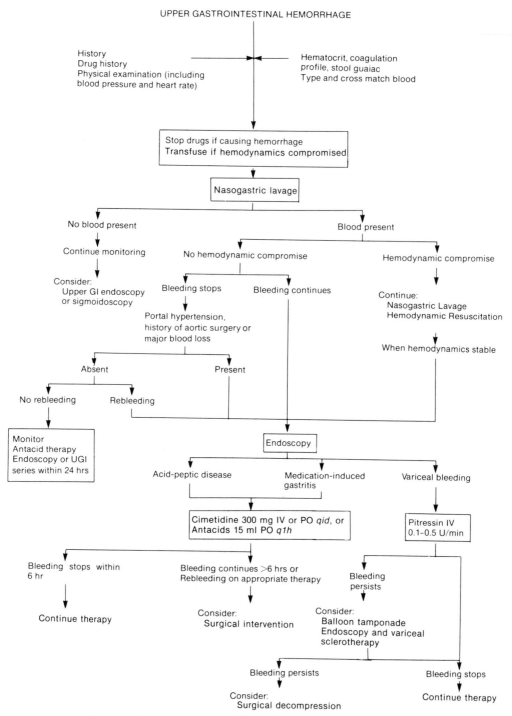

Figure 6–4. Treatment for suspected upper gastrointestinal hemorrhage. (GI, gastrointestinal; NG, nasogastric; UGI, upper gastrointestinal; LGI, lower gastrointestinal.) (From Don H (ed): Decision Making in Critical Care. Philadelphia: BC Decker Inc., 1985.)

The majority of patients stop bleeding without direct intervention. Hemodynamically stable patients who stop bleeding promptly should be treated empirically with antacids, H₂-receptor blocking agents, or a combination of the two. These patients can be investigated with endoscopy or upper gastrointestinal barium radiograms within 24 hours. Barium should be avoided if a lower gastrointestinal source is suspected. Emergent endoscopy is indicated in (1) patients who continue bleeding or who have been hemodynamically unstable, (2) patients with evidence of cirrhosis or portal hypotension because a different therapeutic approach is required for variceal hemorrhage, and (3) patients with aortic grafts because of the importance of identifying an aortoenteric fistula. Surgery should be considered in patients who require transfusion of more than 1500 ml of blood in 24 hours or who bleed again on medical therapy (Fig. 6–4).

Causes of Upper Gastrointestinal Bleeding

PEPTIC ULCER DISEASE

Acid and pepsin secreted by the stomach are powerful proteolytic agents. Normally the intestinal lumen is protected against their potential destructive effects by a cytoprotective barrier consisting of mucous, bicarbonate, and other poorly understood components. Ulcers are thought to occur when there is an imbalance between acid-peptic secretion and gastric cytoprotection. This imbalance occurs at some point in up to 5% of adults and is a major cause of abdominal pain and gastrointestinal hemorrhage.

Clinical Presentation. Nearly 90% of ulcers are found in the proximal duodenum, pylorus, or gastric antrum. Pathologically ulcers appear as sharply demarcated breaks in the normal mucosa, often surrounded by an area of gastritis or duodenitis. Pain is the cardinal clinical feature of ulcers. It is usually localized to the midepigastrium and is described as a gnawing or hungry sensation and may be relieved by eating. In addition to pain and bleeding, ulcers may perforate through the bowel wall and cause peritonitis or gastric outlet obstruction from closure of the pylorus due to surrounding edema. Gastric outlet obstruction generally causes recurrent nausea and vomiting.

Diagnosis. In patients suspected of having peptic ulcer disease, the choice of diagnostic procedures depends on the clinical condition and on the available facilities. Ulcers cannot usually be distinguished from gastritis on the basis of clinical symptoms. Occasionally the pain may mimic esophageal reflux, gallstones, or pancreatitis. In the young, stable patient with suspicious abdominal pain and no evidence of bleeding, it is often appropriate to treat empirically for ulcer disease and to perform other diagnostic tests if the patient does not improve. All patients with severe pain or intestinal bleeding need a precise etiologic diagnosis. Barium contrast radiograph of the upper gastrointestinal tract detects 50 to 90% of the ulcers found by flexible fiberoptic endoscopy. Despite the greater sensitivity of endoscopy, it has not replaced radiographic studies because of the risks of sedation and aspiration and its greater expense.

Treatment. Patients with documented peptic ulcer disease should avoid aspirin, alcohol, and NSAIDs. Approximately 40% of ulcers heal spontaneously after 6 weeks. Antacids have a time-honored place in treatment and increase the resolution rate to 70 to 80%. Unfortunately, antacids need to be taken 7 times per day (30 ml by mouth [PO] 1 and 3 hours after eating, and at bedtime). Magnesium-containing antacids can cause diarrhea, and aluminum-containing antacids can cause constipation. Constipation and diarrhea can generally be controlled by alternating magnesium-containing antacids with aluminum-containing ones. However, these factors have led to poor long-term compliance.

A number of potent suppressors of acid secretion, which heal approximately 70 to 80% of ulcers after 6 weeks of therapy, have been introduced. Cimetidine and ranitidine work by blocking the histamine (H₂) receptor on parietal cells. This receptor mediates acid secretion by a number of potent secretagogues. These drugs are taken less often than antacids (cimetidine, 300 mg PC four times a day [qid]; ranitidine, 150 mg PO twice a day [bid]) and rarely cause diarrhea or constipation. Patient compliance is greatly improved. Histamine receptor antagonists are generally safe and well-tolerated. However, rare cases of leukopenia and confusion have been reported with cimetidine.

There is increasing evidence that ulcer formation is a chronic disease. Even among patients whose ulcers heal after a course of therapy, 50 to 80% have recurrent ulcers in the year following therapy. In patients at risk, recurrence can usually be prevented by cimetidine (400 mg) or ranitidine (150 mg) taken once a day at bedtime. The most common preventable causes of recurrent disease are cigarette smoking and poor compliance with prescribed medication.

GASTRITIS

Gastritis is characterized by inflammation of the mucosal cells that line the stomach and is another common cause of nausea, abdominal pain, and gastrointestinal bleeding in the podiatric patient. The most important causes in hospitalized patients are stress and medication. This differs from acid-induced gastritis, which is usually located in the fundus of the stomach rather than in the pylorus or duodenum, and is generally a self-limited illness. Withdrawal of toxic medications and appropriate use of antacids are the preferred treatment.

Causes and Treatment. Acute gastritis that occurs in the setting of hypotension, sepsis, or surgery is referred to as stress gastritis. The etiology is not known, but it is postulated that mucosal ischemia causes abnormalities of the mucosal cytoprotection. When bleeding occurs in these patients, there is a high mortality because of the underlying illness. The incidence of stress gastritis can be decreased by prophylactic antacid therapy. The ideal regimen has not been established but 15 ml every 2 hours has been shown to be effective. The role of H_2-blocking agents in prevention of stress gastritis is uncertain. Some workers do not believe that cimetidine is as effective as antacids. Consequently, patients at risk for stress gastritis, including those with prolonged fasting, pain, and protracted illness, should generally receive prophylactic antacid therapy.

Drug ingestion is another common cause of acute gastritis. Alcohol is the most common offender, but aspirin and NSAIDs are more often found in clinical settings. Erythromycin and other antibiotics are occasional offenders. The exact pathogenesis of this disorder is not known. Alcohol may serve as a direct mucosal toxin, or it may alter the mucosal cytoprotection. Endogenous prostaglandins are thought to be important for normal cytoprotection, and aspirin and other NSAIDs are potent inhibitors of prostaglandin synthesis. Consequently, these agents may diminish the cytoprotective barrier. There is, however, no direct evidence that prostaglandin inhibition is a cause of gastritis. Drug-induced gastritis usually resolves within 24 to 48 hours after the offending agent is withdrawn. Antacid therapy during this period is recommended to provide symptomatic relief.

OTHER CAUSES OF UPPER GASTROINTESTINAL BLEEDING

Mallory-Weiss Syndrome. The Mallory-Weiss syndrome accounts for approximately 10% of cases of upper gastrointestinal hemorrage. Classically there is a history of repeated severe retching, followed by sudden hematemesis, or vomiting of bright red blood. This results from a mucosal tear at the gastroesophageal junction from the shear force at that site caused by vomiting. However, some patients have no history of vomiting. Endoscopy is usually required for accurate diagnosis because the mucosal tear is rarely seen on upper gastrointestinal series. The bleeding is generally self-limited, and only supportive therapy is needed.

Cirrhosis and Portal Hypertension. Patients with cirrhosis and portal hypertension are at extreme risk of serious gastrointestinal bleeding from esophageal varices. As noted previously, cirrhosis causes an increase in portal venous pressure. When the esophageal vessels are engorged, they are referred to as esophageal varices. These vessels are easily torn or damaged, and the hemorrhage that results is often torrential because of the high portal venous pressure and the coagulopathy frequently seen in liver disease. Consequently patients with gastrointestinal hemorrhage in whom there is a suspicion of portal hypertension should have early endoscopy to document the site of bleeding. Bleeding varices can be injected with a sclerosing agent to stop the bleeding at the time of endoscopy.

These patients are at great risk for complications and require transfer to an appropriate unit for intensive specialized medical and surgical therapy.

Lower Gastrointestinal Bleeding

Lower gastrointestinal hemorrhage is not as common in the hospitalized patient. Although upper tract hemorrhage may result in rectal bleeding or dark, tarry (melenic) stool, findings that point to the lower gastrointestinal tract as a more likely cause of hemorrhage include a history of rectal bleeding, a recent change in stool caliber, acute abdominal pain with frank hematochezia, and recurrent or bloody diarrhea. Rectal examination for hemorrhoids, fissures, or palpable masses is important. The most common causes of lower gastrointestinal bleeding include hemorrhoids, anal fissure, diverticulosis, and ischemic bowel disease. Cancer or polyps generally cause intermittent occult bleeding and anemia but may also cause frank bleeding (Table 6–5).

Diagnosis and Treatment. Sigmoidoscopy can detect lesions involving the lower 20 to 60 cm of the colon, such as hemorrhoids, polyps, inflammatory bowel disease, and cancer. Colonoscopy, angiography, and radionuclide scanning are other modalities used to detect these and other sources of lower gastrointestinal bleeding, located more proximally in the colon, including diverticulosis and polyps.

Initial treatment of lower gastrointestinal bleeding involves hemodynamic stabilization of the patient with parenteral fluids, blood products, or both before and during the diagnostic evaluation. Further treatment depends on identification of the bleeding site and may involve several modalities, including observation only if the bleeding seems to be resolving spontaneously, appropriate surgery, and selected intra-arterial infusion of vasopressors into the affected site.

Abdominal Pain in the Postoperative Period

When evaluating a patient with abdominal pain, the first responsibility is to assure that the patient is hemodynamically stable. If not stable, intravenous saline should be started immediately and vital signs monitored frequently while other tests are pending. The physical examination should focus on evidence for peritonitis or bleeding, and careful attention should be paid to the presence or absence of bowel sounds. Next, a hematocrit and white blood cell count should be performed to screen for hemorrhage or inflammatory processes. Other tests that may be of benefit include serum amylase, urinalysis, and liver function. A nasogastric tube is often helpful in decompressing the upper intestinal tract in a patient with excessive nausea and vomiting or in evaluating a patient with guaiac-positive stools.

Causes of Abdominal Pain

Gastritis or exacerbation of ulcer disease is commonly encountered in the perioperative period as previously described. Other causes of abdominal pain likely to be encountered postoperatively include the following disorders.

ADYNAMIC ILEUS

The normal peristaltic pattern of the small and large intestine can be temporarily impaired by stress, anesthesia, and medications. Typically this results in abdominal distention from the intraluminal accumulation of fluid and gases. Symptoms range from vague discomfort and constipation to severe pain with nausea, vomiting, and obstipation. Generally the abdomen is distended, and bowel sounds are diminished or absent. A kidney, ureter, and bladder (KUB) radiograph shows intestinal gas distributed throughout the

Table 6–5. MAJOR CAUSES OF LOWER GASTROINTESTINAL BLEEDING

Minimal	Moderate	Severe (Transfuse)
Local conditions: hemorrhoids, fissures or prolapse	Colon cancer	Diverticular disease
Colonic polyps	Diverticular disease	Vascular malformation
Colon cancer	Ulcerative colitis	Colon cancer
Inflammatory bowel disease	Colonic polyps	Duodenal ulcer Small bowel diverticula

small and large intestine with no suggestion of focal obstruction. Adynamic ileus is not associated with fever, leukocytosis, or intestinal bleeding. If these are present it indicates that other processes are responsible and further evaluation is warranted. Most patients with adynamic ileus have gradual resolution of their symptoms over 2 to 3 days. They should be managed conservatively, with intravenous hydration and kept NPO (nothing by mouth). Nasogastric suction should be given if there is associated vomiting. Strict avoidance of agents known to decrease bowel motility, including narcotics, should be enforced when possible.

SMALL BOWEL OBSTRUCTION

Mechanical obstruction of the small intestine in the perioperative period is uncommon but usually occurs in patients who have had prior abdominal surgery. Presumably the changes in motility facilitate looping of the intestine around fibrous peritoneal scars from previous surgery. The result is an accumulation of fluid and gas proximal to the obstruction site. The physical examination is similar to that used for adynamic ileus except that a scar from prior abdominal surgery is generally present; bowel sounds are usually increased, in intensity; and a KUB radiograph suggests a focal region of obstruction with little or no gas distal to the site.

Most patients can be managed conservatively, as for adynamic ileus. However, intestinal ischemia may mimic obstruction, or obstruction may lead to ischemia. Consequently suspected obstruction associated with fever, severe pain, or bleeding requires urgent attention.

INTESTINAL ISCHEMIA

The small and large intestines are richly vascularized by a densely interconnecting arterial and venous plexus, and symptoms referable to intestinal ischemia are uncommon. However, older patients may have atherosclerotic involvement of the arterial system, and hypotension related to anesthesia or bleeding may produce ischemia or infarct of the intestine. Ischemia, produces few findings, and the pain often seems out of proportion to the physical findings. Intestinal ischemia should be considered whenever abdominal pain develops following a hypotensive episode. Infarct results in severe abdominal pain and is often associated with hypotension and metabolic acidosis. Guaiac-positive stools, fever, leukocytosis, peritonitis, and metabolic acidosis are also found. Generally invasive procedures such as colonoscopy, arteriography and surgery are required.

Jaundice

Jaundice is usually detected when the skin, sclerae, or urine turns abnormally yellow from an accumulation of conjugated bilirubin . This results from hepatobiliary disease in most cases (Fig. 6–5). Unconjugated hyperbilirubinemia may occur with intravascular hemolysis, as in patients with congenital abnormalities of bilirubin metabolism. The most common congenital abnormality is Gilbert's syndrome, which results in impaired bilirubin glucuronidation. It is important to recognize Gilbert's syndrome since it occurs in 3 to 7% of the population and is not associated with other liver function abnormalities or diseases of the liver.

Unconjugated hyperbilirubinemia is generally classified as intrahepatic or extrahepatic. Intrahepatic causes include hepatitis or cirrhosis, in which there is insufficient cellular mass to conjugate circulating bilirubin. Extrahepatic causes include gallstones in the common bile duct, strictures, and other disorders that impair normal biliary drainage. Rapid identification of extrahepatic biliary tract obstruction is imperative because biliary decompression is frequently necessary. Features suggesting intrahepatic disease include a history of blood transfusions; an exposure to known hepatotoxic agents (Table 6–6); an enlarged, tender liver; and an elevation of the hepatocellular enzymes (AST, ALT) out of proportion to the alkaline phosphatase and bilirubin. Extrahepatic obstruction is suggested by a prior history of gallstones or biliary tract surgery and elevation of the alkaline phosphatase and bilirubin out of proportion to the hepatocellular enzymes. Sonographic examination of the biliary tree provides a safe and accurate assessment of obstruction. Enlargement of the common bile duct to > 10 mm in diameter is presumptive evi-

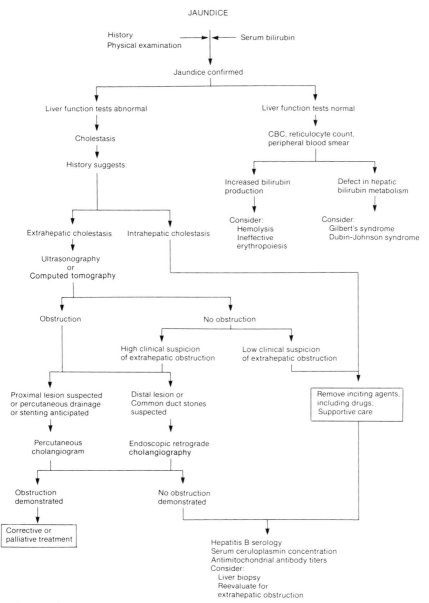

Figure 6–5. Evaluation of jaundice. (CBC, complete blood count; LFT, liver function test.) (From Don H (ed): Decision Making in Critical Care. Philadelphia: BC Decker Inc., 1985.)

dence of ductal obstruction. More invasive techniques (e.g., endoscopic retrograde cholangiography and percutaneous cholangiography) may be necessary in selected patients.

Special Risks. Patients with severe liver disease are at special risk for bleeding, hypoglycemia, and altered mental status. *Bleeding* may result from prolongation of the prothrombin time. Vitamin K–dependent clotting factors (II, VII, IX, X) and other procoagulants are synthesized in the liver, and their deficiency is detected by measuring the prothrombin time. Vitamin K (10 mg subcutaneously every day for 3 days) should be given whenever the prothrombin time is prolonged, since vitamin K deficiency also occurs in liver disease. A repeat clotting time should be determined within 24 hours. *Hypoglycemia* may result from depletion of hepatic glycogen stores and requires frequent serum glucose determinations and intravenous glucose to maintain adequate levels. *Altered mental status* results from failure of the diseased liver to clear circulating metabolic neuro-

Table 6–6. CLASSIFICATION OF DRUG-INDUCED LIVER DISEASE

Category	Example
Hepatotoxins with zonal necrosis	Acetaminophen, carbon tetrachloride
Nonspecific hepatitis	Aspirin, oxicillin
Viral hepatitis–like reaction	Halothane, isoniazid, phenytoin
Cholestasis:	
Noninflammatory	Estrogen, steroids
Inflammatory	Chlorpromazine, antithyroid agents
Fatty liver:	
Large droplet	Alcohol, corticosteroids
Small droplet	Tetracycline, valproic acid
Granulomas	Phenylbutazone, allopurinol
Chronic hepatitis	Methyldopa, nitrofurantoin
Tumors	Estrogen, vinyl chloride
Vascular lesions	6-Thioguanine, anabolic steroids

toxins. This can be treated with dietary protein restriction and administration of lactulose to induce acid diarrhea. Coagulopathy, hypoglycemia, or encephalopathy that results from liver disease is associated with a poor prognosis. Patients with significant liver disease should not receive medications or undergo surgery unless they have been fully evaluated.

Causes of Jaundice

INTRAHEPATIC CHOLESTASIS

Alcoholic Liver Disease. Alcoholic liver disease deserves special recognition as a cause of drug-induced liver disease because of its prevalence in society. It is not a problem limited to chronic alcoholics. Alcoholic liver disease results in three general clinical presentations. Acute fatty liver can occur after a weekend of immodest drinking and generally results in nausea, vomiting, and vague right upper quadrant tenderness.

Alcoholic hepatitis is more severe and may be accompanied by fever and leukocytosis but can be diagnosed with certainty only by liver biopsy. Laboratory evaluation reveals modest hyperbilirubinemia (levels usually less than 6 mg/dl), modest elevation of the alkaline phosphatase level, and elevated AST and ALT levels. Generally AST is greater than ALT, and values greater than 400 IU/L suggest another etiology. Withdrawal of alcohol is the only therapy required, but empiric thiamine and multivitamin therapy is warranted because nutritional deficiencies are common in this group of patients. The factors that predispose a chronic drinker to alcoholic cirrhosis are not fully known, but continued alcohol use is one of them.

Viral Hepatitis. Viral hepatitis can be caused by a number of agents that differ greatly in route of transmission, clinical course, and long-term consequences (Table 6–7). Types A, B, and non-A, non-B hepatitis are the most common forms recognized clinically. In each case, infection is followed by an asymptomatic incubation period of variable duration during which time the host can transmit the virus to others. Most cases of viral hepatitis are subclinical, and when symptoms do develop they are generally self-limited. Hepatitis B and non-A, non-B hepatitis cause chronic liver disease that can lead to cirrhosis in a

Table 6–7. CAUSES OF ACUTE VIRAL HEPATITIS

	Hepatitis A	Hepatitis B	Non-A, Non-B (2 or more agents)
Causative Agent	27 nm RNA virus	42 nm DNA virus core, surface parts	Unknown
Transmission	Fecal-oral; water	Parenteral inoculation or equivalent, direct contact	Similar to hepatitis B
Incubation	2–6 Weeks	4 Weeks to 6 months	2–20 Weeks
Period of Infectivity	2–3 Weeks; late incubation, early clinical phases	When HBsAg +	Unknown
Massive Hepatic Necrosis	Rare	Uncommon	Uncommon
Carrier	No	Yes	Yes
Chronic	No	Yes	Yes
Prophylaxis	Hygiene, immune serum globulin	Hygiene, hepatitis B immune globulin, vaccine	Hygiene, immune serum globulin, avoid commercial blood

significant number of patients. Because no specific therapy is available, every effort should be made to identify carriers of these viruses and to prevent transmission to others.

The clinical features of acute viral hepatitis are similar, and a specific diagnosis depends on serologic testing. Clinical hepatitis develops in a significant number of those infected. Following a period of incubation, nonspecific lethargy, anorexia, and fatigability mark the onset of the clinical phase. These are followed by nausea and vomiting. Subsequently jaundice, dark urine, and light stools are noticed by the patient. There may be modest elevation of temperature, and examination of the abdomen reveals an enlarged, tender liver.

Liver function tests show elevations of AST and ALT and variable elevations of bilirubin.

All patients should be closely monitored and should have serologic tests to determine the specific cause of the illness. Patients should generally be admitted to the hospital if the nausea is severe enough to prevent oral hydration, if the prothrombin time is prolonged to more than 14 seconds, or if there is doubt about the diagnosis.

Hepatitis A. Hepatitis A is the common cause of outbreaks of hepatitis in the community. It is also referred to as infectious hepatitis and is transmitted by oral-fecal contamination or ingestion of contaminated food. Homosexuality, travel to an underdeveloped country, and ingestion of

raw shellfish are common risk factors. Following a 3- to 6-week incubation period, the patient develops typical viral hepatitis (Fig. 6–6). Viral shedding begins during the incubation period, so the patient may be infectious before the clinical illness. Hepatitis A is usually diagnosed by finding gamma M immunoglobulin anti–hepatitis A virus (IgM anti-HAV) within 2 or 3 weeks of the illness and (IgG) anti-HAV thereafter. Hepatitis A does not cause chronic liver disease. Immune globulin provides effective prophylaxis if given within 1 week of exposure.

Hepatitis B. Unlike hepatitis A, hepatitis B may be associated with a chronic carrier state and chronic liver disease. Intravenous drug use, homosexuality, and work in a day care center are recognized risk factors. Following acute infection with hepatitis B there is a prolonged incubation period that averages 2 to 4 months (Fig. 6–7). The patient usually tests positive for hepatitis B surface antigen (HBsAg) during the late stages of the incubation and is infectious during this period. Up to 15% of patients may develop symptoms referable to circulating immune complex preceding clinical hepatitis by 1 to 4 weeks. This is characterized by symmetric polyarticular arthritis, rash, and low-grade fever during the late incubation period. Most patients with hepatitis B infection have a benign, self-limited illness. A small proportion may progress to fulminant liver disease, but the most worrisome feature is that approxi-

Figure 6–6. Sequence of clinical and laboratory findings in a patient with hepatitis A.

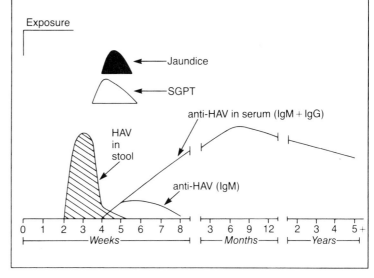

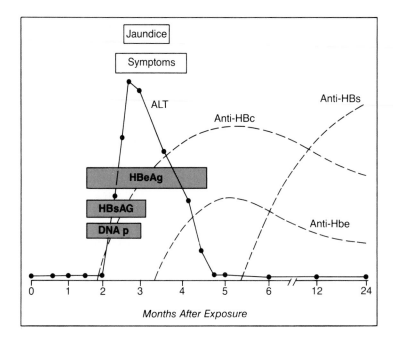

Figure 6–7. Sequence of clinical and laboratory findings in a patient with acute hepatitis B. Approximately 10% of patients fail to clear HBsAg and become chronic carriers (not shown).

mately 10% of those infected never successfully eliminate the virus and become chronic carriers. A carrier is defined as being HBsAg positive more than 6 months after an episode of acute hepatitis. These individuals are usually asymptomatic but may transmit the virus to others and may develop chronic liver disease.

Non-A, Non-B Hepatitis. Non-A, non-B hepatitis accounts for 90% of transfusion-related hepatitis. The infectious agent has not been isolated, and it is not certain whether it is one virus or several related viruses. Clinically non-A, non-B hepatitis has more in common with hepatitis B than hepatitis A. It is transmitted by the parenteral route, has an incubation period from 2 to 12 weeks, and is associated with a prolonged carrier state and progression to chronic liver disease in up to 30% of those infected. Because the causative agent has not been isolated, there is no diagnostic test available for non-A, non-B hepatitis. The diagnosis can be presumed when there is an appropriate history of blood-product exposure, and test results for hepatitis A, hepatitis B, cytomegalovirus (CMV), and other causes of hepatitis are unrevealing.

Drug-Induced Hepatitis. A number of commonly used drugs have been shown to cause acute or chronic hepatitis, including acetaminophen, halothane, alpha-methyl-dopa, isoniazid, phenytoin, and phenothiazines. Symptoms are similar to those seen with viral disease, so a careful history of drug exposure is mandatory in all patients. Most cases of drug-induced hepatitis can be treated simply by withdrawal of the offending agent and supportive care.

A noteworthy exception to this is hepatitis induced by acetaminophen. This drug is widely available and is used routinely in podiatric patients. Unfortunately it is a potentially lethal hepatotoxin when taken accidentally or intentionally in large amounts. It does not usually induce liver disease unless 10 to 15 g have been ingested, but lesser amounts can cause serious injury in alcoholic or malnourished patients. Consequently acetaminophen should be used with caution in patients with known liver disease.

Initially ingestion of toxic amounts of acetaminophen causes few symptoms. As the drug is metabolized by the liver, hepatic glutathione stores are depleted, and toxic metabolites of acetaminophen are formed faster than they can be cleared. These metabolites cause hepatocellular destruction, leading to clinical hepatitis and striking elevation of the AST and ALT levels 18 to 36 hours after ingestion. N-acetylcysteine, if given within 24 hours of drug ingestion (140 mg/kg oral loading dose, then 70 mg/kg by mouth every 4

portive care. Hepatotoxic agents, including alcohol and acetaminophen, should be stopped, and all other medications should be carefully reviewed. Since the liver is an important site of drug metabolism, drug dosage may need to be adjusted and drugs such as diazepam or barbiturates should be used with great care owing to impaired clearance. Fluid retention and ascites can be minimized by restricting dietary sodium (1 to 2/g/day) and by adding diuretics in advanced cases. Similarly, early hepatic encephalopathy can be improved by restriction of dietary protein to 50/g/day or less. All patients should have regular medical evaluations, and consultation is advisable before any surgical procedure or change in medication.

Pancreatitis

Acute pancreatitis refers to acute inflammation of the pancreas with escape of pancreatic enzymes into surrounding tissue. Most cases are related to biliary tract disease or heavy alcohol intake. Other less common causes include hypercalcemia; hyperlipidemia; abdominal trauma, including surgery; drugs such as prednisone and thiazides; vasculitis; and viral infections. Pancreatic inflammation leads to abdominal pain, nausea, and vomiting. The pain is in the midepigastrium and often radiates to the back as a result of the retroperitoneal location of the pancreas. The abdomen is tender in the upper midquadrant and may be distended. Patients may have associated fever, hypotension, and severe shock. The clinical diagnosis is supported by elevated serum amylase and lipid levels. Urine amylase levels are also increased and may confirm a diagnosis in equivocal cases. Sonography or computed tomography shows an enlarged pancreas, and fluid-filled pseudocysts may develop in more advanced cases. Treatment includes withholding food and liquids by mouth, nasogastric suction, pain control, and administration of intravenous fluids.

Acute Diarrhea

Diarrhea is a broad term that may refer to an increase in stool volume, stool liquidity, or frequency. It has many causes, but fortunately, the majority of these episodes are benign and self-limited, so that only supportive care is required. Diarrhea can be a manifestation of severe life-threatening disease. Consequently it is important to have an orderly diagnostic approach so that specific therapy can be instituted when required (Fig. 6–8).

Causes. Diarrhea is caused by an increase in the volume of liquid present in the stool. Under normal circumstances, 1 to 1.5 L of food are ingested each day, and salivary, gastric, biliary, and pancreatic secretions add 7 to 8 L to the volume of liquid presented to the small bowel. As this fluid traverses the intestine, approximately 8 L are resorbed, and the colon resorbs most of the remainder. Normal daily stool volume in the general population of the United States is 200 ml or less. Patients with increased bowel frequency from rectal inflammation or other causes often complain of diarrhea but have normal stool volumes. Consequently an accurate history is necessary. Stool volumes should be measured if necessary.

Diarrhea is generally classified as osmotic or secretory. In *osmotic diarrhea*, there is an increase in poorly absorbable solutes in the intestinal lumen, which trap water in the intestine and result in diarrhea. Lactose intolerance is commonly encountered clinically. In *secretory diarrhea*, there is increased secretion of water and electrolytes that overwhelms the absorptive capacities of the colon. Cholera and other infections may lead to secretory diarrhea. *Abnormal intestinal motility* is seen in hyperthyroidism, stress, and the irritable bowel syndrome. This classification has little clinical utility in the acute setting because most causes of diarrhea have mixed osmotic/secretory features.

Diagnosis. In evaluating patients with diarrhea, it is important to ask for a history of recent travel or exposure because the probability of an infectious etiology is increased (Fig. 6–9). A history of constipation alternating with diarrhea during periods of stress suggests the irritable bowel syndrome. Medications, including magnesium-containing antacids, antibiotics, and NSAIDs, are important causes of diarrhea. Homosexual males are at great risk for a wide variety of enteropathic agents. The physical examination should focus on the presence of fever and hemodynamic instability, which require specific therapy.

An important part of the evaluation of

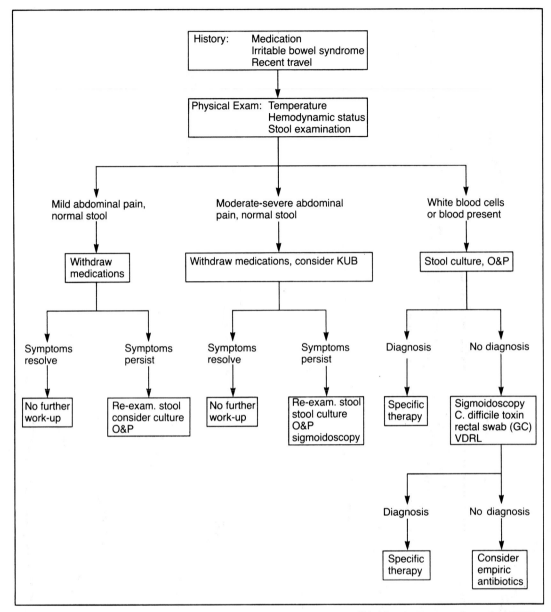

Figure 6–8. Chart for acute diarrhea. (GC, Gonorrhea; KUB, kidney, ureter, and bladder; O&P, ova and parasites; VDRL, Venereal Disease Research Laboratory.)

acute diarrhea is examining the stool for presence of blood and polymorphonuclear leukocytes (Fig. 6–9, Table 6–10). This is done by the stool guaiac test and methylene blue test. The methylene blue test is performed by placing a small sample of stool on a microscope slide with a coverslip. Methylene blue is placed at the edge of the coverslip, and the slide examined under the microscope. If white blood cells are present, they stand out against the background of the methylene blue. The presence of blood or inflammatory cells in-dicates intestinal mucosal invasion or damage and, in general, is associated with a more serious clinical course (Table 6–10).

General Treatment. Most episodes of diarrhea are self-limited and should be treated simply with judicious use of medication. It is essential to eliminate offending agents, such as antacids, antibiotics, and milk products. Oral rehydration with electrolyte solutions, such as broth or juices, is adequate in most patients. Bulk-forming agents such as bran or psyllium hydrophilic mucilloid (Metamucil) absorb

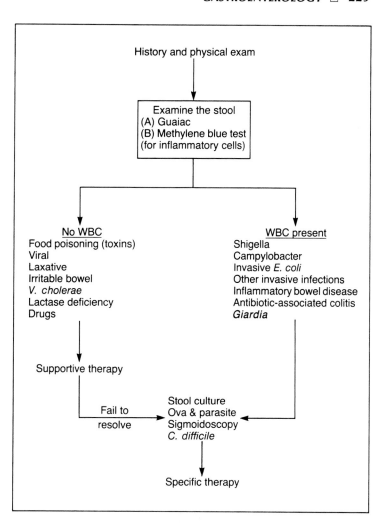

Figure 6–9. Classification of diarrhea by presence or absence of white blood cells.

fluid and are generally beneficial. Nonspecific antidiarrheal agents such as Kaopectate (60 to 90 ml qid before meals and at bedtime) provide symptomatic relief. Narcotic-like agents (e.g., paregoric, opium, codeine, diphenoxylate, and loperamide) are effective, but care should be taken because of their hemodynamic and psychologic effects. A theoretic disadvantage of antidiarrheal agents in infectious diarrhea is that they impair clearance of the microorganism from the intestinal tract and may promote intraluminal proliferation. Consequently care should be used whenever an infectious etiology is considered.

Diarrhea Without Inflammatory Cells

FUNCTIONAL DIARRHEA

Functional diarrhea is attributable to a change in bowel motility during periods of stress. It is common and generally results in several loose, watery bowel movements during periods of stress. Diarrhea in the preoperative period, for example, is frequent. Crampy abdominal pain and mild tenderness are often present, but absence of fever, lack of signs of peritoneal inflammation, and a normal white cell count strongly eliminate diagnosis other than functional diarrhea.

LACTASE INSUFFICIENCY

Lactase is an enzyme located on the luminal surface of intestinal mucosal cells. It cleaves the disaccharide lactose, which is found in high concentrations in milk products, into component monosaccharides. Approximately 20% of white adults and up to 70% of black adults lack this enzyme. Consequently when lactose is ingested in the form of milk, butter, cream, yogurt, or other dairy products, it cannot be absorbed, and symptoms result. These in-

Table 6–10. CAUSES OF DIARRHEA:
CLINICAL CATEGORIES

Acute Diarrhea
Viral, bacterial, parasitic infections
Food poisoning
Drugs (acute or chronic)
Fecal impaction
Traveler's Diarrhea
Bacterial infections (mediated by)
    Enterotoxins: *Escherichia coli,* heat labile or stable
    Invasion (mucosa, inflammation): *E. coli, Shigella, Cam-*
      pylobacter
    Invasion and enterotoxins: *Salmonella*
Chronic and Recurrent Diarrhea
Irritable bowel syndrome
Inflammatory bowel disease
Parasitic infections
Malabsorption syndromes
Lactase deficiency
Drugs (acute or chronic)
Chronic Diarrhea of Unknown Origin
Surreptitious laxative abuse
Irritable bowel syndrome
Unrecognized inflammatory bowel disease
Bile acid and malabsorption

clude bloating, cramping, nausea, and diarrhea. The diagnosis is made by a therapeutic response to withdrawal of lactose-containing foods, the finding of an acid stool, or abnormal results of a breath hydrogen test after ingestion of lactulose. Patients with marginal amounts of lactase may be asymptomatic under normal circumstances, but increased motility from stress can unmask symptoms.

DRUG-INDUCED DIARRHEA

Many commonly used drugs can cause diarrhea as a consequence of changes in fluid secretion, fluid absorption, or changes in colonic bacteria. The most common offenders include antibiotics, magnesium-containing antacids, digitalis, quinidine, and NSAIDs. Whenever drug-induced diarrhea is suspected, the offending agent should be withdrawn. Symptoms usually resolve within 24 to 48 hours.

Bacterial Infections

Certain bacteria produce diarrhea without evidence of mucosal invasion. This diarrhea occurs as a result of synthesis and release of a soluble toxin by the infecting organism that increases fluid secretion and decreases fluid absorption by the small intestine and colon. *Vibrio cholerae* is the best-described toxin-producing bacteria. However, certain strains of *Escherichia coli* are much more common. The diagnosis is made by culture of the stool. Therapy includes replacement of fluids and electrolyte losses. Oral fluids supplemented with electrolytes and glucose are generally adequate, although intravenous saline and antibiotics may be required in severe cases.

Diarrhea With Inflammatory Cells

Other bacteria cause diarrhea by direct mucosal invasion. This results in an inflammatory response and release of white blood cells into the stool. *Shigella, Campylobacter,* enteropathic *E. coli* and *Salmonella* are the most common offenders. These invasions are usually characterized by the abrupt onset of watery diarrhea and crampy abdominal pain. Blood may be present in the stool and systemic fever, chills, and evidence of sepsis are more common. The different organisms produce similar clinical symptoms, and bacterial culture of the stool is the only reliable way to make a definitive diagnosis. Most cases resolve spontaneously even without antibiotic treatment. Antibiotic treatment is usually guided by culture results, but empiric treatment with trimethoprim/sulfamethoxazole is indicated in patients who are severely ill, have protracted symptoms, or have small children at home.

PARASITES

Amebiasis and giardiasis are infectious parasites that result in diarrhea, often with white blood cells in the stool. Parasites are often seen in travelers returning from other countries or campers exposed to water contaminated by animal feces. Each is diagnosed by direct examination of the stool for parasites (three samples are usually required). Amebiasis is treated with diiodohydroxyquin (650 mg three times a day [tid] for 20 days) or metronidazole (750 mg tid for 5 days). Giardiasis often has more upper gastrointestinal symptoms such as nausea and bloating and is treated with quinacrine (100 mg tid for 7 days) or metronidazole (250 mg tid for 10 days). The stool should be re-examined for parasites 2 weeks after completion of therapy to ensure eradication.

PSEUDOMEMBRANOUS COLITIS

Pseudomembranous colitis is a cause of severe diarrhea in occasional patients. It occurs as a result of prior exposure to any of a number of antibiotics, including clindamycin, ampicillin, and erythromycin. These antibiotics suppress the growth of normal colonic bacteria, and overgrowth of *Clostridium difficile*. This bacterium produces a potent toxin that causes intense colonic inflammation and development of a characteristic exudate on the colonic surface called pseudomembranes. Typically patients develop fever, chills, and bloody diarrhea 1 to 2 weeks after exposure to an antibiotic. When these symptoms develop, the stool should be cultured for invasive pathogens and assayed for the *C. difficile* toxin. The characteristic pseudomembrane may be seen on sigmoidoscopy. Treatment consists of stopping the offending antibiotic and administering oral vancomycin (500 mg qid for 10 days) or metronidazole (750 mg tid for 10 days).

Bibliography

Alpers DH: Functional gastrointestinal disorders. Hosp Pract 4:139, 1983.

Alter HJ: The evolution, implications, and application of hepatitis B vaccine. JAMA 247:2272, 1982.

Bartlett JG, Chang TW, Gurwith M, et al: Antibiotics-associated pseudomembranous colitis due to toxin-producing clostridia. N Engl J Med 298:531, 1978.

Dienstag JL: Non-A, non-B hepatitis: Recognition, epidemiology, and clinical features. Gastroenterology 85:439, 1983.

Ginauck R, Macrae FA, Fleisher M: How to perform the fecal occult blood test. CA 34:134, 1984.

Graham DY, Moser SE, Estes MK: The effect of bran on bowel function and constipation. Am J Gastroenterol 77:599, 1982.

Harris JC, Dupont HL, Hornick RB: Fecal leukocytes in diarrheal illness. Ann Intern Med 76:697, 1972.

Ho DD, et al.: Campylobacter enteritis: Early diagnosis with Gram's stain. Arch Intern Med 142:1858, 1982.

Katz L, Spiro H: Gastrointestinal manifestations of diabetes. N Engl J Med 275:1350, 1966.

Levine GM: Postoperative gastrointestinal bleeding. In Brown FH, Goldmann DR (eds): Medical Care of the Surgical Patient: A Problem-Oriented Approach to Management. Philadelphia: JB Lippincott Co, 1982.

Quinn TC, Goodell SE, Fennell C, et al.: The polymicrobial origin of intestinal infections in homosexual men. N Engl J Med 309:576, 1983.

Sleisenger MH, Fordtran J (eds): Gastrointestinal Disease: Pathophysiology, Diagnosis and Management, 2nd ed. Philadelphia: WB Saunders Co, 1978.

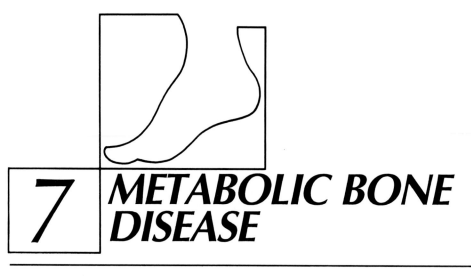

7 METABOLIC BONE DISEASE

GAIL M. GRANDINETTI and JOAN OLOFF-SOLOMON

OVERVIEW

Metabolic bone diseases are classified as such because the common element of these diseases is diffuse skeletal involvement. Although metabolic bone diseases have been known for centuries, their relationship to endocrine disease and calcium and phosphate metabolism disturbances was recognized more recently. Information concerning the causes of metabolic bone disease is either absent or incomplete. Effective therapy is available for only a few of the disorders. Early detection and treatment are essential because after skeletal mass has been lost, it may be difficult or impossible to restore it. This is particularly true of osteoporosis in postmenopausal women and the elderly. It is necessary to develop a high index of suspicion for the presence of metabolic bone disease in patients who are at risk, so that preventive measures and treatment may be instituted early. Any one or a combination of risk factors, especially if accompanied by symptoms such as back pain and muscle weakness and a history of spontaneous bone fractures with or without minimal trauma, should raise the suspicion that the patient may have metabolic bone disease (Table 7–1).

Table 7–1. METABOLIC BONE DISEASE: RISK FACTORS

Physiologic
Nonblack race
Postmenopause
Advanced age
Family history
Inherited low skeletal mass
Dietary
Acid ash diet
High phosphate intake
Anorexia nervosa
Protein starvation diet
Low calcium intake (dietary)
Excessive caffeine intake
Vitamin C deficient
Environmental and Physical
Smoking
Sunlight deprivation
Sedentary living
Immobilization
Drugs
Chronic heparin therapy
Thyroid hormone
Antacids, aluminum type
Cancer chemotherapy
Corticosteroids
Anticonvulsants
Excessive alcohol consumption
Diseases
Hyperparathyroidism
Hyperthyroidism
Sex hormone deficiency
Renal impairment
Renal tubular disorders
Acromegaly
Intestinal malabsorption
Hyperadrenocorticism
Gastric/intestinal resection (malabsorption)
Chronic obstructive biliary disease
Cushing's syndrome
Multiple myeloma

The physician must understand and integrate the anatomy, chemistry, and physiology of the skeletal system to understand the nature of metabolic bone disease. The extent and type of investigation should be determined by the specific metabolic bone disease suspected. The disease process involving the skeleton may be due to more than one pathologic entity. The clinician should evaluate the patient for the presence of all diseases and risk factors that could alter skeletal metabolism and aggravate the bone disease.

BONE FUNCTION AND STRUCTURE

Bone serves four functions. (1) Bones provide rigid support to extremities and body cavities. When bones are defective or weak, erect posture may be impossible, and vital organ function could be compromised, as in cardiopulmonary dysfunction in severe kyphosis. (2) Bones provide levers and sites of attachment for muscles that are an integral part of locomotion. With bone deformities, severe abnormalities of gait develop. (3) Bone houses hemopoietic tissue, which is actively engaged in blood cell production. (4) Bone contains a large reservoir of ions, including calcium, phosphorus, magnesium, and sodium. These ions are necessary for life and are mobilized in bone when the external environment fails to supply them.

Two thirds of bone is mineral; the rest is water and collagen, with other minor organic components, the functions of which are poorly understood. There are two main types of bone mineral, of which hydroxyapatite has the approximate composition $Ca_{10}(PO_4)_6OH_2$ in crystals of varying maturity and is the major form. The other type of bone mineral is amorphous calcium phosphate. One element is a fibrillar protein, which is a collagen substance related to connective tissue. An amorphous ground substance composed of mucopolysaccharides is related to interstitial fluid space. It therefore allows for a ready exchange of ions with the blood. The various ions of the interstitial fluid space are absorbed on the surface of the hydroxyapatite crystals.

Bone is a dynamic substance in which the elements are constantly being exchanged. The exchange is most prevalent at the portions of the bone with the greatest vascularity, such as the epiphyses and cancellous bone. These highly vascular areas of bone often become involved early in metabolic bone pathology.

Bone is rigid, is resistant to force, and is light enough to be moved by coordinated muscle contractions. These characteristics are a function of the strategic location of two major types of bone. *Cortical bone* is the major component of tubular bone; it provides rigidity and is composed of densely packed, mineralized collagen laid down in layers. Defective or scanty cortical bone leads to long bone fractures. *Trabecular (cancellous) bone* provides strength and elasticity; it constitutes the major portion of the axial skeleton and is spongy in appearance. Defective or scanty trabecular bone leads to vertebral fractures. Fractures of the long bone may also occur when normal reinforcement of trabecular bone is lacking.

Mineral Metabolism

Bone mineral is both deposited and maintained as a result of its solubility. In a normal adult, calcium intake equals calcium output. When the ion product of calcium times phosphate exceeds the solubility product of dicalcium phosphate, the substance deposited is hydroxyapatite. This entire process is started by the supersaturated state of the serum with respect to calcium and phosphate ions.

Calcium exists in ionized form as well as in an undissociated complex with protein. Normally the calcium exists in equal amounts in each state. Serum calcium levels depend on a variety of factors. First, an increase in the hydrogen ion concentration, or acidosis, increases bone absorption. The cell responsible for bone absorption is the osteoclast. Increase in bone absorption has the effect of raising the serum ionic calcium level. Secondly, the blood protein level affects certain calcium such that when protein is decreased, so is the serum calcium level. Conversely, serum calcium levels vary inversely to the phosphate ion concentration. In addition, serum calcium levels depend on the amount of calcium absorbed from the in-

terstitial mucosa. It is for this reason that vitamin D plays a role in calcium homeostasis, or regulation of calcium, and has an important effect on both bone deposition and reabsorption.

Vitamin D

Vitamin D is a hormone produced in the skin and found in certain foods. It is not the active substance vitamin D that causes these effects. Vitamin D is really a prohormone and serves as a precursor to a number of biologically active metabolites. Vitamin D must be converted through a succession of reactions in the liver and kidney to achieve biologic potency. Vitamin D is first hydroxylated in the liver to form calcifediol (25-hydroxycholecalciferol [25-OHD]); then this metabolite is further converted in the kidney to a number of other forms, one being calcitriol (1,25-dihydroxycholecalciferol [1,25-$(OH)_2$D cholecalciferol]), and another being 24,25-dihydroxycholecalciferol (24,25-[$OH]_2$D). Calcifediol and calcitriol are both available in drug form to treat disorders of calcium homeostasis. The third metabolite, 24,25-$(OH)_2$D, also shows promise for therapeutic use. This metabolite may affect bone mineralization in uremic patients. However, the precise effect remains to be established.

Vitamin D Metabolism

The vitamin D endocrine system can be divided into three levels of bioavailability. Vitamin D is made available to the body by photogenesis in the skin and absorption from the intestines. The metabolism of vitamin D to its active forms is mainly achieved by renal and hepatic enzymes. The active metabolites act on the target tissue, creating a variety of responses. The three target tissues principally responsible for calcium and phosphate homeostasis are kidney, bone, and intestine. Endocrine tissues also play a role in regulating calcium and phosphorus homeostasis. The parathyroid gland and anterior pituitary are target tissues, and their hormones help regulate vitamin D metabolism. Parathyroid hormone has a direct effect on bone and kidney regulation of calcium and phosphorus. Prolactin (PRL) and growth hormone (GH) help regulate vitamin D metabolism in the kidney.

Parathyroid Hormone

Parathyroid hormone (PTH) has two main actions. It inhibits renal tubular resorption of phosphate, causing a decrease in serum phosphate level, and it also directly affects bone by promoting resorption, with the freeing of calcium into the blood stream. There is a direct relationship between serum calcium levels and parathyroid activity. As serum calcium levels decrease, parathyroid activity increases to further mobilize calcium from the bone to raise the levels. Likewise, normal serum calcium levels cause an inhibitory effect on the parathyroid glands. Parathyroid hormone regulates calcium and phosphate flux across cellular membranes in bone and kidney, resulting in increased serum calcium and decreased serum phosphate. In the kidney, PTH increases the ability of the nephron to reabsorb calcium and magnesium but decreases its ability to reabsorb phosphate, amino acids, bicarbonate, sodium, chloride, and sulfate.

Another important action of PTH on the kidney is its stimulation of $1,25-(OH)_2D$ production. As mentioned, the net effect of PTH is to raise serum calcium and to reduce serum phosphate. The net effect of vitamin D is to raise both. As with other endocrine systems, regulation of calcium and phosphate homeostasis is achieved through a variety of feedback loops. As serum calcium levels rise, PTH secretion falls. Phosphate regulates PTH indirectly by forming complexes with calcium in the serum. Because its ionized concentration of calcium is detected by the parathyroid gland, increases in serum phosphate levels reduce the ionized calcium and lead to stimulation of PTH secretion. The feedback net effect of PTH then is to raise serum calcium and to lower serum phosphate levels. Likewise, both calcium and phosphate at high levels reduce the amount of $1,25-(OH)_2D$ produced by the kidney, increasing serum calcium and phosphorus levels and increasing the amount of $24,25-(OH)_2D$, which has little effect on levels, again giving an appropriate feedback regulation.

Secondary Hormonal Regulators

The secondary hormonal regulators of bone mineral homeostasis are minor compared with PTH and vitamin D. However, a number of these hormones (calcitonin, glucocorticoids, and estrogen) have actions on the bone mineral homeostasis mechanism that can be exploited therapeutically and thus should be remembered.

Availability

Vitamin D is available from the diet and is commonly used as a food supplement in daily products. It is absorbed principally in the jejunum by a process that is facilitated by bile salts, fatty acids, and monoglycerides. Vitamin D and its metabolites circulate in the plasma tightly bound to a carrier protein, mainly an alpha globulin. 1,25-Dihydroxycholecalciferol stimulates intestinal calcium and phosphate transport and bone resorption by acting on the intestine to induce new calcium-binding protein and by modulating calcium flux. The other metabolites of vitamin D are less potent but also stimulate intestinal calcium and phosphate transport and bone resorption.

Measurement

Measurement of vitamin D remains difficult because of its poor solubility in aqueous solutions and modest affinity for the binding proteins used in the assays. Most laboratories generally agree on the measurements of 25-OHD and $1,25-(OH)_2D$. Values differ somewhat from laboratory to laboratory, depending on the methodology and the sunlight exposure and dietary intake of vitamin D in the population studied. Children tend to have higher $1,25-(OH)_2D$ levels than adults.

Disorders Related to Vitamin D

Hypovitaminosis D. Hypovitaminosis D results from insufficient vitamin D in the diet, insufficient production of vitamin D in the skin, inadequate absorption of vitamin D, or abnormal conversion of vitamin D to its bioactive metabolites. Clinically this deficiency appears as rickets in children and osteomalacia in adults.

Hypervitaminosis D. Hypervitaminosis D may occur in three general settings. Hypervitaminosis D may result from (1) excessive consumption of vitamin D, often for therapeutic purposes; (2) abnormal conversion of vitamin D to its biologically active metabolites, as occurs in sarcoidosis and possibly other granulomatous diseases; and (3) change in the sensitivity of the target tissue to vitamin D, as can occur with the remission of a variety of gastrointestinal diseases associated with calcium malabsorption. The initial signs and symptoms of vitamin D intoxication include weakness, lethargy, headache, nausea, and polyuria and are attributed to hypercalcemia and hypercalciuria.

Ectopic calcification may occur, particularly in the kidney. Other sites for ectopic calcification include blood vessels, heart, lungs, and skin. The dose of vitamin D required to produce toxicity varies among patients, reflecting differences in absorption, storage, metabolism of the vitamin, and target tissue response to the active metabolites. An elderly patient with senile osteoporosis can ingest 50,000 IU of vitamin D/day without developing hypercalcemia or hypercalciuria. Such a patient's ability to absorb calcium is reduced, $1,25\text{-}(OH)_2D$ production in the kidney is reduced, and a low bone turnover rate is present. In contrast, in patients of similar age but with osteoporosis related to primary hyperparathyroidism, that amount of vitamin D would almost certainly be harmful. In a patient with primary hyperparathyroidism, the ability of vitamin D to stimulate bone resorption and intestinal calcium absorption is enhanced and related to the greater rate of $1,25\text{-}(OH)_2D$ production and bone turnover.

Patients with sarcoidosis are also prone to vitamin D intoxication due to interruption of normal feedback mechanisms that regulate renal production of $1,25\text{-}(OH)_2D$. This intoxication has been related to the production of $1,25\text{-}(OH)_2D$ in abnormal tissue, which apparently is not subject to the normal feedback mechanisms that regulate renal production $1,25\text{-}(OH)_2D$.

Treatment. Hypervitaminosis is treated by stopping the administration of vitamin D or its analogues or metabolites. Patients with severe hypercalcemia should be placed on a low-calcium diet and given glucocorticoids (prednisone 20 to 40 mg every day [qd]) and generous amounts of fluids. Symptomatic, acute hypercalcemia can be treated with saline and furosemide diuresis. The hypercalcemia of sarcoidosis tends to respond in several days to glucocorticoid therapy. Hypercalcemia lasts only a few days when caused by $1,25\text{-}(OH)_2D$ excess. However, when the cause is related to vitamin D excess, the hypercalcemia may persist for weeks or months.

PRESENTING FEATURES

The podiatric physician may encounter a patient with pedal complaints secondary to a metabolic bone disease or may encounter a disease as a local problem. Recognition of the underlying metabolic disorders is important in treating a local as well as a systemic symptomatology. Surgical therapy may need to be modified, based on recognition of the underlying metabolic process. For example, an implant arthroplasty procedure would necessitate an adequate osseous mineralization for the implant. Failure to recognize a mineralization abnormality prevents a good long-term functional result of surgery.

Symptomatology should not be relied on as the sole indicator of an underlying metabolic disease. Patients may present with a wide range of complaints; they may be completely asymptomatic or may present with painful, deforming skeletal abnormalities. Some patients may present with classic somatic abnormalities, which should clue the clinician to the underlying disease process.

Fractures. Fractures are often encountered in many patients with underlying metabolic bone disease. There is often not a clear history suggesting a traumatic event, yet the patient may indeed present with both clinical and radiographic evidence of such. These types of fractures generally fall into the category of insufficiency type stress fractures, that is, fractures occurring in bone of subnormal strengths subjected to repeated normal stresses. Treatment in these patients could be as simple as controlling the extremity biomechanically to prevent the bones from encountering excessive stress.

Bear in mind that cancer may manifest in bone as pain or pathologic fracture (fractures that occur through regions of localized bone disease in response to trauma that would not cause fracture in normal bone, for example, cancer metastatic to bone). In dealing with insufficiency or pathologic type fractures, the podiatric physician should work closely with the patient's primary care physician to provide a multidisciplinary approach.

ASSESSMENT OF METABOLIC BONE DISEASES

Osteoporosis

Osteoporosis is the most commonly encountered metabolic bone disease and is clinically evident beginning in middle life. Although men develop symptomatic osteoporosis between 50 and 70 years of age, it is predominantly a disease of postmenopausal women. For this reason, primary osteoporosis is also called postmenopausal or senile osteoporosis.

Essential to diagnosis of osteoporosis is the characteristic of an absolute decrease in the amount of bone mass per unit volume, with the defect in the mineralization of the organic phase of bone. Bone strength is proportional to its density, and as its mass declines, the mechanical support is affected. In osteoporosis, bone mass declines to a level below that which is capable of maintaining the structural integrity of the skeleton. Bone formation is usually normal histologically and chemically, with bone reabsorption rate increased. A primary feature of osteoporosis is trabecular bone loss greater than compact bone, which accounts for the signs and symptoms of the disease.

Osteoporosis may be associated with low, normal, or high bone turnover. All three mechanisms have been observed in the various types of osteoporosis. There must be an absolute or relative increase in bone resorption over bone formation. The bone remodeling sequence normally takes about 3 months for completion but may take longer in osteoporotic patients. Osteoclast activity or duration of action may be increased, leading to a larger resorption space in bone remodeling. Incomplete filling of the resorption space may also occur because of decreased osteoblast activity or duration of action.

Epidemiology

Osteoporotic fractures, particularly in women, present a major health problem in the United States, with expenditure in excess of 7 billion dollars annually. Each year in the United States about 1 million fractures are attributed to osteoporosis. By extreme old age, one woman in three and one man in six will have experienced hip fracture. Approximately 150,000 hip fractures occur annually in women older than age 65, with 15% to 25% associated with mortality or needing long-term nursing home care. Of women older than 65, 25% have one or more vertebral fractures caused by osteoporosis. Falls are the leading cause of death in the elderly, primarily because of hip fractures.

Contributing Factors

Skeletal mass is usually maximal by age 35 and declines in women after age 40 and in men after age 50. The etiology of osteoporosis may involve estrogen's enhancing calcium absorption by increasing 1,25-$(OH)_2$. Other influencing or risk factors for osteoporosis are low calcium intake, family history of osteoporosis, fair skin, excessive alcohol consumption, smoking, and sedentary living. Risk factors for bone loss are cumulative and may be multiple in any given patient (Table 7–2).

Osteoporosis may be secondary to an underlying disorder in which laboratory findings may be helpful in the diagnosis. Hy-

Table 7–2. OSTEOPOROSIS: CONTRIBUTING FACTORS

Family history	IDDM (poorly controlled)
Fair skin	Inherited low skeletal mass
Smoking	Sedentary living
Chronic heparin therapy	Low calcium intake (dietary)
Thyrotoxicosis	Excessive alcohol consumption
High phosphate intake	Impaired calcium absorption
	Lack of estrogen
Acid ash diet	Developmental disturbances
Hyperprolactinemia	Hyperparathyroidism
Cushing's syndrome	Increased calcitonin secretion
Anorexia nervosa	Deficient 1,25-$(OH)_2D$
Protein starvation diet	Vitamin C deficient
	Chronic renal calciuria
Hypopituitarism	Multiple myeloma
Acromegaly	Excessive caffeine intake
Leukemia	European extraction

IDDM, Insulin-dependent diabetes mellitus; 1,25-$(OH)_2D$, 1,25-dihydroxycholecalciferol.

Table 7–3 OSTEOPOROSIS: CLASSIFICATION OF CAUSES

Primary Osteoporosis	Endocrine	Bone Marrow	Connective Tissue	Gastrointestinal Diseases
Juvenile	Hypogonadism	Multiple myeloma and	Osteogenesis imperfecta	Subtotal gastrectomy
Idiopathic (young adults)	Ovarian agenesis	related disorders	Ehlers-Danlos syndrome	Malabsorption syndromes
Involutional	Hyperadrenocorticism	Disseminated carcinoma	Marfan's syndrome	Chronic obstructive jaundice
	Hyperparathyroidism	Systemic mastocytosis	Homocystinuria	Primary biliary cirrhosis
	Hyperthyroidism			Severe malnutrition
	Diabetes mellitus			Alactasia

perparathyroidism, hyperthyroidism, and hematologic malignancies may be responsible for the rapid progression of osteoporosis. Recognition of these underlying disorders is essential because the progression of bone loss may be slowed by treatment of the associated disease. The association of diabetes with poor skeletal growth and osteoporosis has been emphasized. The loss of bone marrow appears to be more severe in insulin-dependent patients than in those with noninsulin-dependent diabetes. Decreased bone mass has also been noted in chronic alcoholics and in patients treated with antineoplastic agents such as methotrexate. Osteoporosis may, in fact, be associated with any chronic disease state. The etiology may be due to the disease itself, the treatment of the disease, or immobility.

In summary, general circumstances that increase the risk for osteoporosis are
1. Phenomena of age-related bone loss.
2. Insufficient accumulation of skeletal mass in young adulthood, explained partly by race and sexual differences.
3. Bioavailability of calcium.
4. Menopause.
5. Endocrine abnormalities.
6. Various environmental factors.

Osteoporosis Syndromes

As stated, osteoporosis may be associated with a large number of disorders as a secondary manifestation (Table 7–3). However, the majority of cases of osteoporosis occur in middle-aged and older persons without any secondary abnormality. This common primary form of the disease has been named involutional osteoporosis and occurs in 60% of the cases in men and 80% of the cases in women.

INVOLUTIONAL OSTEOPOROSIS

Primary osteoporosis is most commonly described as postmenopausal or senile osteoporosis. It has become increasingly clear that these may be two distinct syndromes.

Type I. Type I postmenopausal osteoporosis is the classic form of the disease, occurring in women between 51 and 65 years of age who have been postmenopausal for about 15 years. Less frequently, a similar syndrome occurs in men, also between 51 and 65 years of age. Vertebral fracture is the main clinical manifestation, with frequent occurrence of Colles' fracture of the distal radius. Both these sites contain large amounts of trabecular bone. Measurements of bone density have clearly established accelerated loss of trabecular bone in type I involutional osteoporosis. Cortical bone is normal or only slightly less than age-matched normal subjects. Accelerated bone loss leads to decreased PTH secretion, resulting in decreased $1,25\text{-}(OH)_2D$, which causes impaired calcium absorption. This impaired calcium absorption may further increase bone loss.

Estrogen has been implicated as an etiologic factor in osteoporosis because women are predisposed to the disorder, with onset in proximity to menopause. All post-menopausal women are deficient in estrogen, but investigators have found no difference in those with or without type I osteoporosis. Therefore some factor or factors other than menopause must determine susceptibility.

Type II. Type II senile osteoporosis occurs in patients 75 years of age or older and is manifested mainly by hip fracture and vertebral fracture. Other fractures that may also occur include fractures of the proximal humerus, proximal tibia, and pelvis. Densitometric values for the proximal femur, vertebrae, and bones of the appendicular skeleton are in normal range and show proportionate loss of both cortical and trabecular bone at a rate of loss similar to that of the general population.

There may be two causes of type II osteoporosis, impaired bone formation and secondary hyperparathyroidism. From the age of 30 on, less bone is formed than is resorbed, and this imbalance increases with age. Parathyroid function increases with age and may be associated with the age-related decrease in calcium absorption. Overall bone turnover among women may increase with aging, as assessed by measurement of serum bone biochemical markers. Secondary hyperparathyroidism may increase the number of remodeling units in the individual bone and thus increase bone turnover, which results in extended bone loss.

JUVENILE OSTEOPOROSIS

Juvenile osteoporosis is a rare syndrome that occurs in prepubertal children between 8 and 14 years of age. On radiograph, the features are indistinguishable from those of involutional osteoporosis (Fig. 7–1). Bone resorption is strikingly increased. Juvenile osteoporosis has an acute onset with multiple vertebral fractures, which have occurred over a period of 2 to 4 years. There is spontaneous remission and resumption of bone growth. Protection of the spine is imperative until remission occurs. Steroids are contraindicated because they may cause early epiphyseal plate closure.

Other syndromes must be excluded when diagnosing juvenile osteoporosis. Osteogenesis imperfecta can be ruled out by lack of blue sclera, no long bone fractures and other stigmata, and no positive family history for bone disease. Cushing's syndrome can be excluded by adrenal function test results.

The etiology of juvenile osteoporosis is unknown, but the relationship to puberty suggests hormonal factors may be influential.

IDIOPATHIC OSTEOPOROSIS

Idiopathic osteoporosis is a relatively uncommon occurrence of osteoporosis in younger men and premenopausal women. No etiologic factor has been found, but idiopathic osteoporosis undoubtedly is heterogeneous. Some patients with idiopathic osteoporosis present with symptoms similar to those of involutional osteoporosis. In other patients, idiopathic osteoporosis is rapidly progressive and may cause severe disability or even death. Bone biopsy helps to differentiate this syndrome from osteogenesis imperfecta tarda, which has low bone turnover as opposed to the high turnover in idiopathic osteoporosis.

ENDOCRINE DISEASES

A number of endocrine dysfunction syndromes are associated with osteoporosis. *Hypogonadism* in either sex leads to an increased incidence of osteoporosis and is thought to be the main cause of osteoporosis associated with ovarian agenesis

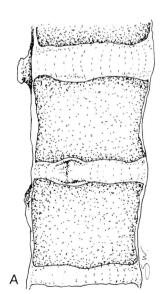
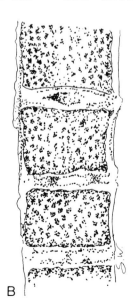
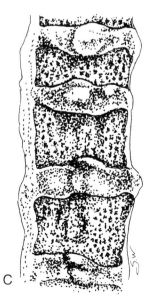

A B C

Figure 7–1. Normal and osteoporotic vertebrae. *A,* Normal vertebrae. *B,* Moderate osteoporosis with shape of vertebrae preserved with disk degeneration. *C,* Severe osteoporosis with vertebrae compressed by bulging disks.

(*Turner's syndrome*). A genetic abnormality in bone maturation may also be present in Turner's syndrome. Osteoporosis associated with *acromegaly* is rare but when present is the result of a concomitant hypogonadism. Most patients with acromegaly have an increase in both trabecular and cortical bone mass because of the anabolic effect of GH. Rapid bone loss is seen in endogenous or exogenous *hyperadrenocorticism*, which is associated with increased bone resorption and decreased bone formation. Patients with increased glucocorticoids have impaired calcium absorption, which is reversed by administration of vitamin D or its active metabolite. *Hyperthyroidism* increases bone turnover, but formation and resorption remain coupled. Osteoporosis with hyperthyroidism is unusual, but it is seen in postmenopausal women. Osteitis fibrosa is the skeletal deformity usually associated with *hyperparathyroidism*, but about 5% of patients do present with osteopenia and vertebral compression fractures, mostly postmenopausal women. Although controversial, it has been suggested that patients with juvenile-onset or adult-onset *diabetes mellitus* have an increased risk for osteoporosis.

Gastrointestinal Diseases

Osteoporosis, osteomalacia, or both are seen in gastrointestinal diseases. About 5% of patients with *subtotal gastrectomy* develop bone disease. Osteomalacia occurs in *malabsorption syndromes*, which are related to impaired absorption of calcium and vitamin D. If the impaired absorption is very mild, however, the primary lesion may be osteoporosis. *Severe malnutrition* and *anorexia nervosa*, involving both calcium and protein deficiency, may cause osteoporosis. *Alactasia* has been reported in 30% of osteoporotic patients and may be a risk factor for osteoporosis because of milk intolerance and associated low calcium intake. Osteomalacia has appeared in *primary biliary cirrhosis* and may be associated with impaired enterohepatic circulation of vitamin D metabolites.

Proliferative Disorders

In *multiple myeloma*, a rise in local production of osteoclast activating factor by bone marrow cells occurs and is thought to be responsible for the diffuse osteoporosis seen in about 10% of patients. This increase of osteoclast activity also occurs in other myeloproliferative disorders but to a lesser extent. Diffuse osteoporosis may also appear when *disseminated carcinoma* involves the bone marrow.

Connective Tissue Diseases

A severe form of osteoporosis may occur in *osteogenesis imperfecta*, an autosomal dominant disease with blue sclera, deafness, thin skin, and impaired type I collagen synthesis. *Marfan's syndrome* and *Ehlers-Danlos syndrome* may also be associated with spinal osteopenia, but with fewer vertebral fractures. Patients with *homocystinuria* commonly present with osteoporosis.

Other Causes

Total *immobilization* related to paralysis and prolonged bed rest results in a loss of up to 1% of bone per month, especially in the trabecular bone of the axial skeleton. Bone loss is associated with increased bone resorption and depressed bone formation. *Alcoholics* have been shown to have thinner bones. Osteoporosis is also seen with pulmonary disease. *Tobacco* is believed to be a bone toxin, and this may be the cause of osteoporosis in patients with *chronic obstructive pulmonary disease*, who are usually tobacco users. It is not known if smoking or pulmonary disease itself is responsible for osteoporosis in these patients. Severe bone loss and spontaneous fractures also occur in patients who are receiving *long-term heparin therapy*.

Clinical Manifestations

Mild osteoporosis may be asymptomatic, with the first suspicion of the disorder occurring after radiographs are taken for an unrelated problem. As mentioned previously, recognition of this disease is imperative in preoperative planning. The most common clinical presentation is that of a spinal compression fracture that occurs with no or minimal trauma, such as stepping from a curb, coughing, or sneezing. Stress fractures may also be apparent in the lower extremities in these patients. Stress fractures under these circumstances are the insufficiency type, as compared with fatigue fractures in normal bone mass. Common areas of stress fractures in the foot include cancellous areas of the metatarsals, the calcaneus, and the navicular bone. These patients are at a much greater risk to develop stress fracture following surgery because of their altered gait patterns. The association of lesser metatarsal stress fractures has previously been reported. I have seen one case of a stress fracture of the distal tibia that occurred 3 months following an arthroplasty of the second digit. Underlying osteoporosis made this patient more susceptible to an insufficiency fracture.

Essential clinical presentations of osteoporosis include mild to severe backache; spontaneous fractures and collapse of vertebrae without spinal cord compression, often discovered accidentally on radiograph; loss of height; spinal deformity such as kyphosis; fractures of the hip, the wrist, and occasionally other bones; and normal levels of serum calcium, phosphorus, and alkaline phosphate. In general, older women commonly develop substantial dorsal kyphosis and cervical lordosis, the so-called dowager's hump, with no significant pain. Half the hip fractures in elderly men and women are spontaneous, and half are associated with falls, as previously mentioned.

Primary osteoporosis is the only metabolic bone disease in which normal serum calcium and phosphorus levels are encountered. The only exception to this is the elevated serum calcium levels that are occasionally observed with a very rapid loss of bone density, such as with prolonged

Table 7–4. OSTEOPOROSIS: SUMMARY OF CLINICAL PRESENTATIONS

History	Loss of height, spontaneous fractures
Pain	Asymptomatic to severe
Fractures	Femur neck, vertebrae (crush), distal radius
Laboratory Values	Normal serum calcium, phosphorus, PTH alkaline, phosphatase (slight increase if recent fracture), urinary hydroxyproline (increased in active osteoporosis)
Radiograph	Demineralization spine, pelvis, especially femoral head and neck; vertebral compression; kyphosis; loss of horizontal trabeculae; biconcave "codfish" vertebrae

PTH, Parathyroid hormone.

cast immobilization or with reflex sympathetic dystrophy syndrome. The serum alkaline phosphate level in osteoporosis is either normal or low; however, it may be slightly elevated if a recent fracture has occurred (Table 7–4).

Radiographic Characteristics

Although there is some controversy concerning the role of plain radiography in the evaluation of osteoporosis, it still provides useful information. Osteopenia is a radiologic term that indicates a reduced amount of bone, including osteomalacia and osteoporosis. The two characteristic findings in osteoporosis are (1) thinning of the cortices and (2) loss of horizontal vertebral trabecular bone, accentuating the end-plates and vertical trabeculae and resulting in biconcave, "codfish'" vertebrae. There is also a loss in contrast between the interior of the vertebral body and adjacent soft tissue. Vertebral deformity may take the form of collapse, anterior wedging, ballooning from biconcave compression of the end-plates of the intervertebral disks, and localized herniation of the nucleus pulposus (Fig. 7–2). Osteoporosis related to glucocorticoid excess should be considered when there is associated osteoporosis of the skull, fractures of the ribs and pelvic rami, and prominent partially mineralized callus at the sites of fracture or osteotomy site.

In the absence of pseudofractures, it may be difficult to distinguish osteomalacia from osteoporosis. However, osteomalacia usually has a "ground-glass" appearance, whereas osteoporosis usually has a "clear-glass" appearance. Unfortunately variations in radiograph techniques prevent these features from being quantitative diagnostic tools. In addition, the loss of bone is evident on plain films only after 30% or more of bone mass has been lost. Evaluation of the spine may prove to be a useful adjunct, as it is recognized that bone loss is more rapid in the axial skeleton. In fact, some patients demonstrate only axial osteoporosis and never appendicular osteoporosis. The converse situation, however, would be extremely rare.

Because 30% or more of bone loss is necessary before plain radiography detects osteoporosis, more sensitive techniques have been developed to detect lesser amounts of bone loss. Osteoporosis results in loss of

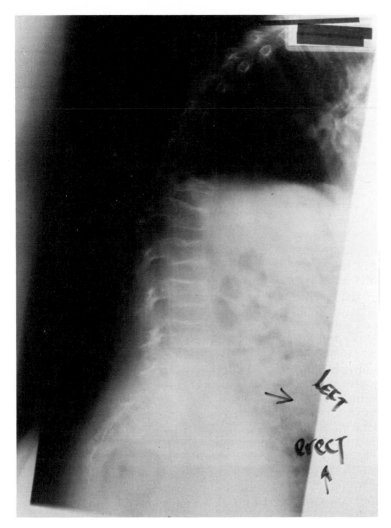

Figure 7–2. Severe spinal osteoporosis demonstrating cortical thinning and compression of vertebral bodies.

cancellous bone. The distal radius is a commonly used reference because it is 25% cancellous bone and is easily accessible. Single-photon absorptiometry using radioisotopes of iodine and americium is a simple and widely available method of quantitation. The information obtained by single-photon absorptiometry is valuable to podiatric surgeons in accessing bone mass in the extremities.

As mentioned previously, osteoporosis may be mild in the appendicular skeleton yet more severe in the axial skeleton. For this reason, a dual-photon technique has been developed to directly access the axial skeleton. An isotope is used that emits photons at two different energy levels and allows differentiation between bone and soft tissue. This differentiation is particularly important in the axial skeleton, which has

a higher marrow content than the appendicular skeleton.

Evaluation

A patient suspected of having newly discovered osteoporosis should be referred to his or her primary care physician for general medical evaluation to rule out secondary causes and disease processes (Table 7–5). As stated, serum calcium and phosphorus levels should be normal in primary osteoporosis. The serum alkaline phosphatase level may be transiently elevated during fracture healing or a new fracture, but if sustained in the absence of liver disease osteomalacia or a destructive skeletal process should be considered. Transiliac bone biopsy may be needed to exclude osteomalacia or to stage the

Table 7–5. DIFFERENTIAL DIAGNOSES IN OSTEOPOROSIS

Osteomalacia	Rickets
Paget's disease	Vitamin D intoxication
Hyperphosphatemia	Hyperparathyroidism
Metastatic disease	Osteogenesis imperfecta
Multiple myeloma	Acute bone atrophy
Hyperthyroidism	Osteopetrosis
Hypophosphatemia	

abnormality in bone remodeling. Severity of osteoporosis can also be assessed by the number of vertebral fractures and by loss of height.

A more precise evaluation of osteoporosis may be accomplished by measuring vertebral density, using dual-photon absorptiometry or quantitative CT. Cross-sectional CT scans of the spine are compared with standardized sample scans, showing normal fat, soft tissue, and mineral content. Unfortunately, the bones of the foot are too small to allow for quantitation of CT scans directly. Single-photon absorptiometry of the forearm assesses cortical bone, dual-photon absorptiometry of the spine assesses cortical and trabecular bone, and CT scans of the spine assess trabecular bone. Computed tomographic scans and dual-photon absorptiometry of bone density are good predictors of osteoporosis.

Hip fractures, the most morbid pathologic fracture, do not correlate well with CT and dual-photon bone densitometric measurements. Vertebral fractures are uncommon when vertebral bone density is greater than 1 g/cm^2 by dual-photon absorptiometry or 100 to 110 mg/cm^3 by quantitative CT scanning. Both absorptiometry and CT scan methods are noninvasive and given an accurate evaluation of cancellous bone mass. These noninvasive methods can be repeated and allow one to follow progression of disease or response to therapy. Absorptiometry and CT scan techniques, therefore, are replacing iliac bone biopsies in standard evaluation of osteoporosis. The tests are safe and acceptable to patients.

Noninvasive assessment of bone density and greater awareness of consequences of osteoporosis have led to screening of asymptomatic women. Women at an above-average risk for development of osteoporosis can be monitored if rapidly declining bone density would lead to initiation of estrogen therapy.

Treatment

Prevention. Prevention is certainly the easiest method of attacking the problem of osteoporosis. Combined hormone therapy, adequate calcium intake, and exercise are particularly useful methods in prevention. Effectiveness is in preventing bone loss, however, not in increasing bone mass. Specific treatment varies with the etiology (Table 7–6).

Estrogen. Estrogen replacement has proved to be particularly useful in the treatment of osteoporosis. Estrogen is more effective than calcium, but it has significant side effects.

There are associated problems with estrogen therapy. Before beginning estrogen therapy in a postmenopausal woman, a pelvic examination to rule out neoplasm or other abnormality should be performed by the primary care physician or gynecologist. The patient or family member should be informed that vaginal bleeding may occur, similar to a light to moderate menstrual period. An elevation in blood lipids that has been associated with an increased risk of cardiovascular disease may also be observed.

Estrogen should be administered daily except for the first 5 to 7 calendar days of each month, then the cycle should be repeated. Estrone sulfate and conjugated estrogenic substances (e.g., Amnestrogen and Premarin) are well tolerated and widely used. Transdermal estrogen

Table 7–6. OSTEOPOROSIS: SUMMARY OF TREATMENT

Causes	Specific Measures
Postmenopausal	Estrogen-progesterone, calcitonin (if estrogen contraindicated or not tolerated)
Senile	Testosterone and estrogen
Idiopathic	Testosterone, estrogen, or sodium fluoride
Dietary	Adequate diet, hormonal supplement as necessary
Multiple myeloma	Phosphate supplement with calcium
Refractory osteoporosis	Sodium fluoride (experimental) combined with vitamin D and calcium

Table 7–7. CALCIUM COMPOUNDS USED IN TREATMENT OF OSTEOPOROSIS

Compound	Route	Effect on Plasma Calcium
Calcium gluconate	IV, IM, or oral	Immediate of short duration
Calcium chloride	IV	Immediate of short duration
Calcium lactate	Oral	Immediate of short duration
Dihydrotachysterol	Oral	Delayed onset; peaks: 48–96 hrs, prolonged effect
Calciferol*	Oral	Delayed onset, prolonged effect
Parathyroid	IM or subcu	Moderate rapid onset, peaks 8–18 hrs

* Vitamin D_2.
IM, Intramuscularly; IV, intravenously; subcu, subcutaneously.

patches are available for treatment of postmenopausal symptoms; however, no data are available on their use for osteoporosis. For extensive disease, especially in women within 15 years of menopause, low-dose estrogen therapy (conjugated estrogen 0.625 mg to 1.25 mg/day or ethinyl estradiol 0.025 mg qd) may be used. Dangerous complications of estrogen therapy include increased incidence of endometrial carcinoma, increased growth of estrogen-dependent tumors of the breast and uterus, phlebitis, and pulmonary edema. Progestin (medroxyprogesterone acetate [Provera] 10 mg qd for the last 7 to 10 days of each estrogen cycle) may reduce side effects and reduce the risk of endometrial carcinoma by causing periodic sloughing of the endometrium. Even women who have undergone hysterectomy should receive cyclic therapy. If fractures continue on this regimen doses of both estrogen and progestin should be doubled. Elderly women may prefer synthetic anabolic steroids to estrogens.

Calcium. Calcium supplementation has also been utilized and appears to decrease bone resorption, although probably not as effectively as estrogens (Table 7–7). Calcium supplements are usually given in conjunction with small amounts of vitamin D to enhance intestinal absorption of the calcium.

Sodium Fluoride. Sodium fluoride therapy has been tried in refractory osteoporosis, but it must still be considered experimental. Given with both calcium and vitamin D, sodium fluoride appears to enhance bone formation and increases bone mass. The long-term safety of this therapy is not yet known.

Calcitonin. Calcitonin (100 IU/day) has been approved by the Food and Drug Administration (FDA) for treatment of osteoporosis. It is an effective antiresorption agent but must be supplemented with calcium concurrently to prevent secondary hyperparathyroidism. Calcitonin must be used parenterally (intramuscular or subcutaneous). Calcitonin is very expensive and another disadvantage is the development of neutralizing antibodies in some patients. Calcitonin can be used as an alternative to estrogen therapy when estrogen is not tolerated or is contraindicated. However, no study has reported a decreased fracture incidence, reflecting either the relatively short duration of treatment or the insufficiency of increased bone density to prevent fractures. Further controlled trials are needed.

General measures with calcitonin therapy include a diet adequate in protein, calcium, and vitamin D. Supplemental calcium salts such as calcium carbonate are advisable (up to 1 to 4 g/day 1 to 3 hours after meals and at bedtime). Vitamin D (2000 to 5000 IU/d) may be needed if there is an associated malabsorption or osteomalacia. This dosage should be individualized to maintain a serum calcium level of 9 to 10 mg/dl. Rarely, a patient may require $1,25\text{-}(OH)_2D$. Patients should be kept active; bedridden patients should be given active or passive exercises. Rigid or excessive immobilization must be avoided. The podiatrist must integrate this into his or her treatment plan for any patient who is at high risk for osteoporosis.

Parathyroid Hormone. Parathyroid hormone in combination with $1,25\text{-}(OH)_2D$ stimulates new bone formation without hypercalcemia. This combination is under investigation as an effective treatment approach for osteoporosis.

Exercise. Exercise is an important component of preventive therapy for osteoporosis. Bone mass in women premenopausally may be significant in the development of osteoporosis later in life, as evidenced by the low incidence of osteoporosis in black women and men, who have a greater skeletal mass than white women. Physical activity and exercise have been shown to increase skeletal mass and to increase total body calcium. Taking 1500 mg of calcium and 400 IU of vitamin D daily in conjunction with exercise offers the best hope for increasing skeletal mass during skeletal growth.

Osteomalacia and Rickets

Osteomalacia and rickets are a result of vitamin D deficiency, which can occur because of insufficient dietary intake, lack of sun exposure, malabsorption, or defective metabolism. These conditions differ only in that rickets occurs in the presence of active bone growth and osteomalacia in the absence of active bone growth. Rickets begins in childhood, although its manifestations may persist throughout adult life. Osteomalacia begins after skeletal growth is completed (Table 7–8).

Rickets in the child or osteomalacia in the adult is characterized by a deficiency of calcium salt or phosphorus deposition, or both, in the bone tissue matrix, an excess of poorly mineralized osteoid tissue. The most common causes of these disorders include vitamin D deficiency, as mentioned, from poor nutrition, lack of sun exposure (as in home-bound patients), disorders of vitamin D metabolism, and malabsorption from gastrointestinal or hepatobiliary disease. Other causes include systemic acidosis and phosphate depletion, resulting from impaired renal tubular phosphate reabsorption or excess aluminum hydroxide ingestion. The serum calcium level is usually low, and the phosphorus level is low or normal. Almost all forms of osteomalacia are associated with compensatory, secondary hyperparathyroidism initiated by the low calcium level, which accounts for the only slightly low serum calcium levels in compensated osteoporosis.

Osteomalacia should be suspected in patients with hypocalcemia or hypophosphatemia, urinary calcium excretion of less than 100 mg/24 hours (unless the patient is taking thiazide diuretics), low 25-OHD levels, elevated PTH, elevated alkaline phosphatase (unless the patient has a recent fracture), and premature osteopenia. Osteomalacia should also be suspected in osteopenic patients who are receiving anticonvulsant therapy.

In osteomalacia, too little bone mineral is precipitated into the bone matrix. This abnormal bone is less resistant to stress and strain. As a result, there is a compensatory overproduction of osteoid by the osteoblasts. Therefore, the serum alkaline phosphatase level is increased.

Epidemiology

Vitamin D enrichment of animal and human food has effectively prevented rickets so that the disease in its florid forms has become a rarity in technically advanced countries. Rickets has persisted in Africa and other underdeveloped areas and is still in urban areas of the United Kingdom, where migratory populations from the West Indies and Pakistan have come from a sunny to a cloudy climate and do not use preventive measures.

Osteomalacia is uncommon in developed and developing countries and is common in countries experiencing famine, affecting especially women. Women from northern China and Muslim countries de-

Table 7–8. OSTEOMALACIC SYNDROMES

Disorders in the Vitamin D Endocrine System
1. Decreased bioavailability: decreased sunlight exposure, lack of vitamin D, urinary loss (nephrotic syndrome), fecal loss (malabsorption)
2. Abnormal metabolism: liver disease, chronic renal failure, type 1 rickets (vitamin D dependent), hypophosphatemia (tumor), X-linked hypophosphatemia, anticonvulsants, chronic acidosis
3. Abnormal target tissue response: type 2 rickets (vitamin D dependent), gastrointestinal disorders

Disorders of Phosphate Homeostasis
1. Decreased intestinal absorption: malnutrition, malabsorption, aluminum hydroxide antacids
2. Increased renal loss

Calcium Deficiency
1. Dietary insufficiency
2. Excessive renal loss
3. Malabsorption of calcium

Primary Disorders of Bone Matrix
1. Hypophosphatasia
2. Fibrogenesis imperfecta ossium
3. Axial osteomalacia

Inhibitors of Mineralization
1. Aluminum: chronic renal failure, total parenteral nutrition
2. Etidronate disodium

Table 7–9. CHEMICAL FEATURES OF DISEASES WITH DISTURBED PLASMA CALCIUM AND PHOSPHATE

	Serum			Urine	
Disease	*Calcium*	*Phosphate*	*Alkaline Phosphatase*	*Calcium*	*Phosphate*
Hypoparathyroidism	Dec	Inc	Nl	Dec	Dec
Osteomalacia	Dec or nl	Dec	Inc	Dec	Dec
Osteoporosis	Nl	Nl	Nl	Nl	Nl
Multiple myeloma	Nl to inc	Nl	Nl	Nl to inc	Nl to dec
Renal insufficiency	Dec	Inc	Nl or inc	Dec	Dec

Dec, Decreased; Inc, increased; Nl, normal.

velop osteomalacia more commonly as a result of low calcium intake, insufficient sunlight exposure, and many pregnancies.

Virtually all cases of osteomalacia in the Western world have been attributed to some factor related to abnormal vitamin D or calcium and phosphorus metabolism, such as poor absorption, excessive intestinal loss, disordered metabolic turnover, or increased renal excretion.

Pathogenesis

Kidneys, intestines, and parathyroid glands all participate in vitamin D metabolism and in the maintenance of normal calcium and phosphate levels in the serum (Table 7–9); thus all are involved in bone mineralization. Consequently there are many forms of rickets and osteomalacia; 30 subtypes have been identified.

Rickets is defined as a disease of the developing skeleton characterized by defective mineralization of the organic matrices of the cartilage and bone. In osteomalacia, the defective mineralization is in the bone matrix. Both are most commonly due to lack of vitamin D specifically. Vitamin D, through its biologically active metabolites, ensures that calcium and phosphate concentrations in the extracellular fluid are adequate for mineralization to occur. Vitamin D also may permit osteoblasts to produce a bone matrix that can be mineralized, which then allows normal mineralization. Phosphate deficiency is another condition that can cause defective mineralization. Phosphate deficiency may act independently or in conjunction with other abnormalities. Most hypophosphatemia disorders associated with rickets and osteomalacia also affect the vitamin D endocrine system. Dietary calcium deficiency has also been identified as a cause of rickets; this deficiency may also contribute to osteoporosis and osteomalacia in the elderly patient.

Rickets and osteomalacia may develop even with normal levels of calcium, phosphate, and vitamin D. The bone matrix may not be able to undergo normal mineralization, as seen in alkaline phosphatase deficiency with hypophosphatasia. Drugs such as etidronate and heavy metals such as aluminum also interfere with mineralization and lead to osteomalacia or rickets.

Disorders in the vitamin D endocrine system are the leading causes of rickets and osteomalacia through decreased bioavailability of vitamin D, abnormal metabolism of vitamin D, and abnormal response of target tissues to the biologically active vitamin D metabolites.

Classification

RICKETS

Rickets has been classified in various ways. One of the simplest classifies two main types according to their pathogenesis. *Type 1* rickets involves an abnormality in vitamin D metabolism, leading to a deficiency of active vitamin D. The chemical transformation of vitamin D occurs at a number of sites in the body, such as the skin, liver, and kidneys. Therefore interference with this process at any of these sites can lead to type 1 rickets. Anticonvulsant therapy, especially combinations of phenobarbital and phenytoin (Dilantin), has also been linked to type 1 rickets. *Type 2* rickets is caused by a target tissue abnormality, specifically, renal tubular disorders characterized by a defective renal tubular absorption of phosphate.

Clinical Manifestations

RICKETS

Rickets involves a greater range of histologic changes than does osteomalacia. The histologic changes of rickets are characteristically seen in premature infants breast-fed without supplementation. In all children, clinical manifestation of rickets occurs only after a long period of vitamin D insufficiency. The clinical presentation depends on the age of the patient and the etiology. In patients with rickets, there is a delay in suture and fontanelle closure of the skull, and frontal thickening becomes evident. The enamel of the teeth may be defective. The long bones are enlarged and weak, with unstable shafts. Weight bearing and normal muscle tension produce bending, rotation, and distortion of many bones.

Severe tibial torsion and femoral bowing may lead to a waddling gait. Deformities of the vertebral bodies may be observed. Enlarged costochondral junctions form the visible prominences known as the rachitic rosary. Pelvic growth may also be compromised. The gross skeletal deformities depend to a great extent on the stress to which each bone is subjected, which is also related to the child's age and activity. The nonambulatory child places greatest stress upon the head and chest. Craniotabes, buckling of the abnormally soft cranium under pressure and recoiling back into position with pressure release, is a clinical sign of rickets. Another clinical sign is a squared appearance of the head, which is the result of excess of osteoid tissue's producing frontal bossing. Chest malformations include the rachitic rosary, caused by overgrowth of osteoid tissue at the costochondral junctions, and the pigeon breast deformity, a result of the collapse of the ribs with protrusion of the sternum. Additional deformities occur in the spine, pelvis, and long bone when the child with full-blown rickets begins to ambulate. Lumbar lordosis and bowing of the legs are common.

The affected infant and young child may exhibit apathy, listlessness, weakness, hypotonia, and poor growth. Hypotonia may result in a pronounced pot belly and a wad-dling gait. The limbs may become bowed, with joint swelling related to flaring at the ends of long bones, including phalanges and metacarpals. Pathologic fractures may appear in patients with florid rickets.

In type 2 rickets, skeletal deformities of the head, spine, and pelvis are less marked. Skeletal deformities of the lower extremities are characteristic.

OSTEOMALACIA

Osteomalacia in adults results in changes similar to those of rickets, but they are confined to defects in membranous bone formation. The inadequate mineralization leads to an excess of osteoid matrix. The bony structure is more coarse but abnormally weak.

Deformities of weight-bearing bones are common. Although pathologic fractures occur, they are often incomplete because of the decreased brittleness of the bones. Other clinical features include bone pain and muscle weakness. Subjective complaints include constant, dull bone aches and proximal muscle weakness, with inability to walk resulting in severely affected patients. These patients often experience hip fractures. However, it is difficult to diagnose osteomalacia on clinical grounds only.

DIFFERENTIAL DIAGNOSIS

One must recognize osteomalacia and consider it in the differential diagnosis of bone disease because it is a potentially curable disease. Rickets may be mistaken for osteogenesis imperfecta or other nonmetabolic bone disorders. Long-standing disease enters into the differential diagnosis of any metabolic or generalized nonmetabolic bone disease. Pseudofracture is often the only outstanding sign of latent osteomalacia. Osteoporosis may exist as well and may obscure the osteomalacia. The diagnosis can be confirmed by a rise and subsequent fall of the serum alkaline phosphatse level after treatment with vitamin D and calcium. Renal tubular acidosis is a cause of renal stone formation and nephrocalcinosis and must be considered in the differential diagnosis of kidney calcifications with bone disease, such as hyperparathyroidism. The prognosis is usually excellent in absorption disorders if diagnosed early. This does not hold for certain vitamin D–resistant forms of osteomalacia or rickets, which respond slowly or not at all unless large amounts of vitamin D are given. In these forms of osteomalacia or rickets, characteristically the serum alkaline phosphatase level is elevated because of the osteoblastic activity. Serum calcium and phosphorus levels may be normal or low. Excessive intake of vitamin D causes hypercalcemia and has been known to be fatal.

Radiographic Characteristics

Radiographic evaluation is of value in patients with rickets and osteomalacia and can be quite striking especially in the young child. Involvement of the pelvis and long bones, with demineralization and bowing, is apparent. Less often, the spine and skull are involved as well. Radiolucent epiphyses are wide and flared, with irregular epiphyseal-metaphyseal junctions in the growing bones. Long bone cortices are often indistinct. Occasionally signs of secondary hyperparathyroidism, signs of subperiosteal resorption in the phalanges and metacarpals, and signs of erosion of the distal ends of the clavicles are observed. Fractures are rare except for pseudofractures, also known as Looser's zones, which are uncommon but almost pathognomonic for rickets and osteomalacia. Pseudofractures are the result of unhealed microfractures at points of stress or entry points of blood vessels into bone. They are radiolucent lines often found along the concave side of the femoral neck the pubic rami, the ribs, and the lateral scapulae. These fractures may go unrecognized and may lead to substantial deformity and disability. One should look for not just one finding but a combination of findings to confirm clinical suspicions. These findings include an ill-defined cortex; a coarse, indistinct appearance of the bone due to the absorption of secondary trabeculae; and a poor mineralization of the primary trabeculae. Secondary bowing deformities due to bone softening may be seen.

If an immature skeleton is involved in addition to the aforementioned findings one may note cupping and fraying of the metaphyses. Widening, an irregularity of the zone of provisional calcification, may be noted. Nephrocalcinosis may appear in patients with renal tubular acidosis. Mineralization changes are often subtle and not readily distinguishable from osteoporosis in adults with normal renal function.

Bone scintiscan may show increased uptake of tracer material and may locate lesions not visualized on conventional radiographs, such as pseudofractures. Bone-density studies are not reliable indicators of osteomalacia. Bone density can be decreased in patients with vitamin D deficiency or increased in patients with chronic renal failure.

Treatment

The goal of treatment of rickets and osteomalacia is to normalize the clinical, biochemical, and radiologic abnormalities without producing hypercalcemia, hyperphosphatemia, hypercalciuria, nephrolithiasis, or ectopic calcification. As the bone lesions heal or the underlying disease improves, the dose of vitamin D, calcium, or phosphate needs to be adjusted to avoid such complications.

Minimum requirements for prevention of rickets is 400 IU of vitamin D/day. Once rickets is overt, the treatment for simple dietary vitamin D deficiency consists of 600,000 IU of vitamin D parenterally in one or more dosages over 24 hours. An alternative method of administration is oral dosages of 2000 to 4000 IU of vitamin D/day for several months, followed by replacement dosages of 400 IU/day orally. The serum calcium, phosphate, and alkaline phosphate levels should be monitored. This is necessary both for detection of possible hypocalcemia and hypercalcemia during bone recalcification and for evidence of complete healing, reflected in a normal serum alkaline phosphatase level. If the patient fails to respond to treatment, other causes should be considered. Patients with hepatic disease and intestinal malabsorption may require 25,000 to 100,000 IU of vitamin D/day orally or may require parenteral administration of the vitamin if large oral doses fail to raise circulating levels of 25-OHD to normal range. In addition, calcium carbonate (1 to 3 g/day) should be supplemented because only osteomalacia responds to vitamin D, osteoporosis does not. Patients are carefully monitored, and histomorphometric evaluation of bone biopsy specimen may be very useful. Adequate treatment of calcium deficiency may be monitored by urinary calcium level and serum calcium and PTH levels.

Most patients with renal disease respond to 1,25-(OH)$_2$D, calcitriol (0.5 to 1.0 μg/day) or dihydrotachysterol (DHT) (0.25 to 0.5 mg qd), a sterol that does not require renal hydroxylation for activation, or 1,25-(OH)$_2$D (0.5 to 1.0 μg qd) and a phosphate-restricted diet supplemented with aluminum hydroxide, a phosphate binder, or any facsimile. This regimen treats osteitis fibrosa more effectively than osteomalacia. Active vitamin D may be more beneficial for osteomalacia, with removal of aluminum. Use of aluminum is being restricted to patients with renal osteodystrophy to prevent phosphate binding and aluminum-related osteomalacia. Hypophosphatemia responds to a combination of phosphate (1 to 3 g/day) and large doses of vitamin D (25,000 to 100,000 IU). Oral phosphate has a laxative action and may be poorly tolerated. If acidosis is present with hypophosphatemia correction with bicarbonate may improve associated metabolic disease.

Renal Osteodystrophy

Renal osteodystrophy describes bone lesions that are present in many patients with advanced renal failure. All the biomechanical morphology abnormalities of kidney dysfunction are seen in renal osteodystrophy. Parathyroid hormone excess occurs early in renal failure. Although skeletal abnormalities appear early in renal failure, the most dramatic changes are in patients with end-stage kidney disease who are on hemodialysis. With advancing renal insufficiency, the tubules lose their capacity to respond to PTH, leading to hyperphosphatemia, persistent hypocalcemia, and severe hyperparathyroidism. Finally, the kidney fails to synthesize 1,25-(OH)$_2$D, resulting in diminished intestinal absorption of calcium. High levels of inorganic phosphate favor entry of serum calcium into bone. Both diminished intestinal absorption of calcium and entry of serum calcium into bone contribute to hypocalcemia, which in turn leads to secondary hyperparathyroidism.

The manifestations of renal osteodystrophy include a combination of osteitis fibrosa and hyperparathyroid bone disease; osteomalacia, a condition secondary in part to alterations in vitamin D metabolism; osteosclerosis, localized areas of woven bone that appear as increased bone density on radiograph; and osteoporosis, an infrequent, minor component (Fig. 7–3). The specific manifestations are greatly influenced by geography, with hyperparathyroid dystrophy predominant in the United States and osteomalacia in the United Kingdom.

Osteitis Fibrosa. Secondary hyperparathyroidism is a common complication of chronic renal disease that has been associated with phosphate retention, altered vitamin D metabolism, skeletal resistance

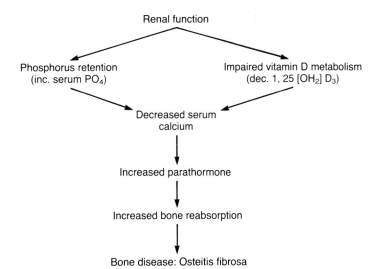

Figure 7–3. Impaired renal function resulting in secondary bone disease. (Inc., increased; dec., decreased.)

Renal function

Phosphorus retention
(inc. serum PO$_4$)

Impaired vitamin D metabolism
(dec. 1, 25 [OH$_2$] D$_3$)

Decreased serum calcium

Increased parathormone

Increased bone reabsorption

Bone disease: Osteitis fibrosa

to calcemic action of PTH, impaired PTH breakdown, and altered feedback regulation between calcium and PTH. Skeletal manifestations of hyperparathyroidism are included in the group of changes known as osteitis fibrosa, which is a histologic entity that reflects increased bone turnover. These skeletal manifestations may be seen in other states of accelerated remodeling, such as hyperthyroidism and Paget's disease. The basic anatomic changes in osteitis fibrosa are osteoclastic resorption of bone with fibrous replacement and microscopic and gross cysts forming in the fibrous tissue. The radiographic cysts are actually soft tissue masses referred to as brown tumors. These lesions resemble giant cell tumors of bone but are non-neoplastic and better referred to as reparative giant cell granuloma. A return to a euparathyroid state may be followed by an amazing reversal to normal bone, but some cystic lesions may persist.

Osteomalacia. An increase of osteoid seam width is seen in osteomalacia, accompanied by decreased mineralization. Impaired mineralizaton of bone matrix is the primary characteristic of osteomalacia, and if calcium continues to be inadequate production of bone matrix also decreases. Normal adult bone is continually being remodeled; as bone is removed by osteoclasts, it is replaced by osteoid laid down by osteoblasts, which is promptly calcified. If calcification fails to occur, the bone largely consists of osteoid, and this is known as osteomalacia, or softening of bone. Altered vitamin D metabolism leads to impaired mineralization, but only a small fraction of patients with severe renal disease present with osteomalacia. Other factors, alone or in combination, that may contribute to the development of osteomalacia include hypophosphatemia, altered collagen synthesis and maturation, defective bone crystallization, increased bone magnesium, elevated pyrophosphate, and diminished calcium carbonate levels. Acidosis also contributes to skeletal disease. In chronic renal insufficiency, the skeleton is an integral part of the buffering system.

Another type of osteomalacia characteristically displays a low level of PTH and does not respond to any metabolite of vitamin D. This type of osteomalacia is associated with aluminum, which has a toxic effect on osteoblast. The patient complains of severe bone pain and has pathologic fractures. The source of aluminum may be from high content in the water, ingestion of phosphate binders containing aluminum, or both.

Clinical Manifestations

Biochemical abnormalities may be present early in the course of renal insufficiency and may allow the physician to introduce preventive treatment measures. Many symptoms of renal osteodystrophy appear only in advanced disease. Bone pain may become so severe as to confine the patient to bed. This pain occurs in both osteitis fibrosa and osteomalacia. Bone pain is generally vague and located in the lower back, hips, knees, and legs, with physical findings usually lacking. Muscular weakness usually has a gradual onset, is proximal, and progresses with time. Muscle enzymes are usually normal. Pruritus is related to calcium deposits in the skin and is common in uremic patients with severe secondary hyperparathyroidism.

Peripheral necrosis and vascular calcification, which may involve the tips of the toes and fingers, may also occur. The skin becomes violaceous, and ulcerations and scars appear. Calcific periarthritis caused by hydroxyapatite crystals exists with acute pain and swelling around one or more joints. Skeletal deformities are common in azotemic children who are still growing. Bowing of the femur and tibia and slipped epiphyses are not uncommon. Typical radiographic findings of vitamin D deficiency are sometimes seen in children with renal rickets (defined in the following section). Growth retardation is also apparent in young children on maintenance renal dialysis. Skeletal abnormalities in adults with renal failure, especially those with osteomalacia, include lumbar scoliosis, thoracic kyphosis, and deformity of the thoracic cage.

Radiographic Characteristics

The development of renal osteodystrophy appears to be determined by the rate of skeletal growth and the chronicity of the renal failure. Renal osteodystrophy is more common in children and in patients with congenital anomalies of the kidney and with slowly progressive renal disease such as chronic pyelonephritis with normal blood pressure. Radiographic changes in bone are general types:

1. Widening of osteoid seams at the growing ends, as in rickets (hence the term renal rickets).

2. Erosive and cystic changes of osteitis fibrosa, as in hyperparathyroidism, the earliest of signs being subperiosteal resorption in the phalanges and long bones.

3. Hyperostosis or osteosclerosis.

The development of osteitis fibrosa cystica appears radiographically as subperiosteal bone resorption. These lesions are most commonly seen in the middle phalanges of the hands and feet, distal ends of the clavicle, and proximal ends of the tibia and neck of the femur. The trabeculae may have a fuzzy, coarse, indistinct appearance or a ground-glass appearance. There is a generalized cortical thinning.

The formation of true cysts and pseudocysts filled with osteoclasts and fibrous tissue, erosion that occurs in conjunction with new bone formation, may be apparent. These cysts are called brown tumors or osteoclastomas. The cysts are characteristic of primary hyperparathyroidism but are noted in hyperparathyroidism also.

Osteosclerosis is another interesting radiographic feature of renal osteodystrophy. This is associated with increased density of bone and is most frequently seen in the vertebrae. The etiology of this bone abnormality has been poorly defined but is thought to be another feature of osteitis fibrosa. The radiographic features of osteomalacia are less distinct but include pseudofracture (Looser's zone). Pseudofractures are pathognomonic findings of osteomalacia in adults. Uremic patients with osteomalacia commonly have secondary hyperparathyroidism with radiographic features of the latter. A certain diagnosis of osteomalacia rests on histologic examinations.

Soft tissue calcification has been associated with renal osteodystrophy, which has been related to increased calcium phosphate production in plasma, to secondary hyperparathyroidism, to alkalosis, and to local tissue injury. Identified areas include medium-sized arteries, articular or tumoral calcifications, and visceral calcifications affecting the heart, lung, and kidney.

Treatment

Azotemic renal osteodystrophy may be treated with vitamin D (50,000 to 200,000 IU daily). This dosage commonly would cause hypercalcemia in the normal individual, but with postulated resistance to vitamin D in the gut and on bone in the uremic patient, this dosage is warranted. Calcium lactate or citrate (10 to 20 g daily) may be given to supplement dietary calcium. Aluminum hydroxide gel (30 to 60 ml with each meal) is given when hyperphosphatemia is present to reduce phosphate absorption.

In many cases, treatment of secondary hyperparathyroidism in advanced renal insufficiency may be accomplished with vitamin D or phosphate-binding antacids and the administration of calcium carbonate. With continuous control of calcium and phosphorus levels in the serum, the level of circulating PTH decreases, and radiographically observed bone lesions may result. If this therapeutic approach is not successful subtotal parathyroidectomy is the treatment of choice (Table 7–10).

Table 7–10. RENAL OSTEODYSTROPHY TREATMENT GUIDELINES

Serum Phosphate Control (3.5–5.0 mg/dl)
Diet restriction: 600–800 mg/day
Phosphate-binding antacids: 1–4 capsules or 30–60 ml with each meal
Predialysis phosphorus: 4.5–5.5 mg/dl
Avoid hypophosphatemia
Adequate Calcium Intake
Calcium supplements when serum phosphorus is controlled, providing 1–2 g/day (e.g., Os-Cal, Titralac)
Vitamin D Sterol
Vitamin D_2 or D_3: 50,000–250,000 IU (1.25–6.25 mg)
Parathyroidectomy
Severe secondary hyperparathyroidism with bone erosion and increased PTH plus any of the following:
1. Persistent serum calcium > 11.5–12.0 mg/dl
2. Recalcitrant pruritus
3. Extraskeletal calcification (progressive or symptomatic)
4. Calciphylaxis (ischemic ulcers and necrosis)
5. Renal transplantation with symptomatic hypercalcemia

PTH, Parathyroid hormone.

Hypoparathyroidism

Hypoparathyroidism is a common cause of symptomatic hypocalcemia. Hypoparathyroidism may also be functional or idiopathic, may result from surgery, or may occur with magnesium deficiency. The most common cause is accidental surgical removal of parathyroid glands in the course of a thyroidectomy. More rarely, hypoparathyroidism occurs following surgery for a parathyroid tumor. Parathyroid hormone deficiency may be of a transient nature, with eventual recovery. Less often, PTH deficiency is idiopathic, affecting children more often than adults and females twice as often as males, with some familial predisposition. Etiology and pathogenesis are unknown, but there is speculation that idiopathic hypoparathyroidism is related to an autoimmune phenomenon. Hypomagnesemia may cause failure of release of PTH and resistance to hormonal action on bone, resulting in hypocalcemia reversible by magnesium repletion.

Clinical Manifestations

Acute hypoparathyroidism causes tetany, with muscle cramps, irritability, carpopedal spasm, convulsions, stridor, wheezing, dyspnea, photophobia and diplopia, abdominal cramps, and urinary frequency. Symptoms of the chronic disease are increased neuromuscular excitability, sometimes with episodes of tetany; cataracts, with blurring of vision; fragility of fingernails; lethargy; personality changes; state of anxiety; thickening of skull; and calcification in the basal ganglia of the brain, sometimes with seizures and mental retardation. Patients initially present with tetany, usually manifested by carpopedal spasm and Chvostek's sign, a facial muscle contraction on tapping the facial nerve near the angle of the jaw. Trousseau's phenomenon, carpal spasm after application and inflation of a blood pressure cuff, is also present. The skin is dry and scaly at times, with fungal infection, usually candidiasis, and loss of eyebrow hair. Hyperactive deep tendon reflexes are apparent. Teeth may be defective with stunting of growth if the onset of the disease occurs in childhood and the disease is chronic. Laboratory findings include low serum calcium levels, high serum phosphate levels, low urinary phosphate levels, low to absent urinary calcium levels, and normal alkaline phosphatase levels. Creatinine clearance is normal, and PTH levels are low or absent in idiopathic or postsurgical hypoparathyroidism.

Radiographic Characteristics

Resnick states that osteosclerosis, or an increase in bony density, is the most common skeletal finding of hypoparathyroidism. The skull may show calcification in the basal ganglia, which may be either generalized or localized. In long bones, one may note bandlike areas of osteosclerosis within the metaphyseal regions. One may also see an increased density of the iliac crest as well as marginal sclerosis of the vertebral body. Within the skull, one may observe thickening of the calvaria. Hypoplastic dentition may also be noted. One may notice calcification of the spinal ligaments along with osteophytic production. Within the soft tissue, subcutaneous calcification may be apparent. Basal ganglion calcification is observed with hypoparathyroidism as well as pseudohypoparathyroidism.

Treatment

The goal of treatment of hypoparathyroidism is to maintain the serum calcium level at approximately normal. Immediate correction of hypocalcemia may be accomplished by intravenous injection of calcium gluconate or calcium chloride. The effect is transitory, and additional calcium must be administered. Parathyroid extract may be substituted along with the administration of calcium, and this combination provides a more prolonged action. Dihydrotachysterol should be administered in dosages of 1.25 to 3.75 mg tid by mouth; the dose is adjusted to maintain a normal serum calcium level. Treatment may be continued with dihydrotachysterol or with a less expensive preparation of calciferol. Supplemental calcium should be given as soon as possible after diagnosis. Calcium chloride is most effective.

The objective of therapy in chronic hypoparathyroidism is to reduce the plasma phosphate and to raise the plasma calcium levels. This is accomplished by a combination of dietary (high-calcium and low-phosphate) and drug therapy.

Pseudohypoparathyroidism and Pseudopseudohypoparathyroidism

Pseudohypoparathyroidism (PHP) was first described by Albright and his associates in 1942. Patients with PHP present with the same clinical and chemical features as hypoparathyroidism except that patients with PHP have round faces and short, thick figures. Pseudohypoparathyroidism differs from hypoparathyroidism in that it involves end-organ resistance to circulating PTH. There is no deficiency in PTH.

Laboratory findings are similar to those of hypoparathyroidism, including evidence of hypocalcemia and hyperphosphatemia. The renal resistance to PTH was discovered by Albright and his associates, who demonstrated the inadequate response to exogenous PTH. The skeletal resistance is due to impaired hydroxylation or activation of 25-OHD. This activation step in vitamin D metabolism occurs only in the kidney. Therefore, a single defect in the kidney would explain both the skeletal and the renal resistance to PTH. This finding of a defect does not, however, rule out other organ involvement in PHP. The renal involvement does not account for other somatic, pituitary, and thyroid abnormalities that may be seen. There appears to be a hereditary transmission to PHP, as an X-linked dominant trait.

Pseudopseudohypoparathyroidism (PPHP) also appears to have a hereditary transmission. In fact, it is often noted in individuals in the same family as patients with PHP. Pseudopseudohypoparathyroidism is merely the normocalcemic form of PHP. The other somatic abnormalities discussed with PHP are seen with PPHP.

Clinical Manifestations

Clinical manifestations of PHP include a characteristic shortening of the metacarpal and metatarsal bones (brachydactyly) with absence of knuckles when making a fist; obesity; and, in many patients, a degree of mental deficiency. Not all characteristics are necessarily present; one or a combination of them may be found. Patients may present with cramping of the extremities because they frequently demonstrate tetany and hyperexcitability. Ectopic soft tissue calcification may be seen and felt. The biochemical picture is identical to idiopathic hypoparathyroidism except that the administration of PTH fails to correct the abnormality. The relative resistance to parathyroid extract, as measured by failure to produce a phosphate diuresis, serves to distinguish PHP from hypoparathyroidism. Pseudopseudohypoparathyroidism has similar structural abnormalities as PHP but with normal calcium and phosphorus levels.

Radiographic Characteristics

Soft tissue calcification is even more extensive in PHP and PPHP than in hypoparathyroidism. This calcification appears plaquelike, is distributed asymmetrically, and is located beneath the skin surface. Soft tissue ossification may even be demonstrated and is usually periarticular in distribution. In the foot, metatarsal shortening is the most obvious skeletal abnormality. This metatarsal shortening shows a predisposition for the fourth and the first metatarsals. Brachymetatarsia is rarely seen as an isolated skeletal abnormality in PHP or PPHP. Shortening of the metacarpals is frequent. Metacarpal shortening shows a predisposition for the first, fourth, and fifth digits. In addition, the phalanges appear to be short and wide, demonstrating cone-shaped epiphyses with premature fusion. Additional abnormalities of the long bones may include bowing deformities of the extremities, or exostoses. These exostoses appear to be centrally located and are directed perpendicular to the bone. These exostoses are in contrast to multiple hereditary exostoses, which tend to grow away from the joint areas. Other findings are similar to hypoparathyroidism, including calcification in the basal ganglia and thickening of the calvaria. In both PHP and PPHP, bony density may vary from being decreased, normal, or increased.

Treatment

The therapy for PHP and PPHP is the same as that given under chronic hypoparathyroidism.

Paget's Disease

Paget's disease (osteitis deformans) is another disease of unknown etiology characterized by continuous excessive destruction of bone and its simultaneous replacement by a soft, poorly mineralized matrix. Paget's disease is a common bone disorder and is usually mild and asymptomatic in the 0.1 to 3.0% of elderly adults whom it affects. Advanced cases produce intense pain in the involved bones. Paget's disease is detected after 40 years of age and has a slight male preponderance. Theories on etiology include a genetically determined defect in connective tissue metabolism; a virus, with viral-type inclusions having been seen in osteoclasts; and possibly a primary endocrine or vascular disorder. Therapy must be directed toward reducing osteoclastic activity by administration of agents such as calcitonin.

Epidemiology

Paget's disease is commonly diagnosed in the United Kingdom and in the countries their citizens migrate to, including the United States, Canada, South Africa, Australia, and New Zealand. The disease is also common in France, Italy, and Germany. There is no major predisposition for either sex. In 50% of the cases, patients reported that at least one relative also had the disease.

Pathogenesis

In the majority of patients with Paget's disease, most of the skeleton is uninvolved. However, this disease can affect one or many bones. Paget's disease may be polyostotic or monostotic. The pelvis and sacrum are generally the first sites affected; the skull, femur, spine, tibia, humerus, and scapula may then be affected. The monostotic form affects the tibia most often. The lesions of Paget's disease evolve through three phases. First, there is an osteolytic phase, with intense focal bone resorption by osteoclasts and the beginning of osteoblast response. Next, there is a mixed osteolytic and osteoblastic phase, with the osteoblasts lining the bony trabeculae that have been partially eroded by osteoclasts. The marrow spaces are filled with highly vascular connective tissue and later by new lamellar bone. Third, there is an osteoblastic, sclerotic, "burnt-out" phase. Mineralization of new osteoid lags; osteoid seams persist at the margin of the newly laid-down bone to create a tilelike

or mosaic-like pattern that is pathognomonic of Paget's disease. All three phases may be present in a single bone. After many years, the osteoclastic phase wanes and osteoblastic activity predominates. The neo-osteogenesis may eventually increase bone thickness or size, which is laid down haphazardly. Structural strength is lacking, the bone is porous and soft, and mineralization is poor. Light microscopy allows differentiation from osteomyelitis, primary hyperparathyroidism, and osteomalacia.

Etiology

Although further proof is still needed, it has been suggested that a "slow" viral infection may cause Paget's disease. Other speculations include an abnormality of hormone secretion, a neoplastic state, a vascular anomaly, an autoimmune state, an inborn error of connective tissue biosynthesis, an inflammatory state, and possible role of parathyroid hormone.

Clinical Manifestations

Paget's disease is often discovered accidentally during a routine evaluation or an assessment of an unrelated problem. Skeletal deformities and musculoskeletal pain are the most common patient complaints. The clavicle, long bones of the lower extremities, and cranium are the most likely bones to appear abnormal on physical examination. Increased skin temperature is usually present over the bone with disease activity. Bone tumors such as osteosarcoma and giant cell tumor may develop in lesions of Paget's disease and may appear as a mass or a worsening of bone pain. The skull is markedly thickened. Complications associated with skull lesions include hearing loss, vertigo, tinnitus, and headache. Compression of the brain may occur with severe enlargement of the skull and ensuing symptoms indicative of the impressed areas. The weight-bearing bones are bowed. Ambulation may be impaired when significant lateral and anterior bowing of the femur or tibia develops, which also makes bone prone to pathologic fracture. Back pain may be severe and of complex origin, owing to the increased incidence of degenerative arthritis and discogenic disease in elderly patients. If back pain is of sudden onset a compression fracture must be considered.

Computed tomography of the spine is a useful means of evaluating the detailed anatomy and neurologic complications in the patient with back pain. After a long sclerotic phase, the bone may be abnormally dense. New bone formation and bone resorption occur simultaneously, and serum calcium and inorganic phosphate levels are normal. An elevated serum calcium level is seen, however, when the patient has a malignancy, has primary hyperparathyroidism, or is bedridden. Hyperuricemia with or without clinical gout can appear and may indicate increase in purine metabolism. High rates of urinary hydroxyproline excretion occur from excessive bone matrix degradation. Serum alkaline phosphatase levels are markedly elevated from new bone formation. Serum alkaline phosphatase activity, an index of osteoblastic activity, and urinary hydrox-

yproline level, an index of bone matrix resorption, correlate reasonably well with extent and activity of Paget's disease (Table 7–11).

Radiographic Characteristics

A bone biopsy is rarely needed to diagnose Paget's disease because the radiographic presentations are so characteristic. Radiographs show the affected bones to be enlarged and relatively radiolucent. The ends of long bones and the skull initially show localized osteolytic lesions. The long bones usually demonstrate progression of the lytic lesion about 1 cm/year in a sharply defined V shape. The convex surface of the long bones may demonstrate linear cortical radiolucencies, especially in the femur or tibia, which may be precursors of fractures. Osteolytic disease in the vertebral bodies is associated with sclerotic margins, giving a "picture-frame" ap-

Table 7–11. CLINICAL FEATURES IN METABOLIC BONE DISEASE

Disease	Pain	Fractures	Deformity	Weakness
Spinal osteoporosis	Acute, episodic, severe; spontaneous improvement in 1–2 months; chronic low back pain, iliac crest impingement	Trabecular, compression from minor trauma; vertebral body: marked deformity; anterior wedging, cortical buckling, asymmetric hip, wrist	Common: loss of height; dorsal kyphosis; reduced ratio: upper to lower segment	Pseudoweakness, disuse atrophy; features of underlying conditions: Cushing's syndrome, thyrotoxicosis, alcohol excess
Osteomalacia	Chronic, persistent, aching pains; bony tenderness; lower extremity, pelvis, ribs, bilateral involvement	Cortical: secondary hyperparathyroidism, appendicular skeleton, "codfish vertebrae"; pseudofractures	Occasional bowing deformity, cortical fractures, residual signs of rickets.	Diffuse muscle weakness; often proximal, waddling gait
Osteitis fibrosa (hyperparathyroidism)	Vague, generalized aches; local pain from giant cell tumors, bone cysts, pathologic fractures	Cortical, pathologic (common in secondary hyperparathyroidism), insufficiency fracture	Uncommon with primary hyperparathyroidism, digital pseudoclubbing (secondary hyperparathyroidism), bone cysts, giant cell tumors.	Diffuse muscle weakness (may be proximal)
Osteitis deformans (Paget's disease)	Less than 10% of cases dull, deepseated; pelvis, hip, femur, skull; increased bone warmth, rarely tender; local pain: pathologic fracture or osteosarcoma and DJD	Pathologic: through involved bone, pseudofractures; long bone: transverse	Common; bowing, bony enlargement, pathologic fractures, DJD	Neuropathies: bony compression; cranial nerves, nerve root, cerebellar ataxia

DJD, Degenerative joint disease.

pearance and making the bodies prone to compression fractures.

The osteoblastic activity that occurs after osteolysis is not seen on radiograph until the patient has had Paget's disease for years or even decades. Cardiac enlargement and frank congestive heart failure may be manifestations of increased cardiac output, which is related to increased vascularity of affected bones.

Advanced involvement of the skull, with marked thickening of the entire cranial vault; areas of osteolysis; and patchy new bone formation result in a "cotton-wool" appearance. The "brim sign" is the thickening of the iliopectineal line in the pelvis and is nearly pathognomonic of Paget's disease. Enlargement of the ischial and pubic bones is also typical. Bone scanning is the most sensitive means to detect active lesions of Paget's disease. Although bone scanning is not a specific diagnostic test, it demonstrates increased uptake of the radiolabeled scanning agent when standard films may not demonstrate an early lesion.

Treatment

Many patients do not require treatment for Paget's disease, or they just require analgesics, such as aspirin or another nonsteroidal anti-inflammatory drug (NSAID). Calcitonin provides safe, effective therapy for Paget's disease. The recommended dosage is 50 to 100 MRC* IU (0.25 to 0.5 ml) daily via subcutaneous injections. After initial response, often about 1 month, the drug may be tapered to 50 MRC IU every other day and then to twice or once weekly. Biochemical parameters have been reduced up to 50%, with relief of bone pain; healing of osteolytic lesions; reduction of elevated cardiac output, which is related to the increased vascularity of involved bones; reduction of elevated skin temperature; and reversal of various neurologic deficits, all of which have been documented during long-term therapy. Patients with active osteolytic lesions may need treatment for years.

Etidronate disodium is given 5 to 10 mg/kg/day orally in a single dose for an initial treatment usually of 6 months. Large doses should be avoided because of etidronate

---

* Medical Research Council.

disodium's interference in mineralization of bone, which increases fracture risk. Benefits of etidronate disodium are similar to those of calcitonin. Etidronate disodium's oral route of administration is a definite advantage over calcitonin. However, healing of osteolytic lesions is not substantially documented. The effectiveness of medical therapy can be monitored through serum alkaline phosphatase activity measured every 2 to 4 months.

Selected patients benefit from surgery, which is an important adjunct to medical therapy. Patients demonstrating neurologic signs associated with skull lesions, severe skull enlargement, and vertebral lesions greatly benefit from surgical repair. Podiatric and orthopedic procedures are required to enable more normal ambulation in patients with pelvic and lower-extremity disease. It is recommended that 1 to 3 months of medical therapy be administered preoperatively to reduce the amount of bleeding intraoperatively and postoperatively and to prevent immobilization and hypercalcemia postoperatively.

Other Disorders of Bone

Fibrous Dysplasia

Fibrous dysplasia is an uncommon disorder that is characterized by focal areas of fibrous replacement of bone. The etiology is unknown but has been related to disturbance in skeletal growth and possibly to an error in formation that results in progressive replacement of bone by fibrous tissue. No familial or hereditary pattern has been established. Individual lesions are composed of dense fibrous tissue in medullary bone interspersed with thin bone trabeculae.

The monostotic lesion of fibrous dysplasia affects males slightly more often than females and appears between infancy and middle age, with a median age of 14 years. Occasionally fibrous dysplasia is polyostotic. In a very small number of patients, fibrous dysplasia is associated with café au lait spots and sexual precocity; this is known as Albright's syndrome and occurs primarily in females. Fibrous dysplasia may involve over 50% of the skeleton and frequently produces "shepherd's-crook" deformity of the femur, resulting in limb length discrepancies and skull involvement that may cause facial disfigurement. Fractures are common. Serum chemistry findings are frequently normal except for elevation of the alkaline phosphate level.

When symptomatic, patients with fibrous dysplasia can be managed by a variety of orthopedic procedures, such as curettage, bone grafting, and osteotomy. Indications for these procedures include progressive deformities, nonunion of fractures, and persistent pain that does not respond to conservative therapy.

Osteonecrosis

Osteonecrosis describes infarction of bone presumably caused by ischemia and is synonymous with aseptic or vascular necrosis of bone. The most common cause of osteonecrosis is fracture or dislocation of the femoral neck. Other bones susceptible to post-traumatic osteonecrosis are the proximal pole of the carpal scaphoid and the body of the talus.

ETIOLOGY

Osteonecrosis is seen in sickle-cell disease, caused by vascular compromise associated with sludging of sickled erythrocytes; in caisson disease; in gas-bubble emboli; and in obstruction by histiocytes in Gaucher's disease. Other important etiologies are hemophilia, polycythemia vera, glucocorticoid therapy, cytotoxic chemotherapy, radiation injury, and renal transplantation. Various reports have stated that the prevalence of osteonecrosis after renal transplantation ranges from 3 to 41%. Osteonecrosis is associated with alcoholism, chronic pancreatitis, hyperuricemia, and diabetes mellitus.

The epiphyseal regions of growing bones in children are also susceptible to osteonecrosis, with the roles of trauma and constitutional factors being poorly defined.

CLINICAL MANIFESTATION

The presentation of infarcts occurring in the shaft of bone, as seen in sickle-cell disease and caisson disease, is usually asymptomatic, or pain is self-limited. Greater morbidity occurs with infarcts of subarticular bone, especially in the femoral head. Other common sites of nontraumatic osteonecrosis include the femoral condyles, distal tibia, humeral head, and talus. Pain occurs in these sites, often of acute onset.

RADIOGRAPHIC CHARACTERISTICS

Diagnosis of osteonecrosis by radiograph may be delayed for weeks or months. Living and dead bone are indistinguishable, and the slow reparative processes are visualized radiographically. Patchy lucencies reflect resorption, and linear subchondral lucencies reflect collapse of bone. Patchy sclerosis indicates growth of new bone over the scaffolding of dead trabeculae. Healing occurs if fragmentation and collapse of weakened bone does not supervene.

TREATMENT

Initial therapy for osteonecrosis consists of keeping the affected limb from bearing weight. Surgery such as transpositional osteotomy, arthrotomy with removal of fragments, or arthroplasty, may be required.

Bone Tumors

Bone tumors form a complex group. Although uncommon, bone tumors are important because they are most frequently seen in the young (the teens to the thirties), which is attributed to the propensity of the tumors to arise in actively growing bones, and they tend to be very malignant, at a ratio of approximately 3 to 1.

Bone tumors occur randomly but have been associated with genetic disorders, radiation injury, Paget's disease, bone infarct, and chronic osteomyelitis. Primary tumors may arise from any one of the components of bone, such as cartilage, fibrous tissue, hematopoietic elements, fibrous tissue, and osteoid tissue. The four most common malignant tumors of bone in descending order of frequency are osteogenic sarcoma, chondrosarcoma, Ewing's sarcoma, and malignant giant cell tumors.

Benign bone tumors usually occur as a mass or deformity detectable on physical examination, as an incidental finding on radiograph, or occasionally as a pathologic fracture. Most lesions are small and painless and on radiograph show well-defined cortical margins, absence of a soft tissue mass, and sclerotic bony margination separating the lesion from the normal tissue. Some lesions may require biopsy for definition. Treatment may be required if the integrity of the skeleton is threatened.

Malignant primary bone tumors are rare, the most common being multiple myeloma. Other primary malignant tumors in order of diminishing frequency are osteosarcoma, chondrosarcoma, round cell tumors (Ewing's sarcoma and primary lymphoma of bone), giant cell tumors, and malignant fibrous tumors.

CLASSIFICATION AND STAGING

Both benign and malignant tumors may be classified according to cell type as osseous, cartilaginous, fibrous, vascular, neural, marrow, lipid, and of unspecified origin. Prior to treatment, all primary bone tumors must be staged in order to assess the local extent of the lesion (T), the grade of the tumor (G), and the presence or absence of distant metastases (M). The determination of T is best accomplished through physical examination, radiographs, and special imaging studies, such as arteriography, CT, bone scintigraphy, magnetic resonance imaging, and technetium scanning. Tumor grading is determined by study of a biopsy specimen, using both standard and specialized techniques. Most bone tumors metastasize to the lungs and occasionally to other bones. To establish M, full lung tomograms or CT of the chest and a bone scan are required.

Bone-Forming (Osteoblastic) Tumors

Osteoma. An osteoma is an infrequent and totally benign growth that is composed of dense normal bone. The tumor is of little clinical significance and is removed only for cosmetic reasons or interference with function.

Osteoid Osteoma. An osteoid osteoma is a small, benign neoplasm that involves the diaphyses of long bones. Osteoid osteomas usually occur in patients under the age of 30 and occur in males twice as often as in females. Any bone may be involved, but the femur and tibia are the most common sites. The tumor arises within cortical bone and erodes the underlying normal bone, creating a red-brown nodule rarely over 1 cm in size. The nodule is surrounded by a zone of dense sclerotic bone and appears as a distinct lytic lesion. It is extremely painful and may necessitate surgical removal.

Osteosarcoma (Osteogenic Sarcoma). The tumor of osteosarcoma is characterized by osteoblastic differentiation of the neoplastic cells, with formation of osteoid directly by the tumor cells. This formation of osteoid is a hallmark of osteosarcoma. Some osteosarcomas also contain cartilage and collagen, which is related to the common origin of osteoblasts, chondroblasts, and fibroblasts. Osteosarcomas must be differentiated from chondrosarcomas and fibrosarcomas, which also arise in the bone. The tumor has a predilection for the distal femur or proximal tibia of the rapidly growing child and appears more frequently in males. The greater majority of patients afflicted by this neoplasm are between the ages of 10 and 25 years. A second smaller peak of instance of osteosarcoma is seen in patients older than age 50, with a very high percentage of patients with pre-existing Paget's disease; osteosarcoma in this age group is also associated with irradiation injury of bone or a bone infarct.

Unlike most other tumors, pain is often an early manifestation, accompanied by local swelling and fever. The patient may be diagnosed as having the comparatively less innocuous osteomyelitis. Tumor growth is rapid. Visible changes in the tumor mass occur rapidly. The serum alkaline phosphatase level is typically elevated. Radiograph shows Codman's triangle and areas of bone destruction as well as soft tissue radiodensity representing new bone formation. The clinical and radiographic findings are best confirmed by biopsy because treatment for osteosarcoma is amputation or a limb-salvage procedure, with use of chemotherapeutic agents such as doxorubicin, high-dose methotrexate with citrovorum factor, and cisplatin. One fourth of the patients have metastases to the lungs at the time of the initial examination or shortly thereafter. If left untreated the course of osteosarcoma is fulminant with a rapid progression of the tumor, widespread metastases, and death in less than a year. Aggressive chemotherapy appears to be successful in effecting cure in more than 20% of the patients so treated.

Chondroma (Cartilaginous) Tumors

Exostosis (Exostosis Cartilaginea). Exostosis is a benign bony neoplasm that is knobby and protrudes from the metaphyseal surface of long bones, mostly the lower femur or upper tibia, and is capped by growing cartilage. Exostosis develops commonly in children and adolescents and has a very indolent course, sometimes with cessation of growth followed by complete ossification. The podiatrist may see a patient with exostosis who presents with a limb-length discrepancy.

Multiple exostoses occur as a hereditary disorder. Hereditary multiple exostoses usually appear earlier than the isolated lesions. Irregular bony excrescences protrude from the expanded metaphyses of the long bones. These osteocartilaginous exostoses arise from the growth plate and grow as the bone does. Growth ceases in adulthood. Disability results principally from limb-length discrepancies; linear bone growth decreases as the bone grows transversely. Less common are syndromes involving nerve, spinal cord, and vascular compression. The clinical significance of these lesions is their propensity to malignant transformation to a chondrosarcoma or an osteogenic sarcoma in 3 to 10% of affected individuals. This must be suspected when a lesion enlarges rapidly, especially during adulthood.

Enchondroma. Unlike exostosis, enchondroma is a benign cartilaginous tumor deep within the bone. The small bones of the hands and feet are the most frequently involved areas. This is a sporadic condition that becomes symptomatic in childhood. Enchondroma produces swelling and interferes with linear bone growth. Pathologic fractures of the involved bone may also appear. However, the lesion may remain completely silent. As with cartilaginous exostoses, enchodromas arise from the growth plate, and growth ceases at puberty.

Grossly enchondromas appear as firm, slightly lobulated, glassy, gray-blue, translucent lesions that abutt on and erode the overlying cortical bone. A thin outer bony shell is usually maintained by the reactive bone formation. On radiograph, enchondromas are seen as radiolucent defects in the metaphyseal area of the tubular and flat bones, wtih central calcific stippling often seen. Thinning of the cortex of the affected area occurs with expansion of the lesion. Hereditary enchondromatosis and fibrous dysplasia must be considered in this presentation.

Multiple enchondromas, or enchondromatosis, may occur in childhood. This condition is known as Ollier's disease. When enchondroma is seen with hemangioma of the skin, the involvement is termed Maffucci's syndrome. As with exostosis, a malignant transformation has been reported, particularly in the multiple patterns of enchondroma. In Maffucci's syndrome, the enchondromas or hemangiomas undergo malignant transformation in 15% of cases.

Chondrosarcoma. Chondrosarcoma is a malignant tumor of chondroblasts and is as frequent as osteosarcoma. The clinical presentation varies. Chondrosarcomas occur in an older group, with most tumors arising after 35 years of age. Their growth is much slower, and the prognosis is better. Chondrosarcomas tend to involve the bones of the trunk, including the pelvic bones, ribs, and vertebrae, and proximal portions of the appendicular skeleton. Some tumors arise from malignant transformation of enchondromas and multiple exostoses, but the majority of tumors arise de novo. Accurate staging and surgical intervention may produce a cure in up to 85% of patients with chondrosarcoma. Radiation and chemotherapy are relatively ineffective, especially for large tumors, and radical excision is the treatment of choice.

Chondromyxoid Fibroma. Chondromyxoid fibroma is a rare benign lesion that is often misinterpreted as malignant and is important for that primary reason. Chondromyxoid fibroma usually arises within the marrow cavity of the upper metaphysis of the tibia or lower metaphysis of the femur. Grossly the lesion appears firm and gray-white and tends to erode overlying cortex, causing pain. The presence of ominous, scattered multinucleated giant cells leads to the frequent misdiagnosis of these tumors as chondrosarcomas or giant cell tumors.

Other Tumors of Bone

Multiple Myeloma. Multiple myeloma, the most common malignant tumor of bone, arises from hemopoietic cells proliferating in the bone marrow, disrupting normal function as well as invading the adjacent bone. The disease is frequently associated with extensive skeletal destruction, hypercalcemia, anemia, impaired renal function, immunodeficiency, and increased susceptibility to infection. Multiple myeloma is most frequently seen in middle-aged and elderly persons, with a median age of 60, and incidence increases with age. Multiple myeloma is slightly more common in males than in females. A rare case in a younger person has been reported in all races. Presenting symptoms not infrequently seen are back pain, anemia, and a very high sedimentation rate in an older person. Patients may have pallor or bone pain, but there are no characteristic physical findings. Laboratory confirmation with evidence of invasiveness, with lytic bone on radiograph being the best sign of invasion, is required for the diagnosis of multiple myeloma. Some patients have an indolent disease, but the majority of patients have significant disease and require active treatment. The two areas of importance in treatment are systemic chemotherapy and supportive care for management of complications. Survival is influenced by clinical stage, degree of renal function, and response to chemotherapy. Patients who respond well to therapy have survived for up to 5 years and longer.

Ewing's Sarcoma (Round Cell Tumor). Ewing's sarcoma, a rare and highly malignant tumor of unknown cytogenesis, arises within the marrow cavity of bone. It primarily affects adolescents and young adults, with a male preponderance. The two major sites of involvement are the metaphyses of long bones, often the femur and the pelvis. Ewing's sarcoma grows rapidly, and the patient may present with both local and systemic signs. Symptoms include local pain, swelling, and a palpable mass, with areas of necrosis and hemorrhage from invasion of the surrounding soft tissue after eroding the cortex. Systemic findings include fever, malaise, chills, and a rapid sedimentation rate. This disease produces a very destructive lytic tumor. In about 50% of the patients, reactive new bone formation creates a concentric "onionskin" layering about the tumor. The prognosis is very poor without treatment, but the combination of local radiation and chemotherapy provides a long survival rate exceeding 60%. Histologically the totally undifferentiated nature of the basic cells may result in confusion with metastatic disease. Hodgkin's lymphoma may appear as a bony focus and is difficult to distinguish radiographically and histologically from Ewing's sarcoma. Patients with Ewing's sarcoma must be staged to be certain that the bony tumor is solitary rather than an osseous focus of diffuse disease.

Giant Cell Tumors (Osteoclastoma). Giant cell tumors begin in the epiphyses and progressively expand outward, often reaching but not eroding the articular cartilage, which produces a clublike deformity of the end of bone. The most frequently involved sites are the ends of the long bones, particularly the lower femur, upper tibia, and lower radius. The tumor is gray-brown, firm, and friable, with scattered foci of hemorrhage and necrosis. Microscopically scattered giant cells resembling osteoclasts are seen and are classified as grade 1, 2, or 3, from benign to malignant, based on stromal components. Histology and clinical behavior do not always correlate. Obviously anaplastic lesions may behave as cancer, and a clearly well-differentiated tumor may behave as a benign lesion. However, between these extremes, prognosis is guarded. Most patients are over the age of 20, and there is no sex preponderance. The clinical presentation is nonspecific, with pain, tenderness, an occasional pathologic fracture, and sometimes a palpable mass. Radiographically one sees a distinctive but not pathognomonic soap-bubble appearance, that is, large cystic areas of bone rarefaction traversed by strands of calcification and surrounded by a thin shell of bone. Statistically 50% of these tumors are benign, 35% tend to recur after excision, and 15% are aggressively malignant from onset. There is a 5-year survival rate in about 25% of patients.

Bibliography

Aloia JF, et al.: Risk factors for postmenopausal osteoporosis. Am J Med 78:95, 1985.

Altman RD: Paget's disease of bone (osteitis deformans). Bull Rheum Dis 34:1, 1984.

Aviolo LV (ed): Vitamin D metabolites: The clinical importance. Arch Intern Med 138:835[Special Issue], 1978.

Bilezikian JP: The medical management of primary hyperparathyroidism. Ann Intern Med 96:198, 1982.

Boskey AL, Posner AS: Bone structure, composition, and mineralization. Clin Podiatr Med Surg 2(4):709, 1985.

Burnstein MI, et al.: Metabolic bone disease in pseudo-hypoparathyroidism: Radiologic features. Radiology 155:351, 1985.

Fairbairn JF, II, Juergens JL: Principles of medical treatment. In Juergens JL, Spittell JA, Jr, Fairbairn JF, II (eds): Peripheral Vascular Diseases, 5th ed. Philadelphia: WB Saunders Co, 1980.

Frame B, Marel G: Paget's disease revisited. Radiology 145:21, 1981.

Goldman DR, et al. (eds): Medical Care of the Surgical Patient: A Problem-Oriented Approach to Management. Philadelphia: JB Lippincott Co, 1982.

Harrison HE, Harrison HC: Rickets then and now. J Pediatr 87:1144, 1975.

Haussler MR, Cordy PE: Metabolites and analogues of vitamin D: Which for what? JAMA 247:841, 1982.

Health and Public Policy Committee, American College of Physicians: Radiologic methods to evaluate bone mineral content. Ann Intern Med 100:908, 1984.

Huvos AG: Bone Tumors, Diagnosis, Treatment and Progress. Philadelphia: WB Saunders Co, 1979.

Kleerekoper M, Sudhaker D, Rao DS, Frame B: Occult Cushing's syndrome presenting with osteoporosis. Henry Ford Hosp Med J 28:132, 1980.

Levy RN (ed): Metastatic disease of bone. Clin Orthop 169:38, 1982.

Meredith SC, Rosenberg IH: Gastrointestinal-hepatic disorders and osteomalacia. Clin Endocrinol Metab 9:131, 1980.

Resnick D, Niwayama G: Diagnosis of Bone and Joint Disorders, 2nd ed. Philadelphia: WB Saunders Co, 1988.

Sakhaee K, et al.: Postmenopausal osteoporosis as a manifestation of renal hypercalciuria with secondary hyperparathyroidism. J Clin Endocrinol Metab 61:368, 1985.

Schajowicz F, Santini AE, Berenstein M: Sarcoma complicating Paget's disease of bone: A clinicopathological study of 62 cases. J Bone Joint Surg [Br] 65:299, 1983.

Sweetnam R: Osteosarcoma. (2 parts) Br J Hosp Med 28:112, 1982.

Vigorita VJ: The tissue pathologic features of metabolic bone disease. Clin Podiatr Med Surg 2(4):725, 1985.

Walker GS, et al.: Dialysate aluminum concentration and renal bone disease. Kidney Int 21:411, 1982.

Wyngaarden JB, Smith LH (eds): Cecil Textbook of Medicine. Philadelphia: WB Saunders Co, 1985.

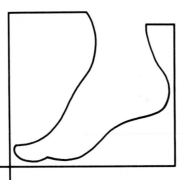

8 *RENAL DISEASE*

WESLEY H. JAN

OVERVIEW

A knowledge of renal function and disease is essential for the podiatrist, as for any practitioner in the health fields, because the kidney is the organ that regulates the body's electrolyte and fluid balance. An approach to renal pathophysiology necessitates a review of renal physiology because only by understanding how the kidney normally functions can one appreciate the ways in which the kidney may malfunction (Table 8–1). The practitioner should have a knowledge of renal physiology and should be familiar with those laboratory tests that are pertinent to renal performance. The practitioner should be able to recognize a number of common renal syndromes, such as hematuria, proteinuria, dysuria, and renal failure, and to take the necessary steps for appropriate management. An understanding of fluid and electrolyte therapy, in both routine and special circumstances, permits the practitioner to provide rational, appropriate, and safe intravenous fluid therapy for patients.

PHYSIOLOGY

One approach to renal physiology is to consider the sequence of events that leads to the formation of urine. Up to 144 L of blood are filtered by the kidney's glomeruli each day. Yet the daily volume of urine that is ultimately produced averages only 2 L. Between the initial filtration and the final appearance of urine in the bladder, a remarkable series of both active and passive, reabsorptive and secretory processes occurs.

Filtration (Fig. 8-1)

Urine first begins to take form in the renal glomerulus, which is a tuft of specially permeable capillaries. The process of filtration depends on differences in hydrostatic or perfusion pressures as well as differences in oncotic pressures across the capillary wall. In addition, the capillaries impose a size and charge restraint and therefore act as molecular sieves to exclude most of the plasma proteins from the glomerular filtrate.

The glomerular filtrate then flows into the proximal tubule, where much of the filtered salts and water as well as amino acids and glucose are reabsorbed. In addition, the secretion of some substances, such as hydrogen ion, takes place. Although more than 50% of the glomerular filtrate can be reabsorbed in the proximal tubules, the filtrate so reabsorbed remains isosmotic to plasma at this level of the nephron. Henle's loop is the next major anatomic division that the urine must traverse. Basically Henle's loop and its surrounding medullary interstitium are the key sites for generating a dilute or concentrated urine.

Table 8–1. SEGMENTAL FUNCTIONS OF THE RENAL TUBULES

Segment	Functions
Proximal tubule	Reabsorption 70% filtered H_2O and NaCl Glucose Urea Uric acid Amino acids K^+, Mg^+, Ca^+, HPO^- Secretion Organic acids and bases H^+ and NH_3
Henle's loop	Reabsorption via countercurrent multiplier NaCl in excess of H_2O
Distal tubule	Reabsorption Filtered H_2O and NaCl (small fraction only) Secretion H^+, NH_3, K^+
Collecting ducts	Reabsorption NaCl H_2O (depends on ADH concentration) Urea K^+ (depends on aldosterone concentration) Secretion H^+, NH_3 (pH of urine may be reduced to 4.5–5.0) K^+ (depends on aldosterone concentration)

ADH, Antidiuretic hormone.
(From Groer ME, et al.: Basic Pathophysiology: A Conceptual Approach. St. Louis: CV Mosby Co, 1979.)

Distal Convoluted Tubule and Collecting Duct

The distal convoluted tubule and the collecting duct are the final regulators of urinary composition. In the absence of antidiuretic hormone (ADH), the dilute urine formed by Henle's loop is maintained, and the tubular fluid is actually diluted even

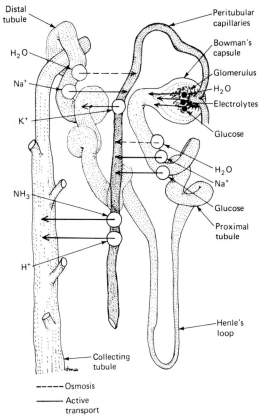

Figure 8–1. Diagram of glomerular filtration, tubular reabsorption, and tubular secretion. (From Scipien GM, et al.: Comprehensive Pediatric Nursing. New York: McGraw-Hill Book Co, 1975.)

further by the additional reabsorption of salt. In the presence of ADH, the collecting duct epithelium becomes permeable to water, and the urine becomes concentrated as it passes through the hyperosmolar gradient of the medulla.

The distal convoluted tubule and collecting duct are also the normal sites for the secretion of potassium and net generation of acid, which are essential functions of the kidney in maintaining electrolyte and acid-base balance. These terminal segments of the nephron are some of the few identifiable sites where an extrarenal agent, in this case aldosterone, is known to modulate renal excretory function.

PRESENTING FEATURES

History

There are a number of symptoms that should prompt the practitioner to consider the possibility of renal disease in a patient. These symptoms include generalized complaints of weakness, fatigue, anorexia, and nausea and more specific complaints of blood in the urine (hematuria), pain on urination (dysuria), and urinary frequency. Alterations in urinary volume, such as large urine volume (polyuria), diminished urine volume (oliguria), and minimal urine volume (anuria), are generally difficult to assess in a patient unless there has been a dramatic change because few patients can reliably quantitate their 24-hour urine output. In comparison, renal disease can frequently be present and not produce any symptoms. Thus the absence of any of these symptoms cannot be taken to exclude the presence of a renal or fluid and electrolyte disorder. The presence of symptoms mandates a more detailed investigation.

Physical Examination

Physical findings of hypertension and evidence of fluid excess, such as edema, may indicate an underlying renal disease, such as nephrosis, glomerulonephritis, or renal failure (Table 8–2). Palpable kidneys suggest a renal tumor or polycystic disease. However, as with the history, abnormalities uncovered by the physical examination are typically not specific for renal disease. For example, a patient with hypertension is more likely to have essential hypertension than glomerulonephritis, and a patient with edema is more likely to have congestive heart disease than nephrosis (Fig. 8–2). Therefore, in both the history and physical examination, there are signs and symptoms that should alert the practitioner to the possibility of renal disease, but confirmation of kidney disease usually requires further laboratory investigation.

Laboratory and Physiologic Data

Although a direct measurement of individual nephron and tubular function is not possible except in the research laboratory, there are readily available tools with which the practitioner can gauge the performance of the whole kidney.

Table 8–2. ETIOLOGY OF EDEMA

Etiologic Factors	Associated Conditions
Increased capillary permeability	Inflammatory reactions
	Burns
	Trauma
	Allergic reactions
Increased capillary hydrostatic pressure	
Na⁺ retention and increased blood volume	Congestive heart failure
	Trauma and stress
	Renal failure
	Refeeding edema
	Adrenocortical hormone secretion
	Drugs: estrogen, phenylbutazone
Venous obstruction	Local obstruction
	Hepatic obstruction
	Pulmonary edema
Decreased plasma oncotic pressure	
Decreased synthesis of plasma proteins	Liver disease
	Malnutrition
Increased loss of plasma proteins	Nephrotic syndrome
	Burns
	Protein-losing enteropathy
Increased interstitial pressure (plasma protein lost to interstitium)	Lymphatic obstruction
	Increased capillary permeability

(From Groer ME, et al.: Basic Pathophysiology: A Conceptual Approach. St. Louis: CV Mosby Co, 1979.)

Urinalysis

The classic measurement of renal performance is the urinalysis (Table 8–3). The urinalysis is typically divided into a dipstick segment and a microscopic segment. The urinary specific gravity and the macroscopic appearance of the urine are also

Table 8–3. NORMAL FINDINGS IN A ROUTINE URINALYSIS

Component	Values
Color	Pale yellow to deep amber
Opacity	Clear
Specific gravity	1.002–1.035
pH	4.5–8
Glucose	Negative
Ketones	Negative
Protein	Negative
Bilirubin	Negative
Red blood cells	None to 3
White blood cells	None to 4
Bacteria	None
Casts	None
Crystals	None

(From Luckmann J, Sorensen KC: Medical-Surgical Nursing: A Psychophysiological Approach, 2nd ed. Philadelphia: WB Saunders Co, 1980.)

part of the urinalysis. Depending on the sophistication of the dipstick, a qualitative measurement of urinary pH, glucose, protein, and heme is usually available, with the newer dipsticks also indicating the presence of white blood cells (WBCs) and bacteria in the urine. The findings of glucose, protein, heme, WBCs, and bacteria in the urine are abnormal and deserve further investigation. The microscopic examination of the urine not only permits quantitation of red blood cells (RBCs) and WBCs but may also disclose the presence of urinary casts. A cast is an admixture of proteins, cells, and cellular debris and, with the exception of a hyaline cast, implies renal pathology. Abnormal casts include

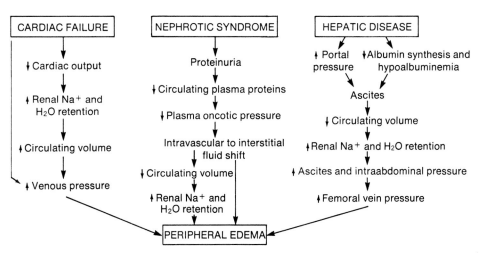

Figure 8–2. Interaction of disrupted capillary hemodynamics and Na⁺ and water retention in three conditions that include edema as a chief manifestation. (From Groer ME, et al.: Basic Pathophysiology: A Conceptual Approach. St. Louis: CV Mosby Co, 1979.)

RBC and WBC casts as well as granular, waxy, and fatty casts.

Blood Urea Nitrogen and Serum Creatinine Tests

Although the urinalysis is indispensable for identifying states of proteinuria, hematuria, and leukocyturia, it is an insensitive assay of renal filtration. The importance of measuring the magnitude of renal filtration lies in the fact that renal disorders may be life threatening when renal filtration has been severely compromised. The tests of blood urea nitrogen (BUN) and serum creatinine are normally employed to estimate the glomerular filtration rate (GFR). A BUN measurement greater than 100 mg/dl or a serum creatinine level greater than 5 mg/dl indicates major renal impairment. An even more specific estimate of GFR is the calculation of the creatinine clearance (see box). This is accomplished by obtaining a 24-hour urine collection and dividing the total excretion of urinary creatinine in 1 day by the steady-state serum creatinine concentration. A normal value for the creatinine clearance is above 80 ml/minute. A creatinine clearance below 15 ml/minute represents severe renal failure.

SERUM CREATININE– CREATININE CLEARANCE TEST*

For an accurate test, report, to the minute, the exact time the test begins and ends. The following formula indicates why this accuracy is so important:

$$\frac{urine\ creatinine}{serum\ creatinine} \times \frac{urine\ volume}{minutes}$$
$$\times \frac{1.73}{area} = blood$$

(ml) cleared of creatinine per minute (glomerular filtration rate)

Normal creatinine clearance is 100 to 130 ml/minute.

---

*Data from Stroot VR, et al.: Fluids and Electrolytes: A Practical Approach, 2nd ed. Philadelphia: FA Davis Co, 1978.

Intravenous Pyelogram

The intravenous pyelogram (IVP) takes advantage of the fact that the radiocontrast material undergoes glomerular filtration. Thus in the normal individual, there is both a nephrogram phase, which is due to the accumulation of the contrast material within the renal tubules, and an excretory phase, when the contrast material fills the collecting system, renal calyces, ureters, and bladder. The entire anatomy of the kidney can be outlined, with attention to the size, shape, and position of the various renal and excretory structures.

Other Tests and Scans

Besides the aforementioned tests, imaging the kidneys by ultrasonography, radionuclides, computerized tomography (CT), and magnetic resonance imaging (MRI) can aid the practitioner in investigating the form and function of the kidneys. All these tests provide the practitioner with anatomic details of the kidneys, and some provide a gross measure of the symmetry of renal function.

A *renal ultrasonogram* cannot measure any of the functional aspects of the kidney, but it is a safe, noninvasive tool for measuring kidney size and for evaluating the presence of cysts, tumors, and hydronephrosis. In addition, ultrasonography avoids the potential for nephrotoxicity, which can result from the contrast material used in the IVP.

The *renal nuclear medicine scan* provides some information about anatomy and function of the kidney. Depending on the radionuclide chosen, there is a certain degree of excretion such that some of the excretory pathway can be identified. Usually, however, there is neither the detail that can be achieved with an IVP nor the simplicity of the ultrasonographic procedure. A nuclear medicine scan may be appropriate as an initial examination when renal function needs to be assessed, and there is some contraindication to doing an IVP.

Computed tomography and *MRI* can be used in certain special circumstances to obtain additional details of renal structures.

ASSESSMENT OF RENAL DISEASES

Hematuria

Gross hematuria can be one of the most obvious of renal disorders. However, if it remains persistently microscopic, hematuria can defy detection until an incidental urinalysis is performed. In any event, the presence of either microscopic or macroscopic hematuria signifies an abnormality somewhere along the urinary tract. Although the degree of hematuria usually has little relevance, the duration is clearly important. Transient, microscopic hematuria can probably be ignored if the patient is otherwise asymptomatic. If the hematuria persists beyond three visits a work-up to localize the site and to identify the cause of the bleeding is in order. This work-up ordinarily consists of a cystoscopy and an IVP.

Causes

Although not always successful, a work-up for hematuria may identify the bleeding site to be of renal, ureteral, vesical, or urethral origin. Hematuria of renal origin can be from idiopathic glomerulonephritis, such as idiopathic membranoproliferative glomerulonephritis, or from glomerulonephritis that is associated with a systemic disease, such as systemic lupus erythematosus (SLE), bacterial endocarditis, or Goodpasture's syndrome. An intrinsic renal infection from tuberculosis or pyelonephritis is rare as a cause of hematuria unless there is some papillary necrosis as well. Intrinsic renal neoplasms, such as renal cell carcinoma or transitional cell carcinoma of the renal pelvis, may have hematuria as the only manifestation. Of the hereditary diseases that are associated with renal hematuria, sickle-cell disease and sickle cell trait are common, but Alport's syndrome, medullary sponge kidney, polycystic renal disease, and tuberous sclerosis are other diagnostic possibilities.

Renal trauma and surgery must be considered as potential causes of renal hematuria, as should renal infarction, systemic bleeding disorders, and blood dyscrasias. Bleeding and hematuria of ureteral origin can stem from a malignancy, stone, or trauma. Bleeding from the bladder should raise questions of infection, neoplasms, trauma, and stones or other foreign bodies. Finally, bleeding from the urethra implies urethritis, a foreign body, trauma, or, in males, a prostate abnormality.

Treatment

Treatment of hematuria is usually supportive and directed against the primary disease.

Proteinuria

Unlike the patient with gross hematuria, the patient with proteinuria rarely presents with symptoms unless the degree of proteinuria is so great that the nephrotic syndrome develops. Transient proteinuria, similar to transient hematuria, can be ignored, but persistent proteinuria needs to be investigated.

Orthostatic Proteinuria

When the presence of continued proteinuria is established, the first step is to determine if there is an orthostatic component. This is done by having the patient bring in two urine specimens. The first one is obtained when the patient arises in the morning, and the second one is obtained after the patient has been ambulatory for 3 or 4 hours. If there is protein in the second specimen but not the first the patient has orthostatic proteinuria. In the absence of any other abnormality, no further work-up is required. The prognosis is good because isolated orthostatic proteinuria is benign.

Quantitation

If the proteinuria is not orthostatic in character or if other urinary abnormalities besides the proteinuria are present, the next step should be to quantitate the degree of proteinuria. This is typically done by ordering a 24-hour urine collection for protein and creatinine, with the latter test being ordered to provide a measurement of the creatinine clearance level as well as the adequacy of the urine collection. There are formulas that predict the amount of creatinine that a patient of a given age, sex, and weight should excrete per day. A protein excretion of greater than 2.5 g/day is considered in the nephrotic range and has a whole scope of possible etiologies, which are discussed subsequently in this chapter. In comparison, protein excretion of less than 2.5 g/day has an even larger differential diagnosis, although typically this does not portend such serious renal disease as the excretion of larger amounts of protein.

Glomerular, Tubular, and Overflow Types of Proteinuria

If there is less than 2.5 g of protein per day it is not possible to say that the protein must derive from a glomerular abnormality. It is frequently helpful then to obtain a urine protein electrophoresis to try to separate the proteinuria into glomerular, tubular, and overflow types. In *glomerular* proteinuria, there is damage to the filtering mechanism so that the proteins that appear in the urine are the same as those in the serum, and consequently the urine electrophoresis resembles the serum electrophoresis. *Tubular* proteinuria stems not from a defect in the filtering apparatus but from a defect in tubular function. Low molecular weight plasma proteins that normally pass through the glomerulus are not reabsorbed by the tubules and escape into the urine. With a tubular disease process, such as Fanconi's syndrome, the urine electrophoresis pattern is dominated by alpha and beta proteins.

The final type of proteinuria, *overflow* or preglomerular proteinuria, originates from an abnormal excess of plasma protein, which as a result of the increase in filtered load appears in the urine. The most common example of this is monoclonal gammopathy.

Treatment

The therapy for these states is directed at the cause of the proteinuria. When under 2.5 g of protein are excreted, the loss of the protein itself is usually of minor consequence.

Dysuria

Dysuria means difficulty or pain in urination. Although traditionally equated with urinary tract infection, there are a number of other causes of dysuria.

Dysuria in Men

In men, dysuria can be caused by a gonococcal or chlamydial urethritis, a foreign body, or a urinary tract infection. Urinary tract infections are more common in older men because most of these infections are related to prostatic disease. A man with urinary tract infection should undergo a full urologic investigation. Treatment for urinary tract infection in men may require prolonged antibiotic therapy lasting 4 to 6 weeks because a prostatic focus may prove difficult to eradicate.

Dysuria in Women

In women, dysuria is most frequently caused by urinary tract infection, but urethritis and vaginitis can also be responsible. Ideally in the investigation of urinary tract infection in women, the practitioner wants to identify the causative organism, the site of the infection, and the optimal duration of treatment. The standard approach has been to obtain a urine sample for culture and sensitivity. If there are greater than 100,000 bacteria/ml it is standard to give a 7- to 14-day course of an appropriate antibiotic.

This standard approach had been modified as follows. First, a colony count of greater than 100,000 bacteria is no longer necessary before antibiotic therapy is considered warranted. In fact, in women who are symptomatic and infected with coliforms, a bacterial count of greater than 100 bacteria/ml is deemed sufficient evidence of infection. Second, for lower urinary tract infection, a single dose of antibiotic, (amoxicillin 3 g by mouth or sulfisoxazole 2 g by mouth) is as effective as the traditional 7- to 14-day course.

RECURRENT URINARY TRACT INFECTION

Repeated urinary tract infections can be from the same organism or from a new organism, with a new organism accounting for the vast majority of repeated infections in women. Intrinsic, possibly genetically determined host factors, such as increased uroepithelial cell adherence of *Escherichia coli* due to increased uroepithelial cell receptors, may explain the frequency of urinary tract infections in some women. Behavioral factors such as sexual intercourse, deliberate deferral of urination, and decreased fluid intake also seem to predispose women to recurrent infection.

In women who have frequent reinfections with no apparent behavioral contributor, IVP and cystoscopy have previously been used as important diagnostic procedures in the work-up. However, a number of studies show that the yield of these procedures is quite low (less than 1 to 3%) in uncovering any correctable lesion. For the majority of women with three or more infections a year, the only recourse may be 6 to 12 months of antimicrobial prophylaxis (half a regular-strength trimethoprim-sulfamethoxazole tablet each evening). During prophylactic therapy, urinary tract infections do not recur. When the prophylaxis is stopped, urinary tract infections typically return.

RENAL INFECTION

Women who have relapsing infections with the same organisms may have a renal focus of infection. These patients are often identified because they have a relapse of infection after oral antibiotic therapy. Of these patients, 10 to 50% have a relapse of infection after the 7- to 14-day traditional therapy, and 30 to 70% have a relapse after single-dose therapy. The optimal antimicrobial regimen for patients who relapse has not been established. A 6-week course of therapy may be appropriate.

PYELONEPHRITIS

Another cause of dysuria is pyelonephritis. In this circumstance, the dysuria is typically associated with fever, vomiting, flank pain, and tenderness. Intravenous antibiotics followed by oral antibiotics for a total of 10 to 14 days is the treatment of choice.

URETHRITIS

Some women who appear to have lower urinary tract infections may have chlamydial urethritis. The patient with *Chlamydia* typically has dysuria and pyuria but a sterile urine culture. This patient and her sexual partner can be cured by 10 days of therapy with doxycycline (100 mg twice a day).

VAGINITIS

Dysuria associated with vaginitis is generally accompanied by a vaginal discharge. The dysuria is typically described as being external rather than internal.

Nephrotic Syndrome

Nephrotic syndrome is defined by the presence of more than 2.5 g of protein in the urine per day. Associated with the urinary protein loss may be peripheral and facial edema, hyperlipidemia, and lipiduria. A drop in plasma oncotic pressure from a lowered serum albumin is perhaps partly the cause of the edema. Other proteins besides albumin are lost in the urine as well. The loss of complement may be responsible for impaired resistance to certain bacterial infections, and the loss of antithrombin III may contribute to the tendency for thromboembolism in nephrotic syndrome.

Glomerulonephropathy

The causes of nephrotic syndrome are many, but the underlying pathology is always some form of glomerular disorder because proteinuria greater than 2.5 g/day does not develop unless the glomeruli are abnormally permeable to the plasma proteins. A glomerulonephropathy can develop either from a systemic disease or from a primary idiopathic renal process (Table 8–4). Although an immune complex–related mechanism has been implicated as the most likely cause for many forms of glomerulonephropathy, there is still considerable uncertainty about the pathogenesis of the lesions. Consequently only a limited number of proven therapies exist.

Idiopathic Types

Idiopathic types of nephrotic syndrome include minimal change disease, focal glomerular sclerosis, membranous glomerulopathy, mesangial proliferative glo-

Table 8–4. ETIOLOGY AND CLINICAL MANIFESTATIONS OF SPECIFIC RENAL DISORDERS*

Condition	Etiology	Clinical Manifestations
Acute glomerulonephritis	Usually follows an infection such as beta-hemolytic streptococcal infection	Lethargy, malaise, anorexia, weakness, hypertension, circulatory congestion, hematuria; edema of face and eyelids common
Chronic glomerulonephritis	May occur after acute glomerulonephritis; frequently, etiology unknown	Proteinuria, edema; may have hypertension and associated headache; anemia; as disease progresses, azotemia and uremia occur
Nephrotic syndrome	May occur during chronic glomerulonephritis, metabolic diseases, systemic sensitivity diseases	Edema; massive proteinuria with decreased serum albumin and increased cholesterol
Polycystic kidney disease	Familial disease in which cysts develop in the parenchyma of both kidneys; mean age of onset, 40 yrs	Hypertension, intermittent hematuria, slight proteinuria, lumbar pain, tenderness, or both, pyuria, and bacteruria may be present; palpable renal mass
Acute chronic pyelonephritis	May follow urinary tract infection or be due to obstruction	Chills, fever, abdominal pain, backache, nausea, vomiting, urinary frequency, dysuria
Fanconi's syndrome	May be inherited or acquired; proximal renal tubular transport function impaired; substances usually absorbed by the proximal tubule lost	Failure to reabsorb phosphate, with hypophosphatemia; renal rickets; glycosuria; aminoaciduria
Cystinosis	Genetic metabolic anomaly affecting renal transport; cystine deposited in organs	Similar to Fanconi's syndrome
Renal tubular acidosis	Defective urinary acidification or reabsorption of bicarbonate; etiology unknown	Hypokalemia; osteomalacia may be present; hypophosphatemia, hypercalciuria
Chronic potassium depletion	May result from renal tubular disorders, Cushing's syndrome, aldosteronism; most common abnormality is kidney's inability to concentrate urine	Nocturia, polyuria, polydypsia, slight proteinuria
Tuberculosis of the kidney	Bacterial infection of the kidney via the bloodstream; can result in renal scarring and destruction	Frequently no clinical manifestations; may be dysuria and intermittent hematuria

* Partial listing of known renal disorders.
(From Howard RB, et al.: Nutrition in Clinical Care, 2nd ed. New York: McGraw Hill Book Co, 1982.)

merulonephritis, membranoproliferative glomerulonephritis, and crescentic glomerulonephritis. Although there are general clinical characteristics to each of these lesions, one cannot usually arrive at any of these diagnoses without performing a renal biopsy. Unfortunately, because of the limited therapeutic options that are available, a renal biopsy is not that helpful in guiding therapy or in predicting outcome, and there can be justification for simply starting empiric therapy, usually with steroids.

Systemic Disorders

If nephrotic syndrome is from some systemic disorder treating the primary disease where possible may be successful in correcting the renal process. Proteinuria in pre-eclampsia almost invariably resolves with the delivery of the infant. Nephrotic syndrome associated with Hodgkin's disease usually resolves when chemotherapy is successful. Systemic lupus erythematosus is a common cause of renal disease and nephrosis, but the results of therapy on the renal process are less certain. Nephrotic syndrome associated with diabetes mellitus is not reversible. Other systemic causes of nephrosis, all of which may require therapy directed at the underlying illness, include bacterial endocarditis; syphilis; hepatitis B; malaria; schistosomiasis; carcinomas of the colon, lung, and stomach; gold or penicillamine therapy; amyloidosis; serum sickness; and malignant hypertension.

Acute Renal Failure

The causes of acute renal failure are multiple, but some diagnostic clarity can be achieved by separating those causes of acute renal failure that act directly on the kidney from those that have actions "upstream" or "downstream" of the kidney (Fig. 8–3). This separation is important not just for diagnostic purposes but because both prerenal and postrenal causes of acute renal failure should be treatable.

Volume Depletion

Prerenal azotemia can be defined as a circumstance in which the drop in GFR is proximate to a decrease in renal perfusion pressure, an intense renal vasoconstriction, or both (Table 8–5). The kidneys themselves are functioning normally. The

Table 8–5. CAUSES AND ALTERED FUNCTIONS OF PRERENAL FAILURE

Cause	Altered Function
Hypovolemia	Decreased fluid volume reduces renal blood flow and GFR
Decreased cardiac output	Kidneys not receiving the normal cardiac output (N25% of the body's blood)
Vascular failure Vasogenic shock Neurogenic shock	Interference with vascular elasticity by vascular collapse or pooling of the blood (vascular dilatation)
Hepatorenal syndrome	Diseased liver causes body to falsely sense a volume deficit, thus retaining fluids; liver becomes grossly edematous

GFR, Glomerular filtration rate.
(From Stroot VR, et al.: Fluids and Electrolytes: A Practical Approach, 2nd ed. Philadelphia: FA Davis Co, 1978.)

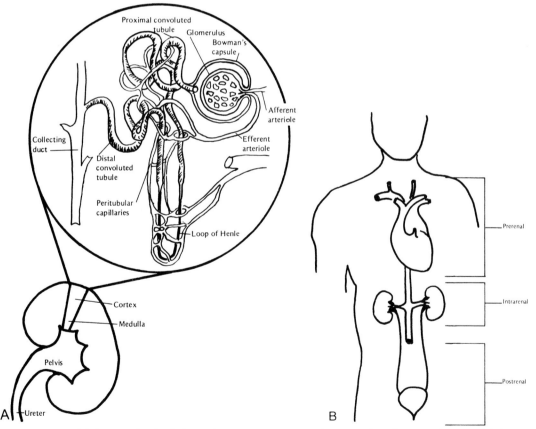

Figure 8–3. Renal failure can be divided into three categories: prerenal, postrenal, and intrarenal. Prerenal failure is caused by events that take place before the blood reaches the kidneys and involves the subsequent reaction of normal kidneys to these stimuli. Postrenal failure may result from an obstruction in the system that leads away from the kidney. Intrarenal failure may be due to primary parenchymal damage, or it may be a sequela of pre- or postrenal failure. *A*, Nephron; *B*, types of renal failure. (From Stroot VR, et al.: Fluids and Electrolytes: A Practical Approach, 2nd ed. Philadelphia: FA Davis Co, 1978.)

consequent oliguria and azotemia develop because of a change in renal hemodynamics and not because of any direct structural destruction or damage to the kidney. The typical cause of prerenal azotemia is volume depletion, which may be from actual volume depletion, such as in hemorrhage, excessive diuresis, and third-space losses, or from diminished effective intravascular volume. Decrease in effective intravascular volume can be seen in congestive heart failure, cirrhosis, and nephrosis. Hypotension from sepsis and antihypertensive medications can also induce prerenal azotemia as can the hepatorenal syndrome and prostaglandin inhibitors. With these last two causes, the mechanism of the azotemia appears to be a redistribution of renal blood flow or an unbalanced stimulus to renal vasoconstriction such that the glomeruli receive less blood for filtration.

Because volume depletion is readily treatable, the practitioner should always rule out volume depletion in any patient with acute azotemia. The simplest way to do this is to administer a volume challenge to the patient of perhaps 200 to 400 ml of normal saline intravenously over 30 minutes and to look for any increase in urine output. Central venous line or pulmonary capillary wedge monitoring can also be of assistance in ruling out volume depletion in the acutely azotemic patient.

Obstruction

Postrenal azotemia stems from any obstruction to urine flow beyond the kidneys themselves (Table 8–6). The site of the obstruction can be the urethra, the bladder neck, or the ureters. In general, significant renal failure from ureteral obstruction occurs only if the obstruction is bilateral or if there is only one functioning kidney with unilateral obstruction. In men, benign prostatic hypertrophy is a common cause of obstruction. In women cervical cancer with extension should be considered. Bladder or prostatic tumors, stones, and retroperitoneal fibrosis are other causes of postrenal azotemia. To rule out the presence of obstruction as a cause of renal failure, a renal ultrasonogram to look for hydronephrosis can be ordered. This test has a diagnostic sensitivity of almost 100% unless the patient is volume depleted or the collecting system is encased in tumors and

Table 8–6. CAUSES AND ALTERED FUNCTIONS OF POSTRENAL FAILURE

Cause	Altered Function
Urethral obstruction (prostatism, tumors)	Complete obstruction causes anuria; partial obstruction usually causes anuria alternating with polyuria
Ureteral obstruction (calculi, tumors, trauma)	Complete obstruction causes anuria; partial obstruction usually causes anuria alternating with polyuria; edema following instrumentation
Sulfate or urate precipitation	Blockage due to precipitation or crystal formation
Anticholinergic drugs and ganglionic blocking agents	Acute urinary retention possible because nerves not adequately stimulated; however, this is unusual

(From Stroot VR, et al.: Fluids and Electrolytes: A Practical Approach, 2nd ed. Philadelphia: FA Davis Co, 1978.)

unable to dilate. Depending on degree and duration of obstruction, relief of obstruction should lead to return of renal function.

Renal Causes

If volume depletion and obstruction can be ruled out in the acutely oliguric patient the cause of the renal failure is most likely intrarenal (Table 8–7). Prolonged volume depletion or obstruction can produce intrinsic renal damage, but renal ischemia, nephrotoxins, interstitial nephritis, and systemic disease are more common causes of intrinsic renal failure. The acute renal failure that stems from renal ischemia, sometimes called acute tubular necrosis or acute vasomotor nephropathy, shares many of the same causes as the volume-depleted forms of acute renal failure. The difference is that blood flow to the kidneys is reduced to such a degree that renal viability is compromised and there is actual renal damage. Nephrotoxic agents include aminoglycoside antibiotics; iodinated contrast agents; and heavy metals such as gold, platinum, lead, and mercury. Acute renal failure may be seen when there is an allergic interstitial nephritis from drugs, such as methicillin, rifampin, sulfonamides, diuretics, and allopurinol. Finally, both systemic diseases and primary renal

Table 8–7. CAUSES AND ALTERED FUNCTIONS OF INTRARENAL FAILURE

Cause	Altered Function
Acute tubular necrosis	
Ischemia	Shock decreases renal perfusion, causing circulatory insufficiency; resultant hypoxia causes tissue death
Drugs, poisons, metals	Nephrotoxic substances cause tissue injury and scarring
Hemolysis	Mismatched blood transfusion causes agglutination of red blood cells, which obstruct tubules
Hypercalcemic crisis	Excess calcium crystallizes in tubules, causing obstruction; condition varies according to pH of urine
Trauma	Burns and crushing injuries result in ECF deficit, causing insufficient tissue perfusion; myoglobin causes sludging in tubules
Acute glomerulonephritis	
Poststreptococcal infection	Antigen-antibody reaction in glomerulus causes inflammation and decreased glomerular blood flow
Vascular	
Renal arterial thrombosis	Thrombi in renal vessels cause occlusion
Acute cortical necrosis	
Pregnancy (abruptio placenta)	Intravascular coagulation possibly due to amniotic fluid in the plasma; anuria without obstruction
Sepsis (especially in pregnant women and patients on steroid therapy)	White blood cells fail to handle toxins as they would under normal conditions
Papillary necrosis	
Urinary tract infection	Papillae slough; particles obstruct the tubules
Intrarenal precipitation	
Urates and sulfonamides	Precipitation and crystal formation cause obstruction
Multiple myeloma	Precipitation of myeloma protein into kidney
Pyelonephritis	Infection of kidney causes scarring of tubular system

ECF, Extracellular fluid.
(From Stroot VR, et al.: Fluids and Electrolytes: A Practical Approach, 2nd ed. Philadelphia: FA Davis Co, 1978.)

diseases can produce acute renal failure. Examples include malignant hypertension, SLE, acute poststreptococcal glomerulonephritis, vasculitis, and postpartum renal failure.

Treatment

The approach to a patient with acute renal failure is to rule out volume depletion and obstruction and then to search for one of the aforementioned causes of renal failure. In the absence of any treatable disease, the management of acute renal failure must be expectant and supportive, including maintaining the patient in fluid and electrolyte balance. In general, fluids are restricted to the replacement of insensible losses plus urine output, and administration of potassium should be avoided. The serum sodium level is maintained by adjusting the amount of free water that the patient receives, and if the patient has a significant metabolic acidosis from the renal failure administration of bicarbonate may be in order as well.

Dialysis

If with time and optimal fluid and electrolyte management the azotemia worsens or the fluid status cannot be balanced, dialysis may be necessary. There are no strict guidelines about when to start dialysis, but a BUN measurement greater than 150 mg/dl, life-threatening pulmonary edema, pericarditis, and unmanageable hyperkalemia would all be reasonable indications. The forms of acute dialysis can be either hemodialysis or peritoneal dialysis, with the choice dependent on the availability of equipment and the patient's hemodynamic and abdominal status. Acute renal failure is by definition short-lived (it should not exceed 2 months), so if the patient can be supported he or she will likely recover renal function. Unfortunately because of the nature of the diseases that can lead to acute renal failure, mortality still approaches 50%.

Chronic Renal Failure

Chronic renal failure is analogous to acute renal failure in that the diagnostic work-up and management are similar.

However, the etiology of chronic renal failure is more frequently in primary renal disease, although systemic diseases, such as diabetes mellitus, hypertension, multiple myeloma, and SLE, can also be causative (Table 8–8). Hereditary renal diseases, such as polycystic kidney disease and Alport's syndrome, can also cause chronic renal failure, as can undetected, prolonged urinary tract obstruction.

Table 8–8. CAUSES AND ALTERED FUNCTIONS OF CHRONIC RENAL INSUFFICIENCY

Cause	Altered Function
Glomerulonephritis	
Proliferative	Diffuse increased cellularity of glomeruli; lesions due to antigen-antibody reaction; inflammation and dysfunction of glomerulus; most commonly seen in poststreptococcal glomerulonephritis; frequently a recoverable lesion
Membranous	Thickening of the basement membrane; usually idiopathic (also seen in diabetic renal disease); leads to heavy loss of protein; nephrotic state
Focal	Nondiffuse scattered lesions of proliferative, membranous, or membranous-proliferative type; frequently benign; most common symptom is hematuria
Nephrosclerosis	Hardening of renal tissues resulting in narrowing or occlusion of vessels; arteriosclerosis related to aging process, which is accelerated in uncontrolled hypertension
Pyelonephritis	Kidney damage attributed to chronic infection with micro-organisms, beginning in the renal pelvis and proceeding to renal parenchyma
Papillary necrosis	Obstruction and sloughing of the papillae may be related to diabetes, infection, analgesic drug abuse, urinary obstruction
Uric acid nephropathy	Uric acid causes blockage of tubules

Table 8–8. (*continued*)

Cause	Altered Function
Nephrocalcinosis	High concentration of calcium in the blood causes calcium deposits with subsequent renal damage; seen in many diseases, such as hyperparathyroidism and sarcoidosis
SLE	A collagen-vascular disease; no set pattern of events; renal involvement most often focal but can cause proliferative or membranous glomerulonephritis
Acute renal failure	Incomplete recovery can lead to chronic renal failure
Sickle cell anemia	Hereditary S-shaped hemoglobin cells cause sloughing into and plugging of the glomeruli; significant to the black race
Polycystic kidney disease	Congenital hereditary disease causes formation of cysts, enlargement of which causes pressure and atrophy of functioning glomeruli

SLE, Systemic lupus erythematosus.
(From Stroot VR, et al.: Fluids and Electrolytes: A Practical Approach, 2nd ed. Philadelphia: FA Davis Co, 1978.)

When the patient is first examined, the practitioner cannot tell if the patient has chronic or acute renal disease, so the initial work-up to rule out volume depletion and obstruction is still essential. Determination of renal size by ultrasonography may be helpful in that if the kidneys are small the renal failure is likely to be chronic. The presence of anemia, hyperphosphatemia, and renal osteodystrophy also generally indicates chronic renal failure.

Anemia

Anemia associated with chronic renal failure is multifactorial and does not show any uniform relationship to the level of renal impairment, although typically anemia is not noted until more than 50% of kidney function has been lost. The cause of anemia is a decrease in renal erythropoietin production, from decreased renal functional mass and the accumulation of unidentified substances in the uremic plasma that retard erythropoiesis and shorten red blood cell survival.

Hyperphosphatemia

Hyperphosphatemia in chronic renal failure is primarily a consequence of the direct loss of phosphate filtration capacity.

Renal Osteodystrophy

Renal osteodystrophy of chronic renal failure is multifactorial, with contributions from hyperphosphatemia as well as from decreased production of the active vitamin D metabolite 1,25-dihydroxycholecalciferol. Hyperphosphatemia occurs because of the reduction in GFR. This reduction in renal function causes a drop in serum calcium level and the development of secondary hyperparathyroidism and bone disease (Fig. 8–4). Decreased production of 1,25-dihydroxycholecalciferol occurs because of a loss of renal mass. The kidney is the site where vitamin D is transformed to its biologically active form. In chronic renal failure, with the loss of renal mass, there is less conversion of vitamin D to its active form. Absence of the active vitamin D metabolite leads to reduced intestinal absorption of calcium and reduced bony responsiveness to parathyroid hormone, both of which lead to increased parathyroid hormone secretion and to metabolic bone disease (Fig. 8–5).

Treatment

Because chronic renal failure is typically progressive, management must change over time. The practitioner needs to remember that all the causes of acute renal failure can be superimposed on chronic renal failure in a given patient. Thus if the patient's renal function deteriorates unexpectedly a search for an acute process must be performed. A helpful way to follow the patient with chronic renal failure is to plot the reciprocal of the serum creatinine level or the logarithm of the serum creatinine level against time. This plot is typically linear and thus can be used to identify the rate of progression of the disease as well as any variance from linearity.

When the patient with chronic renal failure exhibits symptoms, which usually happens when the BUN measurement is greater than 100 to 120 mg/dl, diet is the

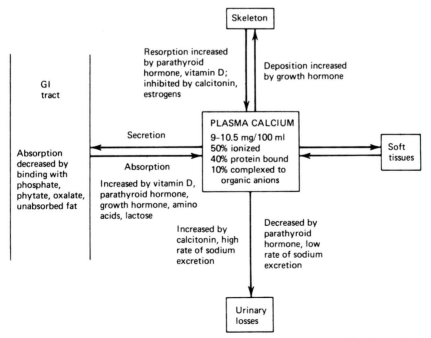

Figure 8–4. Summary of calcium metabolism. (From Muir BL: Pathophysiology: An Introduction to the Mechanism of Disease. New York: John Wiley & Sons, Inc, 1980.)

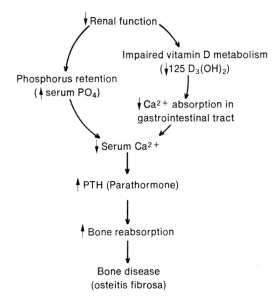

Figure 8–5. Consequences of disease on nutritional status. Secondary hyperparathyroidism and bone disease occur in acute renal failure when there is retention of phosphorus, decreased absorption of calcium, and impacted vitamin D metabolism. (From Howard R, Herbold N: Nutrition in Clinical Care. New York: McGraw-Hill Book Co, 1978.)

mainstay of conservative therapy (Table 8–9). A reduction in BUN level by restricting protein intake is the major goal. Sodium, fluids, potassium, and phosphorus also need to be limited. Bicarbonate supplementation may be needed for metabolic acidosis, and diuretics and potassium exchange resins may be needed to help keep fluid and electrolyte balance. With all these restrictions, it is frequently difficult to ensure adequate caloric intake, and the

Table 8–9. GOALS OF NUTRITIONAL MANAGEMENT OF THE RENAL PATIENT

Nutritional Goal	Nutrients Altered to Achieve Goal
To minimize protein catabolism (adults and children)	Protein

To promote anabolism, i.e., growth (children)	Energy
	  Carbohydrates
	  Fats

To maintain fluid balance (adults and children)	Sodium, water (fluids)
To maintain electrolyte balance (adults and children)	Sodium, potassium, phosphorus (and calcium), water (fluids)

(From Howard RB, et al.: Nutrition in Clinical Care, 2nd ed. New York: McGraw-Hill Book Co, 1982.)

practitioner must try to avoid producing nutritional depletion in the patient.

DRUG THERAPY

Because of the limited renal reserve, potentially nephrotoxic agents should be avoided, and drugs that require renal excretion need to have their dosage modified. Examples of this latter group of drugs include aminoglycosides, digoxin, procainamide, and cimetidine. In making adjustments in drug dosages in renal failure, general guidelines can be followed.

1. The level of renal function must be measured or estimated.

2. The pharmacokinetics of the drug in question must be ascertained to learn to what extent the drug or its metabolites depend on renal excretion.

3. If the drug's half-life of elimination is markedly prolonged because of the renal failure a loading dose may need to be given. This is a result of the fact that a steady-state concentration of any drug requires 3.3 drug elimination half-lives before 90% of the steady-state level is reached.

4. A maintenance dose of the drug must be decided on. This can be accomplished either by lengthening the interval between doses to adjust for the delayed excretion of the drug or by reducing the amount of each dose while maintaining the customary interval.

5. If serum drug levels are available for the drug in question, the levels should be measured to determine that the levels are in the therapeutic and nontoxic ranges (Table 8–10).

DIET

Even before the patient develops symptoms from uremia, some nephrologists would argue that the patient should be placed on a protein-restricted diet. The reason for this recommendation is that large dietary protein loads may increase the work of the kidney and that paradoxically this increased workload can actually accelerate the rate of renal failure. The magnitude of ideal protein restriction has not been established, but a value per day of 0.8 g of protein/kg of body weight seems reasonable.

DIALYSIS

The major indication for starting dialysis in the patient with chronic renal insufficiency is the failure of conservative therapy to keep the patient comfortable without significant malnutrition. There is no doubt that the need for dialysis can be delayed by rigid dietary proscription, but if this is accompanied by significant weight loss there is little to be gained by continuing to withhold dialysis. The forms of therapy available for the management of end-stage renal disease include hemodialysis, peritoneal dialysis, and renal transplantation.

Hemodialysis can be performed either at a hemodialysis outpatient center or in the patient's home if in-home assistance is available. *Peritoneal dialysis* is usually performed at home. Long-term peritoneal dialysis differs from acute peritoneal dialysis. With chronic peritoneal dialysis, a permanent peritoneal catheter is placed, and the patient usually handles all the dialysate exchanges without assistance. The forms of peritoneal dialysis that are available for the patient with chronic disease include continuous ambulatory peritoneal dialysis (CAPD) and continuous cyclic peritoneal dialysis (CCPD). In CAPD, the patient makes the exchanges during the day while ambulatory, whereas in CCPD, the patient makes the exchanges at night with the assistance of a mechanical exchange device. *Renal transplantation* comes closest to completely restoring renal function and can be accomplished through transplantation of either cadaver kidneys or kidneys from living related donors. Each of these three modalities has its own merits and drawbacks, but all are efficacious in treating the uremic condition.

Gouty Nephropathy

Uric acid is considered to be involved with the kidney in (1) uric acid–induced acute renal failure, (2) uric acid nephrolithiasis, and (3) chronic gouty nephropathy. The relationship between asymptomatic hyperuricemia and renal function is under debate.

Uric Acid–Induced Acute Renal Failure

In uric acid–induced acute renal failure, the amount of uric acid that is presented to the kidney for filtration and excretion is enormous. The high concentration of uric acid in the tubular lumen is thought to result in intratubular obstruction from uric acid microcrystallization. The typical clinical setting in which this occurs is in the patient with a large tumor mass, usually a lymphoproliferative malignancy, who receives chemotherapy that causes the rapid destruction of the tumor. Often called tumor lysis syndrome, the destruction of the tumor leads to the release of endogenous nucleotides, which are enzymatically broken down to uric acid that is then presented to the kidneys for excretion. Attempts to avoid tumor lysis syndrome by pretreating the patient with allopurinol, saline infusion, and sodium bicarbonate to alkalize the urine are usually successful. Even when acute renal failure does develop, efforts to promote diuresis and reduce the uric acid burden are still worthwhile. If the patient goes into complete renal shutdown dialysis is usually necessary to remove the uric acid from the body.

Uric Acid Nephrolithiasis

Uric acid nephrolithiasis has many etiologies and may be associated with neither hyperuricemia nor hyperuricosuria. Although high uric acid concentration in the urine would certainly be expected to be a risk factor for uric acid stones, it is likely that a low urine pH and a low urine volume also play important roles. Uric acid stones may be seen in gout and the Lesch-Nyhan syndrome, a rare inherited disorder in which an enzymatic defect leads to massive overproduction of uric acid. Living in a warm climate, which tends to cause low urine volumes and high urine concentrations, can also be associated with uric acid stone formation. The nonsurgical management of these stones includes high fluid intake, urinary alkalization, and administration of allopurinol.

Chronic Gouty Nephropathy

Chronic gouty nephropathy seems to be associated with clinically severe gout. With the present highly effective treatment for gout, chronic renal failure from gout is no longer common. It is likely that the damage caused to the kidney is related to the direct deposition of uric acid in the

Text continued on page 282

Table 8–10. GUIDELINES FOR DRUG THERAPY IN PATIENTS WITH IMPAIRED RENAL FUNCTION

Agent	Metabolism and Excretion*	Maintenance Schedule† Based on Creatinine Clearance (ml/min)				Drug Removed by Dialysis§
		>80 (normal)	~50‡	50–10‡	<10‡	
Antimicrobial Agents						
Antimycotic drugs						
Amphotericin B	Nonrenal	q 24 hrs	q 24 hrs	q 24 hrs	0.5 mg/kg q 24 hrs or 1.0 mg/kg q 48 hrs	No (H,P)
5-fluorocytosine	Renal	25–50 mg/kg q 6 hrs	Unch||	25–50 mg/kg q 12–24 hrs	25 mg/kg q 24 hrs	Yes (H,P)
Miconazole	Hepatic	q 8 hrs	Unch	Unch	Unch	No (H)
Antituberculous drugs						
Ethambutol	Renal	15–25 mg/kg/day	Unch	7.5–15 mg/kg/day	5 mg/kg/day	Yes (H,P)
INH	Hepatic, renal	300–400 mg/day	Unch	Unch	200–300 mg/day	Yes (H,P)
PAS	Renal, (hepatic)	q 8 hrs	q 8 hrs	q 12 hrs	Not recommended	Yes (H)
Rifampin	Hepatic	q 24 hrs	Unch	Unch	Unch	No
Aminoglycosides¶						
Amikacin	Renal	5 mg/kg q 8 hrs	5 mg/kg q 12 hrs	3–5 mg/kg q 12 hrs	1–3 mg/kg q 24 hrs	Yes (H,P)
Gentamicin	Renal	1–1.5 mg/kg q 8 hrs	0.5–0.8 mg/kg q 8 hrs	0.3–0.5 mg/kg q 8 hrs	0.2 mg/kg q 8 hrs	Yes (H,P)
Kanamycin	Renal	7.5 mg/kg q 12 hrs	7.5 mg/kg q 18 hrs	0.25 g q 24–48 hrs	7 mg/kg q 5–7 days	Yes (H,P)
Neomycin	Renal	Not recommended for systemic use				Yes (H)
Tobramycin	Renal	1 mg/kg q 8 hrs	0.5–0.75 mg/kg q 8 hrs	0.25–0.5 mg/kg q 8 hrs	0.1–0.2 mg/kg q 8 hrs	Yes (H,P)
Streptomycin	Renal	0.5–1.0 g q 12 hrs	0.5–1.0 mg q 24 hrs	0.5–1.0 g q 2–3 days	0.5 g q 3–4 days	Yes (H)
Cephalosporins						
Cefadroxil	Renal	0.5–1.0 g q 12 hrs	Unch	Unch	500 mg q 36 hrs	Yes (H)
Cefamandole	Renal	1–2 g q 4–6 hrs	0.75–1.5 g q 6 hrs	0.5–1.0 g q 8 hrs	0.25–0.75 g q 12 hrs	Yes (H), No (P)
Cefazolin	Renal	0.5–1.0 g q 8–12 hrs	Unch	250 mg q 6–12 hrs	250 mg q 24–48 hrs	Yes (H), No (P)
Cefoxitin	Renal	1–2 g q 6–8 hrs	1–2 g q 8–12 hrs	1–2 g q 12–24 hrs	0.5–1.0 g q 24–48 hrs	Yes (H), No (P)
Cephalexin	Renal	500 mg q 4–6 hrs	Unch	500 mg q 8–12 hrs	250 mg q 12–24 hrs	Yes (H,P)
Cephalothin	Renal, (hepatic)	1–2 g q 4–6 hrs	Unch	1–2 g q 6–8 hrs	1–2 g q 8–12 hrs	Yes (H,P)
Cephapirin	Renal, hepatic	0.5–1.0 g q 4–6 hrs	Unch	0.5–1.0 g q 8 hrs	7.5–10 mg/kg q 8–12 hrs	Yes (H)
Cephradine	Renal	0.5–1.0 g q 6 hrs	Unch	0.25–0.5 g q 6 hrs	0.25–0.5 g q 12–24 hrs	Yes (H,P)
Chloramphenicol	Hepatic, (renal)	q 6 hrs	Unch	Unch	Unch	Yes (H), No (P)
Clindamycin	Hepatic, (renal)	q 6–8 hrs	Unch	Unch	Unch	No (H,P)
Erythromycin	Hepatic	q 6 hrs	Unch	Unch	Unch	No (H,P)

Drug						
Lincomycin	Hepatic	q 6 hrs	Unch	q 12 hrs	0.5 g q 24–36 hrs	No (H,P)
Metronidazole	Hepatic, renal	q 8 hrs	Unch	q 12 hrs	q 24 hrs	Yes (H)
Penicillins						
Amoxicillin	Renal	q 8 hrs	Unch	q 12 hrs Unch for UTI	q 16 hrs Unch for UTI	Yes (H), No (P)
Ampicillin	Renal, (hepatic)	q 6 hrs	q 6 hrs	q 9 hrs Unch for UTI	5–10 mg/kg q 24 hrs Unch for UTI	Yes (H), No (P)
Carbenicillin	Renal, hepatic	4–6 g q 4 hrs	4–5 g q 4 hrs	2–4 g q 6–12 hrs	2 g q 12 hrs	Yes (H), No (P)
Isoxazolyl penicillins (oxacillin, cloxacillin, dicloxacillin, nafcillin)	Hepatic, renal	q 6 hrs	Unch	Unch	Unch	No (H,P)
Methicillin	Renal, (hepatic)	q 4 hrs	Unch	Unch	1–2 g q 8–12 hrs	No (H,P)
Penicillin G	Renal, (hepatic)	q 8 hrs	Unch	Unch	q 10–12 hrs <10–15 million U/day	Yes (H), No (P)
Ticarcillin	Renal	3 g q 3–6 hrs	2 g q 4 hrs	2 g q 8 hrs	2 g q 12 hrs	Yes (H,P)
Sulfamethoxazole with trimethoprim		q 12 hrs	Unch	q 18 hrs	q 24 hrs	Yes (H,P)
Sulfisoxazole	Renal	q 6 hrs	Unch	q 8–12 hrs Unch for UTI	q 12–24 hrs Unch for UTI	Yes (H,P)
Tetracyclines						
Doxycycline	Hepatic, renal	q 12 hrs	Unch	Unch	Unch	No (H,P)
All others	Renal, hepatic	Varies with agent	Avoid in presence of decreased renal function			No (H,P)
Urinary antiseptics						
Methenamine mandelate	Hepatic, renal	q 6 hrs	Unch	Not recommended		Unknown
Nalidixic acid	Hepatic, renal	q 8 hrs	Unch	Not recommended		Unknown
Nitrofurantoin	Renal	q 8 hrs	Unch	Not recommended		Yes (H)
Vancomycin	Renal	1 g q 12 hrs	1 g 2–3 days	1 g q 3–10 days	1 g 10–20 days	No (H,P)
Sedative, Tranquilizer, and Analgesic Agents						
Acetaminophen	Hepatic	q 4 hrs	Unch	Unch	Unch	Yes (H), No (P)
Aspirin	Renal, hepatic	q 4 hrs	Unch	q 4–6 hrs	Not recommended	Yes (H,P)
Barbiturates						
short-acting (pentobarbital, secobarbital)	Hepatic	qhs#	Unch	Unch	Unch	No (H,P)
long-acting (phenobarbital, amobarbital)	Renal	q 8 hrs	q 8 hrs	q 12 hrs	q 16 hrs	Yes (H,P)
Benzodiazepines						
Clordiazepoxide	Hepatic	q 6–8 hrs	Unch	q 8–12 hrs	q 12–24 hrs	No (H)
Diazepam	Hepatic	q 8 hrs	Unch	Unch	Unch for short-term therapy	No (H)
Flurazepam	Hepatic	qhs	Unch	Unch	Unch	No (H)
Chloral hydrate	Hepatic	qhs	Unch	Unch	Unch	Unknown

Table continued on following page

Table 8–10. (continued)

Agent	Metabolism and Excretion*	Maintenance Schedule† Based on Creatinine Clearance (ml/min)				Drug Removed by Dialysis§
		>80 (normal)	– 50‡	50–10‡	<10‡	
Diphenhydramine	Hepatic	As indicated	Unch	Unch	Unch	Unknown
Haloperidol	Hepatic, (renal)	q 8 hrs	Unch	Unch	Unch	Unknown
Meprobamate	Hepatic, (renal)	q 6 hrs	q 6 hrs	q 8–12 hrs	q 12–18 hrs	Yes (H,P)
Narcotic analgesics						
Codeine	Hepatic	q 4 hrs	Unch	Unch	Unch	Unknown
Meperidine	Hepatic	q 4 hrs	Unch	Unch	Not recommended for repeated use	Unknown
Methadone	Hepatic	As indicated	Unch	Unch	Unch	No (H,P)
Morphine	Hepatic	q 4 hrs	Unch	Unch	Unch	Unknown
Naloxone	Hepatic	IV bolus	Unch	Unch	Unch	Unknown
Pentazocine	Hepatic, (renal)	q 4 hrs	Unch	Unch	Unch	Unknown
Propoxyphene	Hepatic, (renal)	q 4 hrs	Unch	Unch	Unch	No (H,P)
Phenothiazines	Hepatic, (renal)	q 6 hrs	q 6 hrs	q 8–12 hrs	q 12–18 hrs	No (H,P)
Tricyclic antidepressants	Hepatic, (renal)	q 8 hrs	Unch	Unch	Unch	No (H,P)
Miscellaneous Agents						
Anticoagulants						
Heparin	Hepatic	q 4 hrs bolus or IV infusion	Unch	Use with caution because of hemorrhagic tendency in uremia		No, (H,P)
Warfarin	Hepatic	q 24 hrs	Unch			No, (H,P)
Anti-inflammatory drugs						
Colchicine	Renal, (hepatic)	q 12 hrs	Unch	Unch	Avoid prolonged use	No (H,P)
Corticosteroids	Hepatic	As indicated	Unch	Unch	Unch	Unknown
Ibuprofen	Renal	q 6 hrs	Unch	q 8 hrs	q 12 hrs	Unknown
Indomethacin	Hepatic	q 8 hrs	Unch	Unch	Unch	Unknown
Phenylbutazone	Hepatic	q 8 hrs	Unch	Unch	Use with caution	No (H,P)

		300 mg q 6 hrs	Unch	300 mg q 6–8 hrs	300 mg q 8–12 hrs	Yes (H)
Cimetidine	Renal					
Hypoglycemic drugs						
Acetohexamide	Renal, (hepatic)	q 12 hrs	q 12–24 hrs	Not recommended	Not recommended	Unknown
Chlorpropamide	Hepatic, (renal)	q 24 hrs	q 24–36 hrs	Not recommended	Not recommended	No (P)
Insulin (regular)	Hepatic, renal	As indicated	Unch	Insulin requirements decrease in uremia		No (H,P)
Tolbutamide	Hepatic, (renal)	q 8 hrs	Unch	q 8–12 hrs	q 12–24 hrs	No (H)
Hypouricemic agents						
Allopurinol	Renal	q 24 hrs	Unch	Unch	Unch	Probably yes (H,P)
Probenecid	Hepatic, (renal)	q 12 hrs	Unch	Ineffective, not recommended		Unknown
Immunosuppressive drugs						
Azathioprine	Hepatic	q 24 hrs	Unch	Unch	q 24–36 hrs	Probably some (H,P)
Cyclophosphamide	Hepatic, (renal)	q 24 hrs	Unch	Unch	Avoid or use with caution	Yes (H)
Methotrexate	Renal	Once weekly	Unch	75% of normal dose	50% of normal dose	Unknown
Theophylline	Hepatic	Constant IV infusion	Unch	Unch	Unch	Probably yes (H,P)

* Minor modes in parentheses.

+ When no dosage of drug is listed, use the dose conventionally prescribed for the specific indication.

‡ When a range of dosages, intervals, or combined dosages and intervals is listed for a level of renal functional impairment, use the lower dose, a longer maintenance interval, or a combined lower dose with a longer maintenance interval if the patient's creatinine clearance falls at the lower end of the clearance range for that column.

§ H, Hemodialysis; P, peritoneal dialysis.

‖ Unch, dose level and maintenance interval unchanged from normal.

¶ Require usual loading doses at all degrees of renal failure; blood levels are best guide to therapy.

qhs, Every hour of sleep.

INH, Isoniazid; PAS, para-aminosalicylic acid; UTI, urinary tract infection.

(From Molitch ME: Management of Medical Problems in Surgical Patients. Philadelphia: FA Davis Co, 1982.)

renal tissues and that treatment of the hyperuricemic state with allopurinol can lessen this deposition and damage.

Asymptomatic Hyperuricemia

In asymptomatic hyperuricemia, because there is no tissue deposition of uric acid, one might not expect to find any renal dysfunction. Although there is some debate about the effects of asymptomatic hyperuricemia on renal function, many investigators believe that treatment of asymptomatic hyperuricemia is not necessary and that there is no added risk to the kidney from an isolated elevation of uric acid.

Toxic Nephropathy

Toxic nephropathy can result from the ingestion or administration of a wide range of substances. One can categorize nephrotoxins by (1) mechanism of renal damage, (2) clinical manifestation of renal toxicity, and (3) class of agent. Categorizing by class of agent is simplest.

Antibiotics

Because of their high frequency of use, antibiotics are common causes of toxic nephropathy. Aminoglycosides, penicillins, and amphotericin B are most often associated with nephrotoxicity, but cephalosporins, rifampin, and sulfonamides have also been implicated. The nephrotoxicity associated with aminoglycosides, including gentamicin, kanamycin, amikacin, and tobramycin, has been extensively studied, but there remains uncertainty as to the cause.

AMINOGLYCOSIDES

Aminoglycosides are concentrated to high level in the renal cortex, and ultrastructural lesions, myeloid bodies, in the proximal tubules can be observed when this antibiotic is administered to a laboratory animal. Yet there does not seem to be any definite correlation between total cortical drug concentration, presence of myeloid bodies, and serum drug levels with aminoglycoside-induced nephrotoxicity. Typically aminoglycoside nephrotoxicity is of a nonoliguric nature, developing some 5 to 10 days into the course of antibiotic therapy. A variety of tubular syndromes associated with electrolyte wasting have also been observed. In general, the renal failure is reversible when the drug is discontinued. Even though drug levels are not necessarily correlated with degree of renal failure, it is common practice to adjust the dose of the aminoglycoside for the degree of renal failure.

PENICILLINS

Penicillins, particularly methicillin, have the potential to cause an allergic interstitial nephritis. The pathogenesis of the acute interstitial nephritis is not clear. An immunologic basis has been suggested by the finding of eosinophilia, eosinophiluria, fever, arthralgia, and rash and by the occasional renal biopsy finding of immunoglobulin deposition along the tubular basement membrane antibodies. Steroid therapy has been suggested to hasten the recovery of renal function and to reduce the extent of residual renal impairment, but controlled trials have not been done.

OTHER ANTIBIOTICS

Cephalosporins, sulfonamides, erythromycin, rifampin, and tetracyclines are other antibiotics that may produce an acute interstitial nephritis. Direct cellular injury due to the accumulation of the drug within the renal tubular cell is another mechanism for renal toxicity from these drugs.

AMPHOTERICIN B

Amphotericin B is another antibiotic that can cause renal failure. The mechanism of damage is not known, but there may be an effect on membrane permeability to increase the delivery of monovalent ions to the macula densa. This is thought to activate the tubuloglomerular feedback system to decrease renal blood flow and GFR. Because amphotericin B produces a distal type of renal tubular acidosis as well as renal insufficiency, the concept of a membrane effect being responsible for the toxicity is attractive. The renal failure is said to be reversible if the total dose of amphotericin B administered is less than 5 g. There is controversy over whether pretreatment with mannitol or saline lessens the toxicity.

Analgesics

Common analgesics such as aspirin, acetaminophen, naproxen, and ibuprofen have been increasingly implicated as causes of renal failure. Both acute and chronic renal failure have been known to develop from use of these drugs. The mechanisms of renal toxicity have been attributed to allergic interstitial nephritis, altered renal hemodynamics, papillary necrosis, and tubular necrosis. The typical setting in which these drugs cause acute renal failure is in a volume-contracted state with activation of the adrenergic nervous system and the renin angiotensin system. The explanation given is that all these analgesics have a common action of inhibiting cyclooxygenase, a major enzyme in the biosynthesis of prostaglandins. Prostaglandins have a number of different effects on the kidney, but one of their actions is to induce renal vasodilation. In the setting of volume contraction, the usual vasoconstriction is offset in the kidney by the simultaneous stimulation of prostaglandin synthesis. When prostaglandin inhibitors are present, the renal vasoconstriction is not counterbalanced by prostaglandin synthesis and release, and impaired renal perfusion and consequent renal failure result.

The more chronic forms of renal injury from these nonsteroidal anti-inflammatory drugs (NSAIDs) are said to occur from 2 weeks to 18 months after the start of therapy. Here the mechanism is an interstitial process. In cases in which chronic analgesic nephropathy is attributable to the ingestion of aspirin, phenacetin, or both, a cumulative intake of 2 to 3 kg appears necessary.

Contrast Media

Iodinated contrast media for a variety of radiograph studies are also included in the list of nephrotoxins, and consequently, the practitioner must be cautious when ordering radiographs with contrast media. Patients with diabetes mellitus, patients with pre-existing renal failure, elderly patients, and patients who undergo multiple contrast studies are at special risk for this typically reversible form of acute renal failure.

The pathogenesis of this nephrotoxicity remains to be firmly established.

Metals

Heavy metals, including gold and platinum, are nephrotoxic. Filtered gold seems to injure the proximal tubular epithelial cells and to cause the release of a tubular epithelial protein, which can induce the formation of antibody and consequent immune complex and complement, mediated glomerular damage, and nephrotic syndrome. Similarly the administration of the antitumor drug cisplatin can lead to nephrotoxicity. The cellular mechanism is unknown, but the toxicity is dose dependent.

Substances of Abuse

Substances of abuse, such as heroin, amphetamines, cocaine, and ethylene glycol, have all been associated with renal failure.

Summary

The practitioner should always be aware that all drugs have the potential for renal toxicity and that only a few of the more important drugs have been discussed here in detail.

Diabetic Nephropathy

Diabetic nephropathy can be divided into a preclinical phase and a clinical phase.

Preclinical Phase

In the preclinical phase of diabetic nephropathy, there is ordinarily no detectable evidence of renal dysfunction, but there is an increase in the GFR, an increase in kidney size, and most importantly, the presence of microalbuminuria. Microalbuminuria refers to the presence of albumin in the urine that can be demonstrated only by radioimmunoassays and not by the standard urinary dipstick methods. Thus albumin concentrations as low as 30 μ/ml can be detected as compared with a concentration of 300 μ/ml by dipstick. The cause of microalbuminuria is not firmly established, but an elevated blood glucose level is one of several factors that can increase the rate of albumin excretion. The presence of microalbuminuria seems to be predictive of the development of overt diabetic glomerulopathy. Clinical trials are under way to determine whether the reduction of microalbuminuria by tight glucose control will reduce the incidence of diabetic renal disease.

Clinical Phase

The clinical phase of diabetic nephropathy appears when proteinuria can be detected by dipstick. When constant proteinuria appears, a decline in the GFR can be predicted to occur in about 5 years on the average, with the eventual development of signs and symptoms of uremia. Accompanying the clinical phase of diabetic nephropathy is diabetic retinopathy. In fact, if diabetic retinopathy is absent there should be a question as to whether diabetes mellitus is the cause of nephropathy.

The clinical phase of diabetic nephropathy appears an average of 15 to 20 years after the onset of insulin-dependent diabetes mellitus (IDDM). However, only about 50% of insulin-requiring diabetics develop this clinical phase. If an individual with diabetes mellitus has survived for more than 30 years without clinical evidence of diabetic nephropathy, the chances are very slim that he or she will later develop it.

Proteinuria of diabetic nephropathy is usually in the nephrotic range. The degree of proteinuria has been said to correlate with the prognosis for sustained renal function. Red blood cell casts have been reported in the urinary sediment of diabetics, but there is disagreement on whether RBC casts should be accepted as part of the usual clinical picture of diabetic nephropathy.

When a decline in renal function appears, attempts at stricter control of the blood glucose level probably have little success in preserving renal function. However, it is reasonable to assume, although not yet proved, that tight glucose control in the preclinical phase may well prevent the development of diabetic nephropathy.

Treatment

When the need for end-stage renal disease therapy develops in the diabetic, all the options of hemodialysis, peritoneal dialysis, and transplantation are available. There is an increased mortality in the diabetic as compared with the nondiabetic for all treatment modalities. This increased mortality rate reflects the problems the diabetic has with microvascular and macrovascular disease, rather than an adverse effect of dialysis or transplantation on the diabetic state itself.

FLUID AND ELECTROLYTES

The successful management of intravenous fluid and electrolyte therapy is based on the adequate replacement of the body's daily fluid and electrolyte losses. Under normal circumstances, the kidney is the major route through which fluid and electrolytes are lost, and so intravenous replacement can be guided by the magnitude of urinary fluid and electrolyte losses. However, the kidney is not the only route of fluid loss (Table 8–11). Therefore, an absolute minimum of approximately 1000 ml of fluid should be furnished per day, and an average replacement value is 2000 ml per day.

Electrolyte Replacement

Table 8–12 indicates what guidelines can be used with respect to the intravenous electrolyte replacement of urinary losses. Although the normal kidney can reduce urinary sodium losses to less than 5 mEq/day, it is general practice to provide for an

Table 8–11. DAILY FLUID LOSSES (IN ML)

Route of Loss	Average	Minimum	Maximum
Renal	800–1500	500	1400/hr
Lungs	150	150	1500/day
Skin	450	450	1000
Stool	250	0	2500/hr
Sweat	0	0	4000/hr

Normal Overall Fluid Balance: Intake = Output

Intake		Output	
Fluids	1500	Urine	1500
Solid foods	800	Perspiration	600
Oxidation H_2O	300	Lung vapor (insensible)	400
	2600	Feces	100
			2600

Table 8–12. ELECTROLYTE REPLACEMENT MAINTENANCE THERAPY

Sodium	Kidneys can very efficiently conserve sodium
Potassium	Kidneys cannot completely conserve potassium
Replacement	
Sodium	Arbitrary 60–80 mEq/day
Potassium	Minimum of 20 mEq/day and usually 40–60 mEq/day

Table 8–14. ASSESSMENT OF FLUID STATUS

	History	Physical Findings
Volume Depletion	Thirst	Orthostatic hypotension
	Vomiting	Dry mucous membranes
	Diarrhea	Poor skin turgor
	Diuretic usage	Flat neck veins
	Bleeding	
Volume Excess	Swelling	Edema
	Shortness of breath	Ascites
		Rales
	Presence of congestive heart failure, nephrosis, cirrhosis, or renal failure	Full neck veins

ample amount of replacement sodium (60 to 80 mEq/day) as well as 40 to 60 mEq of potassium/day. With these guidelines, sufficient intravenous replacement can be provided by solution (Table 8–13).

The data in Tables 8–11, 8–12, and 8–13 are applicable when there is no pre-existing electrolyte or fluid imbalance or renal insufficiency. When there is a pre-existing problem, the practitioner must be extraordinarily careful in prescription of intravenous fluids. Ideally the cause for the fluid or electrolyte disorder should be identified and corrected. When this is not possible, intravenous fluids need to be given in such a way so as not to aggravate the condition and, if possible, to correct it. To accomplish this, the practitioner must be able to identify the abnormal fluid and electrolyte state. The practitioner needs to rely on the patient's history, physical examination, and laboratory parameters to determine this.

Assessment

An assessment of the patient's fluid status is made primarily from the patient's history and reported symptoms coupled with the physical examination. A history of vomiting, diarrhea, diuretic usage, or bleeding should alert the practitioner to the likelihood of volume depletion (Table 8–14). Associated physical findings include or-

Table 8–13. STANDARD INTRAVENOUS REPLACEMENT

Solution	D5W/½ NS plus 30 mEq KCl/L at 75 ml/hr
Supplies per Day	
Volume	1800 ml
Sodium	131 mEq
Potassium	54 mEq

thostatic hypotension, dry mucous membranes, poor skin turgor, and poorly distensible neck veins. If the patient complains of leg or ankle swelling or shortness of breath or if the patient has a history of ongoing congestive heart failure, nephrosis, cirrhosis, or renal failure, the practitioner should expect a total body excess of fluid. The physical findings of fluid excess include edema, ascites, rales, and prominent neck veins. The assessment of the patient should include a full electrolyte panel, a serum creatinine test, and a urinalysis. A serum glucose level, calcium level, and phosphorus level are also desirable. The laboratory assessment commonly is not very helpful in diagnosing fluid balance disorders but is essential to the diagnosis of renal or electrolyte disorders.

Electrolyte Abnormalities

The remaining sections of this chapter discuss some of the common electrolyte abnormalities that can be uncovered by performing an electrolyte panel.

Hyponatremia

The isolated laboratory report of hyponatremia or hypernatremia cannot be used as a guide to intravenous therapy because an abnormal serum sodium concentration simply reflects an excess or deficit of sodium relative to water. Hyponatremia can be present when there is a total body excess of volume, volume depletion, or apparent volume balance (Table 8–15). The

Table 8–15. DIAGNOSIS OF HYPONATREMIA

	Fluid Status				
	Volume Excess		**Volume Deficit**		**Normal Volume**
Urinary Sodium	Low	High	Low	High	Not a differential point
Disease State	Congestive heart failure Nephrosis Cirrhosis	Renal failure	Vomiting Diarrhea	Diuretics Addison's disease	Hypothyroidism Drugs SIADH

SIADH, Syndrome of inappropriate antidiuretic hormone.

differentiation of these three states of volume balance in the hyponatremic patient depends on the history and physical examination plus a measurement of urine sodium.

CAUSES

In general, when there is hyponatremia and evidence of volume excess by physical examination, congestive heart failure, nephrosis, cirrhosis, and renal failure need to be considered as causes. In the first three diseases, the urine sodium level is low (typically less than 10 mEq/L). When hyponatremia and renal failure occur together, one should expect the urine sodium level to be elevated (usually greater than 25 mEq/L).

When the clinical assessment of the hyponatremic patient reveals a volume deficit, diuretics, Addison's disease, vomiting, and diarrhea need to be considered as possible causes of the hyponatremia. In the first two instances, the urine sodium level is high, and in the last two, the urine sodium level should be low.

Finally, hyponatremia may exist with no apparent excess or deficit of volume in the patient. Here the urine sodium level is not helpful and generally just reflects the dietary intake. The conditions that can cause hyponatremia without apparent volume imbalance include hypothyroidism, various drugs, and the syndrome of inappropriate antidiuretic hormone (SIADH). Some of the drugs that can either stimulate the release of ADH or enhance its action include nicotine, chlorpropamide, tolbutamide, cyclophosphamide, morphine, vincristine, and indomethacin. In addition, carcinoma of the lung, duodenum, or pancreas; pulmonary disorders such as pneumonia, abscess, or tuberculosis; and some central nervous system disorders such as encephalitis, meningitis, stroke, tumor, or hemorrhage can all be associated with SIADH. The diagnosis of SIADH is usually one of exclusion. If the patient has no other cause for hyponatremia and has one of the listed neoplastic pulmonary or central nervous system disorders, the cause of the hyponatremia can be attributed to SIADH.

TREATMENT

The treatment of all forms of hyponatremia include correcting the underlying process where possible and restricting free water intake to correct the relative excess of water over salt. In patients in whom volume depletion exists, normal saline should be given to restore the deficit. In those circumstances in which there appear to be some neurologic effects from the hyponatremia, including stupor, coma, and seizures, or in which the serum sodium level is less than 115 mEq/L, hypertonic saline (3% to 5%) is advisable. Demeclocycline, a tetracycline antibiotic that interferes with the tubular action of ADH, may be given if the serum sodium level remains resistant to correction by all the preceding maneuvers.

Hypernatremia

Hypernatremia is much more unusual in clinical practice than hyponatremia. This reflects the fact that hypernatremia usually strongly stimulates the thirst mechanism. Therefore most patients who have access to water do not become hypernatremic. The same three volume categories can be seen with hypernatremia as with hypona-

Table 8–16. DIAGNOSIS OF HYPERNATREMIA

	Fluid Status		
	Volume Excess	*Volume Deficit*	*Normal Volume*
Disease State	Hypertonic saline administration	Osmotic diuretics	Diabetes insipidus

tremia, but the number of clinical entities is smaller (Table 8–16). Hypernatremia with an excess of fluid is usually observed only when hypertonic saline has been administered to the patient, and hypernatremia with volume depletion is seen only when osmotic diuretics have been given.

Causes

The most common cause of hypernatremia is diabetes insipidus, which has a normal volume status because the defect is one of inadequate water conservation but not inadequate salt conservation by the kidney. The causes of diabetes insipidus are central when there is insufficient release of ADH from the brain, as in trauma, tumors, and encephalitis or nephrogenic when there is adequate ADH release but impaired renal response. Drugs; chronic medullary or interstitial renal diseases; and some immunologic conditions, such as multiple myeloma, amyloidosis, and sarcoidosis can be causes of nephrogenic diabetes insipidus.

Treatment

Treatment of hypernatremia is directed at the underlying condition where possible. Ample water needs to be given to correct the water deficit, and if there is central diabetes insipidus ADH can be administered to the patient.

Hypokalemia

For the patient who demonstrates hypokalemia, the practitioner should try to uncover the cause of the abnormality and take the appropriate steps to correct it (Table 8–17). Hypokalemia can come about because of either an inadequate intake of potassium, which in the isolated circumstance is rare, or enhanced or poorly compensated gastrointestinal or renal losses of potassium. Sources of gastrointestinal potassium loss include vomiting and diarrhea. Renal losses of potassium can be present in patients using diuretics, in patients with renal tubular acidosis, and in patients with states of enhanced mineralocorticoid activity with adequate distal sodium delivery.

Treatment

The treatment of hypokalemia is usually just potassium replacement. Depending on the circumstances, this can be either oral or intravenous replacement. Addressing the primary cause of the hypokalemia should also be done, and in selected instances, the administration of mineralocorticoid inhibitors is employed.

Hyperkalemia

When hyperkalemia occurs from an excess intake, the practitioner needs to con-

Table 8–17. HYPOKALEMIA

Causes	Treatments
Dietary Deficient dietary intake	Replacement: KCl by mouth or IV
Potassium-free IV therapy Prolonged with no food intake	
Gastrointestinal Vomiting Diarrhea	Address primary process (e.g., vomiting, diuretic usage)
Cushing's syndrome Na$^+$ retention, K$^+$ loss	Administer mineralocorticoid inhibitors (when indicated)
Corticosteroid therapy Na$^+$ retention, K$^+$ loss	
Renal Diuretic phase: acute renal failure Diuretic usage Renal tubular acidosis Excessive mineralocorticoid activity K$^+$-losing nephritis	
Diabetic acidosis Diuresis with K$^+$ loss	

sider the ingestion of salt substitutes or the administration of potassium supplements as a cause (Table 8–18). Renal causes of hyperkalemia include potassium-sparing diuretics and a deficiency in amount or action of mineralocorticoids.

TREATMENT

The treatment of hyperkalemia depends on the severity of elevation and the urgency of correction. If the hyperkalemia is causing cardiac conduction disturbances immediate blocking of the potassium effect by administration of calcium is necessary. If calcium is not necessary, but a rapid decrease of potassium is still required, sodium bicarbonate or a combination of glucose and insulin can be given to promote entry of potassium into the cells. For more permanent correction of hyperkalemia, the potassium needs to be removed from the body using either a cation-exchange resin or hemodialysis. When there is a deficit of mineralocorticoid, mineralocorticoid analogue can be given.

Metabolic Acidosis and Alkalosis

The last abnormality that the practitioner can expect to discover on the electrolyte panel is a high or low total carbon dioxide (CO_2) level. Without an accompanying arterial blood gas measurement, it may be difficult to determine if the dis-

turbance is metabolic or respiratory (see Chapter 3 for discussion of respiratory acid-base disorders). If it is a metabolic disturbance it can be either a metabolic acidosis (total CO_2 level low) or a metabolic alkalosis (total CO_2 level high).

METABOLIC ACIDOSIS

A metabolic acidosis stems from either loss of bicarbonate or gain of hydrogen ion (Table 8–19). Bicarbonate can be lost from the body with diarrhea and biliary tract or small bowel drainage and in the presence of renal tubular acidosis. Hydrogen ion may be added to the body in diabetic ketoacidosis, lactic acidosis, methanol poisoning, ethylene glycol poisoning, and salicylate poisoning.

Treatment. The management of a metabolic acidosis is accomplished by the treatment of the cause of the acidosis. Bicarbonate supplementation is sometimes used, but this may not be effective unless the primary disorder can be ameliorated.

METABOLIC ALKALOSIS

A metabolic alkalosis may develop when there is a loss of hydrogen ions or a gain of bicarbonate (Table 8–20). The gain of bicarbonate is rare and requires exogenous bicarbonate administration. The loss of hydrogen ions is a more common cause of metabolic alkalosis. The sites of hydrogen ion loss are typically the stomach and kidney. Because gastric secretions are highly acidic, suctioning or vomiting of the acidic gastric contents can cause metabolic alkalosis. A less appreciated cause is the loss

Table 8–18. HYPERKALEMIA

Causes	Treatments
Dietary	Calcium
Salt substitutes	$NaHCO_3$
KCl supplements	Glucose and insulin
Iatrogenic	Kayexalate*
Rapid IV administration	Dialysis
Renal	Treat primary process
Renal disease	Administer
K^+-sparing diuretics	mineralocorticoids
Mineralocorticoid	(when indicated)
deficiency	
Renal tubular defect	
(mineralocorticoid	
unresponsiveness)	
Adrenal insufficiency	
K^+ retention, Na^+ loss	
Cellular breakdown	
Hemolysis, burns, crush	
injuries	

* Trademark for sodium polystyrene sulfonate.

Table 8–19. CAUSES OF METABOLIC ACIDOSIS (LOW CO_2)*

Loss of Bicarbonate
Diarrhea
Renal tubular acidosis
Biliary or small bowel drainage
Gain of Hydrogen Ion
Diabetic ketoacidosis
Lactic acidosis
Methanol poisoning
Ethylene glycol poisoning
Salicylate poisoning
Renal failure

* An arterial blood gas measurement is needed to determine whether the disturbance is metabolic or respiratory.

Table 8–20. CAUSES OF METABOLIC ALKALOSIS (HIGH CO_2)

Loss of Hydrogen Ion
Nasogastric suction
Vomiting
Enhanced mineralocorticoid activity
Hyperventilation
Diuretics
Cushing's syndrome
Severe hypokalemia
Gain of Bicarbonate
$NaHCO_3$ administration
Excess alkali ingestion
Milk-alkali syndrome

of hydrogen ions through the kidneys when there is enhanced mineralocorticoid activity coupled with ample distal sodium delivery.

Treatment. In a patient with metabolic alkalosis, stopping the loss of hydrogen ions, paradoxically, is only part of the therapy. Many cases of metabolic alkalosis are also associated with volume depletion. Metabolic alkalosis in these circumstances cannot be corrected unless the volume deficit is also corrected.

Podiatric Implications

The perioperative management of the podiatric patient with renal abnormalities requires that the practitioner first identify any degree of renal insufficiency and any associated electrolyte and fluid balance disorders.

Preoperative Considerations. Because renal disorders can be asymptomatic, the only way to adequately identify the patient with renal disease is to measure the BUN and serum creatinine levels and serum electrolytes preoperatively. If the laboratory values are normal and if the physical examination of the patient does not suggest any disorder of volume status, no special attention needs to be directed toward the renal system. However, the finding of an elevated creatinine level or a depressed serum sodium level necessitates some investigation into the management of the renal failure or hyponatremia, as previously outlined. Probably the greatest error in the perioperative management of podiatric patients with respect to the renal system is the failure to detect before surgery any pre-existing fluid and electrolyte or renal problems.

Postoperative Considerations. Postoperatively, because of the stresses that surgery imparts, periodic assessment and surveillance of physical findings of volume status and renal laboratory parameters should be carried out in case these stresses have overwhelmed the body's homeostatic mechanisms.

Bibliography

Abuelo JG: Proteinuria: Diagnostic principles and procedures. Ann Intern Med 98:186, 1983.

Bennett WM, Aronoff GR, Morrison G, et al.: Drug prescribing in renal failure. Am J Kidney Dis 3:155, 1983.

Bowie WR, Alexander ER, Stimson JB, et al.: Therapy for nongonococcal urethritis. Ann Intern Med 95:306, 1981.

Chen BT, Ooi BS, Tan KK, et al.: Causes of recurrent hematuria. Q J Med 41:141, 1972.

Froom P, Ribak J, Benbasset J: Significance of microhematuria in young adults. Br Med J 288:20, 1984.

Goldmann DR, et al. (eds): Medical Care of the Surgical Patient: A Problem-Oriented Approach to Management. Philadelphia: JB Lippincott Co, 1982.

Hurst JW (ed): Medicine for the Practicing Physician. Boston: Butterworth Publishers, 1983.

Madaio MP, Harrington JT: The diagnosis of acute glomerulonephritis. N Engl J Med 309:299, 1983.

McCrary RF, Pitts TO, Puschett JB, et al.: Diabetic Nephropathy. Am J Nephrol 1:206, 1981.

Mohr DN, Offord KP, Owen RA, et al.: Asymptomatic microhematuria and urologic disease. A population-based study. JAMA 256:224, 1986.

Rubenstein E, Federman DD (eds): Scientific American Medicine. New York: Scientific American, Inc. 1987.

Schwartz WB, Kassirer JP: Medical management of chronic renal failure. Am J Med 44:786, 1968.

Stamm WE, Koustsky LA, Benedetti JK, et al.: Chlamydia trachomatis urethral infections in men. Ann Intern Med 100:47, 1984.

Thomas WC, Jr: Medical aspects of renal calculus disease: Treatment and prophylaxis. Urol Clin North Am 1:261, 1974.

Williams ME, Pannill FC: Urinary incontinence in the elderly. Ann Intern Med 97:895, 1982.

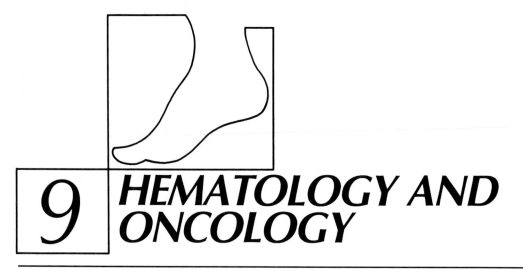

9 HEMATOLOGY AND ONCOLOGY

GAIL M. GRANDINETTI and BENNETT G. ZIER

OVERVIEW

The hematologic system plays an extremely important role in clinical podiatry practice. Preoperative evaluation must address the issues of adequate hemostasis as well as occult anemia in order to ensure a positive surgical outcome. Clinical understanding of lymphadenopathy is necessary to evaluate any associated infection or malignant process.

Podiatric oncology includes recognition of potential skin tumors; nerve tumors; and tumors of muscles, tendons, and joints. Just as important, the podiatric practitioner should be aware of constitutional signs and symptoms of cancer.

PATHOPHYSIOLOGY

The blood circulates continuously throughout the heart and vascular system, performing many vital functions. It transports oxygen to the cells and transports carbon dioxide for removal by the lungs. The blood carries absorbed food products to the tissues and removes metabolic wastes. The blood also carries hormones from endocrine glands to their target organs. White blood cells (WBCs) and antibodies protect the body from injury, inflammation, and infection.

The hematologic system also participates in regulating body temperature, hemostasis, and coagulation. The formation of blood and its constituent cellular elements takes place in the bone marrow, spleen, liver, and lymph nodes. Composition of the blood is 55% plasma, which maintains blood volume, and 45% suspended particles. Cellular elements of the blood are diverse, having in common only an ancestral cell of bone marrow origin. These cellular elements are transported through vessels in plasma. The particles suspended in plasma include erythrocytes, leukocytes, plasma cells, reticuloendothelial cells, and thrombocytes. The blood readily lends itself to biopsy of the bone marrow and to structural, chemical, and functional studies.

Circulating Blood Cells

Erythrocytes. Major functions of the red blood cells (RBCs) involve oxygen and carbon dioxide transport, maintenance of blood viscosity, and bile pigment formation. Hemoglobin, the major constituent of the RBC, is composed of a simple protein globin and heme, a complex molecule containing iron and porphyrin, and is responsible for O_2 transport. Hemoglobin disorders may lead to defective oxygen transport or to premature destruction of the RBC. The biconcave shape of the RBC, essential to its functioning, makes it flexible and elastic. Diseases that affect the shape

of the RBC cause disastrous effects on blood gas efficiency. The abnormally shaped cells fragment and can block capillaries, which provide circulation to the tissues.

A normal erythrocyte is dependent on healthy bone marrow, normal genetics, and proper diet. An erythrocyte lives approximately 120 days and originally arises from a pluripotent stem cell, which is stimulated into differentiation by erythropoietin. On microscopic examination, the erythrocyte may vary in size (anisocytosis), shape (poikilocytosis), staining (normochromic, hypochromic), structure (Heinz's bodies, Howell-Jolly bodies, nuclei, parasites, and so on) and number (polycythemia, anemia).

Leukocytes. The major function of the series of WBCs is defense of the body against potentially harmful foreign substances, infectious and parasitic organisms, and toxic substances. There are two types of leukocytes, granulocytes and agranulocytes. The granulocytes include phagocytic neutrophils, eosinophils, basophils, and monocytes. The agranulocytes include lymphocytes. Normally leukocytes number between 5000 and 10,000/mm^3. A rise in the WBC count over 12,000/mm^3 is called leukocytosis. White blood cells usually increase in response to infection, or, as seen in the leukemias, an abnormal, uncontrolled, destructive proliferation of one type of WBC and its precursors occurs.

A decrease in the WBC count below 4000/mm^3 is called leukopenia and may occur as a result of viral infection, exposure to drugs, or exposure to a myelotoxic agent. Neutropenia is a reduction in the number of circulating polymorphonuclear neutrophils (granulocytes). Agranulocytosis (granulocytopenia, malignant neutropenia) is an acute, potentially fatal blood dyscrasia characterized by profound neutropenia.

Neutrophils. Neutrophils—granulocytic, polymorphonuclear leukocytes—are normally produced in the bone marrow. An enormous number of mature neutrophils are produced daily and divide into a circulating pool and a marginated pool that adheres to the blood vessel walls. The normal production is tightly controlled, and a stimulus, such as a bacterial infection, is needed to cause neutrophils to pour into the blood from the bone marrow. A concomitant proliferating marrow serves to meet the increased demand.

The normal function of the polymorphonuclear neutrophil (PMN) is to destroy microorganisms, which requires chemotaxis, phagocytosis, and microbial killing.

Eosinophils. Eosinophils are weakly phagocytic granulocytes that defend against a variety of multicellular parasites and have an anti-inflammatory role in antigen-antibody mediated disease. Eosinophilia may be seen in parasitic infestations and atopic diseases. The number of eosinophils decreases with age, with glucocorticoid administration, and during acute hypersensitivity reaction. The number of eosinophils increases in chronic myeloproliferative diseases.

Basophils. A basophil is a granulocyte that is the principal source of histamine in the blood and contains heparin. A basophil releases histamine after gamma E immunoglobulin (IgE) binds to its surface.

Monocytes. Monocytes are mononuclear phagocytes that are produced in the bone marrow and rapidly leave to enter the tissues. Monocytes develop into a variety of macrophages: alveolar, pleural, peritoneal, Kupffer's cells, and sinusoidal lining cells of the spleen. These macrophages live in the tissues, in which they perform their main function of phagocytosis and microbial killing. Abnormalities may be genetic, as in enzyme deficiencies, or acquired, as in the rare instance when monocytes are transformed into a malignant state. Abnormalities may be manifested as accumulation of organic debris, defective antibacterial activity, impaired immunity, and malignancy.

Lymphocytes. The maturation and differentiation of lymphocytes are considerably complex. B-cell precursors arise in the marrow, spleen, and lymph nodes. T-cell precursors arise in the marrow, travel to the thymus, further differentiate, and then travel to the spleen, lymph nodes, and marrow, where they perform many of their functions. Circulating lymphocytes represent only a tiny fraction of the total lymphocyte pool. Lymphocytes normally number 20 to 50% of the total WBCs and may increase to 90% in lymphatic leukemia. Various toxins and nutritional deficiencies can seriously damage the orderly progression of undifferentiated progenitor cells.

Plasma Cells. A plasma cell is a mononuclear cell that is the primary producer of gamma globulin. The B lymphocyte differentiates to the plasma cell, which produces humoral immunity. The circulating antibodies are gamma M immunoglobulin (IgM), gamma A immunoglobulin (IgA), gamma G immunoglobulin (IgG), IgE, and gamma D immunoglobulin (IgD).

Hematopoiesis

In the adult, hematopoiesis occurs primarily in the bone marrow. The marrow performs a specific role in providing the correct numbers and types of cells to meet physiologic needs. The hematopoietic cells include pluripotent stem cells, which differentiate into multipotent hematopoietic stem cells and lymphocyte progenitor cells. The multipotent hematopoietic stem cells differentiate into RBCs, WBCs, and platelets (Fig. 9–1). The lymphocyte progenitor cells differentiate into B lymphocytes, plasma cells, and T lymphocytes. The circulating half-life of polymorphonuclear leukocytes is about 6 hours, platelets 8 days, and erythrocytes 120 days. The concept of cell half-life becomes extremely important clinically when noting the effects of drugs on certain cells.

The earliest red stem cells are called erythroblasts. Erythroblasts eventually differentiate into erythrocytes. New erythrocytes released from the bone marrow are called reticulocytes. The earlier WBC precursors are myeloblasts. These stem cells give rise to the neutrophilic, eosinophilic, and basophilic series. Megakaryocytes are the precursors of the platelets. Marrow lymphocytes are mainly of B-cell origin, arising also in the spleen and the lymph nodes. T-cell precursors arise in the marrow and then travel to the thymus, where they undergo further maturation. From the thymus, T-cell precursors travel to the spleen, lymph nodes, and marrow as mature, functional T cells.

The process of growth and development of the stem cells is under the control of humoral substances. Of the humoral mediators that have been identified, erythropoietin is perhaps the most important. Erythropoiesis is under the control of erythropoietin, which is released from the kidney in response to tissue hypoxia. The

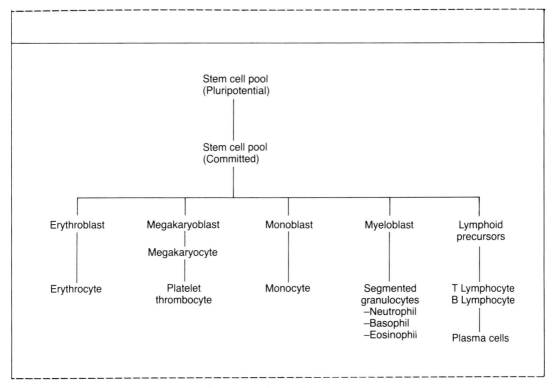

Figure 9–1. Blood cell formation.

number of erythroid precursors increases, enhancing hemoglobin synthesis, and stimulates release of reticulocytes from the marrow. Under homeostatic conditions, production rate precisely equals destruction rate.

Hematopoiesis is dependent on a normal bone marrow as well as the availability of key nutrients, such as iron, folic acid, and vitamin B_{12}. The marrow microenvironment that forms mature differentiated peripheral blood cells is complex and subject to severe dysfunction. It must provide for the normal steady-state rates of renewal of cellular elements of blood. Disorders of the blood and blood-forming organs can be classified according to the cell or mechanism the disorder primarily involves: erythrocytes, leukocytes, platelets, reticuloendothelial cells, and clotting mechanisms.

Hematopoietic Disorders

Hematopoietic disorders involve basic pathophysiologic disturbances of decreased numbers of cells, cytopenia; defects in coagulation mechanism; and over-production of either normal or defective cells.

Anemia, a reduction of oxygen-carrying capacity of the blood, is the result of decreased erythrocytes. Leukopenia, a decrease in WBCs, greatly increases the vulnerability of the patient to infection. A decrease in platelets, or thrombocytopenia, is characterized by a tendency to bleed, to bruise easily, and to develop petechiae. A depletion or absence of one or more of the clotting factors results in persistent bleeding and hemorrhage. This defect includes hemophilias, hypoprothrombinemias, and disseminated intravascular coagulation (DIC). Myeloproliferative diseases, in which a malignant overproduction of bone marrow cells occurs, include polycythemia, an abnormal increase in erythrocytes; leukemia, an increase in abnormal immature leukocytes; and multiple myeloma, an abnormal malignant proliferation of plasma cells. Lymphoproliferative disorders involve overproduction within the lymphatic system. Conditions under this classification include Hodgkin's disease and lymphosarcoma, a malignant proliferation of one form of a reticuloendothelial cell in the lymph nodes. Lymphocytic leukemia, an overproduction of lymphocytes that are released into the blood, is another lymphoproliferative disorder.

The spleen also plays a significant role in hematologic disorders. Enlargement of the spleen, splenomegaly, is associated with numerous blood dyscrasias. *Hypersplenism,* a clinical term that implies overactivity or exaggeration of one or more of the spleen's functions, is characterized by peripheral blood cytopenia. Erythrocytes, granulocytes, and thrombocytes, or any combination, may be involved in this syndrome.

Several other factors can result in disorders of the hematopoietic system. Among these are hemorrhage, dietary deficiencies and malabsorption, metabolic defects, genetic predisposition to abnormal blood cell production, infection, drug toxicity, environmental toxins, malignancies, and immunologic disorders. Disorders of the hematopoietic system can be idiopathic as well.

PRESENTING FEATURES

Disorders of blood or blood-forming organs can affect all organs and tissues. As a result, blood diseases appear in diffuse ways. A careful medical history is essential for determining the cause and severity of anemia. Characteristic of the presenting features are the following signs and symptoms.

Subjective Symptoms

The general medical history must be explored because it is often vague and nonspecific. It is helpful to know if the patient ever had an abnormal blood count. Other areas to explore are any past anemia, the treatment for the anemia, and the patient's response to the treatment. Chronic anemia or recurrent episodes over a period of years suggest a hereditary disease. An anemia of recent onset suggests an acquired disorder. Inquiries should be made about diet, alcohol intake, use of prescribed medications, use of over-the-counter medicines, history of bleeding disorders, response to dental and other surgical procedures, transfusion history, and family history of

bleeding disorders. The presence of bleeding or hematomas hours after surgery suggests a coagulation-factor deficiency. Other questions concern presence of fatigue; dizziness; headache; sensations of pins and needles in fingers and toes; stomatitis; frequent nosebleeds; bleeding into joints; history of splenic, renal, or hepatic disease; heavy flow during menses in the female; and excessive bleeding from a cut during shaving in the male.

Easy Bruising and Bleeding. Tendency to bruise and bleed easily is reported by a surprisingly high percentage of patients. It is important to establish a relationship of trauma to bruising. The physician should ask the patient the amount of time necessary for bleeding to stop when the patient cuts himself or herself inadvertently. Another crucial question to ask is about previous bleeding from any operative procedure, including a tooth extraction. Perhaps the most important question to ask the patient in terms of easy bruisability concerns drug intake. A number of drugs interfere with platelet function. Patients often admit to taking prescription drugs but frequently forget to mention over-the-counter preparations, which frequently contain aspirin or other nonsteroidal anti-inflammatory drugs (NSAIDs). If the answers to all the aforementioned questions are negative, generally no further work-up is necessary. Isolated instances of easy bruising are common and should be pursued only if other features suggest a bleeding disorder. Screening tests for hemostasis should be performed.

Fatigue or Malaise. Fatigue or malaise is a very nonspecific symptom but one that is often encountered in patients with hematologic disease. It is crucial for the physician to obtain a detailed history and to perform an extremely careful physical examination, with specific attention to hematologic organs, when a patient has this symptom.

Dyspnea. Dyspnea is seen in severe anemias, leukemias, and hemorrhagic disorders. Dyspnea is caused by a decrease in erythrocytes, resulting in reduced oxygen-carrying capacity of the blood.

Gastrointestinal Symptoms. Anorexia, weight loss, indigestion, and sore mouth and tongue are often seen in patients with dietary deficient anemias. Drugs and fatigue may also contribute to these symptoms.

Objective Signs

The physical examination aids in quantitation of bleeding. Vital signs are extremely important. Orthostatic changes in pulse and blood pressure indicate an acute blood volume loss of at least 10%.

Splenomegaly. A palpable mass in the left upper quadrant of the abdomen may indicate splenomegaly. Splenomegaly is associated with congestion from overproduction of cells, as in polycythemia and leukemia, or with excessive destruction of RBCs, as in hemolytic anemia.

Splenomegaly implies that the spleen is three times larger than normal and is almost always a pathologic sign. However, 1% of the young adult population has a palpable spleen on routine examination without apparent pathophysiologic significance and without other historical, physical, and laboratory findings. The presence of a palpably enlarged spleen is best considered a physical finding that demands diagnostic evaluation. Additional studies may be required to confirm the physical finding, to establish the magnitude of splenomegaly, and to evaluate the possibility of hypersplenism. Ultrasonography or computed tomography (CT) is often helpful. Generally the etiology of splenomegaly is apparent by history and the physical examination. A further diagnostic approach is dictated by accompanying features, such as hematologic findings, lymphadenopathy, portal hypertension, liver dysfunction, and systemic infection.

Purpura and Petechiae. The presence of purpura implies intradermal bleeding. A petechia is a purpura that is 1 to 3 mm in diameter. An ecchymosis is a purpura that is larger than 3 mm in diameter. Neither ecchymoses nor petechiae blanch with pressure, such as in diascopy, because they are due to extravasation of blood into the tissue. The presence of petechiae may imply drug use, such as aspirin, or a familial bleeding disorder. Petechiae may also be due to abnormalities of platelet number or function.

Hemarthrosis. Patients who have spontaneous bleeding into a joint usually have had a hereditary coagulation abnormality detected in childhood. A first occurrence of hemarthrosis in an adult is usually secondary to local trauma.

Bone Pain and Deformity. Hyperactivity of bone marrow, which produces bone pain and deformity, is seen in myeloproliferative diseases and pathologic fractures that may occur in multiple myeloma.

Lymphadenopathy. Lymphadenopathy is an important physical finding. The accessible areas for enlarged lymph nodes on physical examination include the cervical, submandibular, submental, axillary, epitrochlear, and inguinal lymph nodes. Other areas such as mediastinal and retroperitoneal locations require utilization of radiographs or special invasive contrast studies. Substantial enlargement of lymph nodes should be investigated in the presence of one or more nodes estimated to be equal to or greater than 1 cm in diameter and when the nodes are newly recognized and not known to arise from a previously known cause. Multiple small nodes may also indicate the need for an investigation.

Jaundice. Yellow discoloring of the skin and sclera is the result of rupture and hemolysis of abnormal erythrocytes, which are seen in hemolytic anemia, pernicious anemia, and splenic disease. Bilirubin is released into the circulation, resulting in the yellowing of the skin.

Laboratory and Physiologic Data

The application of diagnostic blood tests is an important component of investigating hematologic and oncologic problems. When used selectively, blood tests can provide not only information to support a given diagnosis but also can provide the basis for ruling out conditions in the differential diagnosis. All these tests should be performed by a qualified laboratory. Laboratory errors are not rare, and most abnormal laboratory values should be checked by repeating the test before alarming the patient with a diagnosis based on one abnormal laboratory test value.

Complete Blood Count

A complete blood count (CBC) provides basic data on RBCs and WBCs, including

RBC count, hemoglobin concentration, hematocrit (packed cell volume), WBC count, and RBC differential. In addition, the laboratory comments on the morphology of the RBCs and WBCs if the cells appear abnormal. The RBC count is invariably reduced in anemias. The count is increased in primary and secondary polycythemia.

Hemoglobin. The blood hemoglobin concentration is reduced in all forms of anemia. Reduction of blood hemoglobin concentration is a measure of the severity of anemia because it reflects the oxygen-transporting capacity of the blood. Hemoglobin concentration is increased in polycythemia.

Hematocrit. The hematocrit is a measure of the combined volume of the RBCs in a sample of blood. Hematocrit is expressed as the percentage of volume occupied by the packed RBCs in a sample of anticoagulated whole blood. Hematocrit is reduced in all types of anemia.

Peripheral Smear. The peripheral smear is a thin, evenly distributed film of blood on a glass slide that is stained for microscopic evaluation. A thorough examination of the peripheral smear is important and should be done in conjunction with RBC indices because they provide complementary information. Peripheral smear and RBC indices are time-tested means of classifying anemias and initiating evaluation. A total of 100 WBCs are counted in an evenly distributed area of the slide. A count is kept on each type of leukocyte identified, and the differential is figured on a percentage basis. The evaluation should routinely include each cell line sequentially for morphologic or numeric change.

Red Blood Cell Morphology

Anisocytosis. Anisocytosis describes excessive variation in the size of RBCs as is seen in megaloblastic anemias, thalassemia major, and spherocytosis.

Poikilocytosis. Poikilocytosis describes excessive variation in the shape of RBCs as is seen in sickle cell anemia, pernicious anemia, thalassemia major, and spherocytosis.

Red Blood Cell Indices. Red blood cell indices are arithmetic ratios derived from the RBC count, the hematocrit, and the hemoglobin concentration. These indices are helpful in the diagnosis of anemia. Red blood cell indices include

- Mean corpuscular volume (MCV)
- Mean corpuscular hemoglobin concentration (MCHC)
- Mean corpuscular hemoglobin (MCH)

Of the three RBC indices, the MCV is most helpful. Mean corpuscular volume is a reflection of hematocrit/RBC count and is a measure of the average volume of the RBCs. The normal value is 82 to 92 μm^3. A value lower than this indicates microcytic anemias, whereas a value higher than this indicates macrocytic anemias. Utilizing MCV and the peripheral blood smear helps to classify anemia as macrocytic, microcytic, or normocytic (Table 9–1).

White Blood Cell Count. Leukopenia is defined as a decreased WBC count, which can result from (1) overwhelming infections, such as noted in septicemia; (2) some viral infections; (3) certain drugs, especially antineoplastic drugs; (4) radiation therapy; and (5) aplastic anemia (pancytopenia). Leukocytosis is defined as an increased WBC count, which can result from (1) acute infections, (2) leukemia, (3) acute hemorrhage, (4) tissue necrosis, and (5) infectious mononucleosis.

Table 9–1. CLASSIFICATION OF ANEMIA BY RED BLOOD CELL MORPHOLOGY

Morphology	Indices	Clinical Correlation
Microcytic	MCV* <80	Iron deficiency†
		Blood loss
		Thalassemia†
Normocytic	MCV 80–100	Anemia of chronic disease†
		Infection, renal disease
		Endocrine disease
		Chronic inflammation
		Bone marrow failure
		Drugs
		Tumors
		Hemolysis
Macrocytic	MCV >100	Folate deficiency
		B$_{12}$ deficiency (pernicious anemia)
		Liver disease
		Anticonvulsant medications

* MCV, Mean corpuscular volume.
† Iron deficiency, thalassemia, and anemia of chronic disease account for 90% of all cases of anemia in the United States.

In addition to the total WBC count, a differential count is made from the peripheral blood smear. The differential WBC count includes

1. Neutrophils, which may be increased in acute systemic or localized infections and in myelogenous leukemia.

2. Lymphocytes, which may be increased in infectious mononucleosis and in lymphocytic leukemia.

3. Monocytes, which may be increased in monocytic leukemia and in protozoan infections.

4. Eosinophils, which may be increased in allergic reactions, in parasitic infections, and in some dermatologic conditions.

5. An increase in nonsegmented neutrophils, otherwise called band forms.

If band forms are noted in the differential WBC count, this may indicate a so-called left shift. A left shift reflects an increase in the percentage of the less mature form of neutrophils plus mature forms of neutrophils, accounting for greater than 80% of the total differential WBC count. A left shift is a sign of increased turnover or demand and is almost always a response to an acute bacterial infection. White blood cell morphology may be described as atypical in such conditions as viral infections (for example, infectious mononucleosis) and leukemia.

Leukocytosis is very common postoperatively. An elevation of the WBC count in the range of 10,000 to 16,000/mm³ is usual for the first 36 to 48 hours. If this count persists for longer than 3 to 5 days one must investigate for other causes, such as occult infection, bleeding, hematoma formation, and necrosis. Medications that cause leukocytosis without a left shift must also be considered. Among these are epinephrine, steroids, and lithium carbonate.

Reticulocyte Count

A reticulocyte count is a measure of those RBCs with inclusions that are fragments of endoplasmic reticulum. The reticulocyte is the most immature type of RBC released into the peripheral blood circulation. The reticulocyte reflects formation of RBCs resulting from hemolysis, hemorrhage, and successful treatment of anemia. In effect, the reticulocyte count is a reflection of bone marrow function (1.8–2.0%).

Erythrocyte Sedimentation Rate

The erythrocyte sedimentation rate (ESR) is a nonspecific test, the primary utility of which is following therapy or progress of infectious, collagen vascular, and malignant diseases. The ESR is a measure of the rate at which anticoagulated RBCs settle out of blood in vitro. The rate increases when plasma proteins, such as fibrinogen and gamma globulin, which cause aggregation of RBCs, are increased. The ESR is not a diagnostic blood test. In fact, utilizing an ESR as a diagnostic tool often leads to an array of time-consuming and expensive tests with no diagnosis being obtained. As stated previously, the primary use of an ESR is following therapy of a known disease.

Tests of Hemostasis

There is a vast array of tests that may be utilized to investigate underlying hemostatic disorders. From a preoperative standpoint, the following four tests give the greatest amount of information and are considered screens for hemostatic disorders.

Platelet Count. The platelet count provides quantification of the amount of mature platelets in the circulation. This test gives no indication of platelet function. The platelet count ranges from 150,000 to 350,000/mm³ but must be very low, less than 25,000, before spontaneous bleeding occurs. High platelet counts, above 1 million, may be associated with malignant disorders.

Prothrombin Time. The prothrombin time provides a laboratory measurement, in plasma, of the extrinsic blood coagulation pathway and of the factors common to both extrinsic and intrinsic pathways (Fig. 9–2). Prothrombin time is prolonged by deficiencies in fibrinogen; prothrombin; and factors V, VII, and X. Prothrombin time measures several coagulation defects and is commonly used to monitor patients taking anticoagulant drugs such as warfarin (Coumadin). Prothrombin time is increased in the following conditions: (1) Vitamin K deficiency; (2) impaired fat ab-

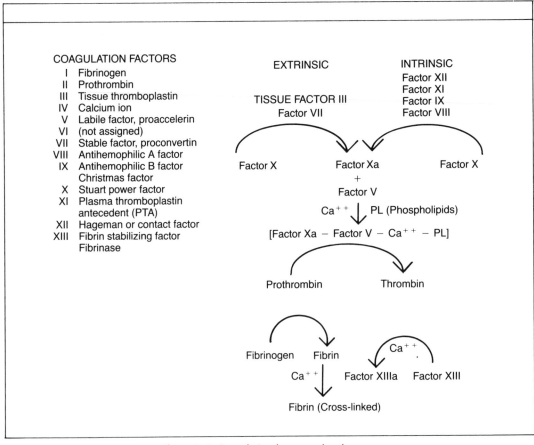

COAGULATION FACTORS

I	Fibrinogen
II	Prothrombin
III	Tissue thromboplastin
IV	Calcium ion
V	Labile factor, proaccelerin
VI	(not assigned)
VII	Stable factor, proconvertin
VIII	Antihemophilic A factor
IX	Antihemophilic B factor
	Christmas factor
X	Stuart power factor
XI	Plasma thromboplastin
	antecedent (PTA)
XII	Hageman or contact factor
XIII	Fibrin stabilizing factor
	Fibrinase

Figure 9–2. Coagulation factors and pathways.

sorption, causing malabsorption of vitamin K; (3) severe liver disease; (4) ingestion of warfarin-type drugs; and (5) circulating anticoagulants. Normal values are reported as a percentage of the control value, which is approximately 11 to 13 seconds. Prothrombin time remains normal in hemophilia A and B and in platelet deficiencies.

Partial Thromboplastin Time. The partial thromboplastin time (PTT) provides a laboratory measurement, in plasma, of the intrinsic blood coagulation pathway and the factors common to both intrinsic and extrinsic pathways. Partial thromboplastin time is the best screening test for disorders of coagulation. Approximately 90% of patients with coagulation disorders show abnormal PTT values. Partial thromboplastin time is prolonged by deficiencies in fibrinogen; prothrombin; and factors V, VIII, IX, and XII. Partial thromboplastin time is increased in the following conditions: (1) Hemophilia A or B, (2) prothrombin complex disorders, and (3) presence of circulating anticoagulants. Normal values are approximately 24 to 36 seconds. Values remain normal with platelet deficiencies or with defects in factors VII and XIII.

Bleeding Time. The bleeding time is a standard in vivo assay measuring the effectiveness of platelet plug formation. Bleeding time is increased if platelet function is abnormal. Normal values are 2 to 9 minutes. Bleeding time remains normal if the hemorrhagic disorder is confined to the coagulation system. This test is usually performed on patients suspected of having a qualitative platelet disorder, such as von Willebrand's disease. From a preoperative standpoint, the bleeding time may be prolonged owing to the use of aspirin or other NSAIDs. Bleeding time is prolonged in thrombocytopenia ($<100,000/\text{mm}^3$). Prolonged bleeding time and a normal platelet count suggest the necessity of obtaining a more thorough history of ingestion of aspirin-containing compounds or other NSAIDs.

Ancillary Tests

Factor Assay. A factor assay is performed to define which particular factor is involved in the defect after the stage of coagulation abnormality is identified through the routine tests for hemorrhagic disorders, as listed previously.

Bone Marrow Aspiration. Bone marrow aspiration is used in the diagnosis of certain blood dyscrasias, such as aplastic anemia, leukemia, pernicious anemia, and thrombocytopenia. Examination of the bone marrow reveals the number, size, and shape of RBCs, WBCs, and platelets as they evolve through their developmental stages. Red blood cells, WBCs, and platelets are studied for various maturation abnormalities.

Blood Typing and Crossmatching. Before a blood transfusion is given, the blood group of the recipient and of the donor must be determined to ensure the similarity of the antigenic and immune properties of the blood. To ensure the safety of blood products to be used for transfusion, testing is also done for the presence of the human immunodeficiency virus (HIV) antigen. Blood is screened in some medical centers for hepatitis through evaluation of antibody levels.

Haptoglobin Level. The haptoglobin level is a sensitive and reliable test of hemolysis. Hemoglobin is released during hemolysis and binds to the alpha globulins called haptoglobin. Thus the level of free haptoglobin falls in the presence of hemolysis. A normal haptoglobin level is 100 mg/dl to 300 mg/dl.

Coombs's Test. Coombs's test is used to detect antiglobulins, immunoglobulins on the surface of the RBCs. Coombs's test is used in diagnosing various hemolytic anemias. The patient's washed RBCs are mixed with Coombs's serum. The mixture is then examined for agglutination, which determines if a specific antibody coats the RBC. A positive test result (direct Coombs's) is found in hemolytic transfusion reactions and in idiopathic acquired hemolytic anemias.

Electrophoresis Tests for Gammopathies

Electrophoresis tests are useful in the analysis of serum protein mixtures, part of which are immunoglobulins in solution.

The normal pattern is diffuse, since no single protein is in excess. The gamma globulins diffuse in the gamma band. However, if a single protein does dominate there is a peak or a spike.

Protein Electrophoresis. Protein electrophoresis is performed first to determine if there is a single dominant protein. This test gives a quantitative numeric value of the amount of protein in each electrophoretic band.

Immunoelectrophoresis. Immunoelectrophoresis is usually performed after the simple serum protein electrophoresis shows a spike in the gamma band. Immunoelectrophoresis is done to classify the type of the excess immunoglobulin (IgG, IgM, IgA, IgD, and IgE).

Hemoglobin Electrophoresis. Hemoglobin electrophoresis is useful for diagnosing hemoglobin abnormalities. This test identifies hemoglobins A, S, C, D, and E. Measurement of hemoglobin A_2 and F is important in the diagnosis of thalassemias, in which both A_2 and F levels may be elevated. Abnormalities of hemoglobin S, which causes sickle-cell disease, and hemoglobin C, which causes a mild hemolytic anemia, are the most common.

Iron Studies

Iron is absorbed in its ferrous form and is in the ferric form in the cell, where it is picked up by transferrin. This binding protein transports the iron to wherever it is needed, such as in hemoglobin production. It is important to understand this concept to identify the cause of the iron deficiency.

Serum Iron. A normal serum iron measurement is 40 to 150 μg/dl. In pure iron deficiency anemia, the serum iron is low, and the total iron-binding capacity (TIBC) is elevated.

Total Iron-Binding Capacity. The plasma has an iron-binding capacity. Transferrin, a beta-globulin, is about one third saturated with iron. The unsaturated transferrin is termed the unsaturated iron-binding capacity, which is the amount of protein that is available for iron transport. Plasma TIBC should be measured at the same time as plasma iron. Normal TIBC measures 250 to 400 μg/dl. Total iron-binding capacity is high in iron deficiency anemia.

Serum Ferritin. Serum ferritin is an iron-phosphorus protein complex containing about 23% iron. Serum ferritin is formed in the intestinal mucosa by the union of ferric iron with a protein, apoferritin. Ferritin is the form in which iron is stored in the tissues. A normal serum ferritin measurement is 5 to 280 μg/dl. Serum ferritin is more commonly measured than iron and TIBC levels and is considered more reliable because iron and TIBC levels can be affected by a number of disease states, such as infection and chronic illnesses.

Lactate Dehydrogenase

Lactate dehydrogenase (LDH) is an enzyme present in nearly all metabolizing cells, including erythrocytes. Damage to nearly any tissue can cause this enzyme to be elevated. Any patient with active hemolytic anemia also has an elevated LDH level. Lactate dehydrogenase can be separated into five isoenzymes, thus specifying its tissue origin. Electrophoresis is used to separate the isoenzymes of LDH, thus determining the tissue source of an elevation.

ASSESSMENT OF COMMON PROBLEMS

Anemia

Anemia presents significant issues in a number of clinical settings for the podiatrist. The ambulatory patient who may have occult anemia as well as the patient with preoperative anemia or postoperative anemia presents a significant challenge in terms of providing excellent treatment outcomes. Anemia is not a disease. Anemia is a syndrome and represents a reduction in the number of circulating RBCs. Anemia exists when hemoglobin content is less than 13 to 14 g/100 ml for males and less than 11 to 12 g/100 ml for females. As noted, males have higher hemoglobin levels than females, primarily as a result of androgens, which stimulate erythropoietin to cause a rise in erythropoiesis. Signs and symptoms of anemia are a function of the rapidity of onset as well as the cardiovascular reserve of the patient. Slowly developing anemias often are asymptomatic, whereas anemias of rapid onset, such as those in which there is acute blood loss, may be reflected by tachycardia, shortness of breath, and even shock. In the United States, one of the most common reasons for anemia is iron loss, most often in premenopausal women from menstrual blood loss. Iron deficiency in men is usually from blood loss through the gastrointestinal or genitourinary tract.

History

A dietary history must be elicited because vitamin B_{12} deficiency or folate deficiency may be a cause of anemia. Specifically folic acid deficiency is a common form of malnutrition, especially in the elderly living alone, and in alcoholics. Family history is extremely important, especially in those with hemolytic anemias; a positive family history of jaundice, splenomegaly, or gallstones may suggest such a condition. Ethnic background is important, especially in the consideration of hemoglobinopathies that are frequent in Mediterranean, African, and Far Eastern populations. Hemolysis may also accompany inherited problems of anemia. Acquired hemolytic anemia is rare, occurring mainly in settings of autoimmune disease and drug ingestion (Fig. 9–3). One must inquire about evidence of toxic exposure or drug ingestion that can cause bone marrow depression and anemia. Lastly, any underlying disease, including chronic inflammatory diseases, renal insufficiency, cancer, and metabolic disease, must be uncovered. Each of these diseases is associated with secondary anemias, otherwise known as anemias of chronic disease.

Laboratory Evaluation

It is important to determine whether the patient is truly anemic. Dilutional anemias may occur when there is increased plasma volume, fluid overload, and congestive heart failure. Once the diagnosis of anemia is established, in addition to a repeat CBC for confirmation, the following tests should be obtained:
1. Peripheral blood smear
2. RBC indices
3. Stool for occult blood
4. Reticulocyte count
5. Urinalysis.

Red blood cell morphology is extremely

ANEMIA
Distribution of causes

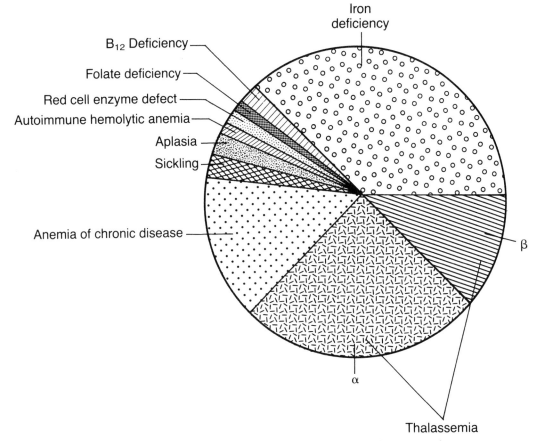

Figure 9–3. Estimate of prevalence of different types of anemia in the U.S. population.

important because it provides a crude classification of the type of anemia. Microcytosis most commonly occurs in iron deficiency and thalassemia trait anemias. Normocytosis accompanies acute blood loss, hemolytic anemias, and anemias of chronic disease. Macrocytosis is characteristic of nutritional anemias, such as folic acid deficiency and vitamin B_{12} deficiency, as well as liver disease and ingestion of certain drugs, such as anticonvulsant medications. The RBC indices give information about the average RBC volume, which is a quantitative expression of RBC morphology. Of the three RBC indices, the MCV is the most useful because it permits separation of microcytic, normocytic, and macrocytic anemias. The reticulocyte count measures the number of newly released erythrocytes in the peripheral circulation. One may assume that an elevated reticulocyte count implies that the bone marrow is responding to the anemia by increasing its erythropoietic activity. A low reticulocyte count may indicate that the bone marrow is not functioning. A nonfunctioning bone marrow may in fact be the source of the anemia. Examination of the stool for occult blood (i.e., a stool guaiac test) and a urinalysis may provide clues as to the source of blood loss in the case of the anemic patient.

Types of Anemia

After establishing that the patient is anemic and obtaining the screening tests' laboratory data, it is important to specify which type of anemia the patient exhibits. The types of anemia fall into three general categories: underproduction, excessive destruction, and blood loss.

UNDERPRODUCTION

Aplastic Anemia. Aplastic anemia is due specifically to bone marrow failure or failure in stem-cell differentiation. Aplastic anemia is characterized by a peripheral pancytopenia that includes not only a low RBC count but also low platelet and low WBC counts. An aplastic anemia may be congenital, as in Fanconi's anemia, but it is often acquired and develops after viral infections or as a reaction to a drug, a chemical agent, ionizing radiation, or an immunologic abnormality. Aplastic anemias can also be idiopathic. Drugs involved in aplastic anemia may include agents used in cancer chemotherapy or agents that induce idiosyncratic marrow aplasia, such as chloramphenicol and phenylbutazone. The anemia is generally normocytic, and the prognosis is determined by the severity of leukopenia and thrombocytopenia.

Red Cell Aplasia. Red cell aplasia is a severe anemia due to an absence of red stem cell precursors in the bone marrow. Red cell aplasia is associated with immunologic-deficiency states such as thymoma. This type of anemia may also be congenital or acquired.

Iron Deficiency Anemia. Iron deficiency is the most common cause of anemia. The RBCs are characteristically microcytic, with an MCV of less than 80 μm^3. The serum iron level is low, and the serum iron-binding capacity is elevated. The serum ferritin level, determined by radioimmunoassay, is also quite low. Bone marrow aspirates show depleted iron stores. The most common cause of iron deficiency in women is menstrual or obstetric blood loss. In men as well as women, evidence of iron deficiency should also bring to mind occult blood loss into the gastrointestinal tract from diverticulosis, aspirin ingestion, peptic ulcer disease, and malignancy. Malabsorption can also lead to iron deficiency. Examples are following a partial gastrectomy or an adult celiac disease.

Anemia of Chronic Disease. Anemia of chronic disease is a mild to moderate anemia related to shortened RBC survival, suboptimal marrow compensation, defective reutilization of iron, and in some cases reduced production of erythropoietin.

This category of anemia includes several diseases. Anemia of chronic disease is seen in a variety of chronic infections, inflammatory conditions, and malignant conditions. Virtually any patient who is chronically ill may develop this type of anemia. The anemia of chronic renal failure is usually more severe than the anemia of chronic disease in other situations.

Regardless of the underlying cause, the presenting history and physical findings are those of the underlying disease. In this type of anemia, the RBCs are morphologically normal, the reticulocyte count is not particularly elevated, and the WBCs are normal. Serum iron levels and iron-binding capacity are low; however, the bone marrow aspirate reveals normal iron stores. The serum ferritin level is normal (12 to 25 $\mu g/ml$). If low, the serum ferritin level implies an element of iron deficiency complicating the anemia of chronic disease. Hemoglobin is seldom less than 9 g/100 ml, and blood transfusions are rarely needed if the anemia responds to correction of the primary disease.

Folic Acid Deficiency. Folic acid deficiency is a megaloblastic type of anemia, with morphologically large RBCs. Folic acid deficiency is seen most commonly in the severe alcoholic because of dietary deficiency brought about by an ethanol-induced block in folate metabolism. Other causes include drugs such as phenytoin and conditions such as nontropical sprue and pregnancy.

Vitamin B_{12} Deficiency. Vitamin B_{12} deficiency impairs DNA synthesis. Vitamin B_{12} deficiency is most commonly apparent as a result of pernicious anemia, prior partial gastrectomy, or small bowel disease of the terminal ileum in which there is a malabsorptive defect. Pernicious anemia involves an atrophic gastritis that leads to deficient intrinsic factor secretion, which impairs vitamin B_{12} absorption. The diagnosis is made from blood smear morphology, a high MCV, and a low plasma level of vitamin B_{12}. Blind loop syndrome is a megaloblastic anemia due to a blind loop or multiple diverticulosis of the jejunum, which becomes infected. The bacteria destroy vitamin B_{12}, resulting in anemia. Treatment includes antibiotics and B_{12} administration, surgical correction of the diverticuli and blind loops, or both.

Pernicious anemia is a chronic macrocytic anemia characterized by achlorhydria, which occurs most commonly in whites in their 30s. Failure of hydrochloric acid (intrinsic factor) secretion by the stomach hinders vitamin B_{12} (extrinsic factor) absorption. Signs of vitamin B_{12} deficiency include weakness, paresthesias of extremities, sore tongue, gastrointestinal symptoms, and pain. It is also known as Addison's anemia and is treated with intramuscular injections of vitamin B_{12}.

EXCESSIVE DESTRUCTION

Hemolytic Anemias. Hemolytic anemias are due to excessive destruction. This is also known as hemolysis and can be separated into two categories, intrinsic and extrinsic. Intrinsic anemias are usually inherited and may be caused by intrinsic defects in the RBC membrane, such as in hereditary spherocytosis. Extrinsic influences include drugs, antibodies, and hypersplenism.

A combination of the two abnormalities may also be responsible for hemolytic anemia. Identification of the abnormality is essential for effective management. Clinical presentation varies according to rate of destruction, compensatory adaptations, and etiology. When the liver is unable to handle the bilirubin excess from hemoglobin breakdown, jaundice occurs, and serum unconjugated bilirubin level rises. Splenomegaly occurs as trapping of damaged RBCs progresses. Severe acute hemolysis is characterized by sudden fever, chills, headache, back and abdominal pain, and hemoglobinuria. The peripheral smear is normochromic and usually normocytic, but it may be macrocytic from release of immature forms in rapid RBC destruction. The reticulocyte count is elevated unless there is a marrow defect. Defects in hemoglobin or hemoglobin production are seen in hemoglobinopathies or enzyme deficiencies, such as glucose-6-phosphate dehydrogenase (G-6-PDH) deficiency. Hemoglobinopathies are the most common. If these problems are suspected a hemoglobin electrophoresis should establish the specific diagnosis. A large number of abnormalities in the hemoglobin molecule have been described, the most common being sickle-cell disease.

Extrinsic Anemias
Acquired: Antibody-Negative Hemolysis. The antibody-negative hemolytic anemias may be due to exposure to inor-

ganic or complex organic toxins, including snake venoms, heavy metals, and infections such as malaria. Red blood cells exposed to excessive mechanical stress intravascularly can undergo fragmentation hemolysis. This type of hemolysis can be seen in patients with abnormally functioning heart valves and in patients who have valve prostheses. Microangiopathic hemolytic anemias result when normal RBCs are fragmented while traversing intravascular fibrin strands in blood vessels that are partially occluded by thrombi. Acute causes of this type of anemia include DIC, thrombotic thrombocytopenic purpura, and hemolytic uremic syndrome. Treatment involves correction of the underlying condition. Blood transfusions are sometimes given to patients with hemoglobin levels below 8 g/100 ml.

Autoimmune: Antibody-Mediated Hemolysis. Antibody-mediated hemolytic anemias represent conditions in which antibodies directed against RBC antigens coat the RBC, and cause hemolysis. Included in this category are autoimmune hemolytic anemias, which are characterized by antibodies directed against the patient's own RBC antigens or antibodies that react with RBCs in cold temperatures, otherwise known as cold antibody–autoimmune hemolytic anemias.

Drug-Induced Hemolysis. Drug-induced immune hemolytic anemia is a relatively common disorder. Three mechanisms have been identified: (1) adsorption to the RBC of drug-antibody complexes, as occurs with quinidine; (2) drug adsorption to the RBC with binding of antidrug antibody, as seen with penicillin; and (3) induction of an RBC autoantibody, as seen with long-term methyldopa use. This third mechanism rarely causes significant hemolysis. The hallmark of the drug-related hemolytic episodes is a positive direct Coombs's test result.

Intrinsic Anemias
Sickle-Cell Disease. Sickle-cell disease results from a single amino-acid substitution on the beta chain of hemoglobin A. The disease is transmitted as an autosomal recessive trait. The heterozygous state, hemoglobin AS, is referred to as sickle cell trait and occurs in about 8% of the black population. Sickle cell trait is asymptomatic, and anemia is absent. Hematuria is sometimes seen owing to sickling in the

hypertonic renal medulla. The peripheral smear is normal except for an occasional target cell. Less than 50% of the hemoglobin detected by electrophoresis is hemoglobin of the S variety.

One of four children of parents who are both carriers will have sickle-cell disease, or hemoglobin SS. The incidence of hemoglobin SS among blacks is approximately 1 in 400 to 600. The anemia is the less benign problem. Painful aplastic crises, which are due to concurrent illness that suppresses erythropoiesis, cause a worsening of the anemia. Leg ulcers, hepatomegaly, hematuria, renal concentrating defects, and mild jaundice can occur. A cardiac flow murmur is common. Painful crises, which are characterized by pain in the lower extremities and pain in the back and abdomen, are often precipitated by stress. The peripheral smear is normochromic. Sickled cells and target cells may be noted. Hemoglobin S is the predominant hemoglobin form detected by electrophoresis.

Thalassemias. The thalassemias, another type of hemoglobinopathy, are due to abnormalities in the rate of synthesis of globin. This abnormality is transmitted as an autosomal recessive trait. The heterozygous state is called thalassemia minor, whereas the homozygous state is called thalassemia major. Abnormalities in the rate of synthesis of alpha chains and beta chains are encountered. Beta thalassemias are common, particularly in people of Mediterranean extraction.

Thalassemia major, the homozygous form, is the most severe type, which is found in children. The earlier thalassemia major is manifested, the more unfavorable the outcome. Thalassemia major is characterized by fatigue, splenomegaly, severe anemia, mongoloid facies, cardiomegaly, and slight jaundice. This thalassemia is also called Cooley's anemia, Mediterranean anemia, erythroblastic anemia, and hereditary leptocytosis.

Thalassemia minor, the heterozygous form, is a mild disease that is usually discovered by chance. Thalassemia minor has an excellent prognosis.

Glucose-6-Phosphate Dehydrogenase Deficiency. Glucose-6-phosphate dehydrogenase deficiency is an enzyme deficiency that makes RBCs more susceptible to hemolysis following the ingestion of drugs and foods classified as chemical oxidants. This inherited disorder is a common problem. Following exposure to one of the 40 or more such drugs and foods, intravascular hemolysis develops and lasts about 7–12 days. The patient suffers from anemia and jaundice during the acute phase. Laboratory findings include hemoglobinemia, elevated bilirubin level, hemoglobinuria, reticulocytosis, and the appearance of Heinz bodies within the RBC. The disease is self-limiting because only the older RBCs are destroyed when in contact with the chemical oxidant. The offending agent must be identified and discontinued or hemolysis will be chronic. A screening test for G-6-PDH deficiency is now available.

Hereditary Spherocytosis. Hereditary spherocytosis is an inherited anemia with the distinct characteristics of abnormal spherical-shaped erythrocytes and an enlarged spleen. Hemoglobin is normal. The defect is in the cell membrane, which allows influx of sodium ions. Spherocytes are thick and relatively inflexible and are easily trapped in the splenic sinusoid. Spherocytes are devoured, and the spleen becomes enlarged because of overwork. The patient suffers from anemia and jaundice as a result of the massive hemolysis of RBCs. Laboratory findings include spherocytosis on blood smear, reticulocytosis, lowered RBC count, lowered hemoglobin value, and osmotic fragility. The condition cannot be completely cured. Blood transfusion may have a short-term benefit for the patient in hemolytic crisis. Most patients undergo splenectomy and experience complete reversal of symptoms.

BLOOD LOSS ANEMIAS

The third causative mechanism for anemia is blood loss. Acute blood loss can result in anemia usually with obvious cause. However, the cause may be occult. This blood loss is ascertained from the history and physical examination, including a stool guaiac test for occult blood and urinalysis. The hemoglobin and hematocrit levels may not accurately reflect the severity of the blood loss until fluid shifts have occurred, usually in 18 to 24 hours. Blood loss that occurs within the body can be due to bleeding into soft tissues. It is not ordinarily difficult to detect large amounts of soft tissue bleeding, as in acute pancreatitis with retroperitoneal hemorrhage, trauma to the hips or legs, and even ectopic pregnancy.

Chronic blood loss usually results in iron deficiency anemia. Nosocomial anemia is a surprisingly frequent complication of prolonged hospitalization. Anemia results from the frequent blood sampling for numerous laboratory tests and often an inadequate reticulocytosis, occurring especially in the seriously ill patient. The key to this problem is prevention through awareness and avoidance of unnecessary blood sampling when anemia does occur.

Podiatric Implications

Anemia in the perioperative period is of major importance. Cardiopulmonary integrity and wound healing are both dependent on tissue oxygen levels, which in turn are dependent on the oxygen-carrying capacity of the blood.

PREOPERATIVE EVALUATION

History. The history is the single most important element in the identification of those patients who do not have normal hematology (Table 9–2). The most important information is the patient's history of bleeding problems. The history has become so reliable that most hospitals do not perform prothrombin times, PTTs, and platelet counts if the patient denies any episodes of bleeding following dental extractions or previous surgery. The following areas must be investigated through specific questions when taking the history to ensure an accurate evaluation. If the history arouses suspicion for any hematologic disorder an explanation must be sought. Extensive investigations are sometimes required to determine the defect and cause.

Fundamental tests for anemia should answer the following to help determine the cause. Is the anemia megaloblastic, microcytic, or normocytic? Is the bone marrow hypoactive? A patient who has a history of prolonged oozing after a surgical procedure or unusual bleeding following a den-

Table 9–2. PREOPERATIVE HISTORY PERTINENT TO HEMATOLOGIC ROS

1. Prolonged bleeding associated with prior surgery (intraoperative or postoperative bleeding), dentistry procedures, or ordinary cuts.
2. History of uncomplicated surgery or trauma versus possibility of clinically silent hemorrhagic disorder, especially of the hereditary variety.
3. Clinical history of spontaneous bleeding, epistaxis or mucosal bleeding, and delayed-onset bleeding after injury (requires detailed evaluation).
4. Family history of bleeding problems.
5. Drug use, current and previous, and OTC drug use. The use of many drugs (ASA, cough syrups) can inhibit platelet function. Other drugs inhibit blood coagulation or induce thrombocytopenia, neutropenia, and anemia (see Table 9–3).
6. History of treatment with warfarin or heparin.
7. History of liver disease or jaundice.
8. History of blood transfusion or administration of blood products.

ASA, Acetylsalicylic acid; OTC, over-the-counter; ROS, review of systems.

tal procedure needs further investigation. The clinical history of spontaneous bruising, epistaxis, and mucosal bleeding requires a detailed evaluation along with a specific evaluation of a family history of bleeding and ethnic background. If the patient has ever received blood or blood products a hemolytic reaction must be considered and ruled out through a coagulopathy screening. Clinically silent hemorrhagic disorders, especially of the hereditary variety; spontaneous bleeding; epistaxis; mucosal bleeding; and delayed onset of bleeding after injury also require detailed evaluation. A history of surgery with no significant postoperative bleeding problems is also an important fact that would support the unlikelihood of a clinically silent hemorrhagic disorder such as hemophilia.

The preoperative history also requires direct questioning of the patient about the use of drugs that are known to interrupt platelet function or to inhibit any phase of coagulation (Table 9–3). Aspirin, other NSAIDs, and some cough syrups and cold preparations can affect platelet function. Other drugs that are prescribed for a therapeutic effect on the coagulation system, such as warfarin, or another disease process also need to be included in this evaluation if they affect or inhibit coagulation in any way. Some drugs cause thrombo-

Table 9–3. DRUGS THAT MAY CAUSE ANEMIA

Bone Marrow Aplasia
Antineoplastic drugs: antimetabolites, alkylating agents
Antibiotics: chloramphenicol
Anticonvulsants: phenylhydantoin
Insecticides
Solvents: benzene
Anti-inflammatories: phenylbutazone

Hemolytic Anemia
Antibiotics: sulfonamides, sulfones
Antimalarials: primaquine
Analgesics: acetanilid
Miscellaneous compounds: methylene blue, naphthalene,
  phenylhydrazine, fava beans, castor beans
Oxidant drugs in G-6-PDH deficiency: chloramine-T
Immune-mediated: penicillin, stibophen, alpha-methyl-
  dopa, quinine, cold agglutinin

Hemodialyzed Wilson's Disease
Copper

Severe Infection
*Diplococcus pneumoniae, Escherichia coli, Staphylococ-
  cus aureus*

Maturation Defects
Alcohol
Folate antagonists: trimethoprim, triamterene, methotrex-
  ate

Hematology Synthesis
INH, lead

Gastrointestinal Blood Loss
Aspirin
NSAIDs

G-6-PDH, Glucose-6-phosphate dehydrogenase; INH,
isoniazid; NSAIDs, nonsteroidal anti-inflammatory drugs;

cytopenia, anemia, and neutropenia. A positive history of treatment with warfarin is obviously important. If the patient is taking aspirin or other NSAIDs he or she should stop for at least 2 weeks prior to surgery. If surgical intervention is necessary for a patient taking warfarin, the drug should be discontinued 3 days prior to surgery. The patient should be given vitamin K and then the warfarin should be restarted 2 days postoperatively.

In summary, if the patient has a history positive for bleeding, is currently taking an anticoagulant drug, has active liver disease, has a history of chronic alcohol consumption, describes cutaneous or mucosal purpura or easy bruisability, or has excessive fatigue, laboratory evaluation of hemostasis is indicated before invasive procedures are performed. The history also helps to determine the impact of anemia on the patient, which is influenced by age, the presence of other disorders that may affect cardiopulmonary compensation, the rate of development of anemia, and the underlying cause. These must all be considered when planning an elective procedure instead of relying on the absolute level of the hematocrit.

Physical Examination. The clinical presentation of the anemic patient depends on the underlying disease as well as the severity and chronicity of the anemia. Most of these signs and symptoms represent cardiovascular and ventilatory compensations for the decrease in RBC mass.

The physical examination and thorough measurement of orthostatic blood pressure and pulse allow for a rapid assessment of the patient's blood volume. Physical findings associated with anemia may include pallor, tachycardia, and wide pulse pressure. Examination of the patient's neck for thyromegaly or increased jugular venous pressure, and of the heart and lungs also helps determine the patient's response to the anemia. A systolic ejection murmur is often heard over the precordium, especially in the pulmonic area. The cardiac findings disappear when the anemia is corrected. Patients with hemolytic anemia often have icterus and splenomegaly and occasionally have superficial skin ulcerations over the malleolus. The skin, joints, and the buccal mucosa are examined for bleeding, bruising, jaundice, petechiae, and ecchymoses. Petechiae or ecchymoses are often associated with quantitative or qualitative platelet disorders, and purpura is associated with coagulation problems. The abdomen is examined for splenomegaly, hepatomegaly, and ascites, which are all clues to the underlying cause. The site of bleeding is very important because if a patient is bleeding from all mucosal surfaces, venipuncture sites as well as the surgical site, DIC should be suspected. Bleeding from drains in the wound is more likely indicative of surgical technique or a hereditary coagulation disorder.

Laboratory Evaluation. The basic laboratory evaluation of the anemic patient consists of a CBC, which includes hemoglobin concentration, hematocrit measurement, RBC count, RBC indices, RBC morphology, platelet count or estimate, and WBC count. A CBC gives an indication of the type of anemia and the morphologic RBC seen in the anemia. The reticulocyte count needs to be corrected for the degree of anemia.

$$\text{reticulocyte index} =$$

$$\frac{\text{reticulocyte count}}{\text{maturation time}} \times \frac{\text{actual hematocrit}}{\text{normal hematocrit}}$$

The maturation time varies inversely with the hematocrit. The following values are used in the formula for maturation time: 1.0 for a hematocrit of 45%, 1.5 for 35%, 2.0 for 25%, and 2.5 for 15%. The normal value for the reticulocyte count and reticulocyte index is 1%. A reticulocyte index is elevated in rapid blood loss or destruction of erythrocytes. The patient should be further evaluated for acute hemorrhage and hemolysis disorder. Serum bilirubin level, haptoglobin level, and LDH level help to establish hemolysis. To pinpoint the cause, a G-6-PDH level, Coombs's test, or hemoglobin electrophoresis can be done. A decreased reticulocyte count is due to depressed bone marrow function with many disorders, including myelophthisic anemia, chronic infection, inflammation, neoplasm, and hypoplastic and aplastic states.

The patient needs to be evaluated for disorders of the thyroid, adrenals, pituitary gland, kidneys, and liver. Presence of chronic infection, inflammation, and neoplasm must also be evaluated. Both serum iron and total iron-binding capacity levels are depressed. A bone marrow aspiration allows for evaluation of cellular maturation and iron stores. Examination of stool for occult blood and urine for blood is helpful in determining active bleeding and source. Further laboratory studies depend on the initial classification of the anemia. As stated, using the morphology on the peripheral smear and RBC indices, one can classify every anemia into one of three categories: microcytic-hypochromic anemias, macrocytic anemias, and normocytic-normochromic anemias.

Postoperative anemia may be present and should be investigated if the patient develops orthostatic signs. It usually takes 24 hours for the hematocrit to equilibrate, and blood should be drawn 24 hours after bleeding has stopped to ensure a more accurate evaluation of blood loss. Specific causes of postoperative anemia include di-

lution anemia, bleeding, hemolysis related to drugs given, and nosocomial anemia from excessive blood sampling. In surgical situations, a hematocrit of <30% may lead to delayed wound healing, and the cardio-pulmonary system of the patient is put under greater stress.

Hemostasis and Blood Coagulation

Hemostasis involves the interaction of the blood vessels, platelets, and coagulation system to form a localized vascular seal. Initially, vessels and platelets interact to form a platelet plug, which is independent of the coagulation system. Within a few minutes, this plug is reinforced by the deposition of fibrin from the coagulation system, producing a blood clot. Eventually during tissue repair, this clot is removed by fibrinolysis. Failure of this complex, rapid, disseminated system may lead either to excessive bleeding or to thrombosis.

Bleeding from small vessels is controlled mainly by vasoconstriction and the formation of platelet plugs. In large vessel injury, however, vasoconstriction and platelet-plug formation are hemostatically inadequate without reinforcement by a fibrin barrier, or blood clot. Injury to a vessel is the usual event that triggers hemostasis. Injury allows platelets to adhere to connective tissue exposed by interruption of the vessel endothelium. This sets off all other phases of the hemostatic system.

Platelets. A platelet is a tissue fragment that plays a critical role in primary hemostasis and coagulation as well as in pathologic thrombosis. Functions of platelets are diverse and hemostatically versatile. Platelets selectively adhere to abnormal surfaces then sequentially secrete, aggregate, fuse, and retract in order to ensure a firm platelet-fibrin plug. This plug assists in the coagulation cascade; synthesizes prostaglandins; and releases adenosine diphosphate (ADP) and other, unknown, substances. If platelets are subnormal in number or defective in function the result is a bleeding tendency characterized by ecchymosis; purpura; and surgical, traumatic, or spontaneous hemorrhage.

Factors in the Coagulation Reaction. The coagulation reaction depends on the presence of several enzymes that transform circulating blood into an insoluble gel. This process is very complicated and results in the conversion of soluble fibrinogen to fibrin by thrombin. Corresponding laboratory tests reveal disorders in each stage of the process and the various blood factors involved. Some of the most important factors are prothrombin, thrombin, thromboplastin, calcium in ionic form, and fibrinogen. The fibrin entraps erythrocytes and platelets. A contractile protein is released and results in a firm insoluble fibrin mass.

Intrinsic and Extrinsic Pathways. The coagulation system can be initiated through either the intrinsic or the extrinsic pathway. Understanding these pathways is helpful in the interpretation of clinical laboratory tests that evaluate the coagulation system.

The intrinsic and extrinsic pathways are complementary and operate concurrently in vivo. Patients with a deficiency in either pathway bleed excessively. Factors in the intrinsic pathway are present in the circulating blood and include factors VIII, IX, XI, and XII. The intrinsic pathway begins with the activation of factor XII. The extrinsic pathway offers a short cut in the usual sequence through the release of tissue factor from damaged cells that allows bypassing of factors VIII, IX, XI, and XII. Activation of the extrinsic pathway also accelerates the intrinsic pathway through conversion of factors V and VIII to more active forms. Hepatocytes synthesize all plasma coagulation factors except for factor VIII (from endothelial cells) and factor XIII (from platelets). Factors I, VII, IX, and X require vitamin K for their synthesis in the liver.

Fibrinolysis. Fibrinolysis is one of the most important mechanisms controlling blood clotting. Clot formation is reversed through enzymatic dissolution of fibrin polymers. Once the clot has served its purpose, it must be dissolved by fibrinolytic or lysis mechanism in order to prevent permanent thrombosis and occlusion of the injured blood vessel. Fragments are the end products of the fibrinolytic process, known as fibrinogen degradation products. Detection of fibrinogen degradation products provides direct evidence of fibrinolysis. This mechanism is activated in less than a day following the formation of a clot.

The two substances involved in the lysis of a clot are plasminogen and plasmin. Aberrations in the fibrinolytic mechanism may occur, resulting in hemorrhage in overactivity and excessive thrombosis of blood vessels in underactivity. Several of the fibrinolytic fragments have significant anticoagulant effects, but under most circumstances the amount of these fragments produced is small enough to have only localized effects. If excessive amounts of fibrinolytic fragments are produced a serious hemorrhagic diathesis can develop, namely, diffuse intravascular coagulation.

Epsilon-aminocaproic acid (EACA) is an important drug that inhibits fibrinolysis by preventing the activation of plasminogen to plasmin. This drug is widely used clinically in the surgical management of patients with inherited defects in their coagulation systems, such as hemophilia A or B, to reduce postoperative bleeding and to reduce the amount of replacement factor needed. Postoperative bleeding from a surgical wound may be due to acquired or congenital defects in hemostasis or to a problem in surgical technique. The diagnosis of hemorrhage related to surgical technique is one of exclusion. Problems of hemostasis must always be ruled out first.

Abnormal Hemostasis

Abnormalities in hemostasis can be caused by one or a combination of general conditions. These conditions include increased vessel fragility, platelet deficiency, platelet dysfunction, and inherited or acquired defects in the coagulation system.

INCREASED VESSEL FRAGILITY

Increased vessel fragility is clinically manifested as purpura, petechiae, or ecchymoses. When purpura occurs and the number of platelets (thrombocytes) remains normal, it is described as a nonthrombocytopenic purpura. Conditions in which nonthrombocytopenic purpura appears include vasculitis, an immunologic injury resulting from drug reactions or allergic response and hypergammaglobulinemia; a vascular injury resulting from rickettsial diseases or bacterial toxins; and an altered blood vessel wall integrity resulting from scurvy, diabetes mellitus, excessive adrenocorticosteroids, and hereditary hemorrhagic telangiectasia. These disorders are poorly understood and generally do not cause serious bleeding. Hemostasis and coagulation laboratory test results are usually normal.

PLATELET DISORDERS

Because platelets are responsible for the initial control of bleeding, their reduction or absence also appears clinically as purpura, known as thrombocytopenic purpura. The number of platelets may be reduced by several different conditions. These conditions include primary idiopathic thrombocytopenia and secondary thrombocytopenia, resulting from bone marrow suppression associated with irradiation, cytotoxic drugs, and drug reactions; bone marrow replacement by leukemia; and disseminated intravascular coagulation.

Thrombocytopenia. Thrombocytopenia, a quantitative platelet disorder, is the most common cause of abnormal bleeding and is the result of decreased platelet production or increased peripheral utilization, destruction, or sequestration. Etiologic distinctions are derived from the history, physical findings, and bone marrow examination. Thrombocytopenia is a common sequel to therapeutic irradiation involving large areas of bone marrow and to generalized marrow depression following administration of systemic cytotoxic drugs. Thrombocytopenia can also be the first sign of an acute leukemia, when marrow is replaced by malignant leukocytes. Laboratory findings include a reduced platelet count, prolonged prothrombin time, and a normal PTT. Clinical bleeding is proportionate to the reduction in platelets. In general, platelet counts in excess of 50,000/mm^3 are not associated with significant bleeding. Prolonged bleeding may occur with platelets below 50,000/mm^3 and spontaneous bleeding with platelets below 25,000/mm^3.

Severe, spontaneous bleeding is rare in patients with platelet counts higher than 20,000/mm^3 in the absence of coagulation factor abnormalities. Platelet transfusions should be reserved for serious hemorrhage and as an adjunct to major surgery to prevent serious postoperative bleeding. Platelets are given as prophylaxis in certain chronic thrombocytopenic states, as in aplastic anemia.

Idiopathic Thrombocytopenic Purpura. Diagnosis of idiopathic thrombocytopenic purpura (ITP) should be made only after exclusion of all other causes of thrombocytopenia. An increase in platelet destruction occurs in ITP, probably caused by an antiplatelet antibody. The peripheral platelet count is low despite the presence of increased numbers of megakaryocytes in the marrow. Idiopathic thrombocytopenic purpura may follow certain infections or the use of certain drugs or may accompany autoimmune diseases such as systemic lupus erythematosus (SLE). Idiopathic thrombocytopenic purpura may appear in an acute self-limiting form, often seen in children following viral infection. Another form is a chronic recurrent disorder not distinctly associated with an initiating event. Prednisone is used in treatment of ITP and gradually withdrawn once the platelet count is above 100,000/mm^3. Lack of response to therapy or rapid recurrence of ITP indicates consideration of a splenectomy.

Thrombocytosis. Thrombocytosis is defined as a platelet count >400,000/mm^3 and occurs in three forms, including a physiologic or transitory form, a relative or secondary form, and an autonomous or primary form. Exercise and stress may cause an increase in platelets. Administration of epinephrine can also cause a mobilization of platelets. Secondary or relative accelerated platelet production occurs in response to hemorrhage, hemolysis, infectious and inflammatory disease, and malignancy. If the underlying disorder is successfully treated platelets return to normal. Primary thrombocytosis is independent of normal regulatory processes. The elevated platelet production is encountered mainly in myeloproliferative disorders, such as polycythemia vera. There also may be alternating episodes of hemorrhage and thrombosis. Death is caused most commonly by thromboembolic phenomena. Results of treatment with heparin and warfarin have not been consistent. Plateletpheresis is recommended for an immediate, though transient result.

Drug-Induced Platelet Disorder. A drug-induced platelet disorder differs from thrombocytosis in that it is not a problem of platelet numbers (quantitative disorder) but of platelet function (qualitative disorder). Platelet dysfunction occurs clinically as prolonged bleeding times despite adequate numbers of platelets. These prolonged bleeding times are associated with various types of clinical conditions. Aspirin and other NSAIDs inhibit ADP release by platelets, which reduces or prevents their aggregation. Platelet adhesion to endothelium is affected also in von Willebrand's disease.

Von Willebrand's Disease. Von Willebrand's disease involves abnormal platelet adhesion, low factor VIII activity, and increased capillary fragility. Mucosal bleeding, ecchymoses, epistaxis, gastrointestinal bleeding, and menorrhagia are common. Hemarthrosis is seen only in severe cases. Laboratory findings include prolonged bleeding time in all cases, prolonged PTT only if factor VIII activity is very low, and normal platelet count and prothrombin time.

Defects in Coagulation System

Acquired Defects

Disseminated Intravascular Coagulation. Disseminated intravascular coagulation, a pathologic form of coagulation, usually appears as diffuse bleeding from many sites. Minimal trauma can cause severe bleeding, or spontaneous ecchymoses, epistaxis, or gastrointestinal hemorrhage may occur. This disorder differs from normal clotting in that it is diffuse not localized, it damages the site of clotting instead of protecting it, and it may consume several clotting factors to the level that diffuse bleeding may occur. Disseminated intravascular coagulation is seen in obstetric catastrophes; in some types of surgeries, particularly those involving the lung, brain, and prostate; and in sepsis syndromes. Deposition of fibrin in small vessels may lead to serious or even fatal tissue necrosis. Other conditions leading to DIC may include malignant tumors, hemolytic transfusion reaction, and hemolytic uremic syndrome in infancy.

These conditions that lead to DIC in part are related to an inability to clear fibrin. Unexpected profuse or uncontrollable bleeding in certain surgical settings suggests acute defibrination, with involve-

ment of multiple coagulation factors. Laboratory findings include reduced platelets, usually 30,000 to 120,000/mm^3, on blood smear; prolonged activated PTT, as much as 100 seconds (normal PTT <35 seconds); and presence of fibrinogen degradation fragments. With marked fibrinogen depletion, <75 mg/dl, the clot that forms in the test tube may be quite flimsy, friable, small, and retracted or not even visible, thus simulating findings of fibrinolysis. A form of hemolytic anemia associated with fragmentation of the RBCs, microangiopathic hemolytic anemia, may also be seen.

The best diagnostic confirmation of DIC is the demonstration of markedly increased fibrin fragments by the latex agglutination test or *Staphylococcus* clumping test. Other conditions in which clots fail to form in vitro occur with the presence of circulating anticoagulants and heparin administration. In vitro clotting may be prolonged to 1 hour or more in the hemophilias and in factor XII deficiency.

Therapy for DIC involves treating the underlying disorder, for example, shock or sepsis. Heparin may be effective in stopping pathologic clotting and may also control the bleeding. If therapy is effective, fibrin degradation products should fall and fibrinogen levels, PTT, prothrombin time, and platelet counts should improve in 24 to 48 hours. Whole blood may be necessary to combat shock. Cryoprecipitate may be given with severe fibrinogen deficiency, and platelet concentrates may be given in severe platelet deficiency.

Inherited Defects

Hemophilia A. Hemophilia A is an X-linked recessive trait disease due to a coagulation factor VIII deficiency. This classic hemophilia disorder is transmitted by unaffected female carriers to male offsprings. The coagulation deficiency can be measured by a standard test, such as PTT.

Hemophilia B. Hemophilia B, or Christmas disease, is a deficiency in the plasma thromboplastin component (factor IX) and accounts for 15% of hemophiliacs. Hemophilia B has the same transmission and clinical manifestations as the classic hemophilia A. Differentiation is done by a specific factor assay and is essential for appropriate treatment. Clinical manifestations rarely involve massive hemorrhage. Bleeding is usually a delayed and prolonged oozing or trickling occurring after minor trauma or surgery. With extravasation of blood, hematomas form in the deep subcutaneous or intramuscular tissue. Joint deformity results from repeated hemorrhage into joint spaces. Gastrointestinal bleeding and hematuria are also prominent. In severe hemophilia, the coagulation time can range from 30 minutes to several hours. The PTT is greatly prolonged. Antihemophilic factor (AHF) is virtually missing from the plasma. Bleeding time (except after aspirin ingestion), platelets, prothrombin time, and fibrinogen content are normal. In mild cases, the coagulation time is normal, but the PTT is prolonged. There are some general treatment measures, which include prevention, elimination of participation in contact sports, and avoidance of physically hazardous occupations.

Before any surgical procedures, the patient should receive appropriate infusions of prophylactic concentrate. Preoperatively, the patient should receive enough concentrate to reach 75% levels; this is given $1\frac{1}{2}$ hours before surgery. Postoperatively, the patient should receive approximately half the preoperative amount of concentrate to keep the AHF at 50% levels. Concentrate is administered every 12 hours for 10 to 14 days. The patient should also avoid any aspirin-containing medications. Treatment is based on raising the level of AHF. Different concentrates are available for factor replacement.

Polycythemias

Polycythemia is defined as an increase in both the number of circulating erythrocytes and the concentration of hemoglobin within the blood. Red blood cells may number as high as 8 to 12 million/mm^3, and the hemoglobin concentration may rise to 25 g/100 ml. There are three forms of polycythemia: polycythemia vera, secondary polycythemia, and relative polycythemia.

Polycythemia Vera

Polycythemia vera, a primary polycythemia, is a myeloproliferative disorder that usually develops in middle age. Polycythemia vera is characterized by an autonomous clonal expansion of erythropoiesis

and often megakaryopoiesis and granulopoiesis. The end result is erythrocytosis, with a variable leukocytosis and thrombocytosis giving increased blood viscosity and total volume.

Secondary Polycythemia

Secondary polycythemia occurs whenever the body must compensate for an increased oxygen demand for any reason. The bone marrow is then forced to produce more erythrocytes to prevent tissue hypoxia. Hypoxia that is prolonged enough to cause a compensatory polycythemia occurs in chronic pulmonary disease; cardiovascular disease; congenital heart disease; high altitude environments; oxygen-transport defects, such as acquired or congenital methemoglobinemia; and inappropriate erythropoietin production, as in hypernephroma, hepatoma, hemangioblastoma, cystic disease of the kidneys, renal arteriostenosis, pheochromocytosis, and other disorders.

Relative Polycythemia

Relative polycythemia occurs whenever the body loses plasma without losing RBCs. The concentration of erythrocytes increases relative to the amount of plasma. Fluid loss and dehydration may occur as a result of insufficient fluid intake, diarrhea, vomiting, burns, and excessive administration of diuretics. Clinical features include dizziness, head fullness, tinnitus, and headache, with lethargy and exertional fatigue often noted. Symptoms related to increased blood viscosity or thrombosis include blurred vision, intermittent claudication, angina, and thrombophlebitis. The clinical course may involve abnormal bleeding and hyperuricemia appearing as gout. Elective surgery is always delayed until the disease is brought under control.

Leukocyte Disorders

Leukopenia

Leukopenia is defined as a reduction in the total number of leukocytes in the blood, usually <4000/mm^3. This laboratory finding is of little significance unless the number of cell types are identified with an accompanying differential count. Because neutrophils are the most common leukocyte, leukopenia usually reflects neutropenia. Neutropenia may be an isolated finding or may be accompanied by lymphopenia, decreased number of other leukocytes, or some combination. Leukopenia is seen in patients with induced or idiopathic aplastic anemia. Reduced numbers of other leukocytes may be detected in other conditions but are not usually detected in routine laboratory examination, especially if the 100-cell differential count is used.

NEUTROPENIA

Neutropenia is a contraindication to surgery if WBCs are <1000/mm^3, with definite risk of infection when WBCs are <500/mm^3. Neutropenia can result from four mechanisms: (1) decrease in size of production pool; (2) ineffective production, with bone marrow cell death; (3) increase in rate of loss of neutrophils so great that the bone marrow cannot compensate; and (4) pseudo/neutropenia, in which there is an increase in the circulating marginal pool ratio. The lower limit of normal for neutrophils is 3000/mm^3. Some of the causes of leukopenia include acute viral infection and congenital and idiopathic acquired defects in WBC maturation. Most commonly, neutropenia is induced by a drug or a physical agent. Irradiation, as used in cancer chemotherapy, and any of a hundred different drugs may account for neutropenia. For example, if the use of chlorpromazine and related compounds is clearly indicated blood counts should be monitored frequently after neutropenia is detected. Aminopyrine and other drugs such as sulfonamides may act as haptens and lead to antineutrophil antibodies. A wide variety of diseases result in neutropenia, including acute leukemias, infection, rheumatoid arthritis, vitamin B$_{12}$ deficiency, and cirrhosis of the liver with congestive splenomegaly. Occasionally patients with rheumatoid arthritis develop splenomegaly and neutropenia, which is called Felty's syndrome.

The only clinical manifestations that can be attributed to neutropenia are bacterial infections and oral ulceration. When neutropenia is very sudden and due to rapid cell destruction, transient chills, fever, and malaise may be present. The frequency and severity of the infection vary markedly and correlate poorly with the severity of the neutropenia. Life-threatening infections usually are found in patients with <500 neutrophils/mm^3. When neutropenia is confirmed, evaluation should determine any and all drugs or potential toxins to which the patient has been exposed; infection history; results of previous blood tests; and clues to underlying diseases associated with neutropenia, such as rheumatoid arthritis, SLE, and infectious mononucleosis. The underlying disease should be treated, and any drug or toxin that may be the offender must be withdrawn. Appropriate antimicrobial treatment of infection is mandatory.

AGRANULOCYTOSIS

Agranulocytosis is an acute disease in which the WBC count drops to extremely low levels with pronounced neutropenia. Clinical manifestations include high fever; chills; sore throat; and necrotic ulcerations of the mouth, rectum, and vagina. Regional lymph nodes become enlarged. Without aggressive therapy or spontaneous remission, death from overwhelming infection ensues. If remission occurs immature granulocytes appear in the circulation before mature cells. Patients with severe neutropenia also have an increased incidence of *Pneumocystis carinii*, cytomegalovirus, and systemic mycoses. Treatment is to discontinue suspected chemical agents or drugs, institute supportive measures, and eliminate documented infections with appropriate antibiotics. It is also imperative to institute reverse isolation to protect the patient with agranulocytosis from exposure to infection.

Leukocytosis

Leukocytosis is defined as persistently elevated WBC counts above 13,000/mm^3. As in leukopenia, it is important to correlate the patient's laboratory findings with the clinical state. If a patient is totally asymptomatic, has a normal physical examination, and has an elevated WBC count with a normal differential, surgery is not necessarily contraindicated. The presence of a history of recurrent infections, an abnormal physical examination, and a left shift on differential together with leukocytosis does require further investigation before surgery is undertaken. Obvious causes of leukocytosis include infection; pregnancy; splenectomy; and certain medications, such as corticosteroids, lithium, and epinephrine.

LEUKEMOID REACTION

The leukemoid reaction is a clinical syndrome that usually appears with an elevated WBC count, but the WBC count may be normal or reduced. The peripheral smear has changes that may suggest leukemia. The difference is that the leukemoid reaction is not an unregulated proliferation of leukocytes. The leukemoid reaction is an expression of a bone marrow response to some underlying cause.

The abnormalities of bone marrow and peripheral blood return to normal when the cause of the leukemoid reaction disappears. In this reaction, any of the WBCs can be involved. The variety of causes includes bacteria, viruses, allergens, inflammatory responses, poisons, toxins, drugs, and malignancies. The leukemoid reaction has also been seen in acute conditions, such as those brought about by physical and emotional stimuli, hemolytic anemias, hemorrhages, and burns. It is unclear why this reaction occurs in some patients and not in others. Eosinophilic leukemoid reactions are observed with parasites, allergies, dermatologic and collagen vascular diseases, and drug reactions.

LEUKEMIAS

The leukemias are a group of blood disorders characterized by uncontrolled proliferation of abnormal WBC progenitors. In some disorders, specific characteristic chromosomal changes are seen, such as in chronic myeloid leukemia. In others, though the disorder is presumed to be related to a defect in DNA, no characteristic chromosomal abnormalities are seen.

In acute leukemia, as mentioned, there is uncontrolled proliferation of abnormal WBC progenitors. In chronic leukemias, mature WBCs as well as immature WBCs may autonomously overproduce. Classically these diseases produce characteristic syndromes with well-defined clinical and laboratory features. However, common to all these diseases are replacement of normal bone marrow with malignant cells, organ infiltration by proliferating WBCs, thrombocytopenia due to lack of platelet-cell production, and anemia secondary to bone marrow failure.

Although it would be unlikely that the podiatrist would make the initial diagnosis of a leukemic state, it must be kept in mind that any patient with signs and symptoms such as new-onset petechiae, recurrent infection, severe fatigue, and unexplained fever may have an underlying hematologic disorder. Obviously any patient whose preoperative CBC reveals unexplained anemia, leukocytosis, or thrombocytopenia must be evaluated for possible hematologic disease before any elective surgery is undertaken.

Acute Lymphocytic Leukemia. Acute lymphocytic leukemia (ALL) comprises 80% of the acute leukemias of childhood and about 20% of acute leukemias of adulthood. In this disorder, there is a proliferation of abnormal immature lymphocytes and their progenitors. Acute lymphocytic leukemia may appear with anemia, thrombocytopenia, or neutropenia. This leukemia is treated initially with combination chemotherapy. Of adults with ALL, 80% achieve complete remission. In children, ALL is much more responsive to treatment, with 95% of patients achieving complete remission.

Acute Nonlymphocytic Leukemia. Acute nonlymphocytic leukemia (ANLL) is chiefly an adult disease, with a median age of presentation of 50 years. There is a proliferation of primitive myeloid cells, or blasts. Most patients present with anemia, bleeding secondary to thrombcytopenia, or infection. Acute nonlymphocytic leukemia is treated with intensive combination chemotherapy. About 70% of adults so affected under age 50 achieve complete remission.

Chronic Lymphocytic Leukemia. Chronic lymphocytic leukemia (CLL) is a lymphoproliferative disorder characterized by proliferation and accumulation of mature-appearing neoplastic lymphocytes. This leukemia is a clonal malignancy of B lymphocytes. Chronic lymphocytic leukemia is slowly progressive and is manifested by immunosuppression, bone marrow failure, and organ infiltration with lymphocytes. Chronic lymphocytic leukemia is a disease of the elderly, with 90% of cases occurring after age 50. Many patients are discovered incidentally from a routine CBC that reveals lymphocytosis. Others present with fatigue and lymphadenopathy. Most patients with early indolent CLL require no specific treatment. If fatigue, anemia, lymphadenopathy, or thrombocytopenia occur chemotherapy is warranted. Mean survival is about 6 years, and 25% of these patients live more than 10 years.

Chronic Granulocytic Leukemia. Chronic granulocytic leukemia, or chronic myelocytic leukemia (CML), is characterized by abnormal proliferation and accumulation of immature granulocytes. These cells retain the capacity for differentiation, and normal bone marrow function is retained in the early phases of the disease. The disease remains stable for years and then transforms to a more malignant phase. Chronic myelocytic leukemia is associated with a characteristic chromosomal abnormality, the Philadelphia chromosome, a reciprocal translocation between the long arms of chromosomes 9 and 22. The presence of the Philadelphia chromosome is important because the small number of those (25%) with CML who lack this chromosome have a much worse prognosis than those with CML who have a Philadelphia chromosome. These patients may present with fever, fatigue, night sweats, pain, and splenomegaly. The usual treatment is palliative. Extreme leukocytosis requires myelosuppressive treatment. Unfortunately median survival is 3 to 4 years.

Lymphomas

The lymphomas are a group of hematologic disorders that represent malignant neoplasms that arise in lymph nodes or lymph tissue. The two major subgroups are Hodgkin's disease and non-Hodgkin's lymphoma. Clinically these diseases most commonly appear with painless lymphadenopathy in more than one body region.

Diagnosis of Hodgkin's disease as well as non-Hodgkin's lymphoma is made by lymph node biopsy. Histology is of absolute importance in terms of diagnosis for these diseases. When a diagnosis is established, staging to define the extent of disease is important (Table 9–4). The most important elements for staging include a careful history, physical examination, CBC, renal

Table 9–4. STAGING OF HODGKIN'S DISEASE

I
Involvement of a single lymph node or a single extra lymphatic site

II
Involvement of two or more lymph node regions on the same side of the diaphragm, which may also include spleen, localized extralymphatic involvement, or both

III
Involvement of the lymph node regions on both sides of the diaphragm, which may also include spleen, localized extralymphatic involvement, or both

IV
Diffuse or disseminated involvement of extralymphatic sites (e.g., bone marrow or liver or multiple pulmonary metastasis); staging is further categorized by absence (**A**) or presence (**B**) of systemic signs and symptoms, such as night sweats, unexplained fever, and unexplained weight loss.

function test, liver function test, chest radiograph, bone marrow aspiration and biopsy, lymphangiogram, abdominal CT scan, and liver biopsy.

Hodgkin's disease usually attacks younger individuals, with a peak incidence between 20 and 35 years of age and a male to female ratio of 2 to 1. Hodgkin's disease is fairly common; about 6000 new cases are detected each year in the United States. Patients usually present with painless lymphadenopathy in the supraclavicular or cervical nodes. About 50% of patients also present with systemic manifestations, such as fever, night sweats, weight loss, and pruritus. Of all lymph node areas, cervical nodes are most commonly involved on presentation. Once a diagnosis is established, staging continues to be extremely important because it has relevance to prognosis and helps to plan further treatment required to cure the disease. Basically treatment of Hodgkin's disease is radiation therapy for early stages and chemotherapy for late stages.

In *non-Hodgkin's lymphoma*, lymphadenopathy is usually the initial complaint. Lymph node biopsy for histologic classification is necessary in terms of diagnosis and treatment. Staging for non-Hodgkin's lymphoma is done in a manner similar to that of Hodgkin's disease. Most of the non-Hodgkin's lymphomas are in an advanced stage when diagnosed. Treatment is usually with chemotherapeutic agents.

Table 9–5. CAUSES OF LYMPHADENOPATHY

Infections
Bacterial
Mycobacterial
Fungal
Viral
Parasitic

Immunologic Disorders
Collagen vascular diseases
Serum sickness
Sarcoidosis
Drug reaction: hydantoin
AIDS/ARC

Malignancies
Hematologic
Nonhematologic

Miscellaneous or Unknown Causes
Angioimmunoblastic lymphadenopathy
Dermatopathic lymphadenopathy
Endocrinopathies: thyrotoxicosis, adrenal insufficiency
Lipoidoses

AIDS, Aquired immune deficiency syndrome; ARC, AIDS-related complex.

Lymphadenopathy

Common causes of lymphadenopathy include local infection, as in streptococcal pharyngitis, and systemic infection, as in infectious mononucleosis (Table 9–5). Lymphadenopathy is also seen in collagen vascular diseases, such as rheumatoid arthritis and SLE; drug reactions; malignancies; and miscellaneous conditions, such as sarcoidosis. Generalized lymphadenopathy may also be an early manifestation of acute HIV infection, the agent of acquired immune deficiency syndrome (AIDS). History, physical examination, and laboratory studies often provide a clinical diagnosis, but if studies are not conclusive or require histologic confirmation, as in lymphoma, a lymph node biopsy should be done. Patients with asymptomatic lymphadenopathy of <1 cm with negative serology and negative blood count findings should be observed. If the nodes enlarge and constitutional symptoms occur biopsy should be done.

BLOOD TRANSFUSION

Human blood is a necessary resource in the therapy of patients who have hemorrhage, severe anemias, and coagulation de-fects. Red blood cells can be transfused as packed RBCs or as whole blood. At one time, whole blood therapy was the only therapy in clinical situations as diverse as acute blood loss, aplastic anemia, and thrombocytopenic hemorrhage. However, advances in technology have permitted the harvesting and selective administration of specific blood components. Blood component therapy has several advantages. The patient is given specifically what is needed, the possibility of circulatory overload is diminished, and unnecessary transfusion of foreign antibodies is avoided. There are very few circumstances in which fresh whole blood is the treatment of choice. Possible exceptions include acute bleeding with a 20% loss of total blood volume. The general indications for transfusion include need for increased oxygen capacity; replacement in acute blood loss, in which case one may consider the use of plasma expanders; and hemorrhage related to platelet disorders, in which case one would use platelet transfusions.

Hazards of Blood Transfusion

The hazards of blood transfusion fall into two main categories. One is transfusion reactions, and the second is transmission of disease by transfused blood components.

Transfusion Reactions

Transfusion reactions include three types of reactions. These are the major hemolytic reactions, or incompatibility, febrile reactions, and allergic reactions. *Major hemolytic reactions* are clinically characterized by shock, back pain, flushing, fever, and intravascular hemolysis. Recognition of this major type of reaction mandates that the transfusion be stopped and the blood be returned to the blood bank, along with a fresh sample of the patient's blood, for typing and crossmatching. These patients need to be hydrated and their blood pressure supported.

The second type of reaction is the *febrile reaction*. This reaction is usually due to sensitization to WBC antibodies. This type of reaction is much more common than hemolytic transfusion reactions. Febrile reactions range in severity from simple fever, to urticaria with fever and chills, to vomiting and hypotension.

The third type of reaction is the *allergic reaction*. This reaction can also be characterized by fever, urticaria, and an anaphylaxis response.

In all instances of suspected reaction to the transfused blood, the transfusion should be stopped immediately and the intravenous line kept open. The compatibility of recipient and donor should be checked. The type of reaction should be evaluated, and appropriate diagnostic and treatment measures should be taken.

Clinically the most common transfusion reaction is fever without hemolysis, produced by sensitivity to donor WBCs in patients who have received multiple transfusions. The transfusion should be stopped, and antipyretics should be administered. If the reaction does not subside or if other symptoms occur, a more serious type of reaction must be considered. In patients with frequent febrile reactions, washed RBCs or washed frozen RBCs, which are both relatively poor in WBCs and platelets, may be used. In both the febrile and allergic reactions, patients may need to be treated with steroids. Minor transfusion reactions can often be avoided if the patient receives acetaminophen (Tylenol, 10 gr by mouth) and diphenhydramine (Benadryl, 25 mg by mouth) 30 minutes before the transfusion is started.

Anaphylaxis with laryngeal edema or vascular collapse is rare. Allergic reactions with urticaria, pruritus, or wheezing are relatively common. The transfusion should be stopped immediately, maintaining the intravenous line. Diphenhydramine (Benadryl, 50 mg intravenously) should be given. Epinephrine and steroids may be required for the more severe transfusion reactions.

Disease Transmission

The second major hazard of blood transfusion is transmission of disease by blood components. Hepatitis transmission remains a serious hazard of blood transfusion despite the reduction in transmission of hepatitis B. Because hepatitis B antigen positivity can be detected, hepatitis B represents only 10% of all cases of post-transfusion hepatitis. However, non-A, non-B hepatitis and delta hepatitis account for the balance of cases. About 7% of patients receiving blood products develop hepatitis, the highest risk being in recipients of commercial coagulation factor concentrates. Transfusion can transmit cytomegalovirus, particularly in patients undergoing organ grafts. Malaria may also be transmitted by transfusion.

Transfusion therapy is further complicated by the explosive spread of AIDS because it has been demonstrated that some cases of this disease are clearly related to transfusions. Concern regarding AIDS transmission by blood components has prompted the screening of potential donors for the presence of antibody to HIV. The risk of transfusion-associated AIDS has certainly increased the frequency of autologous transfusion for elective surgery. In clinical podiatry, transfusions with RBCs are rarely indicated. If a patient is known to have anemia of chronic disease, perhaps secondary to renal failure, and surgery is clearly indicated one might consider the use of packed RBCs, in order to optimize postoperative healing. Because most podiatric surgery is elective, anemia needs to be investigated and corrected by treating the underlying problem rather than by utilizing transfusions. As previously mentioned, the risk of transfusion-associated AIDS makes it imperative that autologous transfusions be considered in elective surgical situations, in which patients may in fact need postoperative transfusions.

PATIENTS TAKING ANTICOAGULANTS

The most common use of anticoagulant drugs is to prevent formation or extension of intravascular clots and related cardiovascular disease. The two most commonly used prothrombin depressants are sodium warfarin and bishydroxycoumarin (Dicumarol). All drugs of this class are well absorbed by the gastrointestinal tract after oral ingestion. Salicylates are weak inhibitors of the liver synthesis of clotting factors and may add to the anticoagulant effect of more potent drugs.

Synthetically prepared anticoagulants have a latent period following oral administration. There is a period of many days before prothrombin concentration returns to normal when a synthetically prepared anticoagulant is discontinued. The maintenance dose is thus decided on an individual basis, as determined by the prothrombin time. The prothrombin time reflects the action of the dose of anticoagulant given 2 days previously except when rapid-acting warfarin is used. Usually the prothrombin time is kept within 2 to 2.5 times normal (normal prothrombin time is 12 to 14 seconds), which is comparable to 20 to 30% of the activity of normal. Heparin acts directly to neutralize any thrombin formed and also inhibits the action of activated factors IX and XI. The most important point is that heparin acts immediately. Duration is dose dependent and brief. The effect is about 50% dissipated in 1 hour. Clotting time is again normal within 4 hours after intravenous injection of a routine dose. Clinically these anticoagulants are used to prevent or treat venous thrombosis, to prevent or treat acute arterial occlusion, to prevent thrombus formations in atrial fibrillation, and to prevent coronary thrombosis.

Surgery. Patients undergoing surgery and taking anticoagulants for a prior or concurrent condition are usually fully anticoagulated with either warfarin agents or heparin. If the indication for anticoagulation appears to have been tenuous or the patient has had nearly a full course of the drug, anticoagulation can be stopped or reversed preoperatively after consulting with the internist.

Heparin. A patient may have been placed on prophylactic low-dose heparin for the prevention of venous thrombosis or thromboembolism. This patient is usually given heparin (5000 U subcutaneously) 2 hours before surgery and then every 12 hours postoperatively. Monitoring of coagulation parameters is not required because this low dose of heparin does not influence such parameters.

There is a general agreement that low-dose heparin reduces the incidence of postoperative venous thrombosis and pulmonary embolism in otherwise hemostatically normal patients after all procedures except major orthopedic procedures and open prostatectomy. Because of bleeding complications, such as wound hematomas and hematuria, it has been suggested that low-dose heparin should be administered to only surgical patients with a high risk of developing venous thromboembolism.

Any patient who has experienced a thromboembolic event should be given a prophylactic dose of low-dose heparin preoperatively.

An internist should be consulted when a patient is taking platelet-active agents such as aspirin within 5 days of surgery. In patients who require full therapeutic anticoagulation, most surgery can be safely performed except for ophthalmic, neurologic, and hepatic surgery. Onset of heparin is immediate, and its effects can be rapidly reversed. Heparin is preferred over warfarin-like agents for the patient who requires anticoagulation at the time of surgery. The effect of warfarin agents can be reversed by vitamin K and, more rapidly, by fresh plasma or fresh frozen plasma. Patients who require anticoagulation in the perioperative period should be carefully controlled on heparin, with the activated PTT maintained well within the therapeutic range. Continuous infusion therapy is desirable to avoid intermittent periods of absolute anticoagulation.

Minor Surgery. In very minor surgery, it is thought that warfarin derivatives do not cause increased bleeding during surgery and avoid problems of re-establishing anticoagulant control later. If postoperative bleeding in the patient taking anticoagulants is life threatening the anticoagulants must be discontinued and reversed. Heparin is reversed by protamine. In less severe bleeding, the degree of anticoagulation should be determined and the dose of heparin lessened to decrease the PTT to the lower end of the therapeutic range. Checks on platelet counts are useful because of the thrombocytopenic effect of heparin. Platelet-active agents must be avoided. An internist should be consulted for any patient who is taking anticoagulants or who is at risk for thromboemboli.

APPROACH TO PODIATRIC PATIENTS WITH SIGNS AND SYMPTOMS OF MALIGNANCY

Although oncologic lesions are not commonly encountered in clinical podiatry, certain pathologies are encountered often enough to warrant the practitioner's having a general overview of podiatric oncology. Statistical data concerning foot tumors and lesions have been reported only sporadically in the podiatry literature. These lesions are placed under the major headings of skin lesions, nerve lesions, and fatty and fibrous lesions. The three most commonly encountered lesions are those of verrucae, Morton's neuroma, and porokeratosis. Verrucae constitute about 48% of all benign lesions, Morton's neuroma constitutes about 15%, and porokeratotic lesions constitute approximately 1%. Tumors of muscle tendon and joint are very rarely encountered, with ganglion cysts being the most frequently seen tumors in this category. Bone lesions make up the fourth largest category and are seen in approximately 2% of all foot lesions and tumors. Of these bone lesions, 92% are exostoses, and the rest are osteochondromas. Primary malignancies of the foot represent less than 1% of all skin lesions and tumors in one study. Kaposi's sarcoma is the most frequent malignant lesion seen in the foot, followed by squamous cell carcinoma, melanoma, basal cell carcinoma, malignant giant cell carcinoma, and sweat gland carcinoma.

Metastases from primary cancers in other regions of the body to the foot are very rare. The most common primary cancers leading to metastases to bones in the foot are from the gastrointestinal, vesical, renal, and uterine areas. A possible explanation for this is the retrograde spread of tumor emboli from the vertebral venous plexus down incompetent leg veins. The radiologic features of peripheral metastases are usually those of purely osteolytic destructive lesions. The neoplasm may expand the cortical shell as it enlarges. In the tarsus, almost total destruction of many bones with destruction of articular cartilage may occur in the late stages of the disease.

The presence of a destructive bony lesion in the extremity of a patient with widespread metastatic disease may produce no difficulty in diagnosis. However, if it is the first indication of an occult cancer the appearance of the lesion may be deceptive. The lesion may resemble soft tissue cellulitis, osteomyelitis, septic arthritis, or tenosynovitis. Clinically the signs of inflammation are often present. Pain, tenderness, swelling, and loss of function may occur. When signs of inflammation are not present, the radiologic differential diagnosis must include such benign lesions as enchondroma, epidermoid cyst, osteoid osteoma, giant cell tumor, and even gout. In an individual over the age of 45 years, any skeletal lesion with a radiologic appearance even remotely suggesting malignancy must always arouse suspicion of a metastatic deposit. A skeletal survey or bone scan may confirm a widespread metastatic process. In cases of a solitary lesion, biopsy usually is required.

It is important also for the podiatric physician to be able to note systemic manifestations of neoplastic disease. Such disturbances include fever, anorexia and weight loss, unexplained anemia, polycythemia, thrombocytopenia or thrombocytosis, and unexplained leukocytosis. Other more subtle laboratory findings may include serum protein abnormalities, such as a polyclonal hypergammaglobulin anemia or a coagulopathy expressed as recurrent venous thrombosis. A severe form of widespread recurrent venous thrombosis has long been associated with gastrointestinal malignancies, mainly pancreatic.

There are a number of neurologic and muscular abnormalities that may be suggestive of an underlying malignancy. These abnormalities include myositis, dermatomyositis, and peripheral neuropathy. The syndrome of pulmonary osteoarthropathy, or clubbing of the fingers, has long been known to be associated with certain neoplasms, especially those arising in the thorax. Herpes zoster has often heralded, or been associated with, neoplasm. The diagnosis of herpes zoster should arouse the clinician's suspicion for possible malignant disease.

Manifestations of Malignancy

Fever

Fever may occur with any malignancy but is more often associated with certain specific malignancies. Fever is seen in Hodgkin's disease and other lymphomas, Ewing's sarcoma, and localized hypernephromas. Contributing to this phenomenon are tumor necrosis, inflammation, toxic product release, and production of endogenous pyrogens.

Anorexia and Weight Loss

Anorexia and weight loss are frequently seen symptoms that may be a direct consequence of the tumor itself or may be an indirect consequence of the physiologic and emotional impact of the malignancy. Other causes include anorexigenic peptides, negative nitrogen balance related to un-neutralized tumor amino acids, uncoupling of oxidative phosphorylation, and impaired glucose tolerance.

Lactic Acidosis

Lactic acidosis, a severe life-threatening or fatal physiologic disturbance, is recognized in patients with advanced malignancy. Excess lactic acid usually occurs in disease processes involving rapid proliferating tumor cells, as in leukemia or in undifferentiated lymphomas. Patients with malignancies and unexplained severe metabolic acidosis need to be evaluated for lactic acidosis. Acid-base balance can often be restored with fluid and electrolyte therapy. This is important because tumors that cause lactic acidosis often respond to chemotherapy, and palliation is effected. A cure may be possible if the life-threatening acidosis is recognized, treated, and reversed.

Bone Marrow Disturbances

Anemia. The principal cause of anemia in malignancies is blood loss due to the direct effect of cancer, such as gastrointestinal ulceration with bleeding and tumor replacement of bone marrow. Other causes of anemia include chemotherapy with myelosuppressive action; abnormal iron metabolism, which results in low serum iron, a decreased iron-binding capacity, and iron sequestration in the liver; shortened RBC life span; ineffective erythropoiesis; hypersplenism; autoimmune hemolysis; microangiopathic RBC destruction; nutrient and vitamin deficiencies; and a rare RBC aplasia associated with thymoma.

Erythrocytosis. Erythrocytosis is an increase in RBC mass that is associated with an increase in erythropoietin or similar substance, produced by hypernephromas, hepatomas, cerebellar hemangiomas, and uterine tumors. This erythrocytosis is not secondary to hypoxemia or a primary panmyelopathy, as in polycythemia vera.

Thrombocytopenia and Thrombocytosis. Unexplained thrombocytopenia may be idiopathic thrombocytopenia purpura, hypersplenism, or DIC. An elevated platelet count is common in a patient with a malignancy and is often due to an unrecognized cancer. This finding should indicate further investigation for an occult neoplasm.

Leukocytosis. Occasionally granulocytosis occurs and is usually associated with tumor-producing necrosis and inflammation or rare leukemia. In marrow metastasis, one would see abnormal RBC morphology, immature granulocytes, and giant platelets.

Coagulopathies. Pancreatic and other neoplasms may occur with a severe form of widespread recurrent venous thrombosis. Disseminated intravascular coagulation, a syndrome with reduced procoagulants, fibrinogen, and platelets, with fibrin-split products in the serum, may occur in patients with advanced cancer. Disseminated intravascular coagulation is seen especially in hepatic metastases. Advanced malignant disease may also appear with nonbacterial thrombotic endocarditis. The associated clots on the cardiac valves, cusps, and leaflets may produce significant emboli, which could be fatal.

Serum Protein Abnormalities. A polyclonal hypergammaglobulinemia may be apparent in patients with malignant disease. Monoclonal gammopathy is usually associated with plasma cell tumors or malignant lymphomas. Monoclonal gammopathy may also be associated with an increase in apparently benign plasma cells in the bone marrow. In the elderly, benign monoclonal gammopathy occurs frequently, and the association of this protein abnormality with cancer could be coincidental. Hypogammaglobulinemia is a characteristic of chronic lymphocytic leukemia and some lymphocytic lymphomas.

Hypercalcemia

Many patients with malignant disease develop significant hypercalcemia as a result of osseous metastases. The bone destruction and calcium release associated with these metastases may not be caused simply by mechanical or destructive effects of cancer cells. Osteoclast activity factor, produced by the tumor in the marrow environment, may be the local cause of the hypercalcemia. Tumors that arise in the kidney, lung, pancreas, and ovary may produce an ectopic parathormone or a parathormone-like substance that results in hypercalcemia. This is a medical emergency and must be dealt with immediately.

Hypercalcemia of Multiple Myeloma. Multiple myeloma is a plasma cell myeloma, which is a disseminated malignancy. A clone of transformed plasma cells proliferates in a malignant fashion in the bone marrow, disrupting its normal function as well as invading adjacent bone. High concentrations of a serum M component, or abnormal immunoglobulins, may lead to blood sludging and hyperviscosity. Rouleau formation is observed on the peripheral blood smear. An increase in the sedimentation rate occurs, which is due to high concentrations of myeloma globulins in the plasma. Myeloma cells also secrete calcium-mobilizing substances, which stimulate local bone resorption by osteoclasts in the vicinity of the myeloma cell focus in the bone marrow. Hypercalcemia can lead to calcium nephropathy and is the most important cause of renal failure in myeloma. Patients with myeloma usually have depressed serum levels of normal immunoglobulins and have a compromised ability to manifest a normal antibody response after antigenic stimulation. Consequently these patients are highly susceptible to infection from pneumococcus.

Presenting symptoms and signs of myeloma include bone pain, which is often an indication of pathologic fractures of the spine or ribs; weakness resulting from anemia; recurrent pneumococcal infection; and hypercalcemia secondary to bone resorption. It is not infrequent for patients to present with back pain, anemia, and a very high sedimentation rate. The diagnosis is made by a monoclonal demonstration of one immunoglobulin as well as an aspirate that shows greater than 20% of plasma cells making up the bone marrow. The treatment of a patient with multiple myeloma requires attention to supportive care, which includes exercise and ambulation, hydration, and administration of chemotherapy.

Neurologic and Muscular Abnormalities

The etiology is largely unknown for the many neurologic and neuromyopathic syndromes associated with malignant disease. Neuromuscular complications must always be distinguished from the direct effects of a neoplasm on the peripheral nerves, the spinal cord, and the brain. Up to 5 to 10% of patients with malignant disease have neuromuscular complications. Over half of these complications are associated with lung cancer, usually of the small-cell or oat-cell type.

Pulmonary Osteoarthropathy

Certain neoplasms, especially those arising in the thorax, have long been associated with the pulmonary osteoarthropathy syndrome and clubbing of the fingers. Occasionally, periosteal reaction and associated pain and tenderness suggest metastases to the bones. Clubbing is more common in nonmalignant disease involving the lungs, congenital heart disease, and certain abdominal disorders. The recent development of clubbing in an adult should lead to further investigation into the possibility of a tumor of the lung or pleura.

Cutaneous Abnormalities

Dermatologic abnormalities associated with malignant disease are not common clinical problems. Hyperpigmentation may occur, ranging from acanthosis migricans to generalized melanin deposits, as in malignant melanoma. Other lesions include neurofibromas, diffuse erythema, erythema multiforme, urticaria, and bullous eruptions. Pruritus is often seen in patients with Hodgkin's disease and with associated biliary obstruction. Management of the underlying condition is the most effective way to treat the pruritus. Kaposi's sarcoma may appear in the lower extremities in immunosuppressed patients and patients with cancer who seek podiatric care.

Bibliography

Adamson JW: Familial polycythemia. Semin Hematol 12:383, 1975.

Bainton D, Finch O: The diagnosis of iron-deficiency anemia. Am J Med 37:62, 1964.

Barber A, Green D, Galluzzo T, et al.: The bleeding time as a preoperative screening test. Am J Med 78:761, 1985.

Berlin NI: Diagnosis and classification of the polcythemias. Semin Hematol 12:339, 1975.

Bessman JD, Gilmer PR, Jr, Gardner FH: Improved classification of anemias by MCV and RDW. Am J Clin Pathol 80:322, 1983.

Burn TR, Saleem A: Idiopathic thrombocytopenic purpura. Am J Med 75:1001, 1983.

Camitta BM, Storb R, Thomas ED: Aplastic anemia: Pathogenesis, diagnosis, treatment and prognosis. N Engl J Med 306:645, 1982.

Cartwright G: The anemia of chronic disorders. Semin Hematol 3:351, 1966.

Cook JD: Clinical evaluation of iron deficiency. Semin Hematol 19:6, 1982.

Crosby WH: Reticulocyte count. Arch Intern Med 141:1747, 1981.

de la Fuente B, Kasper C, Rickles FR, et al.: Response of patients with mild and moderate hemophilia A and von Willebrand's disease to treatment with desmopressin. Ann Intern Med 103:6, 1985.

Elwood PC, Shinton NK, Wilson IL, et al.: Hemoglobin, vitamin B_{12} and folate levels in the elderly. Br J Haematol 21:557, 1971.

Entisham M, Cape R: Diagnosing and treating anemia. Geriatrics 32:99, 1977.

Fairbairn JF, II, Juergens JL: Principles of medical treatment. In Juergens JL, Spittell JA, Jr, Fairbairn JF, II (eds): Peripheral Vascular Diseases, 5th ed. Philadelphia: WB Saunders Co, 1980.

Farfel NR, Noltzman NA: Education, consent, and counseling in sickle cell screening programs: Report of a survey. Am J Public Health 74:373, 1984.

Frank MM, et al.: Pathophysiology of immune hemolytic anemia. Ann Intern Med 87:210, 1977.

Goldmann DR, et al. (eds): Medical Care of the Surgical Patient: A Problem-Oriented Approach to Management. Philadelphia: JB Lippincott Co, 1982.

Hurst JW (ed): Medicine for the Practicing Physician. Boston: Butterworth Publishers, 1983.

Levine PH: The acquired immunodeficiency syndrome in persons with hemophilia. Ann Intern Med 103:723, 1985.

Lind SE: Prolonged bleeding time. Am J Med 77:305, 1984.

Lipschitz D, Cook J, Finch C: A clinical evaluation of serum ferritin as an index of iron stores. N Engl J Med 290:1213, 1974.

Molitch ME: Management of Medical Problems in the Surgical Patient. Philadelphia: FA Davis Co, 1982.

Petrakis NL, Wiesenfeld SL, Sams BJ, et al.: Prevalence of sickle-cell trait and glucose-6-PD-deficiency. N Engl J Med 282:767, 1970.

Rubenstein E, Federman DD (eds): Scientific American Medicine. New York: Scientific American, Inc, 1987.

Stewart JG, Ahlquist DA, McGill DB, et al.: Gastrointestinal blood loss and anemia in runners. Ann Intern Med 100:843, 1984.

Suchman AL, Grinner PF: Diagnostic uses of the activated partial thromboplastin time and prothrombin time. Ann Intern Med 104:810, 1986.

Tudhope G, Wilson G: Anemia in hypothyroidism. Q J Med 29:513, 1960.

Van der Weyden M, Rother M, Firkin B: Metabolic significance of reduced B_{12} in folate deficiency. Blood 40:23, 1972.

Wyngaarden JB, Smith LH (eds): Cecil Textbook of Medicine. Philadelphia: WB Saunders Co, 1985.

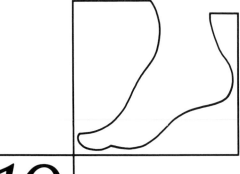

10 INFECTIOUS DISEASE

JULIE L. GERBERDING

OVERVIEW

Despite the proliferation of antimicrobial chemotherapeutic agents and the implementation of global immunization programs in the last 50 years, infectious diseases continue to account for a large proportion of medical practice (Table 10–1). Although considerable progress has been made in controlling many infections, including poliomyelitis, diphtheria, diarrheal illnesses, malaria, and tuberculosis, in developed countries, these diseases continue to contribute to the lowered life expectancy in developing countries. As some pathogens, such as smallpox have been eradicated, new organisms, such as human immunodeficiency virus (HIV), have emerged. In addition, medical advances in organ transplantation, chemotherapy for malignancies, and prolonged survival in persons with a variety of chronic diseases have increased the number of immunocompromised persons at risk for serious infections. Nosocomial infections and the emergence of organisms resistant to antimicrobial drugs have also played an important role in the changing epidemiology of infectious diseases.

PATHOGENESIS

Infection is defined as the presence and replication of organisms in the host. The consequences of infection are varied and depend on the complex interplay among the virulence of the infecting organism, the response of the host to the presence of microbial agent and its products, and the integrity of the host's defense mechanisms, which can be ascertained only by identifying a serologic response to the infection. Pathogens are defined as organisms capable of causing disease, although the distinction between pathogens and nonpathogens is to some degree dependent on the state of the host defenses. For example, *Staphylococcus epidermidis*, usually considered a nonpathogen, may cause serious disease in the immunocompromised host. Colonization indicates that an organism is present in the host and can be recovered in culture, but disease or subclinical consequences of infection are absent. The skin and mucosal surfaces of the host are normally colonized at birth by a variety of organisms. Although these organisms are normally nonpathogenic, some individuals, known as carriers, are colonized with pathogens. Carriers show no evidence of current disease, although disease may develop later or may have been present in the past.

The ultimate outcome of infection is determined by the balance among the virulence of the pathogens and the ability of the host defense to eliminate infection and the repair of the damage produced. Host defense mechanisms together with antimicrobial therapy may eliminate the pathogen, thereby curing the infection. However, when the balance favors the microorganism, tissue damage, systemic toxicity, and even death may occur. Chronic infection is produced when the organism is only partially contained by the host.

Virulence Factor

Virulence factors are properties of a microorganism that confer pathogenicity. Although a variety of virulence factors, which promote invasion, dissemination, proliferation, escape from host defense, and production of the disease state, have been described, knowledge of the complex relationship among these factors and infection is largely incomplete. Toxins directed against other microbes present in the normal flora are termed *bacteriocins*. Bacteriocins may provide a selective advantage by allowing the pathogen to proliferate in sufficient number to cause disease. Enzymes, such as hyaluronidase, protease, collagenase, and mucinase, may also play a role in invasiveness of certain bacteria by disrupting connective tissue barriers to penetration. Factors present on the bacterial surface that promote adhesion of the organism to other surfaces are now recognized to be critically important in the establishment of many infections. Such *adhesins* are thought to contribute to the colonization, proliferation, tissue trophism, and escape from phagocytosis important in the pathogenesis of many bacterial infections. Toxins produced by the pathogen that cause damage in host cells are well-known virulence factors. Exotoxins are protein toxins released from the cell during growth. Examples of exotoxins include tet-

Table 10–1. GUIDE FOR ADULT IMMUNIZATIONS*

Immunobiologic	Schedule	Indications
Toxoids		
Tetanus-diphtheria (TD)	2 doses: IM 4 wks apart; 3rd dose: 6–12 mos after 2nd dose; booster every 10 yrs	All adults;† tetanus prophylaxis in wound management
Live Viruses‡		
Measles	1 dose subcu; no booster	All adults without documentation of positive titer
Mumps	1 dose subcu; no booster	All adults, particularly susceptible males; most adults considered immune
Rubella	1 dose subcu; no booster	All adults without documentation of positive titer
Smallpox	*No indications for the use of smallpox vaccine in the general civilian population*§	
Live-Virus and Inactivated-Virus Vaccines		
Polio (IPV, OPV)‖	3 doses: subcu 4 wks apart; 4th dose: 6–12 mos after 3rd dose; IPV for adult boosters	Incompletely immunized adults and adults in households with children to be immunized; certain health care personnel who travel to areas with endemic or epidemic wild poliovirus
Inactivated-Virus Vaccines		
Hepatitis B (HB)	2 doses: IM 4 wks apart; 3rd dose: 5 months after 2nd dose; need for booster not known	Adults at increased risk of occupational, environmental, social, and family exposure
Influenza (inactivated whole-virus and split-virus)	Annual vaccination with current vaccine	Adults with high-risk condition,¶ residents of nursing homes and chronic care facilities, health care providers, healthy adults 65 yrs and older
Inactivated-Bacteria Vaccines		
Pneumococcal polysaccharide (23 valent)	1 dose; booster not recommended	Adults at high risk for pneumococcal disease and its complications owing to underlying health conditions; healthy adults 65 yrs and older
Immune Globulins		
Immune globulin (IG) Hepatitis A	Hepatitis A prophylaxis: *Pre-exposure*—anticipated risk of 2–3 mos: 1 dose IM 0.02 ml/kg; risk of 5 months: 1 dose IM 0.06 ml/kg (repeat at above dose and intervals if exposure continues) *Post-exposure*—1 dose IM 0.02 ml/kg given within 2 wks of exposure	Household and sexual contacts of persons with hepatitis A; travelers to high-risk areas; day care outbreak: staff, attendees, parents of diapered attendees
Measles	Measles prophylaxis: 1 dose IM 0.25 ml/kg (max 15 ml) given within 6 days of exposure	Exposed susceptible contacts; given within 6 days can prevent or modify measles#
Hepatitis B immune globulin (HBIG)	1 dose IM 0.06 ml/kg as soon as possible, followed by a 2nd dose 1 mo later, unless HB vaccine is given	Following percutaneous or mucous membrane exposure to HBsAG⁺ blood; following sexual exposure or bite from person with acute HBV or an HBV carrier

Table 10–1. (continued)

Immunobiologic	Schedule	Indications
Tetanus immune globulin (TIG)	1 dose 250 units IM	Part of management of dirty, major wound in person with unknown tetanus toxoid status; less than 2 previous doses or 2 previous doses and wound less than 24 hrs old
Varicella-zoster immune globulin (VZIG)	Less than or equal to 50 kg: 1 dose 125 U/10 kg IM Greater than 50 kg: 1 dose 625 U/10 kg IM	Known or likely susceptible immunocompromised patient with close and prolonged contact with infectious person

* Adults aged 18 years and older. A careful history of immunizations should be obtained from all new patients.

† Except women in first trimester of pregnancy. Patients who experience neurologic, immediate hypersensitivity, or Arthus reaction following previous dose should not receive routine or emergency dose of TD for 10 years.

‡ Precautions should be used in pregnant patients, immunocompromised patients, and patients with egg- or neomycin-related anaphylaxis.

§ Laboratory workers involved in production and testing of orthopoxvirus or smallpox vaccine should be vaccinated.

‖ IPV, Inactivated poliovaccine (killed poliovirus); OPV, oral poliovaccine (live poliovirus). IPV is preferred for primary vaccination. When immediate protection is needed, OPV is recommended but not to immunocompromised patients or their family members.

¶ Wait until second or third trimester in pregnant women, if possible. Contraindicated in patients with anaphylaxis hypersensitivity to eggs.

Recipients of IG for measles prophylaxis should receive live measle vaccine 3 months later. IG (0.06 ml/kg) may be used if HBIG is not available.

HBsAG⁺, Hepatitis B surface antigen positivity; HBV, hepatitis B virus; IM, intramuscularly; subcu, subcutaneously.

anus toxin, botulinus toxin, and enterotoxin. Endotoxins are intracellular and cell-surface toxins, including the lipopolysaccharide component of gram-negative organisms.

Virulence factors may also directly interfere with the function of host defense mechanisms. Capsular polysaccharides that interfere with the process of opsonization and phagocytosis are well known to confer pathogenicity to *Streptococcus pneumoniae* as well as many other species of bacteria. Gamma A immunoglobulin (IgA) proteases, which facilitate invasion through mucosal surfaces, are produced by some species of bacteria. Intraphagocytic survival can be improved by a variety of enzyme elaborated by bacteria that interfere with lysosomal function and oxidative killing.

Host Defenses Against Infection

The first lines of defense against invasion by microorganisms are the protective anatomic barriers of the skin and mucous membranes. Bacteria that gain access to the body through the skin or mucous membranes do so via breaks in the epithelial barrier, caused by wounds, foreign bodies, and other tissue disruptions. Organisms capable of invading intact epithelium of the skin are extremely rare, although some bacteria, such as *Salmonella* and *Shigella* species, can directly invade the epithelial lining of the intestine. Indigenous microflora, which colonize the surface epithelium of the skin and gastrointestinal, upper respiratory, and genital tracts, protect against colonization and subsequent invasion by pathogens in several ways, including competition for nutrients, competition for tissue receptors, and production of bacteriocins. Alterations in the normal flora following antibacterial therapy therefore may promote colonization and overgrowth of pathogenic organisms, such as occurs in candidal vaginitis and pseudomembranous colitis, or may enhance invasiveness, as in *Salmonella* bacteremia.

The humoral immune system and the complement system together constitute the second line of defense against infection. Specific antibodies produced in response to invading pathogens or their toxic products are critical in mediating phagocytosis, neutralization, and lysis of many organisms. However, in the absence of performed antibodies or cross-reacting antibodies against the pathogen, antibody-mediated mechanisms do not contribute significantly to defense against infection in the first days or even weeks after invasion. Activation of the complement system with concomitant production of inflammatory mediators is therefore of greatest importance in the early phases of infection. Complement activation directly promotes opsonization, enhances the inflammatory response to infection, initiates lysis, and increases the number of phagocytes available to contain the infection.

The cellular immune system, although involved directly or indirectly in most infections, is particularly important in the defense against certain bacterial pathogens, such as *Listeria monocytogenes* and *Mycobacterium* sp.; viruses; protozoa; and fungi. Activated T lymphocytes, macrophages, and other phagocytes are directly involved in ingestion and intracellular killing of these oganisms. Whether congenital or acquired as a result of chronic debilitating disease, malignancy, antecedent infection, chemotherapy, malnutrition, immunosuppressive drugs, aging, or other nonspecific factors, defects in any of the components of the humoral, complement, and cellular immune systems can render the host susceptible to a variety of infectious diseases. The integrity of the host's defenses should be carefully evaluated when designing the diagnostic, therapeutic, and prophylactic approach to each patient.

PRINCIPLES OF ANTI-INFECTIVE THERAPY

The rapid proliferation of antimicrobial chemotherapy in the last several decades has had a dramatic impact on the practice of medicine. However, as more agents have become available for treating infections, decisions regarding the use of these agents have become increasingly complex. The following sections detail the antibacterial agents that are most commonly used and outline the principles that guide the rational use of these agents. Although the discussion focuses on antibacterial drugs, many of the same therapeutic principles are relevant to antiviral, antifungal, and antiprotozoal agents.

Instituting Antibacterial Therapy

The decision to institute antibacterial therapy requires a careful assessment of the probability of infection; the likely cause of the infection; the probable susceptibilities of the infecting organism to available antibacterial drugs; and host factors likely to influence the presentation, clinical course, and outcome of infection. If infection is not currently present but the clinical circumstances in the host suggest that the risk of infection is high *prophylactic* antimicrobial therapy may be implemented. If infection is suspected but not proved *initial* or empiric therapy is designed to treat the most likely pathogens until a definitive diagnosis is established. If the site and cause of the infection are known, *definitive* therapy specifically targeted against the known pathogens can be utilized.

Identifying the Presence and Site of Infection

The symptoms and signs of infection are myriad and depend on the involved site or sites. In most cases, a careful history and physical examination provide the necessary information to develop a presumptive diagnosis. Laboratory studies, including a complete blood count (CBC) with differential, an erythrocyte sedimentation rate (ESR), and a urinalysis, usually provide additional confirmatory evidence but do not replace clinical evaluation of the patient.

Local Signs

Local signs of infection include erythema, edema, increased temperature of the involved area, and often pain. If fluctuance is present in addition to edema, abscess, gas, or hematoma should be suspected. The presence of suppuration is strongly suggestive of acute infection and may provide a clue to the etiologic agent. A serosanguineous discharge is most often seen with streptococcal infections, whereas a creamy yellow discharge typifies staphylococcal infections. A foul-smelling discharge usually appears with anaerobic infections. Pseudomonal infection confers a blue-green hue to the purulent material, which may fluoresce under Wood's lamp. It is often helpful to outline the involved area to facilitate prospective asessment of the response to therapy. When local infection is suspected in an extremity, the integrity of the vascular supply should be evaluated. Evidence of cyanosis, poor capillary refill, and absent pulses indicate poor tissue perfusion and mandate an immediate aggressive approach to treatment.

Systemic Signs

Systemic signs of infection include fever and its metabolic consequences, tachycardia and tachypnea. Fever is a reliable indicator of infection in many clinical situations. However, fever may be absent in patients with localized infection, in debilitated or elderly patients, in patients with sepsis, in patients receiving immunosuppressive or anti-inflammatory drug therapy, and in immunocompromised patients. The absence of fever therefore does not exclude the diagnosis of infection if the clinical presentation is suggestive.

Sepsis

Sepsis is a systemic illness observed in patients with serious local or bacteremic infections. Aerobic gram-negative bacilli are the most common etiologic organisms, but an identical syndrome can be seen with anaerobic gram-negative bacilli as well as gram-positive aerobes and anaerobes. The hallmarks of sepsis include fever, or less commonly hypothermia; hypotension; tachycardia; tachypnea; and altered mental status. Hypotension is primarily due to peripheral vasodilation and relative volume depletion, so that in the early stages of sepsis, the extremities may appear warm and well perfused. However, as the condition evolves, cardiac output decreases and evidence of hypoperfusion with cyanosis may appear.

Although the pathophysiology of sepsis is complex and not yet clearly defined, endotoxin or similar lipopolysaccharide components of the bacterial cell wall appear to initiate the cascade of inflammation, complement activation, and vascular endothelial events that ultimately produce the signs and symptoms of the disease. Quantitative blood cultures from septic patients indicate that bacteremia is usually inconsistent and of low magnitude. Therefore failure to isolate an organism from the bloodstream does not exclude the diagnosis of sepsis.

Infections of the urinary tract, gastrointestinal tract, and lower respiratory tract are the most prevalent predisposing conditions. Because the most likely etiologic organism depends on the suspected site of infection, the diagnostic approach should include a careful assessment of the aforementioned systems. A chest radiograph, a urinalysis, and an abdominal radiograph are usually performed. If these initial studies do not identify a site of infection further studies, including abdominal ultrasonography, abdominal computed tomography (CT) scan, and echocardiogram may be indicated. In up to 30% of patients, the source of the bacteremia is not identified.

Early recognition of sepsis is imperative. Antimicrobial therapy should be implemented immediately after blood and other appropriate cultures are obtained. The choice of appropriate antimicrobial therapy is dictated by the suspected site of infection and the clinical history of the patient.

Management of Sepsis

It is prudent to utilize a broad-spectrum, combination regimen, with activity against gram-negative bacilli and often staphylococci and anaerobes, if the source of infection is unknown. Antipseudomonal agents should be added if the history suggests an increased likelihood of a pseudomonal agent. In many cases, surgical consultation should be obtained because drainage or relief of obstruction may be necessary to alter the clinical course. Supportive management usually requires intensive nursing care, with careful evaluation of fluid balance, coagulation parameters, hemodynamic status, and renal function.

Identifying the Cause of Infection

In all infections, it is imperative that every effort be made to correctly identify the offending organism before antimicrobial therapy is instituted. Although the diagnostic approach depends in part on knowledge of the most likely sites of the infection, cultures and, whenever possible, Gram's stain of infected material should be performed.

In cutaneous infections, it is important to sample the margins of the involved tissue when obtaining culture material since purulent material may reveal only necrotic debris with negative culture findings. Culture of superficial surfaces may not demonstrate the organism responsible for infection of deep tissue. For example, in osteomyelitis, the organism isolated from cultures of draining sinus tracts may not be the same as the organism isolated from bone biopsy. In patients who have serious infections, in patients who demonstrate systemic toxicity, and in patients who are at increased risk for sepsis, blood cultures should be obtained prior to the institution of therapy. Blood cultures should be obtained with strict attention to aseptic technique and should be timed to maximize the probability of documenting bacteremia. If therapy can be delayed, obtaining consecutive cultures over a period of several hours may improve the diagnostic yield. In severely ill patients with documented bacteremia and in any patient who fails to respond to treatment as expected, blood cultures should be repeated daily to document bacteriologic response and to identify superinfection.

Whenever possible, Gram's stain of infected material should be performed. In patients who have been treated with antimicrobials before cultures were obtained, this test may provide the only clue to diagnosis. Care should be taken to properly process and stain the specimen to avoid misinterpreting the staining characteristics.

Initial Therapy

Initial therapy is guided by knowledge of the likely pathogens in a given clinical situation, the usual suspected organism, and the clinical condition of the patient. For most community-acquired infections, resistant organisms are unusual, and therapy can be directed against the most common offending pathogens. For example, in community-acquired bacterial pneumonia, *S. pneumoniae* is by far the most prevalent pathogen. In a patient with a history of alcoholism, anaerobes from aspiration and gram-negative bacilli may also be etiologic organisms. If the sputum demonstrates intracellular gram-positive diplococci (pneumococcus) and an abundance of polymorphonuclear leukocytes, penicillin would be adequate initial therapy after blood and sputum cultures are obtained. If the sputum Gram's stain does not reveal a predominant organism a broader-spectrum regimen could be employed, such as ampicillin, cefoxitin, or cefuroxime, to adequately cover pneumococci, anaerobes, and *Haemophilus* organisms.

In a patient with suspected cellulitis, initial therapy with a penicillinase-stable penicillin, such as nafcillin, would be effective against staphylococci and streptococci, which are the most common pathogens encountered in this setting. However, if the cutaneous infection was acquired in the hospital, where the prevalence of methicillin-resistant staphylococcal infections is high, vancomycin should be employed. If the patient is a diabetic and the Gram's stain of the margins of the involved area suggests the presence of gram-negative pathogens or anaerobes a broader-spectrum antibiotic, such as cefoxitin, would be appropriate.

In patients with evidence of systemic toxicity or sepsis from nosocomial infection, empiric therapy should include coverage for an even broader range of organisms, depending on the suspected source of the infection, including methicillin-resistant staphylococci, resistant gram-negative bacilli, anaerobes, and in some settings even *pseudomonas* species. Appropriate antibiotic regimens in this situation could include vancomycin, an antipseudomonal penicillin, and an aminoglycoside.

Definitive Therapy

Definitive therapy, specifically directed against the known pathogen or pathogens, should be instituted immediately after diagnosis. A single antimicrobial agent should be used whenever possible to minimize the potential for toxicity and the cost of treatment. If the patient has been receiving initial therapy with a combination of drugs, all drugs not active against the diagnosed organism should be discontinued unless there is reason to suspect polymicrobial infection.

Parenteral therapy is preferable for initial treatment of serious infections. Oral therapy can be implemented after clinical improvement is evident if adequate serum levels of bactericidal antibiotics can be obtained. Oral therapy is preferable for minor infections.

The duration of therapy is dictated by the site and severity of infection, the clinical response of the patient to the drug, and the likelihood of cure after a given time interval. Most documented cutaneous infections in normal hosts require at least 5 days of therapy. Bacteremic infections, pneumonias, genitourinary infections, and other serious deep tissue infections require more than 1 week of therapy. Infections in poorly perfused areas, such as osteomyelitis, or vascular endothelial infections, such as endocarditis, usually require 4 to 6 weeks of treatment with parenteral antibiotics. Infections in immunocompromised patients are treated with longer courses of therapy than would be necessary in immunocompetent hosts.

Lack of Response

The response to antibacterial therapy should be carefully monitored. Lack of improvement could indicate the following:

1. Failure of the drug to kill the infecting organism.

2. Presence of localized infection in poorly perfused areas of abscesses that require surgical drainage.

3. Emergence of resistant organisms.

4. Superinfection.

If the patient fails to respond as expected a careful physical examination should be performed and appropriate specimens obtained. The patient's record should be reviewed to ensure that the drug has actually been administered as prescribed, and the dosage schedule should be re-evaluated. If infection is suspected as the cause of clinical deterioration antimicrobial coverage may need to be broadened, as in empiric treatment of de novo infection, until culture results and sensitivities are available. Occult sources of infection, such as infected intravascular catheter sites, wound infections, decubitus ulcers, and other nosocomial infections, should be systematically evaluated.

Prophylactic Therapy

Prophylactic antimicrobial regimens are employed to prevent the development of infection in situations in which the patient is deemed at risk. Prophylaxis is used in a variety of settings, including the prevention of contagious infectious disease in travelers to areas where infection is endemic, in contacts of persons with infectious diseases at risk for infection, and in persons with valvular heart disease undergoing procedures with a risk of transient bacteremia. However, it is in the prevention of surgical wound infections that prophylaxis is most commonly applied in podiatric medicine (Table 10–2). The risk of developing a surgical wound infection is determined by three main factors: (1) the amount and type of wound contamination, (2) the condition of the wound at the end of the operation, and (3) the susceptibility of the host.

Table 10–2. PREVENTION OF WOUND INFECTION AND SEPSIS IN SURGICAL PATIENTS

Nature of Surgery	Likely Pathogen	Recommended Drug	Preoperative Dosage
		Clean	
Orthopedic: joint implants, internal fixation	*Staphylococcus aureus, S. epidermidis*	Cefazolin or vancomycin	1 g IV/IM
		Dirty	
Traumatic wound, bites	*S. aureus,* group A streptococci, oral anaerobes	Cefazolin Amoxicillin-clavulanic acid or ampicillin sulbactam	1 g q 8 h IM / IV 1 g q 8 h IM / IV

IM, Intramuscularly; IV, intravenously; q, every.

Preoperative Care

The preoperative care of the patient should include measures to minimize surface contamination at the site of the surgical wound. Minimizing the duration of the preoperative hospital stay decreases the possibility of colonization with resistant pathogens acquired in the hospital environment. Use of a preoperative surgical scrub with a broad-spectrum antimicrobial agent, such as povidone-iodine (Betadine) or chlorhexidine gluconate (Hibiclens), can minimize the possibility of contamination. Removing hair with a depilatory rather than a razor and showering with an antibacterial soap can reduce the incidence of surgical infection even when prophylactic antibiotics are not employed.

Surgical Settings

Topical antibiotic irrigation of traumatic surgical wounds is advocated by some to debride loose tissue fragments and to disinfect the wound. Systemic therapy can also reduce the incidence of infection at distant sites seeded during the surgical procedure. Antibiotic prophylaxis is indicated in five surgical settings:

1. In procedures in which the incidence of postoperative infection is unacceptably high.

2. In patients for whom the consequences of infection may be especially severe or lethal.

3. In patients who have a predisposition to developing endocarditis.

4. In patients who have diabetes mellitus and patients who have connective tissue diseases.

5. In patients receiving steroids or other immunosuppressive drugs.

Obesity, extremes of age, venous stasis, malnutrition, alcoholism, and scarring or fibrosis are conditions that may increase the risk of operative infections but that by themselves are not an indication for prophylaxis. Prophylaxis is usually recommended in patients with local inflammatory processes, including abrasions, lacerations, multiple insect bites, and dermatologic disorders.

Prior to surgery, the patient should be screened for the presence of infection at distant sites, including the respiratory tract, urinary tract, skin, and so forth. Elective procedures should be delayed until diagnosed infections are adequately treated. If the procedure cannot be delayed antimicrobial therapy for the diagnosed infection should be administered preoperatively.

Patients undergoing surgeries in which permanent implantable materials, including Silastic implants, fixation devices, stainless-steel wire, Kirschner's wires, staples, and bone grafts, are placed should receive antimicrobial prophylaxis. Fracture repairs involving internal fixation are also indications for prophylaxis. Devitalized tissues or deoxygenated wounds, such as abrasions, lacerations, and hematomas, are more susceptible to wound infections. Tourniquets also increase susceptibility. Most authorities therefore recommend prophylaxis in these settings. If the duration of the procedure is prolonged a second dose of antibiotic should be administered. If the tourniquet is deflated and then reinflated the second dose should be given before reinflation.

Prophylactic therapy should be directed toward the organisms most likely to cause infection in a given setting. An additional factor that must be considered is the expected susceptibility of the organism to antimicrobials. The most likely organism to cause postoperative infection is largely dependent on the site of the surgical procedure. For procedures involving the skin and extremities, *Staphylococcus aureus, S. epidermidis,* and streptococci account for the majority of infections, although *Salmonella* species, gram-negative enteric organisms, anaerobes, and other organisms may occasionally be etiologic factors.

Prophylactic Antibiotics

Ideal prophylactic antibiotics should be active against the most likely etiologic organisms, should be bactericidal, should penetrate bone and soft tissue in concentrations in excess of their minimal inhibitory concentrations (MICs) for potential pathogens, should have a long half-life, should be nontoxic, and should be economical. In most cases, the drug is administered parenterally 30 minutes before the procedure and continued for 24 hours. Therapy for greater than 24 hours is not warranted. For most podiatric infections, antistaphylococcal cephalosporins are the drugs of choice for prophylaxis (Table 10–3). Cefazolin has the advantage of a longer half-life than the other agents in this category. Penicillinase-resistant penicillins, including nafcillin and oxacillin, may also be given, although these agents have shorter half-lives and have little to no activity against other potential pathogens, such as gram-negative bacilli. Vancomycin is used in a patient with a history of serious penicillin allergy or when methicillin-resistant staphylococcal infection is possible.

Antibacterial Agents

Penicillins

Penicillins share a common mechanism of action, similar pharmacologic profiles, and similar toxicities. When employed as indicated, all penicillins are bactericidal by virtue of their ability to inhibit synthe-

Table 10–3. ANTIMICROBIAL PROPHYLAXIS OR TREATMENT IN SURGERY

Prophylaxis Indication

Clean surgery that involves implants and fixation devices
Patients with rheumatic heart disease, prosthetic heart valves, and other cardiac abnormalities

Timing

Single parenteral dose of an antimicrobial 30 min prior to beginning surgery or elevating the cuff

Orthopedic Surgery

Prophylactic antistaphylococcal drugs can decrease the incidence of early and late infection in prosthetic joints; decrease infection rate when fractures are treated with internal fixation

Contaminated Surgery

Compound fracture, animal or human bite, I & D; antimicrobial should be considered treatment not prophylaxis, and continued postoperatively for 5–10 days

Choice of Agent

1. Direct against most likely organism
2. Need not eradicate every potential pathogen
3. Goal is to decrease level below number needed for infection
4. For most procedures, first-generation cephalosporin (cefazolin) should be effective
5. For protracted surgery, repeat dose of first-generation drug or use second-generation cephalosporin that has extended serum half-life (cefonicid)
6. Avoid use of third-generation cephalosporins to prevent emergence of resistance to these valuable agents

I & D, Incision and drainage.

sis of the bacterial cell wall. Approximately 5% of patients who receive penicillin develop a hypersensitivity reaction. Rash, the most common manifestation of hypersensitivity, is usually self-limited when the drug is stopped but may recur with reexposure. Anaphylaxis occurs in about 1 in 10,000 patients who receive penicillin. Although prior sensitization is thought to be the etiology of this life-threatening complication, a history of prior exposure to the drug is not always obtained. The incidence of anaphylaxis is thought to be greater with parenteral administration than with oral ingestion; for this reason, oral therapy is preferable in the outpatient setting.

Penicillin V and Penicillin G

Penicillin G is the drug of choice for treating pneumococcal and most streptococcal infections. Because this drug is readily inactivated by gastric acid, penicillin V, a more stable derivative nearly equal in potency, is the preferred oral agent. Penicillin is excreted by the kidneys, and dosages should be adjusted in patients with severe impairment in renal function. Care should also be taken to avoid administering high concentrations of the potassium or sodium salt of penicillin to anephric patients. Neurotoxicity, primarily seizures, can develop in patients who receive high doses of penicillin, particularly if the meninges are inflamed.

Because most staphylococci produce penicillinase, an enzyme that inactivates penicillin by attacking the beta-lactamase ring essential to its function, penicillin should not be administered to treat infections caused by this organism. The increasing prevalence of beta-lactamase production by many gram-negative organisms, including *Haemophilus influenzae* and some *Neisseria* species, has necessitated the development of new drugs for treating these organisms.

Antistaphylococcal Penicillins

Derivatives of penicillin resistant to inactivation by beta-lactamase include methicillin, oxacillin, nafcillin, cloxacillin, and dicloxacillin. Cloxacillin and dicloxacillin were developed for oral administration and are stable in gastric acid. Nafcillin is the preferred drug for patients with renal failure because it is primarily excreted by the liver. Interstitial nephritis is associated with administration of these drugs in a small percentage of patients, although the incidence of this serious complication appears to be lower in patients receiving nafcillin than in those receiving methicillin. Even though these drugs are active against many gram-positive organisms, they should be reserved for treatment of penicillin-resistant staphylococcal infections.

EXTENDED-SPECTRUM PENICILLINS

Amino-penicillin derivatives, such as ampicillin, amoxicillin, and bacampicillin, are active against many gram-positive organisms as well as many gram-negative organisms, including *Escherichia coli, Proteus* spp. and *H. influenzae.* Amino-penicillin derivatives are therefore important agents for treatment of uncomplicated urinary tract infections, many otolaryngolic infections, and community-acquired bacterial pneumonias. Unfortunately, all agents are sensitive to beta-lactamase, and their use has been progressively limited by the increasing prevalence of this resistance factor in community-acquired isolates. Ampicillin is the most susceptible of these drugs to gastric acid and is associated with the highest incidence of rash of any of the penicillins. Ampicillin is administered four times daily, amoxicillin three times daily, and bacampicillin twice daily. Clavulanic acid and Sulbactam are new beta-lactam drugs that irreversibly bind beta-lactamase. When administered in combination with ampicillin or other beta-lactams, activity against most resistant isolates is restored.

ANTIPSEUDOMONAL PENICILLINS

Agents such as carbenicillin, ticarcillin, piperacillin, mezlocillin, and azlocillin were primarily developed for treatment of infections caused by *Pseudomonas.* Although these agents are active against many other gram-positive and gram-negative organisms, including *E. coli, Serratia* sp., *Klebsiella, Enterobacter,* and *Bacteroides fragilis,* their high cost and sensitivity to beta-lactamase limits their widespread application. In combination with an aminoglycoside, these drugs are synergistic against *Pseudomonas aeruginosa.* Anti-

pseudomonal penicillins are rarely used as a single agent for serious pseudomonal infection because resistant organisms rapidly emerge.

Cephalosporins

Similar to penicillins, cephalosporins interfere with bacterial cell-wall synthesis and are bactericidal. As a class, cephalosporins generally have longer half-lives than penicillins and are usually more expensive. Approximately 5 to 10% of patients with a history of hypersensitivity to penicillin have a similar reaction to cephalosporins. A history of rash from penicillin does not contraindicate the administration of a cephalosporin, but a history of anaphylaxis does. First-generation cephalosporins (e.g., cefazolin, cephalothin) are active against most aerobic gram-positive cocci and community-acquired gram-negative bacilli. Second-generation cephalosporins (e.g., cefoxitin, cefotetan, cefuroxime) are more active against gram-negative bacilli, including *Haemophilus* and some anaerobes, but have less activity against gram-positive cocci. Third-generation cephalosporins (e.g., ceftazidime, ceftriaxone, cefoperazone) are active against most nosocomial gram-negative bacilli. None of the cephalosporins are bactericidal against enterococcus species; in fact, enterococcal superinfections may complicate prolonged cephalosporin therapy.

Rifampin

Although rifampin is primarily used, in combination with other drugs, for the treatment of tuberculosis, it is bactericidal against many other bacterial pathogens. When employed in combination with a cephalosporin or an aminoglycoside, rifampin is effective against methicillin-resistant *S. aureus.* Rifampin's excellent tissue penetration makes it a particularly beneficial agent for soft tissue infections and metastatic abscesses caused by these pathogens. Rifampin is also indicated for prophylaxis in persons exposed to *Neisseria meningitidis* and *H. influenzae.*

Erythromycin

Erythromycin is a bacteriostatic drug that is active against many species of gram-positive organisms. Erythromycin is indicated for oral treatment of streptococcal infections in patients who are allergic to penicillin. Erythromycin is also the drug of choice for *Mycoplasma pneumoniae* and *Legionella* infections as well as many *Chlamydia* and *Campylobacter* infections. Erythromycin often produces gastrointestinal distress when given orally. Parenteral formulations are available, but intravenous administration is frequently accompanied by painful phlebitis.

Tetracyclines

Tetracyclines are inexpensive bacteriostatic drugs that are effective against a wide variety of organisms. Because many organisms are highly resistant, tetracyclines are not usually indicated for serious infections. Tetracyclines are most often prescribed for treatment of chlamydial infections, for prophylaxis of traveler's diarrhea, and for treatment of bacterial bronchitis in patients with chronic lung diseases. Doxycycline is a tetracycline derivative with the advantage of twice-a-day (b.i.d.) dosing. Divalent cations interfere with the intestinal absorption of both tetracycline and doxycycline. Tetracyclines are contraindicated in pregnant women, nursing mothers, and children less than 8 years of age because they are taken up by dental enamel and cause brown discoloration of teeth. Photosensitization to tetracyclines is not uncommon.

Sulfonamides

Sulfonamides are active against a wide array of gram-positive and gram-negative pathogens. Sulfonamides are often additive and sometimes synergistic in combination with other agents. Trimethoprim in combination with sulfamethoxazole is effective against beta-lactamase–producing strains of *H. influenzae*. Because trimethoprim and sulfamethoxazole act at different sites, resistance to this combination is unusual. Sulfonamides are often provided orally for treatment of uncomplicated urinary tract infection. Trimethoprim-sulfamethoxazole is currently the treatment of choice for *Pneumocystis carinii* infection. Allergic reactions, including rash; urticaria; photodermatitis; erythema multiforme; and blood dyscrasias are side effects associated with sulfonamides.

Metronidazole

Metronidazole is indicated for treating *Trichomonas* infection. Metronidazole is also prescribed with increasing frequency for parenteral treatment of serious anaerobic infections produced by gram-negative anaerobes, especially *Bacteroides* spp. Metronidazole penetrates the central nervous system and is efficacious for treating anaerobic brain abscesses. With the exception of disulfiram-like reactions following alcohol consumption, few side effects are associated with metronidazole. Metronidazole is contraindicated in pregnant women.

Clindamycin

Clindamycin is effective against nearly all gram-positive bacteria and most anaerobes, including *Bacteroides*. Clindamycin is bacteriostatic and occupies the same bacterial ribosomal site as erythromycin and chloramphenicol. Therefore when used in combination, these drugs may be antagonistic. Clindamycin is associated with pseudomembranous colitis in a small number of patients. Clindamycin does not cross the blood-brain barrier well.

Chloramphenicol

Chloramphenicol is a broad-spectrum bacteriostatic drug. Chloramphenicol is effective against many anaerobes, including *Bacteroides*, as well as *H. influenzae*. Chloramphenicol crosses the blood-brain barrier well and was the drug of choice for *Haemophilus influenzae* meningitis resistant to ampicillin until the newer third-generation cephalosporins became available. Chloramphenicol is associated with reversible bone marrow suppression and should be discontinued if the white blood cell count decreases to less than $3000/mm^3$. In a small number of patients, the bone marrow suppression is complete and irreversible. For this reason, chloramphenicol is reserved for life-threatening infections resistant to safer antibiotics.

Aminoglycosides

Aminoglycosides are a unique class of antimicrobial agents with a complicated mechanism of action. Aminoglycosides

Table 10–4. ANTIMICROBIAL DRUGS OF CHOICE IN CLINICAL PODIATRY

Infecting Organism	Drug of Choice	Alternative Drugs
Gram-positive Cocci		
Staphylococcus aureus or Staphylococcus epidermidis	Penicillin G or V	First-generation cephalosporins, vancomycin, imipenem, clindamycin
Penicillinase-producing	Cloxicillin or dicloxicillin, methicillin, nafcillin, oxacillin	First-generation cephalosporins, vancomycin, imipenem, clindamycin, amoxicillin-clavulanic acid, ticarcillin-clavulanic acid
Methicillin-resistant	Vancomycin, with or without rifampin, gentamicin, or a combination	Trimethoprim-sulfamethoxazole
Streptococcus pyogenes (Groups A, B, C, G, nonenterococcal group D)	Penicillin G or V	Erythromycin, cephalosporin, vancomycin
Streptococcus viridans	Penicillin G with or without streptomycin or gentamicin	Cephalosporin, vancomycin
Streptococcus faecalis, Streptococcus faecium	Ampicillin or penicillin G with streptomycin	Vancomycin and streptomycin
Streptococcus anaerobes (Peptostreptococcus)	Penicillin G	Clindamycin, chloramphenicol, a first-generation cephalosporin
Gram-negative Cocci		
Neisseria gonorrhea (gonococcus)	Amoxicillin (with probenicid) or ceftriaxone	Penicillin G, ampicillin, cefoxitin, spectinomycin, trimethoprim-sulfamethoxazole, chloramphenicol
Gram-positive Bacilli		
Clostridium perfringens*	Penicillin G, metronidazole	Clindamycin, chloramphenicol
Clostridium difficile	Vancomycin (oral)	Metronidazole, bacitracin
Clostridium tetani†	Penicillin G	Tetracycline
Corynebacterium diphtheriae‡	Erythromycin	Penicillin G
Listeria monocytogenes	Ampicillin with or without gentamicin	Penicillin, trimethoprim-sulfamethoxazole
Enteric Gram-negative Bacilli		
Bacteroides		
Propharyngeal strains	Penicillin G or clindamycin	Cefoxitin, metronidazole
Gastrointestinal strain	Clindamycin or metronidazole	Cefoxitin, imipenem, mezlocillin, ticarcillin, or piperacillin
Campylobacter fetus, subsp jejuni	Erythromycin	Tetracycline or doxycycline
Enterobacter	Cefotaxime, ceftizoxime, ceftazidime	Gentamicin, tobramycin, netilmicin, amikacin, carbenicillin, ticarcillin, piperacillin, imipenem, trimethoprim-sulfamethoxazole, chloramphenicol
Escherichia coli	Ampicillin with or without gentamicin, tobramycin, netilmicin, or amikacin	Second- and third-generation cephalosporin, carbenicillin, ticarcillin, mezlocillin, piperacillin, or azlocillin; gentamicin, tobramycin, netilmicin, or amikacin; amoxicillin-clavulanic acid; imipenem; ticarcillin-clavulanic acid; tetracycline; chloramphenicol

Table 10–4. (continued)

Infecting Organism	Drug of Choice	Alternative Drugs
Klebsiella pneumoniae	A cephalosporin	Gentamicin, tobramycin, netilmicin, or amikacin; amoxicillin-clavulanic acid; imipenem; ticarcillin-clavulanic acid; tetracycline; chloramphenicol, mezlocillin, piperacillin, trimethoprim-sulfamethoxazole
Proteus mirabilis	Ampicillin	A cephalosporin, carbenicillin, ticarcillin, mezlocillin, piperacillin, or azlocillin; gentamicin, tobramycin, netilmicin, or amikacin; chloramphenicol, imipenem, trimethoprim-sulfamethoxazole
Proteus vulgaris (indole-positive)	Third-generation cephalosporin cefotaxime, ceftizoxime, or ceftriaxone	Gentamicin, tobramycin, netilmicin, or amikacin; carbenicillin, mezlocillin, piperacillin, ticarcillin, or azlocillin; amoxicillin-clavulanic acid; imipenem; ticarcillin-clavulanic acid; chloramphenicol, a tetracycline; trimethoprim-sulfamethoxazole
Serratia	Third-generation cephalosporin cefotaxime, ceftizoxime, or ceftriaxone	Gentamicin or amikacin; imipenem; carbenicillin, mezlocillin, ticarcillin, piperacillin or azlocillin; cefoxitin; trimethoprim-sulfamethoxazole
Shigella	Trimethoprim-sulfamethoxazole	Tetracycline, chloramphenicol, ampicillin

Other Gram-negative Bacilli

Acinetobacter	Imipenem	Amikacin; doxycycline, minocycline
Pseudomonas aeruginosa	Carbenicillin, ticarcillin, mezlocillin, piperacillin, or azlocillin plus tobramycin, gentamicin, or amikacin, third-generation antipseud cephalosporin plus aminoglycoside	Imipenem

Acid-fast Bacilli

Mycobacterium tuberculosis	Isoniazid, rifampin, ethambutol and pyrazinamide	Ethambutol, streptomycin, pyrazinamide, capreomycin, para-aminosalicylic acid (PAS), ethionamide, cycloserine
Mycobacterium leprae (leprosy)	Dapsone with or without clofazimine	Acedapsone, ethionamide, propionamide

Actinomycetes

Actinomyces israelii (actinomycosis)	Penicillin G	A tetracycline

* Debride first, large doses of penicillin G, hyperbaric chamber in spreading necrotic type.
† Prophylaxis: tetanus toxoid booster. Some patients require human tetanus immune globulin.
‡ Antitoxin is primary; antimicrobials halt only further toxin production and prevent carrier state.

disrupt the cell membrane by poorly understood mechanisms and also interfere with protein synthesis. Because they require oxidative transport to gain entry into bacteria, aminoglycosides are only active against aerobes. Activity of aminoglycosides is decreased in an acidic environment; these agents are therefore less active for treatment of suppurative infections. Aminoglycosides are often used in combination with a beta-lactam for treatment of serious gram-negative and gram-positive aerobic infections.

Streptomycin is administered primarily in combination with other drugs for treatment of endocarditis and tuberculosis. Gentamicin is employed for serious infections caused by gram-negative enteric organisms and is employed in combination with a semisynthetic penicillin for treatment of *Pseudomonas* infection. Tobramycin is similar to gentamicin, although many strains of *Pseudomonas* are more sensitive to tobramycin. Amikacin is reserved for organisms resistant to the other, less expensive aminoglycosides (Table 10–4).

In general, aminoglycosides penetrate the central nervous system poorly. All aminoglycosides are ototoxic and nephrotoxic. Dosage should be carefully adjusted, and peak and trough drug levels should be monitored during therapy. Renal function, including creatinine clearance level, should be measured at the onset of treatment. Periodic determinations of blood urea nitrogen (BUN), and creatinine levels should be made. If prolonged therapy is anticipated audiometry should also be performed.

ASSESSMENT OF PODIATRIC INFECTIOUS DISEASES

Osteomyelitis

Osteomyelitis is an acute, a subacute, or a chronic infection of the bone commonly encountered in podiatric practice. Bone infection can be caused by a variety of pathogens, including bacteria, mycobacteria, and fungi. Effective treatment of this condition requires prompt diagnosis, prolonged antimicrobial therapy, and often surgical intervention.

Pathophysiology

Acute hematogenous osteomyelitis is thought to be initiated when the involved organism is localized to the metaphyseal arterioles. Because these vessels terminate in large sinusoidal veins at the growth plate, thrombosis readily occurs, which promotes bacterial proliferation. A history of trauma to the involved area is elicited in about one third of cases in children. Direct trauma may promote proliferation by increasing localized thrombus formation. The resultant inflammatory process accounts for the destruction of trabeculae and further thromboses. Infection propagates through haversian and Volkmann's channels to adjacent bone. Isolated units of demineralized dead bone appear radiographically as sequestra. As the infection progresses across the cortex to the periosteal surface, localized areas of radiolucency known as cloacae appear. Inflammation stimulates periosteal growth or involucrum formation. In chronic osteomyelitis, Brodie's abscess, typified by chronic suppuration surrounded by dense fibrous tissue and sclerosis, is often evident.

The age of the patient influences the site and progression of osteomyelitis. In infants, the metaphyseal arterioles perforate the growth plate. Infection can then readily extend into the epiphysis and joint space, resulting in irreversible damage to these structures. Growth inhibition, disorganized growth, and joint damage often occur in this setting even when appropriate treatment is instituted.

The cortex of the shaft of long bones is uniquely predisposed to osteomyelitis in children and produces conspicuous involucrum on radiographs. Permanent damage to the growth plate is less common. However, infection may extend into the hip, shoulder, and ankle joints in older children because the metaphyses of the involved bones remain intra-articular. Acute hematogenous osteomyelitis is uncommon in adults less than 50 years of age. Intravenous drug users are predisposed to infections with staphylococci, *Pseudomonas*, and rarely other enteric pathogens. The axial skeleton and small bones of the wrist and ankle are most commonly involved. Infection may extend to the joint or through the marrow, resulting in chronic osteomyelitis of the entire bone. Involucrum formation and cortical sequestration are less common in adults than in children.

Relative deficiency of phagocytic function in the metaphyseal region is an additional factor that promotes bacterial localization. In patients with sickle-cell disease, impaired phagocytic function more commonly results in medullary diaphyseal infections.

Hematogenous Osteomyelitis. Hematogenous osteomyelitis can follow bacteremic infections from a variety of sites. *Staphylococcus aureus* is the most common offending organism in all age groups, and osteomyelitis is usually due to seeding from a primary suppurative focus, such as abscess, furuncle, paronychia, skin abrasion, or infected heart valve. A primary focus may not be evident at the time of diagnosis. Upper respiratory infections, otitis media, tonsillitis, urinary tract infections, and other primary foci can also be complicated by osteomyelitis. *Hemophilus influenzae* is the second most common pathogen in children less than 2 years old. Patients with sickle-cell disease are predisposed to *Salmonella* osteomyelitis.

Endogenous Osteomyelitis. Endogenous osteomyelitis accounts for more than 50% of all cases of osteomyelitis. Contiguous spread from overlying cutaneous infections is the most common mechanism of infection, followed by direct implantation from puncture wounds or intraoperative contamination. Diabetic ulcerations predispose patients to mixed aerobic and anaerobic osteomyelitis, particularly if vascular insufficiency is present. Burns, hematoma, trauma, and postoperative wound infections are also associated with endogenous osteomyelitis. In addition to staphylococci, a variety of pathogens, including enterococci, group B streptococci, *Pseudomonas*, *E. coli*, and *Candida albicans*, can be isolated.

Chronic Osteomyelitis. Chronic osteomyelitis is associated with sequestrum formation and poor revascularization of infected bone. Impaired host defenses, trauma, and inadequate antibiotic treatment promote the development of chronic osteomyelitis. Occasionally, the etiologic organism is slow growing or of low virulence. Phalanges and metatarsal heads are frequently involved in chronic osteomyelitis. *Staphylococcus aureus* is the most common pathogen in this condition, most

likely because the majority of cases follow acute hematogenous osteomyelitis.

Clinical Presentation and Diagnosis

Prompt diagnosis of osteomyelitis is essential. If treatment is instituted within 72 hours of the onset of symptoms serious sequelae are unusual. In children, symptoms and signs localized to the involved area are common. Warmth over the site of infection; swelling, particularly if suppuration has extended beyond the periosteum; tenderness to palpation; and pseudoparalysis or altered gait suggest the diagnosis. Fever may also be present. Symptoms (e.g., skin infection, otitis media, or tonsillitis) may also suggest the primary focus of hematogenous osteomyelitis. In diabetics with sensory neuropathy, the infection may be entirely asymptomatic. The peripheral white blood cell count is elevated in a minority of patients, but the ESR is usually elevated, especially if the duration of infection is prolonged. Radiographs are usually normal early in the course of infection. The earliest changes on radiograph include localized radiolucency 10 to 14 days after the onset of symptoms, followed by sequestrum, cloaca, and involucrum.

Bone scans are often helpful in diagnosing osteomyelitis. Reactive bone formation surrounding the area of infection produces localized increased uptake. Technetium 99 is the most frequently used nucleotide to establish an early diagnosis. Imaging is performed 3 hours after the dose, and the tracer is renally excreted with a half-life of 6 hours. Gallium 67 can also be used, although imaging is delayed to 48 to 72 hours after dosing to allow time for uptake of the tracer by leukocytes in the region of inflammation. Resolution of bone detail is less with gallium than with technetium. Gallium scanning is theoretically helpful in following the response to therapy since uptake decreases as inflammation resolves. In practice, both gallium and technetium scans can remain positive long after bacteriologic cure because of continued vascular proliferation and bone repair.

Nucleotide scans cannot establish a diagnosis of osteomyelitis with certainty. False-positive results occur with aborted bone infections, overlying cellulitis, and other localized inflammatory conditions. Scanning does not distinguish bone repair from bone inflammation. False-negative results occur in areas of poor perfusion, that is, poor uptake due to necrosis or sequestration. Because of the limitations of bone scanning and other noninvasive studies and the importance of defining the etiologic agent with accuracy, it is essential to obtain bacteriologic confirmation of infection as soon as possible. Because treatment for osteomyelitis is prolonged, exact microbiologic diagnosis is required. Blood cultures should be obtained, and results are more likely to be positive if the primary focus of infection is still evident. Local wound or transcutaneous cultures are unreliable. Even cultures from sinus tracts correlate poorly with the actual causative agent.

Bone cultures should be obtained under sterile conditions through an incision made away from overlying cutaneous infection. Cultures should be processed to allow diagnosis of aerobic and anaerobic bacteria, mycobacteria, and fungi. An intraoperative Gram's stain is often helpful in documenting the suitability of the culture specimen and in suggesting the likely organism so that empiric therapy can be instituted.

Treatment

The appropriate treatment of bacterial osteomyelitis remains controversial. Parenteral antimicrobial therapy with bactericidal drugs alone for 4 to 6 weeks is adequate in some cases, particularly if suppuration and abscess formation are limited and the duration of symptoms prior to diagnosis is short. If a clinical response is not apparent after 48 hours surgical debridement is indicated. A more prolonged trial of antimicrobial therapy may be appropriate if surgical intervention would result in functional disability or neurologic sequelae. Surgical debridement is thought to promote bacteriologic cure and to improve the time to resolution by removing suppuration and necrotic tissue. Most surgeons attempt to remove all of the infected bone tissue when feasible. The appropriate management of contiguous joint infections is debatable. Disarticulation is advocated by most practitioners since the preservation of the cartilaginous surfaces may impede spread to contiguous bone. The wound is packed open after debridement and can be irrigated for 3 to 5 days to facilitate recovery. Parenteral antibiotic therapy is indicated for at least 4 and usually 6 weeks to improve the likelihood of cure. Serial radiographs, gallium scans, and erythrocyte sedimentation rates (ESR) are often helpful in following the resolution of the infection. Peripheral demineralization frequently occurs in the postoperative period owing to osteoclast activation. However, the formation of new sequestra, cloacae, or involucra is evidence of continued infection and mandates evaluation. Delayed primary closure or grafting is performed after complete bacteriologic cure.

Septic Arthritis

Pathophysiology

Septic arthritis is a serious condition with a high potential for complication if it is not recognized and managed appropriately. This condition most commonly occurs in infants and children. Hematogenous infections, associated with bacteremia, account for the vast majority of cases. Contiguous spread from an adjacent osteomyelitis or soft tissue infection and direct penetrating injuries are other mechanisms of infection. Predisposing factors in adults include previous joint damage, underlying debilitating disease, and immunosuppression.

Narcotic addicts are predisposed to infections with unusual organisms, including *Serratia* and *Pseudomonas*. *Staphylococcus aureus* is the most common etiologic organism in all age groups. *Haemophilus influenzae* is the second most common organism, seen in children less than 2 years of age. In sexually active teenagers and young adults, *Neisseria gonorrhea* is a common isolate. In older adults, Enterobacteriaceae and *Pseudomonas* predominate.

Hematogenous infection involves the synovial membrane first and then extends into the joint cavity to underlying bone. Mycobacteria and fungi usually remain confined to the synovial surface. Proteolytic enzymes released by bacteria and inflammatory cells and increased intra-articular pressure combine to produce damage to the articular surface.

Clinical Presentation and Diagnosis

Localized monarticular pain, tenderness, erythema, and swelling are common presenting complaints. The knee, hip, shoulder, and elbow are the most commonly involved joints. A joint effusion may be evident. Joint immobility, pseudoparalysis, and altered gait may be seen. In young children, the symptoms and signs may be indistinguishable from those of osteomyelitis. Fever is usually associated with suppurative septic arthritis but is not a universal finding. Acute onset of symptoms is typical in bacterial septic arthritis. A more insidious presentation and a chronic indolent course suggest mycobacterial or fungal infection.

Laboratory studies may reveal an elevated peripheral white blood cell count, with an increase in immature forms. The ESR is usually elevated. Radiographs may appear normal but often demonstrate soft tissue swelling and joint effusion. Loss of subchondral bone with preservation of underlying trabeculae is strongly suggestive of septic arthritis and argues against osteomyelitis. Blood cultures should always be performed. Joint aspiration is essential for diagnosis. Aspiration should be performed with strict attention to aseptic technique because organisms can readily be introduced into the joint if sterile procedure is violated. The joint fluid should be visually inspected and analyzed for protein content, cell count and differential, presence of crystals, viscosity, and glucose. A Gram's stain should be immediately performed to help guide empiric treatment. A negative Gram's stain in a sexually active adult with an inflammatory synovial aspirate strongly suggests the diagnosis of disseminated gonorrhea. Appropriate cultures to diagnose bacteria, mycobacteria, and fungi should be performed.

Treatment

Parenteral antimicrobial therapy should be implemented after cultures have been obtained. The duration of therapy is controversial and varies with the etiologic organism, the pre-existing status of the joint, and the host's defense mechanisms. Most gram-negative infections are treated for 6 weeks with bactericidal drugs. Infection caused by gonorrhea responds rapidly to treatment and can be treated with 3 to 5 days of parenteral therapy, followed by an additional course of oral therapy for 10 days. Staphylococcal and enterococcal infections are usually cured after 4 weeks of parenteral treatment. In most cases, streptococcal and pneumococcal infections respond to 2 weeks of parenteral treatment.

Adequate drainage of purulent synovial fluid is an important adjuvant to antibiotic treatment. Aspiration may be required as often as two times a day during the early stages of infection. Sequential synovial fluid analysis is helpful in monitoring the response to therapy. In a child with suppurative hip joint infection, open drainage is required to prevent vascular compromise and avascular necrosis of the femoral capital epiphysis. Open drainage is also indicated if serial aspirations do not effectively remove the inflammatory fluid or if loculation and sequestration occur. In previously damaged joints, synovectomy and arthrodesis are frequently required to effect cure. Prosthetic devices present in the involved joint must be removed.

Immobilization is recommended in the acute phases of infection but is not recommended for prolonged periods. Passive range of motion exercises should begin as soon as improvement is evident, but weight bearing is contraindicated until all evidence of inflammation has resolved.

Infection in the Surgical Patient

Infectious diseases continue to present a challenge in surgical practice despite the availability of a multitude of antimicrobial agents and the increasing emphasis on sterile procedures. A surgical infection is an infection that has developed before or as a complication of surgical treatment. Preoperative surgical infections include all infections in which the involved pathogen colonized or infected the host prior to surgical intervention. Intraoperative surgical infections are those in which the pathogen gains access to the body as a direct result of the operative procedure. Preventable intraoperative infections are iatrogenic infections caused by errors in sterile technique or in surgical practice. Nonpreventable intraoperative infections occur when seeding from an infected or a colonized site in the body or from contaminated air currents produces infection despite acceptable surgical practice. Postoperative infections are complications of the surgical procedure or the postoperative management of the patient.

Pulmonary Complications

Fever early in the postoperative period in a patient who was uninfected prior to surgery is frequently due to pulmonary complications. Atelectasis accounts for up to 90% of postoperative pulmonary complications and is nearly ubiquitous after upper abdominal or chest surgery. A variety of factors contribute to atelectasis, including poor inspiratory effort; bronchial obstruction from secretions, blood, and tissue; and decreased surfactant. Factors predisposing the patient to atelectasis include a history of smoking, pre-existing pulmonary disease, decreased cough reflex from anesthesia, postoperative sedation or narcotic analgesia, and obesity. Aspiration of saliva, blood, and gastric contents may also produce fever.

Pneumonia may complicate either aspiration or atelectasis and is suggested by the presence of enlarging infiltrates on chest radiograph and purulent sputum. Anaerobes are the most common etiologic agents, but gram-negative organisms such as *E. coli*, *Pseudomonas*, and *S. aureus* are frequently isolated from debilitated patients and patients with prolonged mechanical ventilation. Early ambulation and pulmonary toilet are advocated to minimize the incidence of postoperative pulmonary complications.

Urinary Tract Infection

Urinary tract infection may also produce fever in the first few days following surgery. Pre-existing cystitis and catheterization are important contributing factors. Elective surgery should be delayed until the urine is sterile whenever possible, and the duration of catheterization should be minimized. Gram-negative enteric organisms and enterococci are the usual organisms isolated from infected urine. If urinary tract infection is suspected as a source of fever parenteral antimicrobial therapy should be promptly implemented after blood and urine cultures are obtained. Catheters should be removed to improve the likelihood of rapid resolution.

Wound Infection

When fever occurs 4 or more days after surgery, wound infection is a probable source. The incidence of wound infection is dependent on the nature of the wound. Clean atraumatic surgical wounds are least likely to become infected unless the gastrointestinal, respiratory, or genitourinary tract was entered. The incidence of infection is increased if the procedure was emergent, if the wound was not primarily closed, or if mechanical drainage was necessary. Traumatic wounds, procedures involving inflamed tissue, and breaks in aseptic technique increase the risk of infection considerably. The highest infection rates are encountered with traumatic wounds and during procedures involving foci of purulent material, abscesses, and perforated viscera.

The status of host defenses also influences infection rates. Important variables include age of the patient; underlying medical conditions, such as diabetes mellitus or malignancy; nutrition; and steroid therapy.

Wounds should be completely uncovered and carefully inspected at regular intervals. Localized pain and tenderness on palpation, erythema, and edema may be apparent. In some cases, a palpable abscess is present. *Staphylococcus aureus* is the most common organism isolated from infected wounds. Gram-negative enteric pathogens may also be isolated, particularly after bowel surgery. Streptococcal and enterococcal infections are less common. If the infection is localized treatment consists of opening the wound, removing cutaneous suture material, and irrigating with sterile saline. Light packing is also usually recommended. Cultures and Gram's stain should be obtained. If the patient has evidence of sepsis, spreading cellulitis, or significant impairment of host defenses (e.g., neutropenia) parenteral antibacterial therapy should be instituted. Surgery may be essential for more severe infections. Antibiotics are also recommended for hemolytic streptococcal infections.

Other Causes of Fever

Other causes of fever in the postoperative period should also be considered. Intravenous catheter sites should be carefully inspected. Localized erythema, edema, and palpable thrombi should prompt an evaluation for septic thrombophlebitis and bacteremia. Sinusitis, otitis media, and bacterial parotitis are unusual postoperative infections that may be overlooked unless a careful history and examination are performed. Intra-abdominal abscess, infected hematoma, and infection of other fluid collections should be considered if the operative history is suggestive. Noninfectious causes of fever may also occur. Pulmonary embolism and drug fever are important causes in the late postoperative period. Finally, albeit rare in postoperative patients, factitious fever should be considered when all other sources have been carefully excluded.

ACQUIRED IMMUNE DEFICIENCY SYNDROME

Acquired immune deficiency syndrome (AIDS) was first recognized in 1981. In less than 2 years, HIV, the etiologic agent of AIDS, was first isolated. Since that time, the spectrum of diseases associated with this pathogen has been expanded to include the diseases treated in almost every medical discipline.

Epidemiology and Transmission

Human immunodeficiency virus is known to be transmitted parenterally during inoculation with infected blood or blood products, sexually during contact with an infected partner, and perinatally to children born to infected women. The virus is not transmitted by casual contact in any environment, by the airborne route, by fomites, or by insects, despite the fact that HIV has been isolated from nearly all body fluids. Blood and semen contain the highest concentrations of virus in most patients. Although HIV can also rarely be detected in saliva, urine, cerebrospinal fluid, tears, breast milk, and cervical/vaginal secretions, the titer of virus present in these fluids is low.

Occupational Transmission of Human Immunodeficiency Virus to Health Care Providers

A small number of health care workers with occupational exposure to blood containing HIV have been infected. The magnitude of risk to health care workers' sustaining accidental needlesticks or other parenteral exposures to the virus is much less than 1% and is at least an order of magnitude less than the risk from similar exposure to hepatitis B virus. Occupational transmission of HIV can be prevented by following infection-control precautions designed to reduce direct contact with blood and body fluids (Table 10–5). The Centers for Disease Control (CDC) recommends utilizing these precautions for all patients since it is not possible to know with certainty, even when screening tests are employed, which patients are infected with transmissible blood-borne pathogens. These precautions include handwashing before and after contact with each patient, wearing gowns or other protective garments when clothing is likely to be soiled with bloody fluids, and wearing masks and protective eyewear when splatter of body fluids is anticipated. Needles and other sharp instruments should be handled safely and disposed of in impervious containers. Needles should never be bent, broken, recapped, or manipulated in any way prior to disposal. Double-gloving is recommended for all operative procedures. Face shields and waterproof garments should be worn when uncontrolled arterial bleeding, bone manipulations, or similar procedures associated with a high risk of blood exposure are performed.

Pathophysiology

Human immunodeficiency virus produces progressive immunodeficiency by selective destruction of a subpopulation of T lymphocytes or helper cells. The virus is a group D retrovirus, which binds to receptors on the surface of susceptible T cells (CD_4 receptors) and is taken up by the cells. After entry, the virus envelope is removed and the viral RNA genome is copied by a unique enzyme, reverse transcrip-

Table 10–5. RECOMMENDED PRECAUTIONS FOR HEPATITIS OR HIV INFECTION
FOR THE PODIATRIST

1. *Wash hands* with an antimicrobial solution that has residual activity before and after contact with *each* patient. Wash hands before and after removing gloves and after sterilizing and disinfecting. End with a cool water wash to close skin pores.
2. Cuts and sores on hands should always *be covered.* Consider double gloving or putting finger cots on a digit before gloving. Keep hands away from eyes, nose, mouth, and hair. Never touch or scratch pimples, cuts, sores, and any open lesions.
3. Jewelry should be removed during patient-contact hours in clinic and on hospital floor and in the perioperative environment. Watches should be completely covered by gloves if worn while giving direct contact care, such as sanding corns, burring nails, and so on.
4. *Wear gloves* during *direct contact* with blood and all other body fluids, when cleaning instruments and environmental surfaces, and when handling specimens. Do not touch unrelated surfaces with contaminated gloves (clean counters, instruments, phone, and so on.)
5. For environmental control of surfaces, counter, walls, chairs, wipe with *benzalkonium chloride* (1:750 or 1:1000).Benzalkonium chloride controls gram-positive organisms, fungi, some but not all viruses; it can support growth of gram-negative organisms). It controls HIV but not HBV. *Glutaraldehyde* or *dilute bleach* may also be used.
6. Use covers of plastic or plasticized paper, which serve as barriers and extra infection-control protection, when doing a procedure that may involve blood, body fluids, or both.
7. Gloves (*latex* and *vinyl* are both effective protective barriers) worn for patient care *should be discarded* after each use.
8. Wear *gowns* or other protective garments when clothing is likely to be soiled with bloody fluids. Garments should not be worn home, to reduce cross-contamination. Wash garments in hot soapy water with bleach.
9. Use *mask* and *protective eyewear* when aerosolization (e.g., nail grinding, sanding hyperkeratotic tissue or nails, and drilling in surgery) or splatter of body fluids is anticipated. *Use vacuum suction when available.*
10. *Face masks* should cover the nose and mouth and should be *discarded when dirty or moist* and after patient treatment that generated a water aerosol spray. If mask is worn between patients do not touch with clean hands and take care to prevent cross-contamination.
11. *Protective eyewear* should be disinfected in active gluteraldehyde solution after each patient.
12. *Decontamination and sterilization of instruments* involves the initial critical step of cleaning with physical removal of oils and protein matter. Smooth instruments used only on the dermis may be wiped clean with alcohol wipes and placed in low-level benzalkonium (1:750 or 1:1000) with rust retardant added, which controls HIV but not gram-negative organisms or HBV.
13. Instruments contaminated with blood or drainage require steam sterilization or terminal disinfection, which is accomplished with a *high-level cold disinfectant* (tuberculocidal and viricidal), such as *glutaraldehyde*, which is reusable for up to 14 days. Instruments must be rinsed well with sterile water before using.
14. When using a *bead sterilizer*, if one must be used as an alternative to terminal sterilization methods, the instrument must be physically cleaned with a wipe (e.g., alcohol) before the tip is immersed in the beads. The sterilizer, operating at 450°F will sterilize in 10–12 seconds.
15. *Syringes, needles, blades,* and *other sharp instruments* should be handled safely and disposed of in impervious containers.
16. *Needles* should *never* be *bent, broken, recapped,* or *manipulated* in any way prior to disposal.
17. *Puncture-proof boxes* should be placed close to the site of use in each examination room. Needle clippers *should not* be used because they cause splatter. Dispose of container before it is full.
18. *Sharp instrument* or *needle punctures* must be cared for immediately. Cleanse wound with a skin antiseptic (iodine product or 79% alcohol) and cover with a bandage or dressing to protect from further injury or contamination. Further immunization management depends on patient status and risk and health worker's status.
19. *Single-dosage vials* are recommended over multi-dosage vials to avoid inadvertent contamination of multi-dosage vials.
20. *Sharp instrument* or *needle punctures* must be reported immediately to a clinician; an incident report must be initiated and then completed by a podiatrist, general physician, or nurse practitioner after treatment has been rendered.
21. *Resuscitation* should be performed using a self-inflating resuscitation device or a two-way device that affords protection to the resuscitator.
22. *Vaccination* may not be appropriate for everyone and must be a matter of individual choice. To help protect ourselves and patients such as the elderly and immunocompromised who are at high risk for complications from contracted diseases, the health care provider may also consider, besides the hepatitis B vaccine, pneumococcal vaccine (Pneumovax), measles vaccine, and influenza vaccine.

HBV, Hepatitis B virus; HIV, human immunodeficiency virus.

tase, to produce a DNA replicate. This DNA is then incorporated into the host cell genome, where it can remain dormant for prolonged periods of time. If the host cell is stimulated to undergo replication the viral genome is replicated along with the host DNA. At some point, viral replication is initiated, and the host cell is lysed. As the number of helper cells is gradually depleted, the cellular immune system is

Table 10–6. CDC* CLASSIFICATION OF HIV INFECTION

Classification	Disease State	Manifestations
Group I	Acute infection	Acute mononucleosis–like syndrome. Transient signs and symptoms of fever 39.4–40°C (103–104°F), macular or papular rash, malaise, diffuse transient lymphadenopathy with mild lymphocytosis or lymphopenia, occasional aseptic meningitis, and seroconversion to HIV
Group II	Asymptomatic infection	Chronically infected, serology positive, virus culture positive with no clinical manifestations, normal physical examination and laboratory test results; "latent state"
Group III	PGL	Palpable enlarged lymph nodes (>1 cm) at 2 or more extrainguinal sites persisting for more than 3 months in the absence of other cause; May have other manifestations of disease; all test results seropositive
Group IV†	Other diseases	Individuals in this group have one or more significant immunodeficiency or central nervous system disease

* CDC, Centers for Disease Control.
† See Table 10–7 for subgroups of Group IV.
HIV, Human immunodeficiency virus; PGL, persistent generalized lymphadenopathy.

irreversibly damaged. As the damage progresses, clinical evidence of cellular immunodeficiency, including reactivation of endogenous opportunistic infections and defective immunosurveillance resulting in malignancies, becomes apparent (Tables 10–6 and 10–7).

Acute Human Immunodeficiency Virus Infection

In some individuals, HIV produces an acute febrile illness 2 to 6 weeks after the initial infection. This illness is believed to correlate with the initial viremic phase of retroviral replication. High fever, diffuse lymphadenopathy, and maculopapular rash following exposure to HIV strongly

Table 10–7. CDC* SUBGROUPS OF GROUP IV HIV CLASSIFICATION

Subgroup	Manifestations
A	Constitutional signs: fever >38.5°C (101°F) for >1 month, >10% baseline weight loss, chronic diarrhea >1 month with no known cause or other current disease
B	Variety of neurologic syndromes: progressive dementia, peripheral myelopathy, peripheral neuropathy with no current disease
C	Infectious diseases indicative of defective cell-mediated immunity
D	Includes secondary cancers

* CDC, Centers for Disease Control.
HIV, Human immunodeficiency virus.

suggest the diagnosis. Splenomegaly, aseptic meningitis, headache, myalgias, and other constitutional symptoms have also been described. The duration of illness is variable but ranges from several days to a few weeks in most patients. Human immunodeficiency virus antigen (p24 antigen) can be detected in the serum during this phase of infection but may disappear as the condition resolves. Human immunodeficiency virus antibody titers are detectable somewhat later and persist, signifying the onset of the latent carrier state.

Chronic Infection

The vast majority of persons infected with HIV remain infected and potentially infectious for life. Although some persons may remain asymptomatic for long periods of time, most eventually develop clinical evidence of immunodeficiency. The risk of progression to clinical disease is higher 5 or more years after the initial infection than it is in the first 5 years. The proportion of infected patients who ultimately develop AIDS is still unknown.

Infection can be documented by measuring antibodies to HIV in the serum. These antibodies usually develop within 6 to 12 weeks after infection, though occasionally their appearance is delayed for up to 6 months. A small minority of patients may never develop measurable antibody. A variety of tests are available to measure antibody. Screening tests are usually performed utilizing a commercial enzyme-linked immunosorbent assay (ELISA) test kit. The tests currently available are extremely sensitive but not entirely specific. Therefore a confirmatory test, such as a Western blot, is usually done to ensure accuracy in diagnosis. A positive result indicates that infection has occurred and that the patient is likely to be infectious. Human immunodeficiency virus can also be cultured from blood and other fluids or tissues, but culture methods are much more time-consuming and expensive, and so their use is primarily limited to research.

AIDS-Related Complex

Many patients with HIV infection develop symptoms and signs that do not meet the diagnostic criteria for AIDS. These conditions constitute the spectrum of illness termed AIDS-related complex (ARC). Diffuse lymphadenopathy is commonly associated with ARC. Fever, weight loss, diarrhea, and weakness are present in the more severe forms of the disease. The presence of mucosal candidiasis; cytopenias; or viral infection of the oral mucosa and tongue, hairy leukoplakia, suggests severe immune impairment and often presages the development of AIDS. A minority of patients die from the consequences of severe ARC.

Acquired immune deficiency syndrome is diagnosed once patients develop a serious opportunistic infection, Kaposi's sarcoma, or other unusual malignancy (see Table 10–6). In general, opportunistic infection in this patient population tends to recur when therapy is discontinued. Most patients require suppressive treatment for life. Once an opportunistic infection is diagnosed, mortality is greater than 50%.

Pulmonary Infections

Pneumocystis carinii pneumonia is the most common serious opportunistic infection associated with AIDS. Patients usually present with dry cough, fever, and shortness of breath. Diffuse interstitial infiltrates are commonly seen on the chest radiograph. Arterial blood gas analysis may demonstrate hypoxemia. Pulmonary function studies are usually but not always abnormal. Although induced sputum demonstrates the organism in a large percentage of cases, bronchoscopy is often required. Approximately 80% of patients respond to trimethoprim-sulfamethoxazole or pentamidine therapy, but relapses are common. Numerous other pulmonary infections, including tuberculosis, histoplasmosis, coccidioidomycosis, and cytomegalovirus can also occur in patients with AIDS. In addition, lymphomas and Kaposi's sarcoma can disseminate to the lungs. These malignancies are more likely to be present when the chest radiograph reveals hilar lymphadenopathy or pleural effusions.

Central Nervous System Infections

The central nervous system is a frequent target organ in AIDS. Human immunodeficiency virus directly invades the neural tissue with a variety of neuropsychiatric outcomes, ranging from mild cognitive dysfunction, dementia, diffuse cerebritis, and aseptic meningitis to florid psychosis. Secondary infections are also common and include cytomegalovirus infection, herpes simplex cerebritis, *Toxoplasma* brain abscess, and cryptococcal meningitis. Central nervous system lymphomas are also seen in these patients (Table 10–8).

Because the prevalence of central nervous involvement is high, any patient with AIDS who has symptoms or signs referable to the central nervous system should be thoroughly evaluated. Headache, fever, focal neurologic findings, seizures, and altered mental status can be seen with any of these disorders. A CT scan should be obtained to exclude mass lesions, such as *Toxoplasma* abscess and lymphoma. A lumbar puncture should also be performed to exclude a diagnosis of bacterial meningitis, cryptococcal meningitis, and lymphoma.

Gastrointestinal Infections

The gastrointestinal tract is also commonly involved in AIDS. In addition to a variety of enteric bacterial and protozoan pathogens associated with diarrhea in normal hosts, two protozoa, *Cryptosporidium* and *Isospora belli*, produce severe chronic

Table 10–8. AIDS: CLINICAL MANIFESTATIONS BY ORGAN SYSTEMS

Skin	Respiratory System	Gastrointestinal Tract	Central Nervous System	Hematologic System
Abscesses	Atypical	Chronic diarrhea with	Brain abscesses	Allergic reactions
Erythroderma	tuberculosis	wasting	Leukoencephalitis	Anemia
Folliculitis	CMV	Disease of the	Meningitis	Bleeding
Kaposi's sarcoma	*Cryptococcus*	appendix	Myelopathy	Bruising
Molluscum	Lymphoid interstitial	Gallbladder disease	Peripheral	Leukopenia
contagiosum	pneumonitis	Necrotizing gingivitis	neuropathies	Lymphadenopathy
Seborrheic	Other fungal	Oral candidiasis	Primary CNS	Lymphopenia
dermatitis	infections	Oral hairy	lymphoma	Non-Hodgkin's
Tinea	*Pneumocystis carinii*	leukoplakia	Profound dementia	lymphoma
Varicella zoster	Pulmonary Kaposi's	Oral Kaposi's	Subacute encephalitis	Spontaneous
(shingles)	sarcoma	sarcoma	Toxoplasmosis of	petechiae
		Other malignancies	brain	Thrombophlebitis
		and ulcers		
		Periodontitis		
		Recurrent *Salmonella*		
		bacterium		

AIDS, Acquired immune deficiency syndrome; CMV, cytomegalovirus; CNS, central nervous system.

diarrhea in AIDS. *Isospora* responds to therapy, but there is no effective treatment for *Cryptosporidium* infection.

Podiatric Implications

Podiatrists may treat patients with cutaneous lesions on the extremities that are associated with AIDS. Kaposi's sarcoma is a unique sarcoma that may disseminate to multiple cutaneous and visceral sites. The lesions have a predilection for the extremities, face, and trunk. Occult sites include the interdigital skin, the intergluteal area, and the oral and rectal mucosa. A variety of forms have been described, but in general lesions appear as slightly raised, violaceous, nontender papules. A biopsy should be performed to confirm the diagnosis if suspect lesions are noticed on physical examination. Patients with Kaposi's sarcoma and no evidence of other opportunistic conditions have a much better prognosis than those diagnosed with opportunistic infections.

Treatment

Considerable progress toward the development of specific antiviral therapy for AIDS has occurred. Drugs currently available or undergoing early clinical trials are at best suppressive and may delay progression of the disease or minimize the se-

verity of the associated opportunistic conditions. Because the virus is incorporated into the genome, developing curative therapy is likely to remain a difficult challenge.

In practice, treatment is usually directed toward minimizing the effects of the opportunistic infections and malignancies in AIDS. The decision to treat must consider the short-term and long-term benefits as well as potential adverse side effects on the overall quality of life for the patient. Outpatient treatment protocols, suppressive therapies, and prophylactic regimens are being developed for many of the common opportunistic infections to minimize the need for hospitalization.

Prevention

Most researchers remain optimistic that a vaccine effective against HIV will become available. In the meantime, prevention depends largely on education. Human immunodeficiency virus infection is preventable by avoidance of high-risk behaviors. Safer sexual practices, including use of condoms, viricidal spermicides, and avoidance of sexual activity with partners at risk for infection, could reduce the incidence of infection in both heterosexual and homosexual populations. Education of intravenous drug users to encourage discontinuation of intravenous drugs altogether or to avoid sharing needles and other drug paraphernalia could also reduce

HIV transmission. Although innovative programs for drug users are being implemented, it is likely that many drug users will continue practices likely to result in HIV transmission. These individuals currently represent one of the most important reservoirs for perpetuating the epidemic in heterosexuals as well as in children in many part of the United States.

Bibliography

Bartlett JG, Chang T, Taylor NS, et al.: Colitis induced by *Clostridium difficile*. Rev Infect Dis 1:370, 1979.

Bodey GP, Bolivar R, Fainstein V, et al.: Infections caused by *Pseudomonas aeruginosa*. Rev Infect Dis 5:279, 1983.

Campbell JM: Sexual guidelines for persons with AIDS and at risk for AIDS. Medical Aspects of Human Sexuality, Special Issue. March 1986.

Cantey JR: Shiga toxin—an expanding role in the pathogenesis of infectious disease. J Infect Dis 151:766, 1985.

Chow AW, Pattern V, Bednorz D: Susceptibility of *Campylobacter fetus* to twenty-two antimicrobial agents. Antimicrob Agents Chemother 13:416, 1978.

Cosimi AB: Surgical aspects of infection in the compromised host. In Rubin RH, Young LS (eds): Clinical Approach to Infection in the Compromised Host. New York: Plenum Publishing Corp, 1981.

Craven DE, Kollisch NR, Hsieh CR, et al.: Vancomycin treatment of bacteremia caused by oxacillin-resistant *Staphylococcus aureus*: comparison with β-lactam antibiotic treatment of bacteremia caused by oxicillin-sensitive *Staphylococcus aureus*. J Infect Dis 147:137, 1983.

Finegold SM: Pathogenic anaerobes. Arch Intern Med 142:1988, 1982.

Finegold SM, Bartlett JG, Chow AW, et al.: Management of anaerobic infections. Ann Intern Med 83:375, 1975.

Fong JW, Tonkins KB. Review of *Pseudomonas aeruginosa* meningitis with special emphasis on treatment with ceftazidime. Rev Infect Dis 7:604, 1985.

Galpin JE, Chow AW, Bayer AS, et al.: Sepsis associated with decubitus ulcers. Am J Med 61:346, 1976.

Giulianso A, Lewis F, Jr, Hadley K, et al.: Bacteriology of necrotizing faciitis. Am J Surg 134:42, 1977.

Goldmann DR, et al. (eds): Medical Care of the Surgical Patient: A Problem-Oriented Approach to Management. Philadelphia: JB Lippincott Co, 1982.

Goldstein EJC, Lewis RP, Sutter VL, et al.: Erythromycin for anaerobic pleuropulmonary and soft-tissue infections. JAMA 242:435, 1979.

Hurst JW (ed): Medicine for the Practicing Physician. Boston: Butterworth Publishers, 1983.

Levy SB: Playing antibiotic pool: Time to tally the score. N Engl J Med 311:663, 1984.

Massell BF: Prophylaxis of streptococcal infections and rheumatic fever. JAMA 241:1589, 1979.

McDonald EC, Weisman MH: Articular manifestations of rheumatic fever in adults. Ann Intern Med 89:917, 1978.

McGowan JE, Jr.: Antimicrobial resistance in hospital organisms and its relation to antibiotic use. Rev Infect Dis 5:1033, 1983.

Ort S, Ryan JL, Barden G, et al.: Pneumococcal pneumonia in hospitalized patients: Clinical and radiological presentation. JAMA 249:214, 1983.

Penicillin-resistant viridans streptococcal endocarditis—North Carolina. MMWR 28:327, 1979.

Reinarz JA, Sanford JP: Human infections caused by non-group A or D streptococci. Medicine (Baltimore) 444:81, 1965.

Rubenstein E, Federman DD (eds): Scientific American Medicine. New York: Scientific American, Inc, 1987.

Snider GE, Jr, Cohn DL, Davidson PT, et al.: Standard therapy for tuberculosis 1985. Chest 87(suppl):117S, 1985.

Steere AC, Mallison GF: Handwashing practices for the prevention of nosocomial infections. Ann Intern Med 83:683, 1975.

Templeton WC, III, Wawrukiewicz A, Melo JC, et al.: Anaerobic osteomyelitis of long bones. Rev Infect Dis 5:692, 1983.

Tuazon CU, Lin MYC, Sheargren JN: In vitro activity of rifampin alone and in combination with nafcillin and vancomycin against pathogenic strains of *Staphylococcus aureus*. Antimicrob Agents Chemother 13:759, 1978.

Tuazon CU, Perez A, Kishaba T, et al.: *Staphylococcus aureus* among insulin-injecting diabetic patients: An increased carrier rate. JAMA 231:1272, 1975.

Watanakunadorn C: Treatment of infections due to methicillin-resistant *Staphylococcus aureus*. Ann Intern Med 97:376, 1982.

Wiernik PH: The management of infection in the cancer patient. JAMA 244:185, 1980.

Wolinski E: Nontuberculosis mycobacteria and associated diseases. Am Rev Respir Dis 119:107, 1979.

Yu VL: Enterococcal superinfection and colonization after therapy with moxalactam, a new broad-spectrum antibiotic. Ann Intern Med 94:784, 1981.

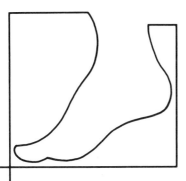

11 NEUROLOGY

ROBERT B. TELFER, MICHAEL S. COHEN, and BENNETT G. ZIER

OVERVIEW

Patients seek podiatric consultations because of a variety of symptoms, and it is not uncommon that a neurologic illness is found to play either a primary or secondary role in the genesis of a problem. Some disorders of the nervous system, such as neuropathies, tend to affect the feet first. The podiatrist is often the first medical professional to see such patients when they report numbness or painful sensations. Disorders of the cerebral cortex, basal ganglia, brain stem, cerebellum, and spinal cord may affect gait and balance as well as sensation, strength, and movement of the feet. In many cases, there is a gradual change of strength, sensation, mobility, and even structure of the feet with time or treatment. Sometimes side effects of treatment, such as neuropathy associated with long-term use of phenytoin (Dilantin), alter podiatric care.

This chapter is a guide to understanding disorders affecting the central and peripheral nervous systems, with special emphasis on manifestations in the lower extremities. Nervous system anatomy, function, and pathophysiology are reviewed. The focus is on practical clinical aspects of examination and treatment. Key observations to aid in the recognition of neurologic dysfunction are presented along with a discussion of how treatment should be combined with continuing podiatric care. The podiatrist who possesses knowledge of these aspects of neurology is able to communicate more effectively with the patient's internist or neurologist.

PATHOPHYSIOLOGY

Cerebral Cortex

Frontal Lobes

Motor regions of the frontal lobes consist of the precentral gyrus and adjacent areas. Electrical stimulation of the primary motor area results in discrete movements of parts on the opposite side of the body. Leg representation is at the medial surface between the hemispheres. Trunk, arm, face, and motor speech areas are located on the lateral aspect from the vertex to the sylvian fissure. Destruction of these areas or their descending pathways leads to contralateral weakness and increased tone. Other frontal lobe areas influence patterned movements, including learned motor tasks and adversive gaze positions. The loss of unilateral frontal lobe tissue leads to gaze toward the involved side and may cause a forced grasp reflex.

Frontal lobe connections contribute to the smoothness and preciseness of movement through the corticopontocerebellar pathways. Behavior, personality, judgment, desire, and anxiety all have some frontal lobe representation.

Parietal Lobes

Similar to the frontal lobes, the parietal lobes have a topographic cortical representation for sensation affecting the opposite side of the body. Sensory input to the legs is transmitted to the medial aspect of the postcentral gyrus, between the two hemispheres. Trunk, arm, and face fibers are represented laterally over the convexity of the surface. Sensory association areas, allowing the identification of the stimulus, are slightly more posterior. A lesion in a sensory association area may lead to agnosia, or inability to identify objects by touch or, at the parieto-occipital juncture, by sight. Taste and vestibular association areas are also represented in the parietal lobes.

Surgery or focal destruction limits interpretation of contralateral sensory data, awareness of body parts, and spatial configurations and even leads to loss of function. A patient may deny that there is anything wrong with a contralateral paralyzed arm (anosognosia) and not recognize it as his or her own body part (autotopagnosia) when he or she sees or feels it. Difficulties in recognizing form or structure of clothing may result in the patient's inability to dress himself or herself.

Temporal Lobes

The temporal lobes are involved in a variety of complex cortical functions. The lower geniculocalcarine visual pathways (i.e., Meyer's loop) pass through the temporal lobe, so that a lesion of one temporal lobe causes a defect in the upper contralateral quadrant of the visual field. Because the temporal lobe is also involved in language processing, lesions of the dominant lobe can result in several types of aphasia. A variety of behavioral disorders, including auditory illusions and hallucinations as well as psychotic behavior, can be seen with unilateral disease; a severe amnestic syndrome, apathy, placidity, and sexual dysfunction may be seen with bilateral disease.

Occipital Lobes

The primary visual cortex of the occipital lobe is responsible for accurate representation of light-stimulating ganglion cells in the retina. Different layers of cortical cells respond to "on" and "off" neurons, others respond to edges or borders, and still others respond to movement across a certain field. Neighboring areas of the occipital and parietal lobes allow a person to identify a particular image. The loss of one occipital lobe results in a contralateral loss of the visual field (homonymous hemianopsia). Loss of the nearby visual association areas may lead to a visual agnosia, or inability to recognize what one sees.

Descending Pathways

Pyramidal or Corticospinal System

The corticospinal pathways are called the pyramidal system because the vast majority of fibers run in the pyramids of the medulla. Some fibers end in direct contact with anterior horn cells, and some terminate on internuncial neurons. These tracts, the largest and most important descending fiber system, consist of neurons that originate in the cerebral cortex, pass down the brain stem, and cross in the pyramids to travel down the spinal cord in the opposite lateral white column; some fibers remain uncrossed, however, and travel in the anterior white column. The fibers are large and myelinated, arising mainly in the motor cortex and make up a major portion of the corona radiata, internal capsule, and cerebral peduncles. These fibers travel with corticobulbar fibers, which mostly cross in the brain stem to end on lower motor nuclei of the cranial nerves.

Corticospinal pathways convey the impulses for voluntary movement. Lesions of the tract usually result in a loss of volitional movement, increased tone with spasticity, hyperactive reflexes, extensor-plantar responses, and loss of abdominal reflexes.

Extrapyramidal System

Motor systems and pathways other than the corticospinal tract compose the extrapyramidal system and are responsible for, among other functions, the refinement and smoothness of voluntary movement. The basal ganglia, which consist of the caudate nucleus, putamen, globus pallidus, substantia nigra, and subthalamic nucleus, are to a large extent responsible for posture and muscle tone and for integration of muscle function for smoothness and efficiency of voluntary movement. Disturbances of this system result in (1) various involuntary movements, such as tremor, athetosis, chorea, and ballism, and (2) interference with muscle tone.

Involuntary movements, or dyskinesias, are thought to be release phenomena resulting from destruction of mechanisms that control or regulate movement. Damage to these mechanisms can cause a tremor or an increase in muscle tone owing to overactivity of a previously inhibited neural system. Additional functions can be lost by impairment of direct neural influences, as expressed in the masklike face of the patient with parkinsonism, infrequent blinking, sialorrhea, oiliness of skin, and slowness of movement, especially gait.

Thalamus and Hypothalamus

The thalamus consists of a number of bilateral nuclear masses of gray matter near the deep midline structures of the brain. These nuclear masses act as relay centers to assimilate diffuse afferent sensory inputs, except olfaction, from the external environment and from other nuclei in the cerebellum, basal ganglia, brain stem, and cortex. The thalamus distributes impulses and information back to most of these centers and especially to all lobes of the cerebral cortex. Lesions of the thalamus impair input to the cerebral cortex not only of information external to the body, such as vision and touch, but also of information about the state of the body, such as posture, fatigue, and vital functions.

The hypothalamus is responsible for regulation of the pituitary gland and the endocrine system. Thalamic and hypothalamic centers are vital for memory and for the experiences of emotion, thirst, hunger, and degrees of pain and feelings of well-being.

Cerebellum

The cerebellum consists of a thin cortex of gray matter, a large white mass of connecting myelinating fibers, and four pairs of deep nuclei. The cerebellum is responsible for the coordination of muscle movement and tone plus the maintenance of equilibrium. The cerebellum is the largest structure in the posterior fossa of the skull and sits just above and posterior to the fourth ventricle and brain stem.

The cerebellum can functionally be divided into three areas:

1. The vestibulocerebellum, consisting primarily of the flucculonodular lobe, is functionally related to the vestibular end-organ and vestibular nuclei.

2. The spinocerebellum, which constitutes the vermis of the anterior lobe as well as the posterior vermis, receives input from the spinal cord (dorsal and ventral spinocerebellar tracts); output of the spinocerebellum goes largely to those areas in the brain stem that form the reticulospinal and vestibulospinal tracts.

3. The pontocerebellum, which is located in the cerebellar hemispheres, receives input from the cerebral cortex by way of the pontine nucleus and sends efferents via the dentate nucleus and thalamus back to the motor cortex.

The cerebellum is not responsible for conscious appreciation of movement or position. The cerebellum receives input from the muscle spindles, the tendon and joint sensors, the vestibular apparatus, the brain stem nuclei, the thalamus, the basal ganglia, and the cerebral cortex. The cerebellum sends information back to most of the same areas, but the main outflow is through the superior cerebellar peduncle to decussate and enter the opposite red nucleus with relays to the ventral lateral nucleus of the thalamus and finally to the motor cortex.

Lesions of the cerebellum lead to ataxia, nystagmus, hypotonia, dyssynergia, and rebound and past pointing phenomena.

The initiation of movement is usually not affected. The smoothness and acceleration or deceleration of movement are altered. Acute loss of the cerebellum, to a larger degree than loss of most other parts of the brain, can be tolerated surprisingly well. With time, other parts of the movement control system seem to compensate. Slowly progressive cerebellar degenerations are much more difficult to overcome.

Brain Stem

The brain stem consists of the midbrain (mesencephalon), pons, and medulla.. The brain stem contains vital centers for respiration, cardiac regulation, balance, vomiting, and autonomic function of the intestines and blood vessels. The central gray matter around the cerebral aqueduct and fourth ventricle contains the reticular activating system responsible for arousal and sleep. The third through twelfth cranial nerve nuclei are contained within the brain stem; all connections to these cranial nerves and to the nerves in the spinal cord from higher centers traverse the brain stem.

A small lesion in the brain stem can have a devastating effect. Any of the vital functions noted previously can be impaired by a tiny vascular occlusion. The medulla contains the paired vertebral arteries for collateral blood supply, but the pons and midbrain must rely on the single basilar artery and perhaps some backflow through cerebellar arteries when the basilar artery is occluded or stenotic. Pressure from a cerebellar mass or from herniation of the medial temporal lobe through the fibrous tentorium causes damage directly or indirectly by distorting the blood supply to the brain stem.

Spinal Cord

The human spinal cord is approximately the diameter of the little finger and extends to the L1 vertebral level in the majority of individuals. The lumbrosacral nerve roots continue downward as a collection known as the cauda equina. The spinal cord carries all the programming from higher centers to the final common pathway of anterior horn cells or, in the case of autonomic activity, to the intermediolateral gray column. The cord contains two principal units: (1) the ascending tracts, conveying information from the periphery (limbs, internal organs, and trunk) to the brain, and (2) the descending motor tract, connecting the brain to the motor neurons. In addition, spinal cord reflexes are relayed locally or within a few root levels within the cord. The cord contains segmental units composed of incoming sensory fibers, interneurons within the gray matter of the cord, and large motor neurons that innervate the musculature of a given segment.

The clinical localization of lesions of the spinal cord depends on knowledge of three important neural pathways:

1. The spinothalamic tract, which carries information about pain and temperature on the opposite side of the body. These sensations are carried by fibers that cross within one or two levels of the entry of the dorsal roots.

2. The posterior white column, which carries information about position, touch, and vibratory sensation on the same side of the body, until the fibers cross at the decussation of the medial lemniscus in the medulla. These sensory fibers enter the posterior white column within a few levels of their dorsal roots.

3. The lateral corticospinal tract, which carries motor commands from the opposite cerebral hemisphere to anterior horn cells on the same side of the body.

Nerve Roots

There are 12 cranial nerves, 8 cervical nerves, 12 thoracic nerves, 5 lumbar nerves, 5 sacral nerves, and 1 coccygeal nerve on each side of the spinal cord. Each nerve exits the nervous system from a small foramen and is particularly susceptible to injury from pressure or torsion near this bony enclosure. The spinal nerves exit the spinal canal below their similarly numbered vertebrae in the thoracic and lumbar spine. In the cervical region, the spinal nerves exit above the same numbered vertebrae except for the eighth cervical nerve.

The anterior portion of the root contains motor fibers with nuclei in the spinal cord, and the dorsal root contains afferent (sensory) information from the appropriate dermatome. Localizing root lesions requires a knowledge of muscle innervation and dermatome distribution plus an awareness that there is a large degree of overlap between adjoining roots and some degree of variation between one person and another.

The most common causes of nerve root compression are the rupture of an intervertebral disk, the encroachment by osteophytic spurs due to degenerative disease of the spine, and both. In the lower extremities, the fifth lumbar and first sacral roots are the nerves most commonly injured.

Peripheral Nerves

After exiting the spinal canal, the nerves to the lower extremities come together in the lumbosacral plexus before forming the peripheral nerve bundles. For the upper extremities, the nerves come together in the brachial plexus. Injuries to the plexus in a relatively small space can result in loss of function in the distribution of multiple nerve roots.

Most peripheral nerves have both motor and sensory fibers. Some, such as the sural and lateral femoral cutaneous nerves, are purely sensory. Nerves that appear to have motor function almost exclusively, such as the gluteal nerves, also carry afferent information from muscle spindles and proprioceptors.

Motor nerve fibers are mostly myelinated and provide rapid transmission to the somatic musculature or, by way of the autonomic ganglia, to the blood vessels, visceral muscle, and glandular epithelium. Some sensory nerve fibers are myelinated and provide fast saltatory conduction; others are unmyelinated and provide slower, more gradual conduction. Some sensory nerve endings, such as Meissner's corpuscles, are specialized for certain stimuli; others, such as free nerve endings, are unspecialized and respond to multiple types of stimulation.

Neuromuscular Junction and Muscle

Each muscle fiber is controlled by a nerve ending, which originates from an anterior horn cell. Transmission of the nerve impulse occurs at the neuromuscular junction (motor end plate) and is carried by the chemical transmitter acetylcholine. Each action potential passing down the axon results in an influx of calcium and a release of acetylcholine from tiny vesicles along the presynaptic membrane. Acetylcholine migrates across the synaptic gap and activates the postsynaptic receptor site, which depolarizes the muscle membrane. Cholinesterase is concentrated postsynaptically and deactivates acetylcholine.

Groups of muscle fibers innervated by a common anterior horn cell are called motor units. An involuntary single contraction of a motor unit in isolation is called a fasciculation and often produces a muscle twitch large enough to be seen. An involuntary firing of a single muscle fiber is called a fibrillation and is too small to be seen.

Conditions affecting the neuromuscular junction include those that block the release of acetylcholine, such as botulism and the Lambert-Eaton syndrome, and those affecting the receptor site, preventing proper chemical transmission of energy, such as myasthenia gravis and ingestion of certain drugs.

Muscle contraction is dependent on a good source of energy provided by creatine phosphate and adenosine triphosphate. Thin muscle protein filaments of myosin and actin, surrounded by endoplasmic reticulum contiguous with the sarcolemma, are pulled along each other to shorten the muscle fiber. The depolarizing electrical signal rapidly becomes internalized, and calcium, which becomes the chemical trigger that initiates contraction, is released from the sarcoplasmic reticulum.

PRESENTING FEATURES

Subjective Symptoms

Neurologic symptoms, such as pain, numbness, tingling, weakness, unsteadiness, and involuntary movements, are difficult for patients to relate to the examiner. The character of these symptoms is often best elicited by asking the patient for a description. The patient may say, for example, "The tingling was like pins and needles," or "My feet feel as though they are burning." Pinpointing the exact location or distribution of the symptoms on the body helps to localize the pathologic process and in many cases narrows the list of differential diagnoses. It is helpful to allow patients who complain of sensory disturbance to map out its distribution. The duration and frequency of symptoms as well as factors that make the symptoms better and worse are also important.

In trying to locate a nervous system malfunction, it is useful to develop a systematic approach. We recommend starting peripherally and moving toward the more central areas, asking such questions as these: Could the lesion be in the peripheral nerves? Could it be local to the toes or foot nerves? Could it be in the muscle or in the neuromuscular junction? Could it be a nerve injury more proximal in the leg or at the nerve root level as it enters or exits the spinal canal? Could it be in the spinal canal, either in the cord or cauda equina? Could it be in the brain stem, cerebellum, basal ganglia, or cortex, or is there diffuse or multifocal involvement? Finding the site of the lesion is extremely useful in diagnosing the cause. Once a possible location or locations have been identified, one can review a checklist of disease processes, such as traumatic, vascular, infectious, metabolic, immunologic, neoplastic, and inherited problems, that may be responsible.

Neurologic disorders should always be considered when patients present with any of the following problems:

1. A foot deformity. About 50% of cases of pes cavus are associated with a familial neurologic disease.

2. Leg or foot weakness. Such affected patients are usually found to have a peripheral nervous system disorder, such as motor neuron disease, peripheral neuropathy, muscle disease, or rarely a disorder of neuromuscular transmission. Some patients with spasticity or extrapyramidal disorders also complain of leg heaviness or weakness even if no weakness is found on examination.

3. Difficulty in walking. This complaint often occurs in patients with disorders of the upper motor neuron, basal ganglia, and cerebellum. Spasticity is produced by upper motor neuron lesions, such as spinal cord lesions, causing paraparesis or quadriparesis, or cerebral hemisphere lesions, causing hemiparesis. Basal ganglia disor-

ders, such as Parkinson's disease, cause a shuffling, short-strided gait. Cerebellar disorders produce a wide-based, unsteady, and reeling ataxic gait. Occasionally, patients with lower motor neuron lesions also present with the chief complaint of difficulty in walking. An equine or a steppage gait is seen in some neuropathies. A waddling gait is characteristic of muscle disorders. The severely unsteady gait of sensory ataxia is due to loss of proprioception in some neuropathies.

4. Pain or paresthesias in the legs. These symptoms point to a peripheral neuropathy, lumbosacral plexus lesion, or spinal nerve root lesion. Sometimes patients with central nervous system lesions, especially in the spinal cord, also complain of painful sensations of the lower extremities.

Objective Signs

Physical Examination

The neurologic history and examination supplement a general medical history and physical examination. The neurologic history should include the chief complaint, detailed history of the present illness, past medical history, family history, and social history.

A screening neurologic examination takes a few minutes (Table 11–1). More time may be required to evaluate the areas that the history suggests are the major problems. After a careful history and ex-

Table 11–1. SUMMARY OF NEUROLOGIC EXAMINATION

Mental Status
  Mood, language, memory, intellect, thought process
Stance and Gait
Cranial Nerves
Motor System
  Strength, tone, bulk, adventitious movements
Sensory System
  Light touch, superficial/deep pain, sharp/dull pain, position, vibratory
Cerebellar Function
  Balance and coordination
Reflexes
  Deep tendon, plantar
Autonomic Function
  Blood pressure, sphincter
Vascular System
  Carotid pulse and bruits, peripheral pulses

amination, the examiner should then be able to isolate the involved areas of the nervous system and, from his or her knowledge of neurologic diseases, arrive at a diagnosis. Until a differential diagnosis is arrived at, it is highly unlikely that any diagnostic testing will be of much benefit. It has often been said that the most important neurologic test after a complete neurologic examination is a second complete neurologic examination.

The neurologic examination consists of an assessment of the patient's mental status, cranial nerves, motor system, sensory system, reflexes, stance, gait, and coordination (cerebellar function). In addition, the carotid arteries, aorta, and peripheral pulses should be palpated and auscultated for evidence of vascular disease.

Mental Status. Assessment of the mental status begins with the patient's orientation to person, place, and time. Even patients with severe dementia are able to give their names; therefore, the apparent inability to remember one's name is usually a sign of malingering or psychiatric illness. Orientation to place is ascertained by asking for the patient's present location and what type of building he or she is in (e.g., hospital or clinic). Orientation to time is tested by asking the patient to state the present date. Language function is tested by listening to the patient's spontaneous speech for abnormal words (paraphasias) and degree of fluency. Comprehension, repetition of phrases, naming, reading, and writing should all be assessed. Abnormalities in these areas of language function define the different types of language disorders, known as aphasias.

The remainder of the mental status examination consists of tests for memory and cognition. Memory is tested for short-term (ability to recall three objects after 5 minutes or the events of the day), immediate (digit span), and long-term recall. The ability to carry out various learned tasks on command, such as combing the hair or brushing the teeth, tests for apraxia. Arithmetic ability can be assessed by having the patient perform serial sevens (e.g., subtracting 7 sequentially starting from 100). Cognitive functioning is further assessed by testing for interpretation of simple proverbs and by similarity testing. Constructional apraxia, often a sign of nondominant parietal lobe dysfunction, may be tested by asking the patient to copy various figures. The patient's emotional state as well as evidence of thought disorders, including hallucinations and delusions, should also be noted.

Cranial Nerves. Evaluation of the first cranial nerve, the olfactory nerve, consists of presenting various odors (e.g., oil of cloves or coffee) to the patient and testing each nostril separately both for the patient's ability to perceive an odor and to name it. The most common neurologic cause of anosmia is head injury, although brain tumors, primarily subfrontal meningiomas, may also be implicated. Non-neurologic causes, such as rhinitis, are more common.

Testing of the second cranial nerve, or optic nerve, includes recording of visual acuity, testing of visual fields, and ophthalmoscopy. The oculomotor system, consisting of the third, fourth, and sixth cranial nerves, is then assessed. The pupils are checked for size, shape, degree of equality, constriction to light, and accommodation. External ocular movements should normally be full and equal in all directions. The presence of abnormalities, such as nystagmus, is noted. The eyelids should be observed for drooping (ptosis) and the degree noted.

Testing of the fifth cranial nerve, or trigeminal nerve, includes assessment of the corneal reflexes, evaluation of sensation of the face, and assessment of the mastication muscles. When testing the seventh cranial nerve, or facial nerve, asymmetry of the facial muscles should be observed at rest, during voluntary movement, and with emotional expression. If a peripheral facial palsy is present, taste on the anterior two thirds of the tongue should also be checked. The eighth cranial nerve, or vestibulocochlear nerve, is assessed by testing acoustic and vestibular functioning.

The patient should be observed for signs of abnormal functioning in areas controlled by the ninth and tenth cranial nerves, or vagus and glossopharyngeal nerves, such as phonation, gag reflex, soft palatal and pharyngeal functioning, and sensation of the posterior pharynx. The eleventh cranial nerve, or the spinal accessory nerve, innervates the sternocleidomastoid and upper trapezius muscles, which control turning the head right or left and shoulder shrugging. Finally, the twelfth cranial nerve, or hypoglossal nerve, is assessed by having the patient protrude the tongue in the midline and looking for signs of atrophy and fibrillation.

Motor System. The motor system should be tested in an organized manner. First, the patient is observed for the presence of abnormal movements, such as tremors, chorea, and dystonia. The muscles are inspected and palpated for signs of atrophy, twitching (fasciculations), hypertrophy, and tenderness, and nerve trunks are examined for enlargement.

The muscle tone, which refers to the resistance to passive stretch, is assessed next. It is common to find diminished tone in patients with lower motor neuron illnesses as well as in patients with cerebellar disorders. Rigidity, as seen in parkinsonism, is characterized by a uniformly increased tone throughout the range of movement about a joint (similar to bending a lead pipe). Spasticity, often associated with increased deep tendon reflexes, is characterized by an increased tone that is dependent on both velocity and length, giving rise to the classic clasp-knife phenomenon.

Muscle strength is then tested in the main muscle groups of the upper and lower limbs. The distribution of any weakness (e.g., proximal, distal, hemiplegic pattern, paraplegic pattern) is noted. Rapid and discrete movements of the hands and feet should also be noted because they are

Table 11–2. CHARACTERISTICS OF MOTOR ABNORMALITIES

Characteristics	Upper Motor Neuron Paralysis	Lower Motor Neuron Paralysis
Distribution of weakness	Several muscle groups	May be focal
Presence of atrophy	Mild or none	Prominent
Fasciculations	Absent	May be present
Spasticity	Present	Absent
Reflexes	Increased	Decreased
Extensor plantar reflex	Present	Absent
Nerve conduction	Normal	Often slow
Denervation potentials (EMG)	None	Present (fibrillations, fasciculations, positive waves)

EMG, Electromyogram.

often the most subtle signs of upper motor neuron dysfunction. Distinguishing characteristics of motor abnormalities of upper and lower neuron lesions are listed in Table 11–2.

Stance and Gait. If possible, the part of the examination assessing stance and gait should be done with the patient at least partially undressed without shoes to allow for assessing alignment of the spine, thighs, knees, lower legs, and feet as well as the angle and base of gait. The assessment should include the following:

Have the Patient:	Observe:
Turn briskly	Arm swing
Walk on heels	Coordination
Walk on toes	Muscle strength
Deep-knee bend	Motor ability
Tandem walk	Abnormal involuntary movements
Ambulate casually	Angle and base of gait

Sensory System. The majority of patients with acquired lesions involving the sensory system complain of abnormalities including tingling; numbness, or paresthesias; and painful perceptions, or dysesthesias. Minor sensory abnormalities found during examination in patients without sensory complaints can therefore often be discarded as an artifact of the examination procedure. Subtle sensory signs or reflex asymmetry may reflect hyperdiscrimination and false interpretation on the part of anxious patients.

Primary modalities, including perception of pain, temperature, touch, and vibration, are tested. Proprioception, evaluated by testing for joint position sense, is also checked. Tests for cortical sensory functioning include stereognosis, the ability to name objects such as a coin or safety pin placed in the hand with the eyes closed; two-point discrimination; graphesthesia, the ability to name letters or numbers traced on the fingertips; and localization. Patterns of sensory loss, such as the stocking-glove loss in neuropathies, dermatomal loss in nerve root lesions, and so-called dissociated sensory loss (loss of pain

and temperature on one side of the body with loss of vibration and position sense on the opposite side) in spinal cord syndromes, are noted.

Deep Tendon Reflexes. Deep tendon reflexes commonly tested include the biceps and brachioradialis (C5 and C6 nerve roots), triceps (C7 and C8 roots), patellar (L2, L3, and L4 nerve roots), and ankle (S1 root). The superficial abdominal reflex as well as the cremasteric reflex should be tested in most patients. The response to noxious plantar stimulation is observed; a normal response is indicated by flexion of the large toe, an abnormal or Babinski's response by extension of the large toe and fanning of the other toes. It is important to note right/left asymmetries and the degree of activity of the reflexes, which may range from complete absence (zero) to sustained clonus (five) on a scale of zero to five.

Cerebellar Function. Balance is assessed through gait evaluation and Romberg's test. Coordination is assessed by having the patient demonstrate finger-to-nose, heel-to-shin, and rapid alternating motions as well as tandem walking.

Laboratory and Physiologic Data

A clinical diagnosis, as in the case of Parkinson's disease when there is no practical confirmatory laboratory test, is made strictly by history and physical examination. In many instances, however, the laboratory evaluation narrows the field, helping to exclude important alternatives or confirming the diagnosis. Often blood chemistries and counts or routine radiographic examinations are all that are necessary. At other times, one or more of the following tests may be helpful.

Lumbar Puncture. In lumbar puncture, using aseptic technique, a needle is inserted between the spinous processes of L3 and L4. Other sites, such as the second cervical interspace, may be used but are more dangerous. The cerebrospinal fluid (CSF) pressure is measured with a manometer, and the fluid is then allowed to drip into test tubes.

The CSF cell count is abnormal if more than five cells are present, in which case meningeal inflammation or sometimes carcinoma can be diagnosed. Cytologic examination of the cells is often helpful. The glucose level is reduced in the CSF of patients with bacterial and fungal infections or carcinomatous meningitis but seldom in those with subarachnoid hemorrhage or viral meningitis. The CSF protein level is elevated in patients with demyelinating neuropathies, infections, lesions that block the flow of CSF, and epidural disease processes. The presence of specific proteins, such as determined by the Venereal Disease Research Laboratory (VDRL), leads to the diagnosis of syphilis. Increased gamma globulins with typical electrophoretic patterns in bands can be seen in the CSF of patients with multiple sclerosis, subacute sclerosing panencephalitis, and syphilis.

Radiographic Examinations. With and without contrast media, radiographic examinations help define normal and pathologic anatomy. Arteriograms utilize an iodinated protein solution to outline the lumen of vessels, which can show the circulation of tumors, infarcts, and arteriovenous malformations, including aneurysms. Myelograms use a similar fluid to outline the CSF pathways around the nerve roots, spinal canal, and basilar cisterns of the brain. The dye is inserted into the CSF by lumbar puncture. Air or radionucleotides may also be injected into the CSF and serve to outline these spaces for a pneumoencephalogram or cisternogram.

Computed Tomography Scan. Computed tomography (CT) is an image produced when a computer is connected to the radiograph apparatus. Pictures of the brain or spine can be obtained in any body plane. Dense structures, such as bone, produce greater radiograph diffraction and cause a light image. Less dense structures, such as CSF, produce a dark image. Tumors or vascular abnormalities and sometimes degenerative diseases produce characteristic patterns or displace normal structures in an identifiable pattern.

Magnetic Resonance Imaging. Magnetic resonance imaging (MRI) is obtained with a computer-produced image of changes in magnetic fields triggered by radio frequencies. These images show about 10 times better definition of brain tissues and avoid the distortion produced by bone on CT scan. There is no irradiation of the patient.

Electroencephalograms. An electroencephalogram (EEG) measures electrical activity of the outermost 3 to 4 mm of the cerebral cortex. An EEG can be helpful in diagnosing seizure and sleep disorders as well as focal structural abnormalities.

Electromyograms. An electromyogram (EMG) measures nerve conduction of peripheral nerves and electrical activity of muscle cells. An EMG is helpful in diagnosing peripheral neuropathies, neuromuscular junction diseases, and myopathies.

Evoked Response Measurements. Evoked response measurements provide information about the conduction of visual, auditory, and somatosensory stimuli from the peripheral neuron to the cerebral cortex. These tests help to localize conduction blocks in the central nervous system and sometimes in the peripheral nerves. Evoked response measurements are particularly helpful in the diagnosis of multiple sclerosis and optic, or eighth cranial, nerve lesions.

ASSESSMENT OF COMMON CLINICAL PROBLEMS

Seizure Disorders

A seizure is a sudden disturbance of cerebral function due to a paroxysmal neuronal discharge in the brain. The clinical appearance depends on the part of the brain involved. The term epilepsy implies a chronic condition of recurring seizures. Status epilepticus is the occurrence of several seizures, one following another without full recovery from the preceding seizure. The etiology of seizures may be metabolic, as in the case of hypoglycemia, hypocalcemia, phenylketonuria, drug toxicity, and drug withdrawal, or a focal structural abnormality of the brain, as in trauma, congenital malformation, tumor, and stroke.

If only a small number of neurons are involved in the abnormal discharge there may be no clinical expression, and the seizure may go undetected by the patient and observers. However, if the neuronal discharge spreads to enough surrounding neurons there is a clinically detectable symptom, depending on which nerve cells are firing. If the motor strip of the cortex is involved there is probably twitching of the appropriate part of the opposite side of the body. If neurons affecting level of consciousness are involved the patient loses awareness of his or her surroundings.

It is helpful in the diagnosis of seizures to describe the time sequence of events that can be recalled by the patient or observers.

- The *prodrome* is the time preceding a seizure when a patient feels unwell or uneasy and often suspects that a seizure is coming. The prodrome lasts minutes to hours.
- The *aura* is a symptom or sign signaling the beginning of the seizure. The aura lasts only seconds and by its nature indicates the part of the brain where the seizure begins.
- The *postictal* period lasts from minutes to hours after the seizure while the patient returns to normal. There is usually a feeling of fatigue, weakness, and sometimes soreness and confusion. The patient often sleeps for several hours.

The International Classification of Epilepsy recognizes two basic groups of seizures.

1. *Generalized seizures.* The cerebral cortex appears to be bilaterally involved in paroxysmal activity from the start. The most common generalized seizures are grand mal, with tonic-clonic convulsions, and petit mal, with no significant convulsive activity. There is almost always a loss of consciousness or awareness.

2. *Partial seizures.* The paroxysmal activity begins focally and unilaterally. Partial seizures may be simple, when there is no loss of consciousness (focal motor or focal sensory seizures), or complex, when there is loss of consciousness (psychomotor or temporal lobe seizures).

The management of a patient with a seizure disorder begins with a careful history and physical examination. If a seizure is observed it is most helpful to recall the exact sequence of events and whether the symptoms seemed to begin focally. As soon as the patient is safe, the clinician should try to write down what happened in detail.

First aid usually requires only protecting the patient from hurting himself or herself. Once the seizure has begun, it is usually too late to protect the patient from biting the tongue by inserting a foreign object between the teeth. This may lead to obstruction of the airway and sometimes further damage to the teeth and gums. The seizure generally stops within 3 to 5 minutes. Maintaining a patent airway and placing the patient on his or her side to prevent aspiration are advised.

If the seizure does not stop within 5 minutes, emergency medical care should be instituted. An intravenous line is started, blood is drawn for chemical evaluations, and glucose is given intravenously as soon as possible. Anticonvulsant medications can then be administered. In the emergency situation, diazepam, phenytoin, and phenobarbital are most frequently administered.

For long-term control of seizures, phenytoin, phenobarbital, carbamazepine, valproate, and ethosuximide are the most effective medications. The choice depends on the type of seizure, blood chemistry results, and EEG results. The goal of treatment is to eliminate seizures without adverse effects of the drug used, but sometimes mild toxic effects of the drugs must be tolerated to achieve freedom from seizures. It is best to treat with one drug until either control is achieved or adverse effects are produced. If some improvement has been obtained without full control a second drug is added, and the dosage is slowly increased until there are no further seizures. If no improvement occurs with the first drug and it has been increased to the point of adverse effects the drug should be stopped.

Control should be achieved with as few anticonvulsants as possible. When more than one medication is being used and an allergic reaction or adverse effect occurs, it may be difficult to determine which drug is at fault. Measuring the serum level of a specific anticonvulsant may be helpful to judge toxicity as well as patient compliance. If all medical therapy fails to control seizures irritative foci in the cortex are sometimes removed surgically.

Cerebrovascular Disorders

Cerebrovascular problems usually appear dramatically with sudden onset and often result in permanent loss of neurologic function. The etiology is often multifactorial, relating to a number of predisposing factors. There are two general types of cerebrovascular injuries, hemorrhagic and ischemic.

Intracranial Hemorrhage

Trauma is a common cause of intracranial hemorrhage. Nontraumatic hemorrhages may be related to hypertension or a weak focus in a blood vessel wall. The weakness may be due to a congenital anomaly, such as an aneurysm or arteriovenous malformation, or to a disease process.

HYPERTENSIVE INTRACEREBRAL HEMORRHAGES

Hypertensive intracerebral hemorrhages almost always begin within the parenchyma of the cerebrum. Approximately 90% of hemorrhages communicate with the CSF, usually by rupture into the ventricular system. After 2 to 6 months, the blood is gradually removed by macrophages, and only a small orange cleft may remain.

The most common sites for intracerebral hemorrhages are the putamen and adjacent internal capsule (50%), subcortical white matter in any lobe (10 to 15%), thalamus (10 to 15%), cerebellar hemisphere (10 to 15%), and pons (10 to 15%). The reason the hemorrhages occur in these areas is not known. It is suspected that a small cryptic vascular anomaly may have been present. The vessel walls may be weakened over the years by hypertension, and finally a rupture occurs. There are usually no warning symptoms. The hemorrhage frequently appears when the patient is up and about, not during sleep. Patients tend to be younger than those with ischemic strokes. The incidence follows that of hypertension and is more common in blacks.

Symptoms are usually quite abrupt, and the patient complains of headache unless or until there is loss of consciousness. The symptoms are maximal within a few minutes, but in some instances of continued bleeding or edema around the site of bleeding, symptoms progress. The exact symptoms and signs depend upon the area in which the hemorrhage has occurred; common findings include hemiparesis, gaze palsies, and decreased level of consciousness. Nuchal rigidity and vomiting are common, and seizures occur in about 10% of cases. The CT scan has been extremely helpful in the diagnosis and localization of these hemorrhages.

The prognosis is generally poor, with about 70% of patients dying 1 to 30 days after the hemorrhage. Surgery should be considered for cerebellar and superficial cortical hemorrhages; deeper hemorrhages are usually too devastating to allow surgery. Medical treatment is limited to attempts to reduce intracranial pressure, such as the use of corticosteroids, diuretics, osmotic agents, and hyperventilation.

RUPTURED ANEURYSMS

Saccular aneurysms are thin-walled balloons or blisters protruding from artery walls, usually around the circle of Willis, a ring of arteries at the base of the brain. Saccular aneurysms are thought to be the result of developmental defects in the arterial wall at bifurcations or in larger arteries.

About 2 to 5% of normal individuals are found to have small aneurysms at routine autopsy; 20% of those with one aneurysm have another. These aneurysms are rarely found in autopsies in children but seem to increase in frequency with age, probably enlarging with time. Mycotic aneurysms are those caused by septic emboli and may occur anywhere in the cerebrovascular system. Mycotic aneurysms are most frequent within the parenchyma of the brain at branching points of the middle cerebral artery.

Symptoms often begin during vigorous physical activity. Patients may complain of headache, neck stiffness, lethargy, and confusion without focal symptoms if the hemorrhage is confined to the subarachnoid space. A massive hemorrhage, especially into the parenchyma, may lead to death within minutes. If the initial increased intracranial pressure is survived later complications include vasospasm secondary to the presence of extravasated blood and hydrocephalus due to blockage of CSF exit pathways.

Treatment usually consists of supportive care during the acute hemorrhage. Antihypertensive medications help to prevent rebleeding. Medications to reduce intracerebral pressure are utilized. Studies suggest that calcium channel blockers reduce vasospasm and that antifibrinolytic agents may reduce rebleeding (but may result in an increased incidence of ischemic deficits). If the patient improves to the point of only minor-to-moderate neurologic deficit and it is believed that the aneurysm can be ligated or trapped to prevent rebleeding, surgery is recommended. There is a high mortality for patients with severe neurologic dysfunction in whom surgery is undertaken. Some aneurysms are in such a position or are of such size that no surgical therapy is feasible.

ARTERIOVENOUS MALFORMATIONS

Arteriovenous malformations (AVMs) are congenital malformations or angiomas, commonly associated with seizure disorders, that are a relatively rare cause of intracranial hemorrhage. Arteriovenous malformations tend to become symptomatic after the age of 10 and are twice as common in males as in females. Huge angiomas may be associated with a gradually progressive neurologic deficit due to a mass effect or a stealing of blood from normal brain tissues. A bruit may be heard over the head, eyes, or carotid vessels. Bleeding is usually less severe than it is with aneurysms, but rebleeding is more frequent. Arteriovenous malformations are difficult to remove because it is difficult to ligate all of the arterial blood supply.

TRAUMATIC INTRACRANIAL HEMORRHAGE

Usually a result of bleeding into the subdural space, traumatic hemorrhage may become apparent acutely or may progress slowly with a chronic subdural hematoma. A cerebral contusion and laceration may also result in a subarachnoid hemorrhage. Epidural hematomas begin with skull fractures that tear meningeal arteries.

HEMORRHAGE SECONDARY TO BRAIN TUMOR

The most common tumors to bleed are choriocarcinoma, malignant melanoma, renal cell carcinoma, and bronchogenic carcinoma. Almost any kind of brain tumor may cause bleeding, even primary glial tumors.

HEMORRHAGIC HEMATOLOGIC DISORDERS

Leukemia, aplastic anemia, thrombocytopenic purpura, anticoagulant therapy, and hemorrhagic syndromes should always be considered when a patient presents with an intracranial hemorrhage. The combination of alcoholism with liver disease and head trauma is a common clinical picture, resulting in a subdural hematoma.

Ischemic Stroke

Ischemic necrosis, or infarction, occurs when brain tissue is deprived of blood and oxygen. Obstruction of the nutrient artery by a thrombus or embolism is the usual cause, but decreased cardiac output or hypotension with resulting hypoperfusion can also produce infarction. An ischemic infarction may become hemorrhagic if there is an extravasation of blood from the necrotic vessels.

Symptoms of an ischemic stroke are usually related to the major artery and its perfusion territory. Various syndromes have been recognized for the internal carotid, middle cerebral, anterior cerebral, posterior cerebral, vertebrobasilar, and cerebellar arteries.

THROMBOTIC STROKE

The onset of thrombotic stroke is often sudden but may progress slowly over a few days. In approximately 80% of cases, the main paralysis or deficit is preceded by minor signs in a stepwise progression. If reversal of the neurologic deficit occurs within 24 hours the episode is called a transient ischemic attack (TIA). A brief TIA is likely to be secondary to carotid thromboembolic disease; a more extended TIA is likely to be due to cardiac emboli. When an ischemic attack is suspected, one should look for evidence of stenosis, which often occurs as a bruit over a carotid artery or a decreased blood flow to one arm, as in the subclavian steal syndrome. An arteritis or a hypercoagulable state should also be considered.

CEREBRAL EMBOLISM

In cerebral embolism, the embolus breaks away from a thombus within the heart, a vegetation on a heart valve, or a small ulceration at an atherosclerotic plaque. Other types of emboli include fat globules, tumor cells, and septic emboli. The most common cardiac irregularity associated with cerebral emboli is atrial fibrillation, but any arrhythmia that interferes with cardiac contractility may be implicated. The loss of contractility after a myocardial infarction may lead to mural thrombi and embolic phenomena. Marantic endocarditis may be associated with carcinomatosis and disseminated intravascular coagulation. Fat emboli are usually widely dispersed, with diffuse cerebral symptoms and multiple cerebral petechial hemorrhages. Air emboli can be complications of surgery on the heart and major vessels.

The prognosis after a stroke is usually dependent on the blood vessel involved and its perfusion territory. Some edema and progression of neurologic signs may occur for 2 to 3 days before improvement begins. The eventual prognosis may not be known for several weeks because improvement often continues for 6 to 12 months. Treatment of underlying medical problems, such as cardiac disorders, blood-clotting dysfunction, diabetes mellitus, hypertension, and vasculitis, should be considered immediately. Anticoagulation may be advisable for thrombotic strokes that are progressing or in cases in which the risk of recurrent emboli is high. Surgical treatment is sometimes warranted for a stenotic or ulcerated lesion of the carotid arteries or removing a thrombus or valvular vegetation from the heart.

Peripheral Neuropathies

In terms of subjective complaints, peripheral neuropathies are the most common causes of foot and toe dysesthesias, commonly called the burning feet syndrome. In addition, patients often complain of distal weakness, muscle atrophy, or both. Whether or not the patient is symptomatic, he or she usually has some degree of hypoflexia or areflexia. The podiatrist may gather further data from the history and physical examination to arrive at a specific diagnosis.

Peripheral nerves provide the anatomic and functional interface between the spinal cord and muscle. In addition to motor function, peripheral nerves are responsible for two other extremely important functions: (1) sensory, which allows the organism to feel its environment, and (2) autonomic, which allows for cardiovascular, thermoregulatory, sexual, micturition, and defecation control. The peripheral nerves are susceptible to injury by a variety of known metabolic, toxic, inflammatory, vascular, physical, and infectious agents.

Neuropathies usually fall into one of three general forms.

1. *Segmental demyelination* refers to destruction of the myelin segments with survival of axons until late in the course of illness. Examples include acute postinfectious polyneuropathy, or Guillain-Barré syndrome; infectious mononucleosis; and diphtheria.

2. *Axonal degeneration* involves destruction of the axon, which often "dies back" from the distal end. Most of the nutritional, metabolic, and toxic neuropathies are of this form.

3. *Wallerian degeneration* occurs when the nerve is injured or severed at a focal point, and the distal segment breaks down and is reabsorbed. Some wallerian degeneration is triggered by a loss of blood supply with nerve infarcts, as in polyarteritis and diabetes mellitus (mononeuropathy multiplex). Other wallerian degeneration is due to a progressive ischemia of the nerve bundle caused by narrowing of feeding blood vessels, as with amyloid deposits and arteriosclerotic changes.

There are multiple ways to classify neuropathies (Table 11–3). They can be classified by the extent of anatomic involvement (mononeuropathy versus polyneuropathy), by the physical findings (degree of areflexia and associated physical findings), and by the etiologic factors (inflammatory, toxic, infectious, and so on). Our discussion and listing of peripheral neuropathies is based on the most common types of neuropathy encountered by the podiatric clinician.

Toxic Etiologies

ALCOHOL NEUROPATHY

It is estimated that about 9 million people in the United States are alcoholics (7% of the adult population). Alcohol is converted to acetaldehyde by alcohol dehydrogenase mainly in the liver. The acetaldehyde is then further oxidized to acetyl coenzyme A and acetate, which are eventually converted to carbon dioxide and water. The toxic effects are probably due to high levels of alcohol and, to a lesser degree, acetaldehyde.

A nutritional deficiency often occurs concomitantly with alcohol toxicity.

Table 11–3. MNEMONIC FOR CAUSES OF PERIPHERAL NEUROPATHIES: "DANG THERAPIST"

D—Diabetic	Polyneuropathy: sensorimotor in the setting of long-standing diabetes mellitus
	Mononeuropathy: abrupt painful onset of third or sixth cranial nerve palsies or subacute asymmetric lumbosacral plexus dysfunction (diabetic amyotrophy)
A—Alcoholic	Sensorimotor neuropathy with multiple nutritional deficiencies
N—Nutritional	Individual B-complex vitamins: thiamine, niacin, B_6, B_{12}
G—Guillain-Barré	Acute form of inflammatory neuropathy: immunologically mediated, chiefly motor, demyelinating, respiratory, facial muscles may be involved, CSF protein often raised without pleocytosis
T—Toxic	Drugs: furantoin, vincristine, cisplatin (sensory), isoniazid (vitamin B_6 antagonism), penicillamine, gold salts, vitamin B_6 (sensory neuropathy following massive doses)
	Metals: lead (radial nerve palsies), arsenic
	Industrial and environmental agents: acrylamide, hexacarbon solvents (industry, glue sniffing), triorthocresyl phosphate
H—Hereditary	Charcot-Marie-Tooth disease: very slowly progressive, predominantly motor, with high arches, stork legs, often nerve enlargement, dominant inheritance
R—Recurrent	Relapsing form of inflammatory neuropathy; often responds to steroids
A—Amyloidosis	All forms include autonomic involvement
P—Porphyric	Chiefly motor neuropathy, may process rapidly; younger patients with acute intermittent form of porphyria
I—Infectious	Diphtheria, leprosy
S—Systemic	Association with collagen diseases, uremia, sarcoidosis
T—Tumor	Carcinomatous neuropathies: pure sensory or sensorimotor neuropathy, may be combined with myopathy

CSF, Cerebrospinal fluid.
From Harvey A, et al.: Principles and Practices of Medicine, 22nd ed. East Norwalk, CT: Appleton & Lange, 1988.

Chronic alcoholism combined with nutritional deficiency can produce a parenchymatous cerebellar degeneration characterized by ataxia, especially of the lower extremities. The peripheral neuropathy seen in chronic alcoholics is a sensorimotor polyneuropathy caused by axonal degeneration. Optic atrophy, and myopathy can also be seen in chronic alcoholics.

Other alcohols, such as the industrial solvents amyl alcohol and isopropyl alcohol, have similar effects to those of ethyl alcohol but are more toxic. Methyl (wood) alcohol may be an adulterant of alcoholic beverages. Methyl alcohol is particularly toxic to the ganglion cells of the retina and produces blindness.

NUTRITIONAL NEUROPATHY

Nutritional deficiency neuropathies usually follow a subacute course, with symptoms occurring over at least a few weeks. These neuropathies include thiamine, vitamin B_{12}, and niacin or tryptophan (pellagra) deficiencies as well as malabsorption syndromes.

DRUG-INDUCED NEUROPATHY

Almost all medications can produce toxic neurologic effects if given in high doses or to patients with impaired metabolic or excretory pathways (i.e., renal or hepatic insufficiencies). Similar to nutritional deficiency neuropathies, drug-induced neuropathies follow a subacute course. These neuropathies include the side effects of isoniazid, ethionamide, hydralazine, nitrofurantoin, disulfiram, carbon disulfide, vincristine, chloramphenicol, phenytoin, amitriptyline, dapsone, stilbamidine, trichloroethylene, thalidomide, nitrous oxide, clioquinol, and megadoses of pyridoxine (vitamin B_6).

Opiates and sedatives may lead to traction or pressure damage to the peripheral nerves, brachial plexus, and lumbosacral plexus. Chemotherapy for cancer often affects normal cells, and in the nervous system it may result in a peripheral neuropathy, as seen in patients on vincristine or cisplatin. Chemotherapy may also result in encephalopathy, as seen in patients on intrathecal (into CSF) methotrexate, or in ataxia, as seen in patients on 5-fluorouracil (5-FU).

BACTERIAL NEUROPATHY

Tetanus, botulism, and diphtheria are the most important clinical examples of bacterially induced neuropathies. The tetanus toxin is formed by *Clostridium tetani* in wounds and produces a strychninelike effect by interfering with postsynaptic inhibition. Generalized, painful muscle spasms are typical. Diphtheria may be associated with a sensorimotor peripheral neuropathy, with segmental demyelination due to a toxin of *Corynebacterium diphtheriae*. Paralysis often occurs first in the pharyngeal muscles. Botulism is the result of an exotoxin released by *C. botulinum*, which interferes with the release of acetylcholine at the neuromuscular junction. There is generalized paralysis involving cranial nerves and extremities.

Leprosy is the most common infectious neuropathy in the world and produces either a diffuse sensory polyneuropathy involving mainly pain and reduction in temperature (lepromatous leprosy) or a multifocal neuropathy (tuberculoid leprosy).

HEAVY METAL–INDUCED NEUROPATHY

Lead is the most common neurotoxin and produces an encephalopathy in children or a motor neuropathy in adults. Mercury produces an encephalopathy with confusion, ataxia, and choreoathetosis. Manganese may produce a Parkinson-like syndrome. Thallium leads to a progressive, painful polyneuropathy with optic atrophy and diffuse alopecia. Organophosphate compounds (mostly insecticides) produce a depolarization blockade at the neuromuscular junction, resulting in weakness and fasciculations.

PLANT-, SNAKE-, AND INSECT-INDUCED NEUROPATHY

Poisonous plants, snakes, and insects may produce paralysis either at the neuromuscular junction or at the peripheral nerve. These organisms may also act as chemical transmitters or vasospastic agents, resulting in seizures, confusion, and autonomic overactivity.

Metabolic and Chronic Neuropathies

Many systemic disorders, such as uremia, diabetes mellitus, hypothyroidism, ischemic vascular disease, sarcoidosis, polyarteritis, and connective tissue diseases, may produce chronic or subacute neuropathy. Amyloidosis, and paraproteinemias, such as myeloma, tend to be more chronic and slowly progressive but may have an undulating course. Treatment is directed at the underlying disease processes or vitamin deficiency, and toxins are avoided. Orthotics and braces are often helpful in addition to a regular exercise program.

PORPHYRIA POLYNEUROPATHY

Porphyria polyneuropathy involves destruction of both axons and myelin sheaths. Symptoms, including leg weakness and pain or numbness, frequently regress. Patients often present with abdominal pain and psychosis. Cerebrospinal fluid is normal.

DIABETIC NEUROPATHIES

Diabetes mellitus is one of the most common chronic diseases in the United States, with over 5 million diagnosed cases and an estimated additional 5 million undiagnosed. Prevalence of diabetes mellitus has increased sixfold during the past 40 years, and it continues to be a major medical problem in the United States. Diabetes mellitus is a disease of variable severity, affecting all age groups and often running a course of many years. Because of its complications, diabetes mellitus is the third leading cause of death by disease in the United States. Fortunately, significant advances in therapy as well as increased emphasis on educating diabetic patients have resulted in a longer life span for the overall diabetic population. However, these additional years have emphasized the devastating magnitude of diabetic complications.

Perhaps nowhere else in the body do we see the effects of vascular disease and neuropathy so clearly as in the foot of the diabetic. Of all lower extremity amputations, 80% occur as a result of vascular disease, with neuropathy as the initiating factor in most cases. More than 35,000 major amputations are performed in the United States every year because of diabetes mellitus.

Diabetics may develop both temporary and permanent neurologic problems during the course of the disease. Diabetic neuropathy is a common and disabling complication of diabetes mellitus, resulting in a great deal of morbidity and a reduced quality of life. The reported incidence of neuropathy among diabetics varies considerably, but it is estimated that at least two thirds of all diabetics show evidence of clinical or subclinical peripheral nerve dysfunction when clinical electrophysiologic techniques are used to evaluate function. Identified causes of diabetic neuropathy include vascular insufficiency and high blood glucose levels, both of which can lead to metabolic disturbances within the neuron itself.

Some patients who maintain a high degree of metabolic control develop lesions early; others who maintain poorer control do not develop lesions even after many years. This tendency probably indicates some element of genetic susceptibility and a multifactorial pathogenesis that may represent a spectrum of operative disorders. The disturbance in the physiology and biochemistry of the peripheral nerve that results from the exposure of this tissue to hyperglycemia may also be affected by metabolic, environmental, vascular, and local mechanical factors. These factors may play an individual role, a cumulative role, or both. There is, however, a strong positive relationship between diabetic control and good nerve conduction, suggesting that hyperglycemia is an influential factor for diabetic neuropathies. Normalization of blood glucose level is therefore important for prevention of diabetic neuropathies.

Peripheral nerve degeneration is a common form of diabetic neuropathy and tends to develop in stages. The patient may present with mononeuropathy or polyneuropathy and can have sensory impairment, motor impairment, or both. At the earliest stage of diabetic neuropathy, the patient usually suffers from episodes of pain and tingling in the extremities, particularly the feet. In later years, the pain becomes more nagging and constant and particularly troublesome at night. The patient may develop a neuropathy characterized by inability to perceive pain 10 to 15 years after the onset of diabetes mellitus. This is a dangerous condition because the patient may be totally unaware of injury, particularly in the lower extremities.

The long-term problems of diabetics are of great concern to the internist, ophthalmologist, and podiatrist. Data indicate that the functional changes that take place during the first 10 to 15 years of diabetes mellitus can be altered with improved control.

After this time, if control is not adequate the changes become structural, permanent, and irreversible. The burden of providing adequate control and prevention is therefore on the shoulders of the health professionals who manage diabetic patients during the critical 15 years after clinical recognition of the disorder.

Symmetric Distal Polyneuropathy. Symmetric distal polyneuropathy usually occurs with a loss of sensation in a stocking-glove distribution that is commonly observed bilaterally in the distal lower extremities but can also affect the upper extremities. Although sensory function is predominantly affected, motor abnormality is not uncommon and may at times be quite severe. In general, this abnormality is associated with metabolic factors. The sensory loss and motor weakness affect the distal portion of the longest nerves first; feet are affected before hands. The decreased sensory perception may result in neuropathic foot ulcers or Charcot's joints. In addition to the lack of sensation, there is frequently associated numbness, tingling, pins-and-needles sensation and burning, cramping, and shooting pains. Burning sensations in the feet should alert the physician to the possibility of a concomitant toxic or deprivational state.

When large fibers are affected early, vibration sense is often preferentially depressed. Pain loss, impaired touch perception, and decreased position sense rapidly supervene. Symmetric motor nerve abnormalities can occur and are often manifested by bilateral wasting of the intrinsic muscles of the hands and feet, particularly in the extensors and flexors of the toes. If atrophy occurs it is often not present until long after the onset of clinical weakness.

Mononeuropathies. An array of mononeuropathies with both cranial and spinal loci is associated with diabetes mellitus. Peripheral mononeuropathy is particularly common in diabetics and may occur after vascular lesions, trauma to superficially placed nerves, and external pressure and entrapment.

Mononeuropathy multiplex involves several nerve trunks simultaneously. Femoral mononeuropathy, which occurs acutely with pain, motor and sensory deficit, and loss of knee jerk, occurs with high frequency in the patient with diabetes mellitus. The likely cause of femoral mononeuropathy is ischemia, which gives the patient an excellent prognosis for complete recovery because of extensive anastomoses of collateral circulation. An isolated sciatic mononeuropathy may occur on a similar basis.

Mononeuropathies can also affect sensory nerves and result in painful dysesthesias and hypesthesias localized to the anatomic distribution of the nerve. These mononeuropathies frequently remit spontaneously within several weeks to months, but recurrence is not uncommon.

Peroneal mononeuropathy typically produces a sudden foot drop, usually without associated pain. In addition to vascular factors, peroneal neuropathy may be due to trauma because of the superficial location at the knee. Ulnar mononeuropathy is probably related to the vulnerable position of the nerve at the elbow. Unlike femoral and peroneal neuropathy, symptoms of ulnar neuropathy usually appear insidiously and may be due to chronic trauma rather than to acute insult to the nerve. Carpal tunnel syndrome (median nerve entrapment at the wrist) is also common among diabetics.

Diabetic mononeuropathies can involve the third, fourth, and sixth cranial nerves; other cranial nerves are rarely affected. Extraocular muscle paralysis results in diplopia. The most common syndrome is diabetic ophthalmoplegia, a third-nerve palsy with sparing of the pupillary reflex. The onset is usually abrupt with pain around the eyes. There is usually full recovery in 3 to 12 months. This suggests that demyelination without significant axonal destruction may be the significant lesion in most cases. Recurrence is not uncommon.

Radiculopathy. Diabetic radiculopathy is an infrequent form of peripheral neuropathy that may arise from ischemic infarction of nerve roots. Pain, deep-seated in the distribution area of one or several dermatomes, may be lancinating or more continuous. When thoracic roots are involved, abdominal pain and weight loss may be the prominent symptoms. A workup for malignancy is not uncommon. The presence of paresthesia or subtle sensory findings in a dermatomal distribution and segmental EMG abnormalities in paraspinal muscles are helpful in identifying this condition.

Prognosis is excellent, and recovery usually occurs in several months. When an arm or leg is involved, a rootlike pattern of sensory and motor deficit may be found, and a compressive lesion such as herniated nucleus pulposus or spondylosis must be considered.

Diabetic Neuromuscular Disease (Amyotrophy). Diabetic proximal motor neuropathy, sometimes called amyotrophy, occurs mainly in elderly men and most commonly with unilateral atrophy and weakness of the large muscle groups of the upper leg and pelvic girdle. Some patients may present with rapidly evolving asymmetric wasting and weakness with little or no sensory impairment. Weakness of the thigh muscle with loss of corresponding patellar reflex and occasional involvement of the lower leg muscles is usually seen. Other patients may present with a more gradual, symmetric evolution of weakness over months and wasting of thigh muscles with loss of both knee jerks. On occasion, the upper extremities may be affected.

Many patients with diabetic neuromuscular disease have hypertriglyceridemia. After 6 to 12 months of good control of both hyperglycemia and hypertriglyceridemia, the neuromuscular abnormalities usually diminish in severity. Severe weight loss, loss of appetite, depression, bladder dysfunction, and other autonomic symptoms may also be manifested. Diagnosis of proximal motor neuropathy is established by history, clinical findings, electromyography, and rarely muscle biopsy. Differential diagnoses include amyotrophic lateral sclerosis and polymyositis.

Autonomic Neuropathies. Diabetic autonomic neuropathies are manifested as heterogeneous and complex combinations of disorders. Visceral neuropathies may be present. Disturbances may be seen in bowel, bladder, and sexual function. Symptoms of autonomic nerve damage include diarrhea, constipation, urinary retention or incontinence, impotence, and decreased sweating. Autonomic neuropathy rarely occurs alone; it is seen with symmetric distal polyneuropathies. The patient presents with dry, cracked, scaly skin from anhidrosis that predisposes the foot to infection.

Genitourinary Symptoms. Impotence or impairment of sexual function occurs in more than 50% of men with long-standing diabetes mellitus and may be the first symptom of the disease. Although this is a common manifestation of autonomic neuropathy, impotence or impairment of sexual function may also be due to other etiologies, such as vascular insufficiency, psychologic causes, and endocrinologic dysfunction. Psychogenic causes for impotence must be excluded because diabetes mellitus does not preclude these relatively more common causes. A characteristic history of progressive loss of penile tumescence, diminution of morning erection, and inability to masturbate with intact libido is highly suggestive of diabetic impotence. Serum testosterone level is usually normal. Cystometrograms should be ordered to rule out bladder neuropathy in these patients. Rigorous control of blood glucose may occasionally re-establish penile function in mild-to-moderate, short-duration impotence. Testosterone replacement, vitamins, and other medications are largely unsuccessful. Penile prosthesis may be considered in advanced cases; penile implants are available and are often successful. Impotence caused by diabetes mellitus is usually not reversible by other means. Sexual dysfunction in females is rarely observed.

Mild-to-severe urinary bladder dysfunction occurs in more than 50% of patients with diabetes mellitus of more than 20 years' duration. A neurogenic bladder with retention and urinary tract infection is typical. Decreased bladder propulsive power and increased residual volume may be observed on a voiding cystometrogram. As increasing paresis of the detrusor muscle occurs, increasing residual volume, asymptomatic bacteriuria, and ultimately overt cystitis develop.

Cholinergic agonists are only partially effective in treatment. A successful strategy has been to urge patients with atonic dilated bladders to void at timed intervals regardless of the perceived need to void by using manual compression of the lower abdomen. In more advanced cases, bladder neck resection may be attempted to reduce the amount of detrusor power required for bladder emptying. Even in the absence of obstruction, this surgery can provide some improvement, but it can also result in permanent urinary incontinence. Urinary diversion may become necessary in a few patients.

Gastrointestinal Symptoms. The entire gastrointestinal tract can be affected by diabetic neuropathy, resulting in a range of disorders from esophageal motility to diabetic gastroparesis, with dysphagia, impaired gastric emptying, and even impaired peristalsis with diabetic diarrhea, constipation, and anal incontinence.

Diabetic diarrhea is the most common and distressing of the gastrointestinal neuropathies. The patient complains of explosive diarrhea, seemingly worse at night. Daytime hyperactivity is also fairly common. The diarrhea may be sufficiently severe and sudden, not being preceded by cramps, to produce the appearance of fecal incontinence. Characteristic radiographic patterns of small bowel motility disorder are sometimes seen. In a small percentage of this patient population, improved control of diabetic hyperglycemia is effective in relieving the diarrhea. Anticholinergics, such as diphenoxylate (Lomotil), and stool-bulking agents have limited utility. Diarrhea may also be treated with codeine (30 to 60 mg four times a day [q.i.d.]), though it often fails to respond. Therapies using oral antibiotics, such as tetracycline, for relative bacterial overgrowth in the small intestinal lumen may be efficacious.

Gastroparesis leads to early satiety and unpredictable gastric emptying, which can result in erratic food absorption. Nausea and vomiting may also occur. All these symptoms of gastroparesis complicate diabetic control. Multiple small feedings of a predominantly liquid, low-fat diet may be effective in maintaining nutrition. Approximately 1 to 3 months of rigorous euglycemia are essential before the symptoms disappear. Metoclopramide may be quite useful in facilitating gastric emptying. Cholinergic agonists in general have limited utility.

Cardiovascular Symptoms. Autonomic neuropathy manifested by orthostatic hypotension is the most common cardiovascular effect of diabetes mellitus and may be disabling. Symptoms include light-headedness, visual disturbance, and syncope on standing. These so-affected patients may not be able to rise from a supine position without a period of 10 to 30 minutes of adaptation to an increasing upright position. The diagnosis is made by demonstrating a decrease of approximately 25 mm Hg in systolic or 10 mm Hg in diastolic blood pressure after 2 minutes of upright posture without a compensatory increase of the heart rate.

Orthostatic hypotension may be alleviated by fludrocortisone (0.1 mg daily) or ephedrine (25 mg three times a day [t.i.d.]) and wearing support hose. If this therapy fails to provide sustained symptomatic relief, the patient may become bedridden.

Neuroarthropathy

Foot Pathology.   Foot ulcers can occur in diabetic patients secondary to large vessel atherosclerosis, microangiopathy, neuropathy, or a combination of these factors. Ulcers secondary to neuropathy characteristically occur in areas of weight bearing and pressure. The average duration of diabetes mellitus in patients with this neuroarthropathy is 12 to 18 years. Most cases occur in the 30s or 40s. The neuropathic joint, also called Charcot's joint, is a disorder characterized by joint disruption and bony dissolution caused by repeated trauma to joints with a compromised protective mechanism (Table 11–4). In the diabetic, Charcot's joint is seen most commonly in the foot, including the tarsometatarsal, lesser tarsus, and metatarsophalangeal joints. The exact etiology of Charcot's joint, with or without perforating ulcers, is unknown.

The best therapy for diabetic foot ulcers is prevention. Meticulous foot care can reduce the incidence of ulcers and gangrene and prevent amputations. Clinical presentation includes cartilage degeneration, formation of loose bodies, and marginal osteophyte formation. Fractures occur in the articular facets, osteophytes, and epicondyles with callus formation and further osteophyte formation. The presence of loose bodies may give the joint a feeling of a "bag of bones" on palpation and range of motion.

A joint disruption occurs, producing instability and possible subluxation of the involved joint. With progression of this disorder, the foot becomes edematous, erythematous, and warm; it also appears shortened with a rocker-bottom deformity. The most common bony deformities in Charcot's foot are medial convexity, plantar deformity with flattening medially, dorsal midfoot deformity, and plantar-flexed metatarsals. Stable ankle joint arthropathy is associated with a persistent limp. The most frequent local complication is soft tissue swelling, which usually responds to elevation of the lower extremity to heart level. Swelling tends to recur.

There is a 20% incidence of bilateral disease in patients who present with unilateral neuroarthropathy. Routine bilateral radiographic films of the patient with one-sided overt disease lead to early diagnosis and possible prevention of advanced destruction on the other side. Differential diagnoses of Charcot's joint include tabes dorsalis, osteomyelitis, congenital insensitivity to pain, leprous neuropathy, and peripheral nerve injuries.

A study at the Joslin Clinic in Boston, Massachusetts, in 1970 demonstrated that diabetic neuroarthropathy was more common than had previously been thought. Any joint deprived of nociperception and subjected to repeated trauma develops arthropathy. It is therefore important to be aware of the salient clinical features, di-

Table 11–4. DIAGNOSIS OF DIABETIC NEUROARTHROPATHY

Duration
Diabetes 15 yrs or more
History
Peripheral neuropathy, lower extremity
Clinical features
Early
  Soft tissue swelling
  Bony foot deformity
  Lisfranc's joint involvement
Sequela to "Burnt-Out" Process
  Arrested: Difficulty with shoe gear
           Infection
           Local complications of bony deformity
Classic Findings
  Bony deformity: medial convexity, dorsal, plantar prominence (any combination)
  Calluses: related to abnormal weight distribution and skeletal derangement
  Blisters: associated with tarsal collapse, rapidly progressing plantar deformity, rocker-bottom
  Callus infection: common in points with MPJ dislocation with plantar flexion of metatarsal head
  Ulcerations: commonest cause of hospitalization, associated with infected callus, treat bony deformity
  Radiograph:
    Mild disease: articular margins irregular, minimal to gross periarticular sclerosis or resorption
    Advanced disease: disorganization with epiphyseal and metaphyseal fragmentation, bony dissolution

MPJ, Metacarpophalangeal joint.

agnosis, and management of Charcot's joint and to be able to identify the patient who is more prone to develop this particular complication. A diabetic with peripheral neuropathy of the lower limbs who presents with any of the aforementioned clinical features should be further examined.

The radiographic features in diabetic neuroarthropathy range from irregularity of the articular margins, with minimal periarticular sclerosis or resorption in mild cases, to gross disorganization with epiphyseal and metaphyseal fragmentation and bony dissolution in advanced cases. Periosteal new bone formation is present in about 50% of cases, whereas healing occurs in 15 to 20%. Resorptive changes and, in some instances, marked bony dissolution, resulting in "penciling" of the metatarsal or phalangeal shafts, are also seen. Other features on radiographic films include fractures within or at a distance from affected joints, soft tissue swelling, and vascular calcification.

Active-stage treatment includes an initial period of 1 to 2 weeks of bed rest followed by nonweight-bearing walking with crutches for soft tissue swelling. This swelling usually subsides in 7 to 10 days, but duration of crutch use depends on clinical and radiographic response. Gradual weight bearing is instituted once stability or arrest is evident on radiographic series (films taken 1 to 2 months apart). A cast may be necessary in some instances. Adequate follow-up is necessary to ensure no further damage to the same or adjacent joints. Whether the neuroarthropathy is stable or healed, management depends on the bony deformity present. Further treatment is directed toward preventing callus formation by the use of local padding, custom-made accommodative inserts, or custom-made shoes that minimize weight bearing on the bony prominences.

Patients with fractures in the lower third of the tibia are prone to develop ankle arthropathy, which frequently is not suspected until 3 to 4 years after the fracture. Careful monitoring is recommended during the first few years after an initial injury. Radiographic examinations every 6 months for 2 to 3 years, then yearly, may help to detect joint changes sufficiently early to institute treatment.

Preventive management is the basis of successful care of insensitive feet. All patients with diabetic neuropathy should be regarded as potential victims of neuroarthropathy, and any injury, no matter how trivial, should be carefully treated. Swelling is treated with elevation and avoidance of weight bearing. Follow-up evaluation, including radiographic examination, is essential. Early joint destruction must be detected and treated immediately.

TREATMENT AND PREVENTION OF DIABETIC NEUROPATHIES

Diabetic teaching centers are of help to patients and physicians. No matter how good the initial teaching, however, most patients require repetition after an interval of time. Contact with others who have the same problems and are undergoing the same experiences is reassuring and helpful to most diabetics.

Neuropathy, once present, is difficult to reverse. Strict metabolic control must be the primary goal. Evidence indicates that the adequacy of control is correlated with the arrest of symptoms and signs of polyneuropathies. In general, good control can help to prevent the neuropathy or at least delay its onset and reduce its severity. Treatment modalities can help the diabetic with neuropathies to lead a normal productive life of better quality (Table 11–5).

Sensory symptoms often are the major source of disability and misery imposed by diabetic neuropathy. Patients with sensory symptoms and muscle tenderness may not be able to bear prosthetic aids. These symptoms may also be a major source of insomnia and significant depression. In general, analgesics are unsatisfactory. Even high doses of narcotics do not control the pain satisfactorily. The risk of addiction must also be considered, especially since the chronic lack of sleep and depression experienced by such patients compounds this risk.

Burning pain and dysesthesia may respond to a combination of amitriptyline (Elavil) at bedtime and a low-dose tranquilizer, such as fluphenazine (Prolixin) (1 mg t.i.d.) or diazepam (Valium) (5 mg t.i.d.). It is recommended to start amitriptyline at a low dose and to increase it gradually. Minor side effects, such as dry

Table 11–5. TREATMENT SUMMARY: DIABETIC
NEUROPATHIES

Signs and Symptoms	Treatment Modalities
Muscle weakness	Supports, splints, modified shoe gear, physical therapy
Burning pain	Amitriptyline 50–150 mg at bedtime, low-dose tranquilizer t.i.d.
Lightninglike pain	Carbamazepine: dose to maintain 4–10 µg/ml blood level
	Phenytoin: dose to maintain 10–20 µg/ml blood level
Itching	Diphenhydramine 25–50 mg t.i.d., mild moisturizer
Entrapment	Accommodative devices, padding, splints, surgery
Autonomic neuropathies	
Orthostatic hypotension	Fludrocortisone 0.1 mg q.d., ephedrine 25 mg t.i.d., or both, digoxin 0.25 mg q.d., support hose
Diarrhea	Codeine 30–60 mg q.i.d., diphenoxylate 1–2 tabs q.i.d.
Impotence	Penile implants, intracavernous papaverine and phentolamine
Atonic, dilated bladder	Void at regular intervals with manual compression; bladder neck resection

q.d., Every day; q.i.d., four times a day; t.i.d., three times a day.

mouth, fatigue, constipation, impotence, and difficulty focusing the eyes, should be explained. Forewarned patients tend to tolerate such side effects better. On this regimen, relief is usually experienced within 3 to 4 days, even before the antidepressant effect is established. If itching is persistent and does not respond to amitriptyline and a tranquilizer, low-to-moderate doses of diphenhydramine and a mild moisturizer may be more successful.

Carbamazepine (Tegretol), phenytoin (Dilantin), or both may be successful in treating lightninglike stabs of pain. Mexiletine, an oral lidocaine analogue, may help. Carpal and tarsal tunnel syndromes may be treated with splints or accommodative devices to attempt reduction of pressure on the involved nerves. If these fail to provide sustained relief surgical decompression is considered; however, surgery may be ineffective or harmful.

Inflammatory Neuropathies

ACUTE POLYNEUROPATHY

Acute polyneuropathy (acute idiopathic polyneuritis or Guillain-Barré syndrome) is characterized by rapid onset of weakness, usually beginning in the lower extremities and ascending to involve all extremities and often the cranial nerves. Mild-to-moderate sensory findings, such as decreased sensations of vibration and touch, frequently indicate involvement of the large myelinated fibers. The greatest danger is paralysis of respiration. Segmental demyelination with focal infiltrates of mononuclear cells are found around the peripheral nerves and roots. This syndrome, which often follows a viral illness, is quite similar to experimental allergic neuritis, suggesting an autoimmune mechanism. Nerve conductions are usually slow. The CSF protein level is elevated in the majority of cases after the first few days, reflecting the inflammatory response around nerve roots. Acute polyneuropathy may also be associated with infectious mononucleosis and is clinically similar to the idiopathic form.

Treatment is supportive, with respirator care if necessary. Physical therapy is utilized to keep muscles active. Evidence suggests that plasmapheresis results in a more rapid recovery, probably by removing antibodies that attack myelin.

CHRONIC IDIOPATHIC INFLAMMATORY POLYNEUROPATHY

Chronic-relapsing inflammatory polyneuropathy is a chronic or relapsing form of demyelinating polyneuropathy; the clinical picture of primarily motor weakness with usually lesser sensory changes is similar to the acute form, described previously. Chronic idiopathic inflammatory polyneuropathy may be difficult to diagnose because a biopsy specimen of a relatively unaffected nerve may show no evidence of the mononuclear cell infiltrate. This neuropathy may respond to corticosteroids, immunosuppressive drugs, or both.

Hereditary Neuropathies

PERONEAL MUSCULAR ATROPHY

Peroneal muscular atrophy, or Charcot-Marie-Tooth disease, is an autosomal-dominant disorder that accounts for 80 to 90% of all hereditary neuropathies. Peroneal muscular atrophy usually begins during childhood or adolescence with mild motor and sensory symptoms in the feet, such as unsteadiness and discomfort, and progresses slowly. Severely affected patients may become wheelchair bound. There is some overlap of this clinical syndrome with Friedreich's ataxia (spinocerebellar degeneration).

Often misdiagnosed, peroneal muscular atrophy is characterized by dramatic clinical variations. Symptoms can range from a minor foot deformity without weakness or sensory change to a major atrophy with stork legs and wasted hands. About a third of all patients have central nervous system involvement expressed in speech defects, involuntary eye movements, and learning disabilities. One clinical survey found peroneal muscular atrophy in 45% of all patients with foot deformities or walking difficulties.

The CSF protein level is usually normal. Nerve conduction velocities are slow, and both axons and myelin sheaths are affected. Late in the process, anterior horn cells and dorsal root ganglion cells are diminished. There is no effective treatment. Orthotics, physical rehabilitation, and sometimes surgery, such as arthrodesis, to correct foot drop may be helpful.

PROGRESSIVE HYPERTROPHIC NEUROPATHY

Progressive hypertrophic neuropathy, or Déjérine-Sottas disease, is characterized by large nerve bundles secondary to multiple regenerations of myelin sheaths, or "onion bulbs." There is a repetitive demyelination and remyelination. The CSF protein level is elevated. Inheritance is usually recessive.

AMYLOIDOSIS

Amyloidosis shows an autosomal dominant pattern. Carpal tunnel syndrome as well as other pressure neuropathies and autonomic involvement is frequently seen.

The CSF protein level is normal or mildly elevated.

Pressure and Entrapment Neuropathies

Pressure and entrapment neuropathies are focal neuropathies that are caused by damage to the myelin sheath by pressure and ischemia. Less often the axons are injured. The superficial position of some nerves combined with the inflexibility of the surrounding anatomy makes some nerves particularly susceptible to injury. Examples are the ulnar nerve at the elbow, the peroneal nerve at the fibular head, and the radial nerve at the upper arm (Saturday night palsy).

Entrapment of the nerve is usually due to thickening of the perineurium and chronic compression. Particularly susceptible are the median nerve at the wrist (carpal tunnel syndrome); the posterior tibial nerve at the ankle (tarsal tunnel syndrome); the lateral femoral cutaneous nerve at the inguinal ligament (meralgia paresthetica); and the median cord of the brachial plexus, compressed by a cervical rib, causing numbness in an ulnar nerve distribution (thoracic outlet syndrome).

Infectious Diseases

Meningitis

Of cases of meningitis, 80 to 90% are caused by three organisms: *Haemophilus influenzae*, *Neisseria meningitidis*, and *Diplococcus pneumoniae*. A marked inflammatory response occurs in the pia-arachnoid and CSF, causing symptoms such as fever; headache; neck stiffness, or nuchal rigidity; disorders of consciousness; and seizures.

Diagnosis is confirmed by lumbar puncture. The CSF is cloudy, and the pressure is usually elevated. The white blood cell count, often over 1000/mm³, consists mostly of polymorphonuclear cells. Protein level is elevated, and glucose level is reduced, usually to less than 40 mg/dl. Gram's stain often helps to identify the bacteria while one is waiting for a culture.

Treatment is usually administration of penicillin G for pneumococcal and meningococcal infections and ampicillin or chloramphenicol for *Haemophilus influen-*

zae. Cefotaxime is a third-generation cephalosporin that penetrates inflamed meninges and is effective against most gram-negative organisms. Obtaining antibiotic sensitivity determinations for the offending organism is essential. Therapy is continued for 10 to 14 days. The mortality is about 10%, and complications include residual brain damage, seizures, hydrocephalus, and hearing loss.

Brain Abscess

Sometimes infections become localized and produce a mass effect within the brain parenchyma. After spreading from sinusitis, otitis media, or septic embolus, the infection gradually becomes walled off with granulomatous tissue and causes a mass effect with increased intracranial pressure. The CT scan shows a lucent center surrounded by a ring of enhancement, and there is often evidence of severe cerebral edema. Treatment with antibiotics alone may be successful, but if there is progressive deterioration surgical drainage or removal of the abscess may be necessary.

Tuberculosis

Tuberculosis produces a thick granulomatous response, especially at the base of the brain, resulting in multiple cranial nerve palsies. A patient with this infection may also present with an epidural abscess and myelopathy, producing back pain and paraparesis. Usually there is evidence of tuberculosis of the lung or miliary spread.

Neurosyphilis

All types of neurosyphilis originate from a syphilitic meningitis, which is usually asymptomatic and occurs in 25% of all patients with syphilis. The CSF white blood cell count is about 200/mm^3, mostly lymphocytes, and the protein level is elevated. The CSF glucose level is normal. The fluorescent treponemal antibody absorption (FTA-ABS) test result is always positive, although results of the VDRL and rapid plasma reagin (RPR) tests may be negative. Penicillin is the treatment of choice.

Tabes dorsalis is a late form of syphilis. Symptoms begin 15 to 20 years after the original infection. There is degeneration of dorsal roots and posterior columns of the spinal cord. Patients most commonly present with leg symptoms, such as sensory ataxia with a loss of position and vibratory sensation and an absence of reflexes. Patients often complain of lightninglike pains and urinary incontinence. Rarely syphilis may be seen with progressive meningomyelitis and progressive spastic paraparesis.

Fungal and Miscellaneous Nonviral Infections

Several types of fungi, the most common being *Cryptococcus neoformans*, may produce a subacute meningitis. A common fungal meningitis in California is coccidioidomycosis. The CSF shows a moderately reduced glucose level associated with a lymphocytic pleocytosis and elevated protein content. Mucormycosis is almost always associated with diabetes mellitus or deficient immune states. Mucormycosis begins with an orbital cellulitis and spreads intracranially. Treatment is with amphotericin B alone or in combination with flucytosine.

Protozoa, rickettsias, and parasites may all be associated with central nervous system infections but are infrequently seen in the United States. The most common cause of seizures in patients from Central and South America is infestation with cysticerci.

Acute Viral Infections

Poliomyelitis, an infectiton of the gray matter of the spinal cord, appears as an influenza-like illness, followed by meningitis and then flaccid paralysis of limbs, trunk, and bulbar muscles. The acute phase, which is rare since the widespread use of polio vaccine, is still seen in undeveloped countries. Many patients are still living who suffer from the chronic changes of polio, including paralysis with atrophy and sometimes contractures and secondary joint degeneration or malformation.

Herpes zoster, or shingles, is an acute inflammation caused by a DNA virus identical to varicella, or chickenpox. Clinical signs include pain in a dermatomal distribution, most commonly thoracic, sometimes with sensory loss, followed by a vesicular eruption in the same distribution. Segmental weakness, myelitis, and encephalitis are rarely seen. An inflammatory reaction occurs in one or several adjacent sensory ganglia. Pain (postherpetic neuralgia) may persist for years and be refractory to all analgesics.

ASEPTIC MENINGITIS

Aseptic meningitis appears with fever, headache, and neck stiffness lasting about 1 week. The CSF shows lymphocytic pleocytosis and normal glucose level. Protein content is normal or slightly elevated. Usually caused by a viral infection, most commonly an enterovirus, such as coxsackie virus, echovirus, or poliovirus, this syndrome may be indistinguishable from early fungal or tubercular meningitis. Mumps or infectious mononucleosis may also be associated with a mononuclear meningitis.

ENCEPHALITIS

Both meningeal and brain parenchyma are involved in the inflammatory response in the syndrome of encephalitis. The patient usually shows a depressed level of consciousness, seizures, and ataxia and may have focal neurologic signs. Arboviruses tend to be responsible for epidemics in summer and early fall when mosquitos and ticks pass the infection to humans. Eastern equine encephalitis is the most severe from. A fourfold rise in antibody titer establishes the diagnosis.

Herpes simplex encephalitis is the most common form of sporadic encephalitis in adults. Herpes simplex encephalitis often produces more serious pathologic changes in the temporal lobes and is frequently associated with focal neurologic signs, such as aphasia, hemiparesis, and focal seizures. Morbidity and mortality are high, more than 30%. Treatment is with acyclovir (Zovirax).

Rabies usually occurs with delirium and hydrophobia due to spasms of the pharyngeal muscles, then coma and death. The incubation period is generally 1 to 4 weeks but may last much longer after contact with the saliva of an infected animal. Rabies is fatal in over 95% of cases once central nervous system symptoms have begun. Prophylactic treatment with rabies immune

serum and human diploid cell rabies vaccine is protective.

Chronic Viral Infections

Subacute sclerosing panencephalitis (SSPE) is a latent central nervous system infection due to measles. Subacute sclerosing panencephalitis remains dormant for years and then is activated usually during childhood or adolescence. The disease generally appears with a progressive dementia and myoclonus, leading to death within months to a few years. The CSF measles antibody and gamma globulin levels are elevated. The EEG shows a characteristic paroxysmal pattern.

Creutzfeldt-Jakob disease is characterized by progressive dementia in adults, parkinsonian features of rigidity and bradykinesia, and myoclonus. There may be muscle atrophy, indicating anterior horn cell involvement, and a steady progression to death usually occurs within 2 years. No treatment is available. The virus has been transmitted to animals and humans by percutaneous exposure to infected brain tissue.

Progressive multifocal leukoencephalopathy (PML) is a progressive demyelinating disease of the central nervous system usually seen in patients with a lymphoproliferative disorder and an impaired immune system. A papovavirus has been isolated.

The majority of patients with acquired immune deficiency syndrome (AIDS) develop a progressive dementing illness thought to be caused by chronic human immunodeficiency virus (HIV) infection of the brain. A large number of opportunistic central nervous system infections also occur in these patients.

Movement Disorders

Diseases characterized by involuntary movement are generally associated with disorders of the extrapyramidal motor system. The basal ganglia are composed of the caudate nucleus, putamen, and globus pallidus along with their connections with other subcortical nuclei, such as the substantia nigra and subthalamic nucleus, as well as the thalamus, cerebral cortex, and brain stem nuclei. There has been a dramatic advancement in understanding the neurochemical basis underlying movement disorders. The following are the most common movement disorders encountered by clinicians.

Parkinson's Disease

The most common disorder of the basal ganglia is Parkinson's disease, which occurs in approximately 100 persons/100,000 population. Pathologic examination shows degeneration with neuronal cell loss of the zona compacta of the substantia nigra. These cells send their axons to the striatum (caudate nucleus and putamen), utilizing dopamine as their neurotransmitter. Parkinson's disease may therefore be thought of as a disorder of dopamine deficiency.

Parkinson's disease is characterized clinically by hypokinesia, tremor, rigidity, and disorders of gait and balance. Hypokinesia refers to a slowing of the initiation and performance of voluntary movements as well as a marked reduction of spontaneous movements, such as blinking and crossing the legs. The characteristic tremor of Parkinson's disease, which has a frequency of approximately 4 to 6 Hz, is present at rest and often produces a "pill-rolling" tremor of the hands. Rigidity of axial as well as limb structures is seen, predominantly in flexor muscle groups. Passive movement may demonstrate a cogwheel rigidity of muscles. The gait is characteristically shuffling, with short steps, absent arm swing, and flexion at all joints. A progressive loss of both postural and righting reflexes causes falling as well as difficulty arising from chairs and turning over in bed. Approximately 10 to 20% of patients have associated dementia.

Several drugs are available for treatment of Parkinson's disease. The loss of dopaminergic activity in the striatum produces a relative cholinergic overactivity. The drugs used to treat parkinsonism act by either decreasing cholinergic activity or by increasing dopaminergic activity. Drugs that decrease cholinergic activity include several anticholinergics, such as trihexyphenidyl, and some antihistamines. Drugs that increase dopaminergic activity include L-dopa, usually combined with carbidopa, a peripheral decarboxylase inhibitor in the form of Sinemet; amantadine; and bromocriptine.

Neuroleptics, such as chlorpromazine and haloperidol, may produce severe difficulties with gait and balance, resulting in a Parkinson-like syndrome, with rigidity, bradykinesia, tremor, and retropulsion, that is indistinguishable from Parkinson's disease. This syndrome usually disappears or abates after withdrawal of the drug. Neuroleptics can also produce an acute dystonic reaction, such as torticollis, or an inner restlessness and constant motion (akathisia). In some cases, a tardive dyskinesia may appear after the patient has been taking the medication for a long time or even after the medication has been stopped. Tardive dyskinesia may persist for years, most often occurring as an involuntary repetitive movement of the face and tongue.

Chorea

A variety of neurologic diseases are associated with chorea, which is characterized by involuntary, purposeless, unpredictable, asymmetric, and abrupt movement, usually affecting the distal extremities more than the proximal. Chorea is often superimposed on voluntary movement. Chorea may be associated with childhood rheumatic fever (Sydenham's chorea); systemic disorders, including hyperthyroidism, hypoparathyroidism, and systemic lupus erythematosus (SLE); certain drugs, such as oral contraceptives; pregnancy (chorea gravidarum); and hereditary disorders, such as Huntington's disease.

Ballismus is similar to chorea but affects proximal limb movement, is more violent, and is usually unilateral. Ballismus is ordinarily caused by an infarction or a hemorrhage of the contralateral subthalamic nucleus.

Huntington's chorea, the most well known of the choreiform disorders, is an autosomal-dominant disorder, affecting 5 to 10 persons/100,000 population. Research has localized the genetic defect to chromosome 4. Pathologic examination reveals a characteristic atrophy of the striatum, particularly the head of the caudate nucleus, and a loss of cortical neurons in certain areas. Neurochemically, there is a marked decrease in the level of gamma-aminobutyric acid (GABA) as well as some other neurotransmitters, such as acetylcholine. Huntington's disease usually begins between the ages of 30 and 40, with progression to death within 20 years. Huntington's disease is manifested by the combination of chorea and dementia with behavioral changes. The chorea affects both limbs and trunk, and the choreiform movements during walking produce a dancinglike gait. There is no known treatment, although phenothiazines have been found to decrease the severity of the abnormal involuntary movements.

Dystonia

Dystonia is a movement disorder likely to be first seen by a podiatrist. Dystonia consists both of slow, sustained contraction of muscle groups, resulting in abnormal postures of the trunk and extremities, and of more rapid, twisting movements. These movements may be absent at rest, which may lead to the erroneous diagnosis of hysteria or malingering.

Dystonia musculorum deformans is a primary hereditary dystonia unassociated with other neurologic symptoms. This disorder begins in childhood, often with action dystonia of one leg. It is typical for the foot to twist into an equinovarus posture when the patient is walking yet to appear normal when he or she is sitting. However, some patients show different patterns of abnormal movement of the lower extremity, such as hyperextension of the knee or flexion of the knee and hip. During its early stages, dystonia may be present only when the patient is walking. Eventually the movements occur at rest as well, with forceful spasms of muscle groups leading to sustained, abnormal postures. Dystonia eventually spreads to all the extremities, the trunk, and the cranial muscles. Treatment of primary dystonia is unsatisfactory, although some patients do respond to anticholinergic medications.

A disorder that may include dystonic movements along with tremor, chorea, dysarthia, and behavioral changes is Wilson's disease, an autosomal-recessive disorder of copper metabolism. Decreased levels of ceruloplasmin and serum copper are found along with increased levels of urinary copper. Atrophy of the striatal portion of the basal ganglion is associated with hepatic cirrhosis. It is important to exclude Wilson's disease in any patient with dystonia

or the other abnormal movements previously noted. Wilson's disease is treatable with penicillamine and a low copper diet. Wilson's disease is fatal if untreated.

Tremor

Essential (postural) tremor is a benign disorder of the nervous system. This disorder is often autosomal dominant and is not associated with other symptoms or signs. Essential tremor is most prominent in the upper extremities, where it is present primarily during action (postural tremor) and is absent at rest. Tremor of the head, voice, trunk, and occasionally legs may also be seen. When the legs are involved, the greatest movement is usually proximal, consisting of alternating flexion and extension at the hip. The treatment of choice for essential tremor is propranolol, a beta-adrenergic antagonist, or primidone, a sedative anticonvulsant.

Tumors

Tumors of the central nervous system are encountered only rarely in podiatric practice. Symptoms depend on the location of the lesion. Focal symptoms are often produced as well as more generalized symptoms due to increased intracranial pressure.

Lesions in the parasagittal region, such as a meningioma, may appear with slowly progressive spasticity and clumsiness of one leg due to pressure on the "leg area" of the precentral gyrus. Lesions in other areas may appear as more profound hemiparesis, language dysfunction, mental dysfunction, and frequently seizures. Signs and symptoms of increased intracranial pressure include optic disk swelling or papilledema, headaches with vomiting, depressed levels of consciousness, and uncal herniation syndromes. Herniation of one temporal lobe through the tentorial opening compresses the third cranial nerve and brain stem circulation, resulting in rapid death.

About 50% of brain tumors in adults are derived from glial tissue. These tumors arise in the white matter, widely infiltrating the nervous system to become oligodendroglioma, astrocytoma, and poorly differentiated glioblastoma multiforme. More than two thirds of gliomas are considered malignant when first diagnosed. The 1-year survival rate of patients with glioblastoma multiforme is only 20%. In comparison, patients with low-grade astrocytomas and oligodendrogliomas have much greater mean survival rates, averaging more than 5 years. Treatment of malignant gliomas includes surgical resection when feasible followed by radiation therapy and chemotherapy. Results of any treatment are very disappointing and never curative.

Ependymoma, which develops from ependymal linings of the ventricular system, often produces hydrocephalus or spinal cord compression. Primary lymphoma of the central nervous system, which occurs frequently in immunosuppressed patients, including patients with acquired immune deficiency syndrome (AIDS), is diagnosed with increasing frequency and fortunately is extremely radiosensitive.

Meningiomas are believed to arise from arachnoidal cells and are considered benign. Meningiomas may grow anywhere but characteristically occur in specific locations. Most important for the podiatrist is the parasagittal-falx region, since a tumor in this area may be associated with slowly progressive leg weakness. Meningiomas do not invade the brain but rather compress the underlying neural tissue. Meningiomas can be cured by surgical removal but may recur.

Some studies indicate that more than 30% of all brain tumors have metastasized from a systemic cancer. These cancers usually originate in the lung, breast, or skin (malignant melanoma) and less commonly in the gastrointestinal tract or kidney. Brain metastases may occur either as a solitary mass lesion or as multiple lesions. The treatment for most metastatic tumors is radiation therapy, although a single metastasis can occasionally be removed surgically.

Trauma

Because patients with acute head injuries never present primarily to the podiatrist, head injuries are only briefly considered here. A closed head injury of significant severity often results in a concussion. This reversible, traumatic paralysis of nervous system function causes brief periods of unresponsiveness and can be associated with both anterograde and retrograde amnesia. The degree of amnesia is the best index of the severity of the injury. Most concussions of short duration are not associated with macroscopic pathologic changes.

Contusions, or bruises on the surface of the brain, usually occur in the frontal or temporal tip. In more severe injuries, large hemorrhages may occur within the brain or outside the brain in the epidural or subdural space.

Chronic subdural hematomas often appear in elderly persons who have either no history of trauma or a trivial one. Patients may present with few or no localizing signs, but fluctuating confusion, apathy, and headache are common.

The syndrome of dementia pugilistica, or traumatic encephalopathy, is recognized more and more frequently in professional boxers. Symptoms, which include various combinations of dementia, dysarthria, ataxia, and parkinsonism, often occur several years after boxers stop fighting.

Demyelinating and Degenerative Diseases

Multiple Sclerosis

The cause of multiple sclerosis is still unknown. The incidence among individuals living in northern parts of Europe and the United States is higher than among those living in the tropics, and the incidence is higher among those who have lived in these areas before the age of 15. One theory holds that an infection occurs in childhood and remains dormant for years. When something triggers activation, an immune-mediated reaction to central nervous system myelin occurs.

Multiple sclerosis is characterized by a remitting and relapsing course of multiple neurologic symptoms, including blindness, diplopia, ataxia, nystagmus, spastic weakness, dysesthesia, and difficulty with bowel and bladder function. The CSF may reveal a few cells, usually mononuclear, plus an elevated gamma globulin level. Electroimmunodiffusion shows migration of gamma G immunoglobulin (IgG) on discrete (oligoclonal) bands. Evoked responses to visual, auditory, and somato-sensory stimuli document a delay in conduction of nerve impulses within the central nervous system. There are numerous scattered lesions throughout the white matter showing focal demyelination with relative sparing of axon cylinders.

There is no specific treatment for multiple sclerosis. Sometimes a course of corticosteroids shortens the duration of acute attacks. Treatment of an accompanying infection (in the urinary tract, for example) often lessens symptoms. Symptomatic treatment and supportive care diminish the effects of pain, disuse atrophy, contractures, and other complications of inactivity.

Motor Neuron Disease—Amyotrophic Lateral Sclerosis

Amyotrophic lateral sclerosis (ALS), a disease of the anterior horn cells or lower motor neurons, may also affect the motor cells of the cortex and brain stem. Progressive weakness, atrophy, and fasciculations occur in a widespread distribution. Fasciculations are thought to be due to irritability of anterior horn cells. Spasticity and hyperreflexia are considered secondary to loss of motor cortex cells.

There is a wide variation of clinical symptoms, with some patients showing more atrophy or more spasticity than others. Sometimes the hands are affected much more than the legs or vice versa. Some patients have almost exclusive cranial nerve involvement (progressive bulbar palsy), with speech and swallowing difficulties. Sensation is normal except for "uncomfortable sensations" and muscle cramps.

Blood chemistry results are normal except for slight creatine phosphokinase (CPK) level elevations in some patients. The electromyogram shows diffuse fasciculations and denervation. Muscle biopsy results demonstrate group fiber atrophy without inflammation.

Of patients with ALS, 90% are 40 to 70 years old. Men outnumber women 2 to 1. The mean survival is 3 to 4 years. A familial form of this disease affects about 10% of patients in the United States but about 57% of patients in Guam.

The etiology of ALS is unknown. Differential diagnoses should include polio-myelitis, cervical cord compression, hyperthyroidism, lead poisoning, and perhaps a paraneoplastic syndrome. There is no specific therapy except for an exercise program and an attempt to maintain good nutrition.

Friedreich's Ataxia

Of the many known cerebellar degenerations, the most important is Friedreich's ataxia. This autosomal-recessive disorder usually begins at puberty. Characteristics of Friedreich's ataxia include progressive gait and limb ataxia, decreased position sense and vibratory sensation in the legs, pyramidal weakness and extensor-plantar responses, absent deep tendon reflexes, dysarthria, and nystagmus. In addition, there is progressive kyphoscoliosis as well as prominent pes cavus and hypertrophic cardiomyopathy. The symptoms reflect pathologic degeneration, which is most prominent in the spinal cord and involves the spinocerebellar tracts, corticospinal tracts, and posterior columns.

Pes Cavus

Pes cavus, the major type of foot deformity associated with neurologic illness, is an exaggeration of the normal longitudinal arch of the foot, usually associated with some clawing of the toes. The mechanism underlying this deformity remains unknown. There are probably multiple causes, varying according to the specific disease with which the deformity is associated. Muscle factors, both intrinsic and extrinsic to the foot, may be operational. In some patients, weakness or dysfunction of intrinsic foot muscles, primarily the lumbricals, interossei, and short flexors, is postulated to cause clawing of the toes, with the cavus deformity being secondary. In other patients, a preponderance of certain muscle groups in the leg may bring about weakness of the antagonists; hypertonus of those muscles themselves; or perhaps some sort of muscle imbalance, as seen with cerebellar disease.

Patients with pes cavus can be divided into four groups:

1. Those with heredofamilial neurologic disease. Examples include the ataxic syndromes of spinocerebellar degenera-

tions, primarily Friedreich's ataxia and also some cases of hereditary olivoponto-cerebellar degeneration, and hereditary neuropathies, including peroneal muscular atrophy, or Charcot-Marie-Tooth disease; hereditary sensory radicular neuropathy; and Refsum's disease, a phytanic acid storage disease producing a peripheral neuropathy, ataxia, and retinitis pigmentosa. Other heredofamilial diseases associated with pes cavus are disorders of the spinal cord, including hereditary spastic paraplegia; developmental disorders, known as dysraphic states, often associated with spina bifida; and rare forms of congenital muscle disorders, such as nemaline and central core myopathy. (Table 11–6).

2. Those who have isolated pes cavus but whose family members have one of the aforementioned heredofamilial neurologic diseases. Families with members who have Friedreich's ataxia or Charcot-Marie-Tooth disease are particularly prone to have members with isolated pes cavus, which is thought to represent a very mild expression of the abnormal gene.

3. Those with isolated, or idiopathic, familial pes cavus with no family history of heredofamilial neurologic disease. Other family members may or may not have pes cavus, but no neurologic disease is found in any member on examination. A family history of pes cavus is found in nearly half of all patients with idiopathic pes cavus.

4. Those with familial pes cavus and

Table 11–6. NEUROLOGIC DISEASES ASSOCIATED WITH PES CAVUS

Spinocerebellar Degenerations

Friedreich's ataxia
Olivopontocerebellar atrophy

Spinal Cord Disorders

Hereditary spastic paraplegia
Spina bifida and other dysraphic states

Peripheral Neuropathies

Charcot-Marie-Tooth disease
Hereditary sensory radicular neuropathy
Refsum's disease

Congenital Myopathies

Central core disease
Nemaline myopathy

lymphedema. This very rare syndrome is not associated with any neurologic illness.

Cerebellar Disorders

Patients with cerebellar disorders occasionally present to the podiatrist because of imbalance and difficulty with walking. There are two broad clinical categories of cerebellar syndromes:

1. The midline syndrome, due to lesions of the spinocerebellum and vestibulocerebellum, consists primarily of severe gait ataxia and truncal instability. Some patients also have truncal tremor, or titubation; head tilt; and nystagmus, especially those with posteriorly located lesions. Lesions confined to midline structures cause little if any limb ataxia.

2. Lateral syndromes, due to lesions of the pontocerebellum, cause limb abnormalities ipsilateral to the side of the cerebellar lesion. These abnormalities include hypotonia; dysmetria, or disturbance of the trajectory of a limb; decomposition of movement; clumsiness of fine movement; postural and intention tremor; and abnormalities of pace and rebound. Dysarthria and various disturbances of extraocular movement are also present. Gait abnormalities, characterized by falling toward the side of the lesion, are observed in the majority of such patients.

Many different disease entities can cause cerebellar symptoms, and the clinical picture depends on their location, etiology, and rate of progression. Heredofamilial degenerative disorders, such as Friedreich's ataxia, have been discussed in a previous section. Various cerebellar anomalies, such as agenesis, Dandy-Walker deformity (association of a fourth ventricular cyst with vermal atresia and usually hydrocephalus), and Arnold-Chiari malformation (displacement of cerebellar tonsils and posterior vermis into the cervical spinal canal), often cause symptoms in infancy or early childhood. A variety of vascular diseases, including infarction and hemorrhage, cause acute onset of cerebellar dysfunction. Infections, including bacterial abscesses and viral meningoencephalitis, may cause ataxic disorders.

Many metabolic derangements produce cerebellar symptoms. These derangements include hypoxic-ischemic insults, hyperthermia, hepatic insufficiency, vitamin deficiency (especially thiamine), hypothyroidism, and hypoparathyroidism. Some inherited amino acid disorders as well as inherited lysosomal storage diseases may be expressed as prominent cerebellar dysfunction. Certain drugs may cause reversible cerebellar dysfunction, especially when taken in overdose. Chronic alcoholism is associated with a classic midline cerebellar syndrome, with degeneration of the superior vermis. Alcoholic cerebellar degeneration appears primarily with ataxia of gait and stance and is thought to relate to the vitamin deficiencies associated with chronic alcohol abuse rather than to the toxic effect of alcohol itself.

Multiple sclerosis frequently includes the cerebellar signs of ataxia, dysarthria, and intention tremor among its multiple symptoms. A subacute cerebellar syndrome is sometimes seen as a remote effect of carcinoma, especially small-cell carcinoma of the lungs. Occasionally, metastatic tumors may spread to the cerebellum. Astrocytomas of childhood and medulloblastomas appear in this location.

Disorders of Muscles and Nerves

Myopathies are disorders of muscle characterized by progressive weakness. The vast majority of myopathic disorders cause weakness that is most intense proximally in the shoulder and hip joints and less intense distally. There is progressive atrophy of muscle and eventual depression of reflexes. Laboratory aids useful in the diagnosis of myopathies include measurement of serum muscle enzymes, including CPK. Many myopathic disorders, however, are associated with normal muscle enzyme levels. Electromyography discloses early recruitment pattern of muscle units, full interference pattern, and fragmented motor units of low amplitude and short duration. Nerve conduction study findings should be normal. Muscle biopsy specimen discloses various changes in the muscle fibers, such as muscle fiber size variability, hyalinization of muscle fiber, internalized nuclei, and degeneration and phagocytosis of muscle fibers.

Muscular Dystrophies

The pathogenesis of muscular dystrophies, inherited disorders of progressive muscle weakness, is unknown, but many researchers believe that at least some cases are due to a genetic dysfunction of the muscle surface membrane. The most important of the muscular dystrophies is Duchenne's muscular dystrophy, an X-linked recessive disorder with a high rate of spontaneous mutation (30%). The incidence is 16 to 25/ 100,000 male births. The onset of symptoms is usually within the first 3 years of life. Walking may or may not be delayed, and the child never runs normally.

The disorder appears as a slowly progressive proximal weakness, beginning in the lower extremities and later involving the upper extremities. This weakness is often associated with early toe walking and causes a waddling gait. There is frequently pseudohypertrophy of the calves. Progressive orthopedic deformities, such as Achilles tendon contractures, contractures of the knee and elbows, and kyphoscoliosis, occur. Electrocardiogram abnormalities (tall right precordial R waves) occur in most patients. Rarely, arrhythmias and heart failure occur. About one third of these so-affected patients have IQs of less than 75. Patients with Duchenne's muscular dystrophy have progressive muscle atrophy and weakness. Patients become wheelchair bound by the age of 12 and succumb in their teens or 20s.

The serum CPK level is markedly elevated early in the course of the disease and declines progressively with age. Genetic screening should be offered to potential female carriers, that is, mothers or sisters of patients with Duchenne's muscular dystrophy; 75% of carriers have elevated serum CPK levels. Such carriers could then be given the option of terminating pregnancy. The location of the abnormal gene on the X chromosome has been identified (Xp21 locus). Dystrophin, a muscle enzyme coded for this genetic region, is absent in Duchenne's muscular dystrophy.

Becker's muscular dystrophy, a more benign form of X-linked muscular dystrophy, is clinically similar to Duchenne's dystrophy and is manifested by progressive proximal limb weakness. The onset in most patients occurs after the age of 7 and in some instances not until the 20s. Such patients are still walking by age 15 and do not become wheechair bound until the 20s to the 50s. About half of all patients with Becker's dystrophy survive beyond the age of 40.

Facioscapulohumeral dystrophy is an autosomal-dominant disorder with variable penetrance. Facioscapulohumeral dystrophy has an insidious onset of weakness between the ages of 7 and 25 and is compatible with a normal life expectancy. The characteristic distribution of weakness involves the shoulder girdle with marked weakness of the scapular muscles and weakness of the biceps and triceps and relative sparing of the forearm muscles (the so-called Popeye arm). This is associated with bilateral facial and leg weakness, the latter being most marked in the anterior muscle compartment, causing a foot drop.

Limb girdle muscular dystrophy refers to a heterogeneous group of disorders characterized by progressive proximal weakness. Most cases are autosomal recessive, although a large number of sporadic cases appear in the literature. The time of onset ranges from childhood to early adulthood.

Myotonic muscular dystrophy is an autosomal-dominant disorder that affects multiple systems. Symptoms involve a combination of weakness and myotonia. Myotonia refers to delayed relaxation of muscle following contraction and is associated with abnormal EMG discharges (sustained, repetitive motor unit potentials that wax and wane, giving a dive-bomber effect). The progressive weakness in myotonic dystrophy involves facial muscles, pharyngeal muscles, and limb muscles. The weakness is most marked distally and is associated with hyporeflexia. Other abnormalities include dysfunction of smooth muscle; hypogonadism and other endocrine dysfunction; mental retardation; cataracts; heart disease, especially conduction defects; and frontal balding.

Myotonic dystrophy must be distinguished from other hereditary disorders associated with myotonia. Most important among these rare disorders is myotonia congenita, an autosomal-dominant or a recessive disorder consisting of severe myotonia with little weakness.

Congenital Myopathies

Congenital myopathies are characterized by onset of weakness at birth or shortly thereafter and delayed motor development. The course is usually nonprogressive or very slowly progressive in contrast to the muscular dystrophies. The serum muscle enzyme levels are either normal or only slightly elevated. The hallmarks of these disorders are the various structural abnormalities seen in muscle biopsy specimens. Congenital myopathies are frequently associated with skeletal anomalies, such as dislocated hip, and pes cavus.

Central core disease, which is transmitted as an autosomal-dominant trait in most reported cases, appears as clinically mild, slightly progressive weakness, especially of the legs, and mild facial weakness. Of these patients, 70% have muscle contracture and pes cavus. The pathology involves a central core in type 1 muscle fibers.

Nemaline myopathy, which is characterized by small, round bodies in muscle fibers, has been reported to occur as an autosomal-dominant inheritance as well as sporadically. There is universal wasting of muscle mass and a variety of skeletal deformities, including high arch palate, kyphosis, pigeon breast, and pes cavus.

Other congenital myopathies are myotubular myopathy, which includes eye-movement weakness; sarcotubular myopathy; fingerprint-body myopathy; reducing-body myopathy; fiber-type disproportion; and other rare disorders characterized by distinctive morphologic abnormalities.

Metabolic Myopathies

Metabolic myopathies appear either as slowly progressive proximal weakness, sometimes resembling muscular dystrophy, or as exercise-induced cramps and myoglobinuria. Two broad categories of metabolic myopathies exist: (1) disorders involving glycogen metabolism, and (2) disorders affecting lipids. The best studied glycogen storage disease is McArdle's disease, or myophosphorylase deficiency, which occurs as exercise-induced contracture and myoglobinuria. Another glycogen storage disease, acid-maltase deficiency, appears as progressive limb girdle weakness either in childhood or adulthood. Intercostal and diaphragmatic muscles are involved relatively early, leading to respiratory failure.

Lipid myopathies include muscle carnitine deficiency, which appears as progressive limb girdle weakness, and carnitine palmitoyl transferase deficiency, which occurs as exercise intolerance and myoglobinuria after prolonged exercise. A few cases of mitochondrial myopathies, a heterogeneous group of disorders characterized by abnormal mitochondria, have been reported. Some myopathies have been shown to be associated with specific defects, including mitochondrial respiratory gas chain enzyme.

Acquired Myopathies

A variety of endocrine disorders may cause slowly progressive and prominent muscle weakness. Hyperthyroidism causes significant proximal muscle weakness in approximately half of all patients. Hypothyroidism may also produce proximal limb weakness, and hyperparathyroidism may produce a distinct syndrome with proximal aching and muscle weakness, at times associated with hyperreflexia. Proximal weakness is a prominent feature of Cushing's syndrome.

A variety of drugs, the most important of which are corticosteroids, may also produce muscle weakness. Antibiotics may occasionally cause weakness as well. Patients who abuse alcohol may present either with an acute, painful, generalized or focal myopathy associated with myoglobinuria, or with a chronic, painless, progressive proximal weakness, which may be at least partly neuropathic. Severe subacute myopathy associated with severe hypokalemia is also frequently seen in alcoholics, especially after prolonged vomiting or diarrhea.

Among the most common acquired myopathies are the inflammatory disorders of polymyositis and dermatomyositis. These disorders appear as subacute symmetric proximal limb and trunk weakness progressing over a period of weeks to months. Dysphagia is common. Dermatomyositis is distinguished by the presence of typical skin lesions. The erythematous rash characteristically occurs over the malar region, eyelids, knuckles, elbows, and knees. The inflammatory myopathies may be associated with other collagen vascular diseases, such as scleroderma, rheumatoid arthritis, and SLE, as well as carcinoma, most commonly bronchogenic. Characteristic laboratory abnormalities include elevated muscle enzyme levels, "myopathic" EMG results, and muscle biopsy results showing destruction and phagocytosis of muscle fibers associated with a mononuclear infiltration. Standard treatment includes high doses of corticosteroids and if this is not effective the addition of immunosuppressive agents. There have been no controlled trials of this treatment.

Fluctuating Muscle Weakness Disorders

Several diseases are responsible for fluctuating muscle weakness. The most common is myasthenia gravis. Myasthenia gravis is an autoimmune disorder caused by serum antibodies directed against the acetylcholine receptor in the postsynaptic region on the muscle membrane and is characterized by fluctuating weakness of voluntary muscles, which fatigue with exercise and are restored to strength with rest. In more than 90% of patients, there is involvement of the cranial muscles, particularly the oculomotor muscles, producing various combinations of ptosis, eye-movement abnormalities, bifacial weakness, and oropharyngeal dysfunction. Limb muscles are involved in a proximal to distal distribution, but reflexes and sensation are intact. The thymus gland is enlarged in 70% of patients, and an actual thymoma is found in 10%.

Laboratory test abnormalities include the presence of antibodies to the acetylcholine receptor in 90% of patients as well as abnormal decremental response to repetitive stimulation on electrodiagnostic testing. Treatment includes the use of anticholinesterases, corticosteroids, immunosuppressive drugs, thymectomy, and plasmapheresis.

The myasthenic syndrome, or Eaton-Lambert syndrome, is frequently associated with an underlying carcinoma, usually small-cell carcinoma of the lung. Eaton-Lambert syndrome, characterized by a decrease in the release of acetylcholine from the presynaptic terminal, appears as progressive weakness, mild atrophy, and fatigability of the proximal limb muscles. Cranial nerve abnormalities are rare in patients with this condition, in contrast to those with myasthenia gravis. Repetitive stimulation on electrodiagnostic testing reveals a dramatic incremental response at fast rates of stimulation. Treatment includes removal of the underlying tumor, administration of guanidine, and plasmapheresis.

The most common of the familial periodic paralyses is familial hypokalemic periodic paralysis, an autosomal-dominant disorder. Familial hypokalemic periodic paralysis appears with attacks of weakness rapidly developing over the course of an hour to involve all four extremities and usually resolving within several hours. During the attack, there is a reduction in the amount of serum potassium passing into the muscle, which becomes inexcitable. The frequency of attacks is quite variable, ranging from one in a lifetime to weekly or daily. Thyrotoxic periodic paralysis is an acquired form of hypokalemic periodic paralysis, occuring primarily in hyperthyroid male Asians and characterized by attacks of weakness associated with hypokalemia.

Familial hyperkalemic periodic paralysis, also an autosomal-dominant disorder, usually has its onset before the age of 10. The attacks are relatively mild, lasting an hour or so, and may be precipitated by the administration of potassium. The serum potassium level usually is elevated during an attack. Myotonic phenomena are seen in some patients.

Disorders of the Spinal Cord and Nerve Roots

Spinal Cord Disorders

The spinal cord is subject to a multitude of diseases and may produce a variety of clinical syndromes, some of which occasionally come to the attention of the podiatrist. The clinician should be able to localize the involved segmental units and the level of tract dysfunction of the spinal cord lesion on examination. Localizing a particular level of a focal lesion is easier if one remembers the Brown-Séquard syndrome (hemisection of one lateral half of the spinal cord). Below the hemisection is weakness and usually spasticity of muscles on the same side. Reaction to touch and vibration and sense of position are severely impaired below the lesion on the same side; pain and temperature are lost on the opposite side. A careful sensory and motor examination shows the site of the lesion, usually within one or two root levels.

Acute spinal cord dysfunction may be caused by trauma, compression, inflammation, infarction, vascular malformation, and hemorrhage. Trauma, usually associated with fracture, dislocation, or both of the vertebral column, leads the list. The most common sites of traumatic injury are at the cervical and the eleventh-thoracic–second lumbar vertebral levels. As is the case in most acute myelopathies, initial examination reveals spinal shock, with flaccid paralysis, areflexia, paralysis of bowel and bladder functions, and a lack of sensation below the level of the lesion. After approximately 2 to 3 weeks, increased tone with spasticity, hyperreflexia, and reflex emptying of bowel and bladder occur.

Compression from metastatic tumor usually arises from vertebral metastasis and appears early with localized back pain, followed by progressive signs of cord dysfunction. Acute epidural cord compression may also be caused by epidural abscess, usually arising from osteomyelitis of the spine; epidural hemorrhage, which sometimes occurs spontaneously; sometimes secondarily to anticoagulation therapy or bleeding in hemophiliacs; and, rarely, cervical and thoracic central disk herniation. Cord compression constitutes a medical emergency, usually necessitating neurosurgical intervention. In the case of epidural compression from known neoplasm, emergency steroids and radiation are indicated. The diagnosis is usually made by MRI or myelography.

When a patient presents with an acute myelopathy and has a normal myelogram, other disorders must be considered. Acute transverse myelitis is an inflammatory spinal cord disorder, probably representing several different etiologies. The most common type of acute transverse myelitis often occurs after a viral infection and is thought to be the result of an autoimmune process. Multiple sclerosis is a rather uncommon cause of acute transverse myelitis, which usually results in a more subacute or chronic myelopathy.

A spinal cord vascular malformation appears either as a subacute myelopathy or as an acute disorder caused by hemorrhage from the malformation. The spinal cord vasculature is very tenuous. The main supply to the anterior two thirds of the cord comes from the anterior spinal artery, which is fed by relatively few radicular arteries. Acute infarction of the spinal cord usually occurs from processes that cut off the blood supply from one or more of the feeding radicular arteries. This infarction can occur after aortic aneurysm surgery or as a result of dissecting aneurysm of the aorta or diseases affecting the small arteries, such as syphilis, diabetes mellitus, and vasculitis.

Chronic spinal cord syndromes are associated with a variety of disorders. In the elderly, cervical spondylosis is the most common etiology. In this condition, degenerative bony and ligamentous changes of the cervical vertebral region slowly compress the cervical spinal cord. Certain benign tumors, primarily meningiomas and schwannomas, also cause chronic syndromes. Nutritional disorders, especially vitamin B_{12} deficiency; some toxins; and some hereditary disorders, such as hereditary spastic paraplegia, are rare causes of chronic myelopathies.

Chronic spinal syndromes are marked primarily by dysfunction of the long tracts, although segmental weakness, pain, and reflex changes may also be present. In addition, there are a variety of disorders that primarily affect the segmental units within the cord. Syringomyelia, a central cavity within the cord, usually occurs in the lower cervical and upper thoracic regions. During early stages, involvement of lower motor neurons at several segments usually produces hand atrophy; the crossing of spinothalamic fibers causes pain and temperature loss in a segmental, often capelike distribution; and reflexes are absent in the involved segments in the upper extremities. Later,if the cavity enlarges, there is pressure and destruction of the long tracts, producing spasticity and a posterior column sensory loss. Although syringomyelic syndromes sometimes occur with intramedullary tumors, arachnoiditis, or following a trauma, syringomyelia is usually associated with maldevelopment of the hindbrain and cerebellar tonsillar herniation (Arnold-Chiari syndrome). Other disorders that primarily affect the lower motor neurons include some forms of motor neuron disease and poliomyelitis.

Radiculopathies

About 400,000 claims for financial compensation for low back pain, one of the most common disorders treated in the practice of medicine, are made annually in the United States. Often a clear diagnosis cannot be reached. Poorly understood injury to the muscles or ligaments, often given labels such as "lumbosacral strain" or "lumbosacral sprain," causes pain and spasm. A variety of other diseases, such as metastatic tumor or osteomyelitis, may also cause back pain.

A common cause of back pain in patients seen by the podiatrist is compression of the lumbosacral nerve roots, which may be secondary to osteoarthritic changes encroaching on the exiting nerve roots in the neural foramina, or disk herniation. Of lumbosacral disk protrusions, 95% occur either at the fourth lumbar-fifth lumbar area, which usually compresses the fifth lumbar nerve root, or at the fifth lumbar-first sacral region, which usually compresses the first sacral nerve root. A fifth lumbar nerve radiculopathy, in addition to back pain, often causes radiating pain down the lateral aspect of the leg, numbness or paresthesias of the lateral calf and dorsum of the foot, and weakness of toe and ankle dorsiflexion. A first sacral nerve radiculopathy characteristically causes radiating pain down the posterior leg associated with sensory changes on the lateral and plantar aspects of the foot, weakness of foot and toe plantar flexion, and absent ankle reflex. So-called mechanical back signs are present with straight leg raising pain, paraspinal muscle spasm, and scoliosis. However, not all the aforementioned symptoms and signs are present in patients with radiculopathy, who often present with leg pain or paresthesias and few objective findings on examination. Diagnosis of the herniated disk may be confirmed by myelography, CT or MRI of the lumbosacral spine, and electromyography.

Disorders of Behavior and Cognition

Confusional States

Some disorders cause acute confusional states in which the sensorium is impaired and varying degrees of inattentiveness, distractibility, delirium, and stupor as well as global impairment of cognitive abilities are featured. Confusional states are largely the neurologic manifestations of medical illnesses. Pulmonary, renal, and hepatic failure can all cause encephalopathies characterized by confusional states, behavioral changes, postural tremors, asterixis, and at times myoclonic jerks. Cardiac arrest can be followed by various degrees of confusional and demented illness, depending on the degree of ischemia and anoxia. Malignant hypertension is also associated with mental status changes, headaches, and sometimes seizures. Acute derangement of mental functions may be caused by a variety of endocrine disorders, including diabetic ketoacidosis, nonketonic hyperosmolar coma, hypoglycemia, hyperthyroidism, hypothyroidism, Cushing's syndrome, Addison's disease, and disorders associated with hypercalcemia. Both elevation and depression of serum sodium levels may be associated with mental status changes.

A variety of hematologic disorders, such as those associated with hyperviscosity states and intravascular coagulation, may produce confusional states along with multifocal neurologic signs. Vasculitides, including SLE, at times cause prominent mental status changes. Neoplasms, either directly through metastatic spread or in association with various paraneoplastic syndromes, may cause behavioral and cognitive changes. Infections of the central nervous system, including meningitis and encephalitis, as well as a variety of deficiency states, such as vitamin B_{12} deficiency, may at times cause mental status changes. Acute confusional states may appear as a prominent part of the neurologic picture in patients with vascular diseases affecting the brain.

Clinical effects of acute alcohol intoxication include euphoria, lack of coordination, and sedation, sometimes to the point of coma or even death. Obvious ataxia occurs at blood alcohol levels of 0.1%; deep anesthesia occurs at about 0.4%. Alcohol withdrawal may produce a syndrome of tremulousness, hallucinosis, seizures, and delirium tremens with autonomic overactivity due to the sudden withdrawal of the sedative effects of alcohol. The biochemical mechanism is unknown. The delirium usually begins 2 to 4 days following the withdrawal of alcohol and lasts about 72 hours or sometimes longer. The morbidity is about 15%. Chronic alcoholism may be associated with dementia, recent-memory

difficulties, ataxia, and oculomotor weakness (Wernicke-Korsakoff syndrome). Both the toxic effects of alcohol and chronic thiamine deficiency are probably responsible for the pathophysiology.

Sedative-hypnotics, such as barbiturates, bromides, chloral hydrate, and benzodiazepines, are particularly dangerous when they produce enough sedation to interfere with respiratory drive and lead to anoxic encephalopathy or death. These agents may also lead to withdrawal seizures and an organic mental syndrome when stopped abruptly after a period of high dosage.

Tricyclic antidepressants (e.g. amitriptyline, imipramine) in overdose may cause coma or confusion, seizures, and cardiac arrhythmias. Monoamine oxidase inhibitors may produce a hypertensive crisis and encephalopathy if taken with tyramine-containing substances. Strychnine is a central nervous system stimulant that interferes with postsynaptic inhibition, causing severe tetanic spasms and altered cognition. Stimulants, such as amphetamines, may cause hypertension, necrotizing vasculitis, and cerebral hemorrhage. Personality changes and schizophrenia may occur with long-term use of stimulants.

Dementia

Conditions characterized by deterioration of cognitive abilities in the presence of a clear sensorium are known as dementias. The most common cause of dementia is Alzheimer's disease. An estimated 10% of the population over age 65 in the United States suffers from Alzheimer's disease. Alzheimer's disease is characterized by early onset of short-term memory problems that steadily progress, gradual disturbance of language and cognitive abilities, and behavioral symptoms. The disease is associated with nerve cell loss and typical microscopic changes, such as neurofibrillar tangles, senile plaques, and granulovacuolar variations. Studies of the neurochemical basis of Alzheimer's disease have found a selective degeneration of a small group of subcortical cells in the nucleus basalis of Meynert, which projects diffusely to the cortex. Acetylcholine is the neurotransmitter. Preliminary trials using medications that increase central acetylcholine levels have been promising. Unfortunately no significant clinical benefits have been derived by any treatment. Ordinarily Alzheimer's disease is inexorably progressive over a period of several years.

Many other diseases may appear as dementias, including other degenerative diseases; some infectious diseases, especially neurosyphilis; and multiple cerebral infarctions. Occasionally patients with some of the disorders that more commonly cause acute confusional states may also present with chronic dementia. Evaluation of such patients includes metabolic evaluation, CT or MRI of the head to exclude tumors or subdural hematomas, and electroencephalography.

Neurologic Complications of Surgery and Anesthesia

Central Nervous System Complications of General Anesthesia and Surgery

The most devastating and feared complication of surgery is anoxic central nervous system injury due to anesthetic accidents. An estimated 60% of anesthetic accidents lead to cerebral hypoxia and death and almost half of these are due to faulty technique, such as esophageal intubation.

Certain anesthetics have direct toxic effects on the central nervous system. Ketamine, for instance, can cause postoperative hallucinations, delirium, and transient cortical blindness; it may also increase seizure activity. Halothane can cause convulsions and tetany. Enflurane (Ethrane) may occasionally cause delayed seizures. As patients awaken from anesthesia in the recovery room, an "emergence" delirium and excitement may occur.

A rare complication of surgery, usually occurring in women, is hyponatremia due to inappropriate antidiuretic hormone secretion. Usually incorrectly diagnosed, this condition may cause otherwise unexplained seizures, confusion, and coma during the postoperative period and may lead to permanent brain damage or death if not promptly treated.

Malignant Hyperthermia

Malignant hyperthermia is a rare but serious complication of volatile anesthetics and depolarizing neuromuscular blocking agents, such as succinylcholine and decamethonium. This complication is characterized by intense contraction of muscle, which results in severe hyperthermia, and is associated with muscle breakdown, myoglobinuria, renal failure, hyperkalemia, lactic acidosis, and shock. Malignant hyperthermia carries a 60 to 70% mortality rate. Those patients who survive have diffusely weak, swollen muscles and extremely high serum CPK values. This syndrome is thought to occur in patients with an underlying muscle disorder, many of whom have persistently high CPK values and a positive family history of similar reactions to anesthesia. The treatment of malignant hyperthermia consists of immediate cessation of anesthesia and the administration of intravenous dantrolene.

Postoperative Apnea

During recovery from anesthesia, an occasional patient exhibits persistent inadequate ventilation, often associated with ocular and bulbar weakness, due to prolonged neuromuscular blockade. Such a situation could occur for the following reasons:

1. Prolonged action of succinylcholine. Certain patients have very low activity of plasma cholinesterase, the enzyme that hydrolyzes and inactivates succinylcholine. In such individuals, the action of succinylcholine is prolonged and may last for several hours. Decreased plasma cholinesterase activity may occur during pregnancy; in patients with hepatic disease or malnutrition; in patients who are taking certain drugs, such as oral contraceptives; and in patients with a genetic variant of the enzyme.

2. Side effects of nonanesthetic drugs. A variety of drugs may interfere with neuromuscular transmission, including antibiotics, such as aminoglycosides; adrenergic-blocking agents; membrane stabilizers, such as quinidine; psychotropic drugs, such as chlorpromazine; and corticosteroids.

3. Latent or previously unrecognized disorders of neuromuscular transmission. Patients with myasthenia gravis or Eaton-Lambert syndrome are very sensitive to the paralyzing effects of *d*-tubocurarine or pancuronium, and prolonged and severe

neuromuscular blockade can result after the use of such agents.

4. Anesthetic errors (e.g., administering excessive doses of neuromuscular blocking agents).

The treatment of postoperative apnea consists of reintubation and support of the patient until spontaneous improvement occurs.

Peripheral Nerve Injuries

A variety of neuropathic injuries, usually caused by stretching or compression of nerves, can occur during surgery. The most common is a brachial plexus neuropathy due to stretching of the plexus when the arm and body are held in certain positions during surgery. The upper brachial plexus is most often involved, but occasionally the lower plexus or the entire plexus is injured. The radial nerve can be compressed at the spiral groove, the ulnar nerve can be compressed at the elbow when the arm is extended and pronated, and, rarely, the median nerve can be injured in the antecubital fossa from intravenous injections. In the lower extremity, the peroneal nerve can be compressed against the fibular head; the sciatic nerve can be injured when the opposite buttock is elevated, especially in a thin, emaciated patient; and the femoral nerve can be injured, especially during surgery in the lithotomy position.

Clinical signs of tourniquet paralysis have become rare since the introduction of the pneumatic tourniquet, which is used during certain surgical procedures to create a bloodless operative field. However, EMG evidence of denervation in muscles distal to the tourniquet are found in two thirds of patients in whom the tourniquet is used. Peripheral neuropathic injuries may also result from direct surgical trauma.

Complications of Spinal Anesthesia

Neurologic complications of epidural and spinal anesthesia are rare. Occasionally the spinal needle can injure a single nerve root directly, and this usually resolves within a few weeks. An acute cauda equina syndrome with areflexic paralysis of legs and bowel and bladder dysfunction due to a direct toxic effect of the spinal anesthetic on the cauda equina has been de-

scribed. Ischemic necrosis of the lumbar spinal cord immediately following epidural anesthesia is a very unusual occurrence. In patients with thrombocytopenia, an epidural or a subdural hemorrhage may be precipitated by spinal or epidural anesthesia, with symptoms of cord or cauda equina compression appearing after a delay of hours or days. Progressive spinal adhesive arachnoiditis (inflammation followed by fibrosis of the arachnoid space surrounding the cord and nerve roots), in which symptoms of a myelopathy and polyradiculopathy occur weeks to months following spinal anesthesia, is now quite rare.

Management of Surgical Patients With Neurologic Illness

The care of surgical patients with chronic neurologic illnesses differs little from the management of other surgical patients, and under most circumstances, special precautions are not necessary except as common sense dictates.

Patients with seizure disorders need to be maintained on anticonvulsants. The majority of such patients undergoing podiatric surgery should not have a prolonged period without oral intake and therefore can be maintained on their regular anticonvulsant regimens. If postoperative ileus or other circumstances preclude oral intake for a prolonged period, parenteral anticonvulsants should be used. The primary anticonvulsants available for parenteral use are phenobarbital and phenytoin. Phenytoin should never be given intramuscularly. The daily parenteral dose of anticonvulsants is the same as the oral dose.

Patients with cerebrovascular disease, including significant carotid stenosis, have not been found to be at significantly increased risk for perioperative stroke. Therefore special precautions and extensive preoperative vascular evaluations are unnecessary.

Patients with multiple sclerosis may have an increased rate of acute exacerbations following spinal anesthesia. These patients do not have an increased rate of acute exacerbations following general anesthesia or surgery by itself.

Patients with myasthenia gravis are at particular risk for prolonged postoperative apnea. Special precautions and meticulous monitoring of such patients are necessary.

Parkinsonian patients as well as many elderly patients who are otherwise neurologically intact may develop severe problems with postural reflexes and ambulation following prolonged bed rest. Early ambulation and physical therapy are important in the management of these patients.

Patients with dementia frequently deteriorate markedly during hospitalization and may become quite confused, agitated, hallucinatory, and very difficult to manage. These patients are frequently worse at night ("sundowning"). This situation of "beclouded dementia" is often multifactorial in origin, with the new environment, sleep deprivation in the hospital setting, medications, and developing metabolic abnormalities all playing a role. Careful review of medications, blood tests, and other evaluations is required. Such patients may benefit from low-dose neuroleptics, such as haloperidol. Patients who develop a florid delirium several days after being admitted to the hospital should also be evaluated for the possibility of alcohol or drug withdrawal.

Bibliography

Adams RD, Victor M: Principles of Neurology, 3rd ed. New York: McGraw-Hill Book Co, 1985.

Baker AB, Baker LH: Clinical Neurology, Philadelphia: Harper & Row Publishers, Inc, 1983.

Harvey AM, Johns RJ, McKusick VA, Owens AH, Ross RS: The Principles and Practice of Medicine. 22nd ed. East Norwalk, CT: Appleton-Century-Crofts, 1988.

Isselbacher KJ, Adams RD, Braunwald E, Petersdorf RG, Wilson JD: Harrison's Principles of Internal Medicine, 10th ed. New York: McGraw-Hill Book Co, 1983.

Layzer RB: Neuromuscular Manifestations of Systemic Disease. Philadelphia: FA Davis Co, 1985.

Merritt HH: A Textbook of Neurology, 7th ed. Philadelphia: Lea & Febiger, 1983.

Mohr JP (ed): Manual of Clinical Problems in Neurology. Boston: Little, Brown, & Co, 1984.

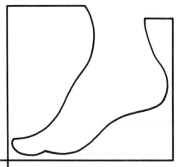

12 DERMATOLOGY

RICHARD B. ODOM, STEVEN BAKER, and ROBERT SHAPS

OVERVIEW

The close relationship between dermatology and podiatry is obvious to those who practice either specialty. It would be an unusual day indeed, in either a general podiatry or dermatology practice, that would not have a significant number of patients whose main complaint concerned the skin of their feet. From the podiatrist's point of view, some surveys estimate 50% of patients' visits are related to dermatology. Despite what would seem to be arduous conditions, skin problems of the foot do not occupy a greater percentage of a dermatologist's practice than would be accounted for by the foot's percentage of body skin. This would indicate that the skin of the foot is well adapted to its often hostile environment. In today's modern industrial societies, this environment usually includes being in shoes, which oftentimes means hot conditions that bring about sweating and contact with chemicals from the shoes. These conditions are conducive to the growth of microorganisms and disruptive to the normal physiology of the skin.

Many of the types of skin problems that bring patients to physicians can be well recognized and treated. To the novice with an untrained eye, a rash is a rash, and everything looks the same. This unfortunate attitude is doubly disappointing when one appreciates how much can really be differentiated by a competent practitioner, a brief history, and a physical examination. The podiatric physician with a strong foundation in dermatology should be able to diagnose and treat a wide variety of skin diseases and also recognize those that should be referred to other specialists.

PATHOPHYSIOLOGY

The skin is obviously designed to "hold us together." Besides this, however, the skin is involved in keeping out harmful elements, whether they are chemical, microbiologic, or environmental. Temperature regulation, adaptation to changing conditions, and other functions are usually taken for granted, although all these processes are in a constant state of equilibrium and require dynamic regulation of changing conditions.

Layers of Skin

The skin of the foot, with certain modifications, shares most of its anatomy with that of the skin of the rest of the body. The skin is composed of three layers: the *epidermis,* or outermost layer; the *dermis,* or supportive layer; and the *subcutaneous fat,* usually quite minimal on the foot, which functions as a cushion and a fat repository. The dermis, which is sometimes grouped with the subcutaneous fat as cutis, is mostly collagen fibers and gives the skin strength and elasticity. Blood vessels and nerves run through the dermis.

Growing down from the epidermis into the dermis are several skin appendages. The pilosebaceous structure consists of a hair follicle with an attached sebaceous, or oil, gland. On a few areas of the face and upper trunk there may be sebaceous glands unassociated with hair follicles, which empty directly onto the surface of the skin. Also piercing the epidermis are tiny ducts from the eccrine sweat glands, which are lodged in the lower dermis and upper subcutaneous tissue. The eccrine glands provide sweat for thermoregulation. In the axillae, groin, and a few other areas, there are also apocrine sweat glands, the ducts of which empty into hair follicles.

The epidermis is the highly differentiated outer layer of skin, which usually consists of four distinct histologic zones. These zones are, starting from the outside, the stratum corneum, or horny or keratin layer; the stratum granulosum, or granular layer; the stratum spinosum, or prickle or spiny layer; and the basal cell layer. Basal cells divide and migrate upward to become prickle cells, then progressively change into granular cells, and finally into cells of the stratum corneum. This migration, from the basal cell layer to the top of the stratum corneum, takes approximately 28 days and is defined as turnover time. It takes 14 days (transit time) for the cell to reach the stratum corneum and another 14 days to be discarded.

In the foot, as in the hand, there is another distinct zone, the stratum lucidum, which is located between the spiny and granular layers. In the epidermis, the basal cells, or bottom-most cells, divide and push living cells upward. At the outer surface, these cells undergo a chemical change into a dead fibrous protein called keratin, which is the body's protective barrier against the environment. There are also specialized cells, such as melanocytes and Langerhans's cells, scattered in the epidermis. Some of the specialized structures and cells throughout the skin are of great importance to skin diseases of the foot (Fig. 12–1).

The epidermis and dermis are bound together by a series of projections that grow up (dermal papillae) and down (rete ridges), which interface with each other. The skin ranges in thickness from $1\frac{1}{2}$ to 4 mm. The epidermis is usually only $\frac{1}{10}$ mm thick. However, the keratin layer may increase this by 1 mm in such areas as the palms and soles. Because the skin is so accessible to biopsy, histopathology plays a great role in diagnosis.

Skin Changes

Skin diseases often appear with distinct histologic pictures. Dermatologists utilize specific terms to describe the various microscopic changes and lesions (Table 12–1). Skin lesions are pathologic changes in normal structures. Each change that one sees during clinical inspection is due to a change in one of the structures mentioned. Elevations of the skin may be due to an increase in thickness of one or all three layers of the skin. The ability of the skin to resist disrupting forces and shearing and the ability of the skin to heal are related to the mechanical properties of the skin. The aging process and defective structural elements from inherited disorders also affect toughness and resistance to forces. Strength and flexibility are essential. For example, the collagen fiber network gives high tensile strength, and the loose meshing allows mobility of joints. As we age, the degradation of the elastin fiber network

Table 12–1. DESCRIPTIVE TERMS OF MICROSCOPIC CHANGES

Hyperkeratosis—thickening of the horny layer (stratum corneum)
Parakeratosis—thickening stratum corneum with nuclei that may be disintegrating
Acanthosis—thickening of the epidermis, particularly the spiny layer
Spongiosis—intercellular edema of the spiny layer
Intraepidermal—from the basement membrane upward
Intradermal—within the dermis

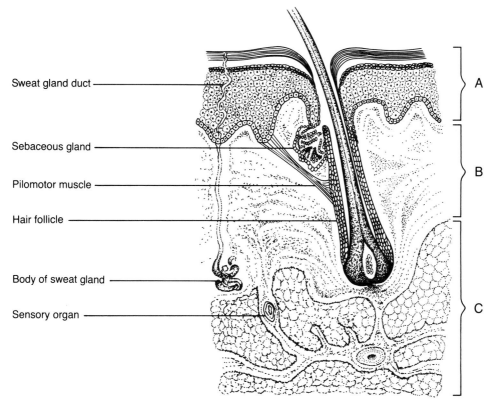

Sweat gland duct

Sebaceous gland

Pilomotor muscle

Hair follicle

Body of sweat gland

Sensory organ

A

B

C

Figure 12–1. Structures of the skin. *A*, Epidermis; *B*, dermis; and *C*, subcutaneous tissue.

leaves the collagen mesh without the support to restore fully its original configuration, and the surface evidence is wrinkled skin. The ground substance, which is not well understood, resists compression and accepts molding, which reduces point pressure on more sensitive skin structures.

The skin cannot survive without oxygen and nutrients. The prime-provider role of blood vessels is well understood through results from disruption in gangrenous toes and leg ulcers that do not heal. Apart from the main role, of nutrition and thermal regulation, dermal blood vessels participate in the inflammatory response and demonstrate pathologic changes in specific diseases. These changes include transient vasoconstriction, as seen with noxious stimuli; increased vessel permeability, resulting in the escape of fluid into the interstitial spaces; vascular proliferation; and, with certain trauma or stimuli, construction or development of complete lesions, as seen in collagen diseases, psoriasis, and lichen planus.

Changes associated with aging include thinning epidermis; atrophy of skin of appendages; sparse hair; and decrease of sebaceous secretions, with dryness, chapping, and fissuring the consequences. The dermis loses elastic and support properties. Sun exposure intensifies and augments the aging process. Actinic damage results in thin, wrinkled, unevenly pigmented, scaly skin. Telangiectatic vessels are seen along with actinic keratoses. Yellow plaques, comedones, and follicular cysts also appear.

APPROACH TO DIAGNOSIS OF DERMATOLOGIC PROBLEMS

Describing the Lesion

Dermatology is primarily a visual specialty. The vocabulary in this specialty centers on visual descriptive terms. The terms in Table 12–2 are the ones used most often and allow a dermatologist or podiatrist to visualize lesions described in a patient's chart or over the telephone.

Lesions are divided into primary and secondary lesions (Table 12–3). Primary

Table 12–2. TERMS USED TO DESCRIBE SKIN
LESIONS

Term	Description
Color	Purple papule (Kaposi's sarcoma), pearly (basal cell carcinoma), red (acne), yellow (xanthoma)
Shape	Linear, annular (ring), oval, polygonal, dome shaped, pointed
Number	Objective way to assess improvement or worsening in some cases
Size	It is always helpful to measure things, to determine growth
Grouping	Discrete (separated), confluent (run together), grouped, dermatomal, scattered, symmetric, asymmetric
Location	Pictures with distances from common landmarks (lateral malleolus, angle of jaw, patella)
Texture	Soft, hard, boggy, firm, cystic
Surface	Smooth, warty, pebbly, granular, oozing, weeping, macerated, lichenified (more prominent skin markings)
Symptoms	Although part of history, may be elicited during the examination. Pruritic (itchy), burning, stinging, painful, tender, asymptomatic

Table 12–3. HOW TO DESCRIBE SKIN LESIONS

Primary Lesions

Macule—a circumscribed change in color of normal skin without elevation or depression; less than 1 cm in diameter; example—freckle
Patch—similar to a macule but greater than 1 cm in diameter
Papule—a circumscribed solid elevation in the skin, most of which is above the plane of the skin; less than 1 cm; example—wart
Nodule—similar to a papule but greater than 1 cm
Tumor—similar to nodule but greater than 2 cm
Plaque—an elevation above the skin surface that occupies a plateaulike surface area; example—psoriasis
Vesicle—a circumscribed elevated lesion containing clear fluid; less than 1 cm in diameter
Pustule—same as a vesicle except that it contains pus
Bulla—same as a vesicle except larger than 1 cm

Secondary Lesions

Scale—an excess of horny material on the skin surface
Crust—scab consisting of dried blood, serum, or pus
Oozing and weeping—fluid drainage

Breaks in Skin Continuity

Fissure—linear
Erosion—a scooped out and shallow break
Ulcer—a deeper lesion involving the dermis

Other Lesions

Atrophy—thinning of skin
Hypertrophy—thickening of skin
Lichenification—thickening of the skin, with attenuation of the skin lines with scaling and hyperpigmentation
Hypopigmentation—loss of normal color
Depigmentation—absence of color

skin lesions arise from a change in pre-existing normal skin. Primary lesions usually involve change in color, shape, hardness, or softness. Secondary lesions are those that arise from pre-existing changes over time. Secondary lesions are caused either by natural progression or by external influences, such as scratching and rubbing. Naturally there are overlaps, as in all biologic classifications. Nevertheless this orientation is extremely helpful in understanding the progression of a skin disease and in making the proper diagnosis. Besides noting the types of lesions, arrangement of lesions is also useful for diagnosis (Fig. 12–2).

A visual picture of the lesion can be created by refining and adding more adjectives to the term primary or secondary. For example, psoriasis and tinea infections are scaly, but even though they share this characteristic, the lesions are not identical. A complete description of all the characteristics of a lesion helps to distinguish between the two diseases. The physician should not just look at the skin and give a diagnosis; he or she should concentrate on describing.

The simplest change in the skin is a *macule*. A macule is a lesion that is completely flat and cannot be distinguished from the surrounding tissue by palpation. Technically macules are 1 to 2 cm in size. Larger macules are called *patches*. A macule is visible only because it differs from the surrounding skin by color. Color of the skin is determined by pigment; melanin, produced in the epidermis by melanocytes or in the dermis by nevus cells; or by a pink or red vascular flush. A macule can be light in color because of decreased pigment or because of blanching from blood diverted from the skin. The skin may be red as a result of dilatation of blood vessels. The skin may be brown if there is increased pigment in the epidermis. If pigment is produced and carried deeper into the dermis the color may appear slate gray or blue-black. External pigments, such as tattoos or particles of gravel, may also impart color to the skin.

If darkened areas of the skin are due to increased melanin this is called hyperpig-

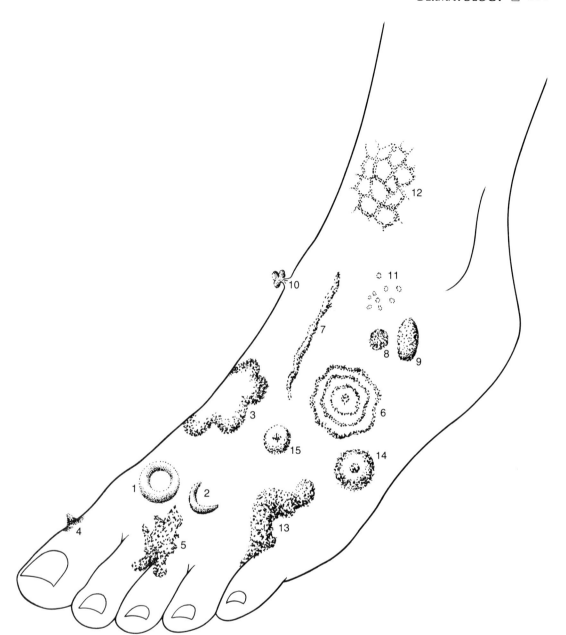

Figure 12–2. Shapes of lesions. *1*, Annular; *2*, arciform; *3*, circinate; *4*, conical; *5*, geographic; *6*, imbricated; *7*, linear; *8*, numular; *9*, oval; *10*, pedunculate; *11*, punctate; *12*, reticulate; *13*, serpiginous; *14*, target; *15*, umbilicated.

mentation. Hypopigmentation is the term used to describe decreased melanin. If melanin is absent, depigmented or amelanotic changes develop. A bluish discoloration caused by vascular congestion is not a hyperpigmentation because it is not due to increased melanin.

Elevated lesions may be due to increased thickness of any or all layers of the skin. Elevated lesions may be caused by cellular growth, infiltration, or inflamma-

tion. Deposition of fluid or material in the tissues should also be considered in the differential diagnosis. The size and shape of the elevation determines what terms are used to describe it. A small elevation, up to 1 cm, is a *papule*. The shape (round or oval), the surface (angular, smooth, flat-topped, or verrucous), and the color of a papule should be described. Lesions elevated 1 to 3 cm are called *nodules*. Very large lesions are called *tumors*. A papule

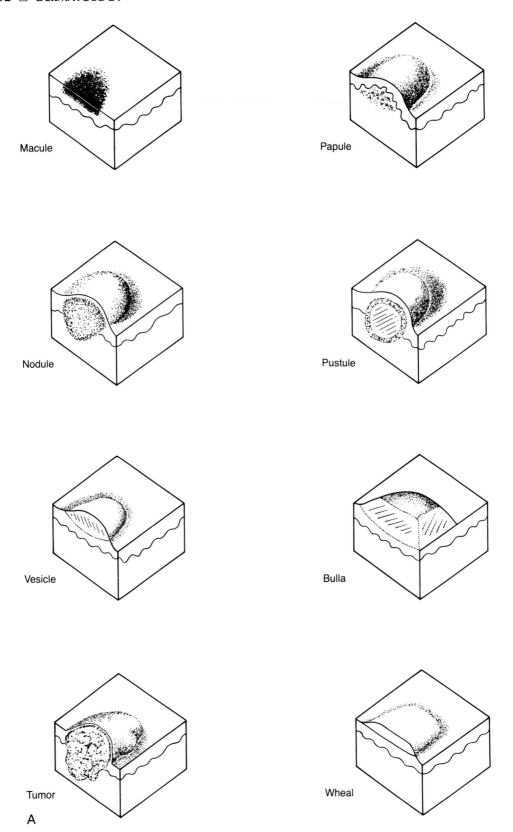

Figure 12–3. *A,* Primary skin lesions.

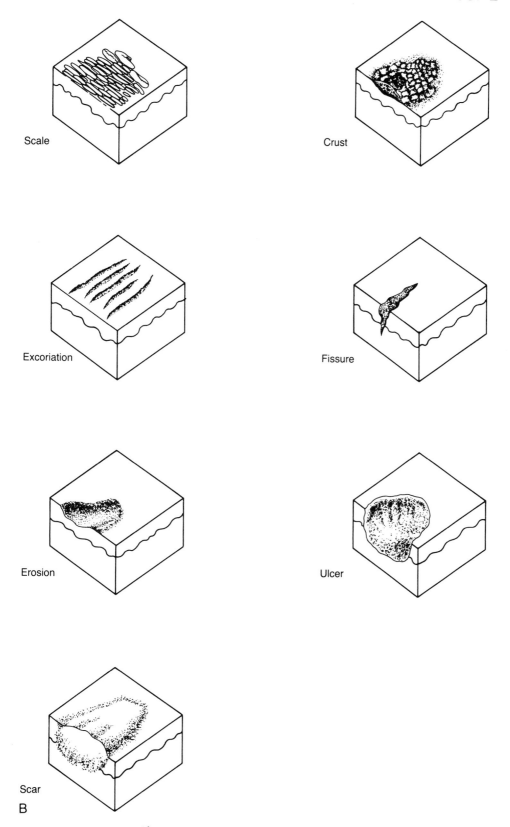

Scale

Crust

Excoriation

Fissure

Erosion

Ulcer

Scar

B

Figure 12–3. *Continued B,* Secondary skin lesions.

or nodule may be a sac for entrapped cellular debris and secretions. A *cyst* is suspected by the palpation of a soft center or firm roundness.

When papules or nodules fuse to form an elevated, plateaulike lesion, *plaque* is used as the descriptive term. A wheal, or hive, is a type of plaque and is due to leakage of serum into the dermis, causing the dermis to swell like a moistened sponge, which is known as urticaria.

Trapped fluid in the skin is called a *vesicle* if the blister is less than 0.5 cm in diameter and a *bulla* if the blister is larger than 0.5 cm. When vesicles are numerous and fuse, they may appear as a weeping denuded area. Superficial bullae rupture easily. Bullae that are deeper, such as friction blisters, can persist and may be overlaid with skin, making them difficult to differentiate from papules.

The fluid in a vesicle may become mixed with blood cells, other tissue cells, or bacteria. Whitish or yellow material is called pus, and the lesion in called a *pustule*. In some diseases, the pustule arises as the initial lesion and is therefore primary, but in other diseases, a pustule develops from a vesicle and is a secondary lesion.

When blood or pus oozes and hardens, it forms a secondary change on the lesion called a *crust,* or scab. If a blister has ruptured and the fluid and crusts are removed one sees a shallow defect. This defect is called an erosion and involves the epidermis only. If there is death and loss of the dermis, subcutaneous tissue, or both there is a much deeper defect called an *ulcer*. A crack in the skin that may extend just through the epidermis or into the dermis is called a *fissure* (Fig. 12–3).

Damaged skin may produce abnormal or too much keratin. This is observed on the surface of the skin as flakes of adherent or loose keratin, called a *scale*. In a wart or callus, the keratin layer may also be greatly thickened but not loose or flaky. This discrete thickening of the keratin layer is called *hyperkeratosis*.

When the epidermis is damaged, it heals without scarring, although there may be temporary or permanent change in pigmentation. When the dermis is damaged, however, it can heal only by formation of a *scar*. Scarring is permanent and is a secondary change in the skin. Some individuals tend to form an exuberant growth of scar tissue that extends beyond the margins of the original injury. This special type of aggressive scar tissue is called a *keloid*.

In addition to thickening of the skin, damage to the tissue may result in thinning. This change is called *atrophy*. It is usually impossible to detect atrophy of the epidermis because the epidermis is so thin. Damage to the dermis may result in formation of paper-thin, atrophic scars. One type of atrophic scarring of the dermis is stretch marks or *striae*. Loss of subcutaneous fat causes a depression in the skin with normal-appearing skin over it. This is referred to as lipoatrophy.

Some pathologic changes appear most commonly or exclusively in the skin. *Alopecia*, the loss of hair, may be localized, with a discrete area of complete hair loss, or may be diffuse, with just fine thinning of hair over an entire area. Alopecia may be due to simple loss of hair follicle function or may be due to damage to and scarring of the skin.

A *comedo*, or blackhead, is another change that occurs in hair follicles. A comedo is shed keratin cells, bacteria, and dried sebum that forms a plug in a hair pore. A saclike growth off the hair follicle is seen as a spheric bulge in the skin and is called a *cyst*. Sometimes tiny cysts are seen very high in the dermis. These little white pinhead-sized cysts are called whiteheads or *milia*. Inflammation and pus formation in follicles is called *folliculitis*. Large inflamed isolated follicles are called *furuncles* or boils. An *abscess* is any encapsulated area of pus, which may or may not be associated with a hair follicle.

Telangiectases are fine, dilated, visible capillaries. Bleeding from vessels into the skin forms rust-colored hemorrhages called *petechiae*. Large areas of hemorrhage are called *ecchymoses* or bruises.

Rubbing or scratching of the skin may cause several types of changes. Rubbing may produce closely set, flat papules that resemble the surface of moss or lichen. *Lichenification* manifests inflammation, crusting, scaling, and a characteristic exaggeration of normal skin markings and skin lines. Scratching, as with the fingernail, often leads to a linear superficial defect in the epidermis called an *excoriation*, or a scratch mark.

If the skin is kept moist for a prolonged period of time the keratin layer swells and becomes white and soft. Fingertips acquire these characteristics after 15 minutes in a bath or swimming pool. Prolonged immersion causes this softened keratin layer to peel off and leave irritated, denuded skin. This entire condition is called *maceration.*

Skin lesions appear in various shapes. A specific vocabulary describes the different presentations and is an important part of defining the lesion and determining the diagnosis (Table 12–4).

Differential Diagnosis

Primary and secondary lesion classification is helpful to understand the pathologic process in skin disease. When a lesion develops without any preceding skin change, it is primary. When a lesion changes from this primary characteristic, whether by natural evolution or by scratching, infection, or other trauma, it becomes secondary. Each lesion then has a primary characteristic and may be modified by secondary changes. However, it is usually not necessary to know whether a lesion is primary or secondary in order to

Table 12–5. DIFFERENTIAL DIAGNOSES

Characteristic	Diagnoses
Pigmented	Freckle, lentigo, lentigo maligna, cafe au lait spot, nevus, dysplastic nevus, melanoma, pigmented basal cell carcinoma, seborrheic keratosis, postinflammatory hyperpigmentation
Scaly	Psoriasis, seborrheic dermatitis, tinea, tinea versicolor, pityriasis rosea, secondary syphilis, atopic dermatitis, stasis dermatitis, irritant dermatitis, allergic dermatitis
Vesicular	Herpes simplex, herpes zoster, varicella, pompholyx (dyshidrotic eczema), acute contact dermatitis, vesicular tinea
Pustular	Acne, bacterial folliculitis, *Candida* (diaper rash), pustular psoriasis
Maculopapular	Drug eruption, viral infection, toxic shock syndrome
Bullous	Impetigo, erythema multiforme, toxic epidermal necrolysis, staphylococcal scalded skin syndrome, pemphigus, pemphigoid
Macular	Vitiligo (loss of pigment), postinflammatory hypopigmentation, tinea versicolor, chemical leukoderma, ash-leaf (tuberous sclerosis), pityriasis alba (atopic dermatitis) port-wine stain

Table 12–4. SHAPE AND ARRANGEMENT OF LESIONS

Annular—round lesion, ringlike; rim is different from center, giving ring-like appearance; usually with a normal center

Linear—long thin lesion or distribution of smaller lesions in a long thin line

Target or Iris—concentric rings like an archer's target, associated with various degrees of inflammation; color of rings can be hues of pink, red, dusky blue

Imbricated—target lesions that have normal skin between abnormal zones; very rare

Serpiginous—snakelike distribution, partially circular and undulating; example—cutaneous larva migrans

Geographic—lesion appears like an outline of a continent on a map

Vegetating—lesion has a surface that grows outward in uneven, fleshy tufts that feel soft

Verrucous—wartlike; tufts of protruding lesion are hyperkeratotic not soft

Zosteriform—conforming to the distribution of a nerve root; example—herpes zoster

Polycyclic or circinate—annular lesions grow together; parts of their circles form a larger lesion

Grouped—several similar lesions located in close proximity surrounded by large area of normal skin

generate a differential diagnosis. Clinically it may sometimes be difficult to decide what is primary and what is secondary.

Some basic differential diagnoses are listed in Table 12–5. These diagnoses are not complete nor are they indisputable. Skin lesions have more than one characteristic. Podiatrists and dermatologists may differ with regard to which characteristics they use in grouping various diseases. One may choose any characteristic, even the distribution or location of a rash, to begin making a differential diagnosis. The point is to have a system for grouping diseases and generating a differential diagnosis. The list given should be modified according to one's experience and inclinations. The dermatologist can generate a great number of complete differential diagnoses that cover many different problems. Therefore the podiatrist must also be able to recognize when a referral is indicated.

PRESENTING FEATURES

Subjective Symptoms

The traditional approach to the medical patient is to elicit the chief complaint and history of the present illness. Elaboration of the history is elicited before supportive clinical findings are obtained, but the dermatologist looks first. The history of the present illness is often written in the skin, including markers of genetic predisposition and indications of the patient's physiologic age and exposure to the elements and to actinic radiation. This visible information may indicate an inflammatory, a metabolic, or even a neoplastic change that is widespread in the body but that comes to focus first in the skin.

Depending on the cause of the problem, symptoms related to the skin of the foot can include pain, itching, burning, foul odor, and sweating. These symptoms can be localized in an area of one foot or can be spread over both feet. The skin has a limited number of ways to express disease symptoms and signs. The aforementioned examples are not exhaustive. Pain can be caused by direct injury to the skin, such as friction blisters, fissuring, and laceration, and muscle or joint disease. Neural inflammation may cause pain, itching, and burning, such as in herpes zoster and metabolic peripheral neuropathy. Burning pain is also a classic component of the poorly understood disease erythromelalgia. Excessive sweating may be secondary to sympathetic nervous system imbalance, emotional stress, and excessive wrapping in a warm environment. Foul smell is usually associated with bacterial overgrowth (e.g., *Corynebacterium* causing pitted keratolysis and excessive moisture). Clues as to diagnosis can be derived from the duration and extent of the problem or the location (e.g., bilateral or localized to one area of one foot). One must consider systemic disease when evaluating cutaneous symptoms.

Objective Signs

General Examination

The golden rule of a general examination is to see *what* is there and *all* that is there.

Good lighting is essential. Nonglaring direct light is best for both lesion configuration and color, but a mix of fluorescent bulbs to simulate daylight is acceptable. The skin should be observed from head to toe in a routine repetitive way so that no orifice or surface area is overlooked. After having surveyed the entire skin surface, generalized observation warrants first notation. A patient may have argyria, the result of silver deposits, but presents with a fungus infection on the feet. Although the pigmentation may be untreatable and permanent, it is still an important part of the dermatologic assessment. The pattern of the problem is significant, such as having a dermatome distribution. The appearance and description are important to the diagnosis as well as for the record, so that other health care providers can follow the patient. Once the examiner is aware of the whole skin and the pattern of the problem, he or she may focus on specific lesions.

Examination of Lower-Extremity Skin

Good lighting, exposure of the whole foot, and occasional use of a magnifying glass cannot be overemphasized in examination of the lower-extremity skin. Gross observation of the skin reveals a wide variety of changes. Because visual observation forms such a large part of a dermatologic examination, it is important to be as precise as possible concerning descriptive terms. Diascopy is another extremely useful technique when examining the skin. Diascopy consists of using a clean microscope slide or any transparent object to press on the lesion. This technique allows one to differentiate an erythematous presentation. Persistence of erythema with diascopy reveals that blood has escaped from the vessels and is free in the dermis. Blanching of erythema indicates that the erythema is due to inflammation or engorged blood vessels, as seen in vasculitis.

Laboratory and Physiologic Data

Much data can be differentiated through the use of relatively simple laboratory procedures. The most important procedures are a potassium hydroxide (KOH) test; a fungal culture; a Tzanck preparation; and a skin biopsy, either punch or excisional.

Potassium Hydroxide Test

The proper use of a KOH preparation can provide immediate confirmation of fungal and yeast infections of either the skin or the nails of the foot. These organisms live in keratin and can easily be identified with a properly prepared specimen.

Various agents are used to dissolve and examine skin for fungi. Potassium hydroxide, in concentrations of 10 to 20%, is the most commonly used agent. Sometimes dimethyl sulfoxide (DMSO) is added to the KOH to facilitate the dissolving action. Stains, such as the lactophenol cotton blue, are sometimes added to help highlight the hyphae. Solutions containing only KOH are usually gently heated to facilitate dissolving, whereas those with DMSO do not have to be heated. It is important to gently heat the slide because a boiled slide is useless for diagnosis (Table 12–6).

Table 12–6. POTASSIUM HYDROXIDE TEST PROCEDURE

Materials: No. 15 scalpel blade, slides, coverslips, heat source, microscope
A. Arrange the patient so that the lesion is vertical and easily accessible. The patient should be comfortable.
B. Taking the specimen is most important. Use the no. 15 blade to collect the specimen.
   1. Dry scaling lesions—gently scrape the advancing edges or furthermost border onto the slide. In mocassin distribution eruption, scrape from the edge.
   2. Macerated inter–toe web infection—spread toes to get moist macerated tissue.
   3. Vesicles and bullae—gently dissect roof. Place the roof on the slide for the specimen.
   4. Nails—cut the nail back and scrape the subungual debris onto the slide.
C. With the specimen on the slide, either add solution directly and cover with a coverslip or cover specimen dry and add a drop of diluant to the side of the coverslip and let it spread by capillary action.
D. Specimen may be gently heated (with a match or alcohol lamp) if KOH only is used. The specimen should not be heated all the way to boiling.
E. Place the slide on the microscope and examine at 10× magnification. The condenser and diaphragm should be set to allow just enough light to see clearly. This light helps to highlight the details. Too much light obscures the image.
F. Hyphae and spores stand out as branching refractile tubes. These tubes have a characteristic birefringence, a greenish brightness that is apparent when the microscope is fine focused. The bright change in color stands out and draws attention to the the fungus. If results are negative wait 10 minutes and then re-examine the slide. If there is still some suspicion several preparations should be done before ruling out fungi.

KOH, Potassium hydroxide.

Fungal Culture

Cultures are extremely useful in diagnosing fungi. Specimens are obtained in the same manner as that for the KOH preparation. Specimens can be transferred to Sabouraud's agar, a glucose medium that contains antibiotics to prevent bacterial overgrowth. Cultures take 2 to 4 weeks to grow and should be examined by someone familiar with fungal cultures. Differentiation from contaminants and saprophytes can be tricky.

One short cut in fungal cultures is the dermatophyte test medium (DTM). This agar turns red in the presence of true dermatophytes within 1 to 3 weeks. Dermatophyte test medium inhibits bacteria and saprophytic molds and contains phenol red, which turns the agar from yellow to bright red when its pH becomes alkaline from dermatophyte growth. Dermatophyte test medium inhibits spores. The morphologic structure of the spores is frequently necessary to determine the species of the fungus. It should be remembered that dermatophytes are aerobic and do not grow in a tightly sealed bottle. Even a cursory description of fungal cultural and microscopic morphology is beyond the scope of this chapter.

Bacterial Culture

Although many variables are involved in the detection of the etiologic agent in infectious disease, a simplified approach is essential in the diagnosis. The best way to isolate the pathogen is through culture. Identification of the pathogens and sensitivity to the offending organism should also be included to ensure effective therapy. Any primary lesion that is a pustule and purulent drainage in a secondary lesion should be cultured.

Viral Culture

There are many different isolations that can be ordered for viral cultures. Clinical data must be applied when determining the type of culture to order. A comprehensive viral profile can be ordered that includes isolation, identification, and serotyping of the following viruses: adenovirus group; cytomegalovirus; enteroviruses, including coxsackievirus A and B, poliovirus, and echovirus; herpes simplex virus 1 and 2; influenza A, B, and C; lymphocytic choriomeningitis; mumps; and varicella. If a particular virus is suspected after a thorough evaluation it is more cost effective to order the test for that particular virus.

Biopsies

A well-done biopsy should produce very little discomfort. The patient should be able to leave the office immediately and resume normal activities in most cases. There are three basic types of skin biopsies: (1) excisional biopsy, (2) punch biopsy, and (3) shave biopsy. A basic knowledge of histopathology and a prebiopsy differential diagnosis help determine the kind of biopsy to be performed. If the pathologic process is epidermal a shave biopsy is usually sufficient. If the process is both epidermal and dermal a punch or excisional biopsy may be necessary. If the process involves subcutaneous fat, such as polyarteritis nodosa or erythema nodosum, a deep excisional biopsy to include an adequate amount of subcutaneous fat is necessary for diagnosis. Biopsies performed without careful consideration of the aforementioned information can be at best inconclusive and at worst misleading.

Generally excisional biopsies are performed in the shape of an ellipse with pointed ends. The long axis of the ellipse should be roughly three times its central, and greatest, width to prevent buckling of the skin, known as "dog ears." Additionally the long axis of the ellipse should be oriented in skin-fold lines or lines of tension to reduce scarring. In large excisions, especially in areas with high skin tension, subcutaneous, buried, interrupted, or dissolving sutures should be used. The skin closure should be done with a suture such as a vertical mattress if possible. Nylon or other nonabsorbable suture is preferable for superficial skin closure. Nonabsorbable nylon sutures last long enough and cause less tissue reaction than absorbable sutures. The patient's return visit for suture removal affords a face-to-face discussion of the biopsy results and a chance to answer any questions the patient may have.

A shave biopsy is appropriate on certain occasions, such as when the lesions appear to be extremely superficial and are not suspicious regarding malignancy. When dealing with pigmented lesions, which might be considered to be malignant, it is advisable to perform a complete excision. This excision should be done during the initial procedure if at all possible. A shave biopsy should never be performed in the case of a pigmented lesion with a suspected diagnosis of malignant melanoma. When performing a biopsy of a large lesion or one of multiple lesions, it is advisable to take either an advancing border of a lesion or an early or fresh lesion. Removing some normal skin with the lesion and marking the orientation of the lesion are also helpful to the pathologist in making the diagnosis. Care should be taken to handle the specimen very gently (Table 12–7).

Table 12–7. PUNCH, EXCISIONAL, AND SHAVE BIOPSY

Materials

Local anesthetic (preferably xylocaine 1% with or without epinephrine)
3 cc syringe with a 25- to 30-gauge needle
A 22 needle (optional) for drawing up xylocaine
A punch biopsy (available in sizes from 2 to 10 mm) or no. 15 scalpel
Needle holder, mosquito clamp, rat tooth forceps, iris scissors
Suture material (preferable 5–0 nylon)
Cautery material, silver nitrate sticks, Monsel's solution, 33% aluminum chloride in isopropyl alcohol, a hyfercator
Dressing

Procedure

Cleanse the area
Mark the lesion with a pen
Inject anesthetic directly into a lesion
After anesthesia has been obtained, use the punch biopsy or the no. 15 blade to excise the lesion; pigmented lesions may be malignant (advisable to excise initially)
Never perform a shave biopsy in the case of a pigmented lesion with suspected malignancy, large lesion, or multiple lesions; take either an advancing border, an early lesion or fresh lesion
Remove normal skin with the lesion
Do not squeeze the specimen with the forceps when removing it
Small punch biopsy (3 mm or less): a cautery is all that is necessary for hemostasis
Otherwise, 2 or 3 sutures are more than sufficient to control hemostasis

Shave Biopsy

Anesthetize the lesion
Pinch the skin
Take a no. 15 blade and shave the lesion; include part of the dermis
Use a chemical cautery for hemostasis

Tzanck's Preparation

If the primary lesion is a vesicle or bulla a rapid cytologic examination known as Tzanck's preparation can be helpful. The vesicle or bulla is unroofed with sterile scissors, and the base is curetted lightly with the blunt side of a scalpel. A smear is made and stained with Wright's or Giemsa's stain to reveal multinucleated epidermal giant cells, which denote a viral infection, or rounded acantholytic cells devoid of their intercellular bridges, a phenomenon present in certain blistering diseases and in viral vesicles.

Diascopy

Diascopy is extremely valuable in examining the skin. Diascopy consists of utilizing a transparent object, such as a microscope slide, to press on a lesion. Blanching of an erythematous lesion on diascopy reveals that the lesion is due to inflamed or engorged blood vessels, as in vasculitis. Persistence of erythema reveals that blood has escaped from the vessels and is free in the dermis.

Wood's Light

Use of a Wood's light is helpful in detecting hair and skin infected with fungi that fluoresce at 360 nm. A Wood's light is important for diagnosis and plucking infected hairs for culture. Inspection under a Wood's light is also useful in differentiating between hypopigmented and depigmented areas of skin and in the diagnosis of erythrasma.

Patch Test

A patch test of a suspected allergen material, for example, from the patient's own shoes, can easily be performed. A small sample of the shoe should be taken and patch tested on the patient's back. There is a shoe contact-dermatitis kit available from Hollister-Stier for this purpose.

GENERAL CONCEPTS OF DERMATOLOGIC TREATMENT

Principles of Topical Therapy

In the presence of irritation or disease, the skin can react in only a small number of ways. These reactions include inflammation, increased keratin production, and infection. Inflammation appears with redness, edema, microvesiculation or macrovesiculation, oozing, crust formation, and lichenification. Increased keratin production appears as scaling. Dryness of the skin is functionally similar to scaling. Infection is the result of bacteria, yeast, viruses, or fungi.

These abnormalities may be combated by topical therapy. Topical agents serve to deliver active medications to the skin; the vehicles for active ingredients are designed in various ways to either stay on the surface of the skin or penetrate deeply.

Wet Dermatoses: Inflammation, Weeping, and Oozing

Drying of wet dermatoses may be accomplished with powders, soaks, and paints.

Powders. Powders are poor for drying wet dermatoses because they merely become caked in the exudate. Powders are best used to decrease friction in moist body folds. Active medications, such as antifungals, are released poorly from powders.

Soaks. Soaks are the basic treatment for wet dermatoses. Soaks may be applied as compresses or baths. In a bath, the body or body part is immersed for 10 to 15 minutes. Often gentle rubbing of the oozing, crusted area during the bath helps debridement. Compresses of clean cotton towel or gauze are dipped into the solution, wrung gently, then applied to the body part. Compresses are removed every 2 to 5 minutes, rinsed in the solution, and reapplied. Total treatment time is 15 to 30 minutes for each session.

Soaking solutions work by defatting keratin and softening and washing off proteinaceous crusts and debris. Oversoaking results in tight, dry, scaly skin. Very significant drying can be achieved with water. By adding astringent materials to water, more drying is achieved, but the increase is very slight. The astringents help to kill bacteria and fungi. Common astringent soaks are aluminum acetate (Burow's solution), magnesium sulfate (Epsom salts), and sodium hypochlorite (Dakin's solution).

Paints. Paints can be applied to small oozing defects in the skin, such as ulcers or fissures (administered twice a day [b.i.d.] or three times a day [t.i.d.]), or on macerated areas, such as the podiatrist often sees in toe webs. The two most common paints are Castellani's (carbol-fuchsin solution) and gentian violet. Alcohol painted on the skin is a drying agent. Active ingredients in alcoholic solutions constitute a tincture, such as tincture of iodine.

Lubrication

Lubrication is usually achieved by fat-containing oils, lotions, creams, and ointments (Table 12–8). Generally the thicker and greasier the material is, the more lubricating it is. Maximum lubrication is achieved by applying the oily material after the keratin layer has been hydrated with bathing. Many effective lubricants are available on the market today. Simple mineral oil and shortening (e.g., Crisco) are excellent and inexpensive lubricants.

Cooling and Soothing

Cooling and soothing are achieved by soaks (evaporation) and alcoholic paints.

Also alcoholic materials, such as phenol, menthol, and camphor, added to creams give a cooling sensation to the skin and slight numbing. Lotions such as calamine are water with alcohol plus a powder, which is not in solution. Calamine must be shaken to get the powder into suspension. On the skin, the powder retards evaporation and prolongs soothing. Other materials such as menthol may be added. Benadryl hydrochloride (Caladryl) is a topical antihistamine added as a slight anesthetic.

Removing Scales and Calluses

Excess keratin in the form of scales and calluses is removed from the skin by hydration or keratolytics, chemicals which loosen or soften keratin (Table 12–9).

Soaps

Soaps remove oil from the skin, thus cleaning it and leaving it dry. Pure soap is

Table 12–8. TOPICAL VEHICLES

Ointment—almost pure grease with very little water added; most occlusive and hydrating; usually steroid effect greater than same concentration in cream or lotion; Use for dry rash (psoriasis, chronic dermatitis); never use on wet rash; use on palms and soles

Cream—grease with more water, so is vanishing; leaves little oily residue; steroid effect weaker; can be drying; Use on dry rash, face, semi-intertriginous areas such as antecubital area

Lotion—little grease with more water (similar to hand lotion); steroid effect weaker; use on scalp, hairy areas, moist areas such as toe webs, armpits, and groin.

Solution—oily liquid of alcohol (propylene glycol); steroid effect strong; fairly drying; burns on dry cracked skin; use on scalp, hairy areas, moist areas such as toe webs, armpits, and groin

Gel—oily gel of propylene glycol; steroid effect is strong as in ointment; drying; use in same places as solution or under occlusion; steroids may cause atrophy in intertriginous areas

Aerosol spray—very expensive, low potency, drying; most useful in scalp surface for steroids (Aeroseb HC or D, Barseb Theraspray)

Occlusion—with plastic wrap over steroid enhances potency 10–100 times; very useful in dry, chronic dermatosis-like psoriasis; enhances infection in moist or oozing lesions

Tape—Cordran tape has steroid built in to adhesive; automatic occlusion system; expensive, excellent for small, dry chronic rash (neurodermatitis); prevents scratching

Table 12–9. AGENTS USED TO REMOVE SCALES AND CALLUSES

Salicylic Acid*

Creams and ointments—2–10% for scaly rashes (Whitfield's)
Oils—5–10% olive oil or Nivea oil
Collodion—10–25% for corns, warts, calluses (Duofilm, occlusal)
Plasters—40% for calluses, corns, warts
Gel—6% (Keralyt)

Urea

Creams—10–20% for scaling or mild hyperkeratosis (Carmol, Aquacare); burns on dry, fissured skin; helps steroid penetration when combined (Carmol–HC)

Lactic Acid†

Lotion—5% for scaly skin; Lacticare lotion
   12% ammonium lactate; Lac-Hydrin
Collodion—combined with salicylic acid for warts
Petrolatum—5–10% for ichthyoses

Tars‡

Ointment—1–5% crude coal tar, most effective, but repugnant
Gels—5%, more acceptable for use, for scaly rashes and scalp (Estar, Psorigel, Aquatar)
Oils and creams—5–10% for scaly rashes
Liquor carbonis detergens—tar derivative, less messy, less effective

* Occlusion enhances effect. Irritating if used in excess. Salicylism can result from total body use.
† Similar to salicylic acid.
‡ Keratolytic, anti-inflammatory, and photo-enhancing.

very drying. Ivory soap is a prime offender and unfortunately is one that is often switched to when a patient notices dry, chapped skin. Oilated or superfatted soaps are less drying but leave one feeling less clean. Alpha keri, Basis, Purpose, and Neutrogena are good "medical" superfatted soaps; Lowila is also good but moderately drying. Dove, which is a bar of cream, is just as effective and is much less expensive. Antibacterial or deodorant soaps do reduce bacteria considerably but are often harsh and drying. Dial is moderately drying. Among the most harsh and drying soaps are Irish Spring and Zest. With dry, cracking feet, harsh soaps, such as deodorant soaps and Ivory, should be avoided. The patient should be advised to wash the feet with lukewarm water and to use gentle soaps, such as Dove.

Other Topical Agents

Steroids. When using steroids in treatment, it is best to start with a high-potency steroid and then decrease potency as the condition improves. General rules should be followed. Patient education is an integral part of the safe use of steroids.

Maximum effect is achieved by the thinnest layer when applying a topical steroid. Thicker is not better, just more expensive. A tiny dab should be applied on the affected area and rubbed in completely. Steroids can be administered b.i.d. or t.i.d. With thin application, one can cover the entire body with 20 g of cream. Approximately 30 g treats a leg b.i.d. for 1 week.

If the skin is very inflamed and itchy, a very potent preparation should be employed. Potent preparations are also needed where there is poor absorption, such as on thickened skin. Mild preparations are adequate for a mild inflammation or where absorption is good, such as the face, the axillae, and the groin. Significant systemic absorption can occur with total body application of the most potent preparations (group 1), especially in children. Group 4 steroids and lower-potency creams are generally safe. Occlusion of large areas (e.g., both legs) may cause systemic absorption in adults. Such absorption usually causes only biochemical abnormalities, not clinical symptoms. Potent steroids, fluorinated or not, can cause an acne rosacea–like rash on the face after

many weeks of use. Short-duration use, such as 2 weeks, is safe. This rash occurs most commonly in young, white women. Atrophy of the skin can occur from prolonged inappropriate administration, such as potent preparations on thin skin (e.g., eyelids and genitals) or unsupervised occlusion. A potent preparation may be used on any area, but the patient must be monitored and switched to a milder preparation as the condition improves (Table 12–10).

Bacterials. Treatment of *Pseudomonas* infections with topical polymyxin (Neosporin) is often effective. Infections with *Corynebacterium minutissimum* can be treated with topical erythromycin, topical clindamycin (Cleocin), or oral erythromycin.

Podophyllin. Podophyllin is a resin of the mandrake root and is beneficial for many different types of warts. For warts on the feet, podophyllin should be prepared in a 20% solution mixed with 20% linseed oil and 60% lanolin. This creates a brownish paste that, after a wart is pared down, can be applied to the wart and covered for 24 hours.

Tape or Moleskin. Many times merely covering a wart with tape or moleskin and occluding it for several days results in a smothering of the wart. This method is painless and quite simple.

Oral Therapy

The appropriate oral antibiotic should be administered for a *Staphylococcus* or *Streptococcus* infection. Antihistamines are also very useful in dermatologic disorders. Antihistamines are employed often for soporific or tranquilizing effects. These agents are helpful in blocking one or more effects of histamine. No single antihistamine blocks all the effects. There are three major groups of antihistamines. If response to one antihistamine is minimal or poor another agent from another group should be added or substituted.

Surgery

Cryosurgery

Cryosurgery with liquid nitrogen is also an extremely beneficial therapy in dermatology. Liquid nitrogen can usually be

Table 12–10. POTENCY RANKING OF COMMONLY USED TOPICAL STEROIDS*

Group	Generic Name	Brand Name	Size
1	Betamethasone dipropionate	Diprolene Ointment 0.05%	15 g, 45 g
	Clobetasol propionate	Temovate Ointment, Cream 0.05%	15 g, 30 g, 45 g
2	Amcinonide	Cyclocort Ointment 0.1%	15 g, 30 g
	Betamethasone dipropionate	Diprosone Ointment 0.05%	15 g, 45 g
	Diflorasone diacetate	Florone Ointment 0.05%	15 g, 30 g, 60 mg
	Halcinonide	Halog Cream 0.1%	15 g, 30 g, 60 mg, 240 mg
	Fluocinonide	Lidex Cream 0.05%	15 g, 30 g, 60 mg, 120 mg
	Fluocinonide	Lidex Gel 0.05%	15 g, 30 g, 60 mg, 120 mg
	Diflorasone diacetate	Maxiflor Ointment 0.05%	15 g, 30 g, 60 mg
	Desoximetasone	Topicort Cream 0.25%	15 g, 60 mg, 120 mg
	Desoximetasone	Topicort Ointment 0.25%	15 g, 60 mg, 120 mg
3	Triamcinolone acetonide	Aristocort Cream (HP) 0.5%	15 g
	Betamethasone dipropionate	Diprosone Cream 0.05%	15 g, 45 g
	Diflorasone diacetate	Florone Cream 0.05%	15 g, 30 g, 60 mg
	Diflorasone diacetate	Maxiflor Cream 0.05%	15 g, 30 g, 60 mg
	Betamethasone valerate	Valisone Ointment 0.01%	15 g, 45 g
4	Triamcinolone acetonide	Aristocort Ointment 0.1%	15 g, 60 g, 240 g
	Betamethasone benzoate	Benisone Ointment 0.025%	15 g, 60 g
	Flurandrenolide	Cordran Ointment 0.05%	15 g, 30 g, 60 g, 225 g
	Triamcinolone acetonide	Kenalog Ointment 0.1%	15 g, 60 g, 80 g
	Fluocinolone acetonide	Synalar (HP) 0.2%	12 g
	Fluocinolone acetonide	Synalar Ointment 0.025%	15 g, 30 g, 60 mg, 120 mg
	Desoximetasone	Topicort LP Cream 0.05%	15 g, 60 mg
5	Betamethasone benzoate	Benisone Cream 0.025%	15 g, 60 g
	Fluradrenolide	Cordran Cream 0.05%	15 g, 30 g, 60 g, 225 g
	Betamethasone dipropionate	Diprosone Lotion 0.1%	20 ml, 60 ml
	Triamcinolone acetonide	Kenalog Cream 0.1%	15 g, 60 g, 80 g, 240 g
	Triamcinolone acetonide	Kenalog Lotion 0.1%	15 ml, 60 ml
	Fluocinolone acetonide	Synalar Cream 0.025%	15 g, 30 g, 60 mg, 120 mg
	Betamethasone valerate	Valisone Cream 0.1%	15 g, 45 g, 110 mg
	Betamethasone valerate	Valisone Lotion 0.1%	15 ml, 60 ml
	Hydrocortisone valerate	Westcort Cream 0.2%	15 g, 45 g, 60 mg, 120 mg
6	Flumethasone pivalate	Locorten Cream 0.03%	15 g, 60 g
	Fluocinolone acetonide	Synalar Solution 0.01%	20 ml, 60 ml
	Desonide	Tridesolon Cream 0.05%	15 g, 60 mg
7	Hydrocortisone	Hytone Cream 1%	30 g, 60 g, 120 g
	Hydrocortisone	Hytone Lotion 1%	30 ml, 120 ml
	Dexamethasone	Hexadrol cream 0.04%	30 g, 60 g
	Hydrocortisone	Cortaid 0.5%	30 g, 60 g

* Group 1 is the most potent, and potency descends with each group. Group 7 is least potent. There is no significant difference among agents within any given group.

kept on a desk in a thermos, which has to be refilled daily. After dipping a cotton-tip swab in the liquid nitrogen, the swab is applied directly to the lesion to be destroyed. A cryosurgical unit can also be utilized for delivery. Destruction with liquid nitrogen is measured by the thaw time. With a bit of practice, it is possible to estimate the amount of time it takes for the ice ball to melt. As a general rule, a thaw time of 5 to 10 seconds is quite sufficient to destroy a lesion of moderate thickness. The patient experiences some pain, but this disappears quickly. Afterward the patient can expect a blister and crust forma-

tion and, it is hoped, a complete resolution of the process within a week. Cryosurgery can be performed on any type of wart but results in a painful blister for plantar warts. Such a blister may make it difficult for the patient to walk for several days.

Electrodesiccation and Surgery

In electrodesiccation and surgery, the wart is first anesthetized, and then fine scissors, a scalpel, or a spatula is used to cut around the wart. A curet can be utilized to shell out the wart, which should come out as a whole. At that time, electrodesiccation of the base for hemostasis and destruction of any residual virus results in destruction of the wart. This method must be used cautiously for plantar warts because it can result in permanent scarring.

Laser Surgery

The use of carbon dioxide lasers for destruction of warts has proved to be quite effective. There is less pain than after standard surgery with electrodesiccation, but healing time is prolonged.

Intralesional Medications

When local, conservative, and topical therapy has been ineffective or very slow in resolving a particular lesion, intradermal or intralesional injections should be considered. Local infiltrative nerve block with a local anesthetic agent may be necessary prior to giving an intralesional injection in the lower extremity. In some cases, the local anesthetic agent may be mixed with the medication to be injected, which minimizes the painful effect. The most frequent intralesional agents employed include local anesthetics, corticosteroids, sclerosing agents, 5-fluorouracil, bleomycin sulfate, and hyaluronidase.

Steroids

Intralesional corticosteroid injections have become a common treatment for lesions that are resistant to topical application of corticosteroids. Clinical conditions for this treatment include bursitis, ganglionic cysts, granuloma annulare, hypertrophic scars, keloids, lichen planus and its variants, pyoderma gangrenosum, recalcitrant plaques of psoriasis, neuromas, eczema, and myxoid cysts.

Sclerosing Agent

The three main types of sclerosing agent in podiatry are 2 or 4% alcohol solution with local anesthetic, 0.4% sodium chloride solution, and 1 or 3% sodium tetradecyl. The following clinical conditions may be treated with intralesional sclerosing solutions. These conditions include bursae, keloids, hypertrophic scars, nerve entrapment, neuroma, piezogenic papules, plantar fibromas, porokeratosis, and intractable plantar keratoses.

Hyaluronidase

Hyaluronidase is a spreading agent that acts to promote diffusion and absorption of fluids into tissues. Hyaluronidase increases the rate and extent of medication diffusion. This agent is used where absorption and diffusion may be difficult, such as in large keloids, plantar fibromas, pyoderma gangrenosum, and hypertrophic lichen planus.

Bleomycin

Bleomycin injected intralesionally in a verruca results in destruction of the wart. This method, however, can be very painful.

ASSESSMENT OF COMMON SKIN DISORDERS

Eczema and Dermatitis

The term eczema is actually a Greek word that means "boiling over." Eczema has come to be known as a grab bag term that has included various conditions. Oftentimes various problems are referred to as eczema or dermatitis for lack of a specific diagnosis. The problem is further complicated by the fact that these conditions can be acute, subacute, and chronic and depending on the etiology have different presentations. Besides classic eczema, contact dermatitis, stasis dermatitis, bacterial infections, irritation from diapers, various immunodeficiency syndromes, and other factors can give rise to an eczema-like picture. Sensitivity to various chemicals and bacteria can appear similar to eczema.

The pathogenesis of atopic dermatitis is unknown, although it is believed to be associated with factors relating to immunity. Elevation in gamma E immunoglobulin (IgE) and T-cell regulatory defects have been shown to exist in atopic dermatitis. Specific eczemas, such as contact dermatitis and stasis dermatitis, do have identifiable etiologies. All of them, though, can appear with similar clincial features.

The real hallmark of the clinical presentation of all the eczemas is the presence of itching. Without this symptom, diagnosis of eczema is doubtful. All conditions can appear in the acute, subacute, and chronic phases, depending on the situation. The acute phase usually consists of small vesicles and papules, which can coalesce to form patches or plaques. These patches or plaques may ooze and crust. Many times dermatitis of the feet appears as pruritic vesicles along the sides of the feet and toes with no apparent cause. This condition can turn into chronic dermatitis in time, showing scaling, hyperpigmentation, and lichenification.

Diagnosis. Obtaining a careful history revealing past cases of eczema in the family or the patient is helpful. Microscopic examination for fungi or presence of psoriasis elsewhere on the body and in other family members also helps the diagnosis. Biopsy results reveal a spongiotic dermatitis compatible with eczema.

Treatment. Treatment depends on identifying a specific etiology, such as a particular allergen or stasis dermatitis. Treatment for eczema of unknown etiology usually consists of topical steroids. It is best to start with a high-potency steroid and then decrease as necessary. Harsh soaps should be avoided, and the patient should be advised to wash the feet with lukewarm water and gentle soaps. As the condition improves, the patient can then use lower-potency corticosteroids.

Eczema

Eczema is a general term. Erythema, vesicles, and weeping with pruritus may be seen. Eczema may be acute, subacute, and chronic. Classic eczema, or atopic dermatitis, is a condition that affects the entire skin. Classic eczema usually goes through three phases, an infantile phase, a childhood phase, and an adolescent or adult phase. Classic eczema is characterized by itching and sensitivity to various environmental factors that cause breakdown of the skin, many times with secondary infections.

Atopic Dermatitis

Atopic dermatitis is usually a genetic disorder, sometimes associated with asthma and allergic rhinitis, or hay fever. Atopic dermatitis usually has multiple positive scratch or prick test results. Frequently immunoglobulin E is increased in serum. Of patients with atopic dermatitis, 35% have a family history of atopy. Skin disease usually starts in infancy. Many children experience resolution after 2 to 6 years. The three phases of atopic dermatitis, as mentioned previously, are infantile, childhood, and adolescent or adult. Sites affected are the face, scalp, diaper areas and buttocks, hands, and antecubital and popliteal fossae. Occasionally atopic dermatitis is generalized. One may see dry skin, hyperlinear plams, and pityriasis alba. The patient is susceptible to viral infections, warts, molluscum contagiosum, herpes, and vaccinia. Frequently the patient develops staphylococcal skin infections.

Aggravating factors include extreme temperature changes, sweating, bacteria, soaps, detergents, and alkalis. Scratching and friction, such as created by wool, and emotional stress also aggravate atopic dermatitis. Treatment includes administration of erythromycin for staphylococcal organisms, topical steroids, antihistamines, and avoidance of allergens and triggering factors.

Nummular Eczema

Nummular, or coin-shaped, eczema is usually not familial. There is no associated atopy. Nummular eczema is intensely pruritic. This form of eczema has a multifactorial etiology.

Hand Eczema

Hand eczema may be a manifestation of atopic dermatitis but is usually unrelated and is secondary to irritants and occasionally allergens.

Dyshidrotic Eczema

Dyshidrotic eczema is a sporadic condition. Vesicles form along sides of fingers. Dyshidrotic eczema may involve the palms and the soles with deep-seated vesicles. This disorder is exacerbated with stress. When making a diagnosis, atopic dermatitis and allergic contact dermatitis must be ruled out.

Lichen Simplex Chronicus

Lichen simplex chronicus, or neurodermatitis, is usually localized, with pruritic, lichenified patches. Lichen simplex chronicus may occur as one or a few patches of chronic dermatitis, with a predilection for the ankles. Commonly affected areas include the posterior scalp line, the pretibial area, and the dorsal area of the hands. The itch-scratch cycle of lichen simplex chronicus must be disrupted.

Xerotic Eczema

Xerotic eczema, or dry skin dermatitis, appears as dry areas of the skin, such as the lower legs, that become intensely pruritic and then inflamed and irritated after scratching. In xerotic eczema, the skin must be hydrated.

Nodular Prurigo

Nodular prurigo appears as localized nodules, frequently located over the arms and legs, that are intensely pruritic. Lesions are quite elevated. Therapy is directed toward reducing itching and scratching with topical and intralesional steroids.

Factitial Dermatitis

Factitial dermatitis is a self-inflicted disorder frequently associated with underlying psychopathology. Lesions are frequently bizarre shapes. Some patients suffer from a psychotic disorder and may feel that there are parasites in the skin (parasitophobia).

Neurotic Excoriations

Patients who have neurotic excoriations are not necessarily psychotic, and they are aware that they scratch themselves. Deep excoriations produce scarring.

Stasis Dermatitis

Stasis dermatitis is the result of venous insufficiency in the lower portion of the legs. Stasis dermatitis appears as erythema and scaling and oozing. This disorder eventually develops into chronic dermatitis. The diagnosis of stasis dermatitis should not be difficult. This dermatitis usually occurs in older individuals, and the presence of edema and hyperpigmentation of stockinglike distribution, along with varicose veins, should be apparent. Stasis dermatitis naturally necessitates therapy directed at the underlying cause. Elevation, support stockings, and diuretics, may be helpful.

Secondary bacterial infection and contact dermatitis are common. Treatment with antibiotics is essential in order to help clear the dermatitis. Sometimes systemic steroids, such as triamcinolone (40 mg intramuscularly) or a short course of prednisone orally, are necessary to control allergic eczematous contact dermatitis from topical medications.

Contact Dermatitis

Allergic eczematous contact dermatitis and irritant contact dermatitis constitute the two types of contact dermatitis. Allergic eczematous contact dermatitis is caused by contact of the skin with a specific substance to which the patient has become specifically sensitized. For patients with dermatitis caused by contact with a box-toe shoe, shoes without box toes are available. Shoes free of dichromates or rubber cement are obtainable from the Alden Shoe Company,* a manufacturer of dermapedic shoes.

Many pruritic eruptions of the feet that appear as either acute or chronic dermatitis are labeled eczema or dermatitis of unknown etiology. It is important to obtain a history to determine if the patient has had true atopic dermatitis at various other locations. True contact dermatitis must be ruled out. Many cases of unknown dermatitis turn out to be allergic contact dermatitis. Two common allergens found in shoes are mercaptobenzothiazole and tetramethylthiuram, which are used in rubber adhesives. Also phenolic resins, leather tanning agents, and formaldehyde have been identified as allergens. It is not uncommon for a problem to be caused, not by new footwear, but by old shoes or sneakers which are in the process of breaking down

---

* Palm Street, Middleboro, Massachusetts.

ing down and are putting the feet into contact with various components of the shoes. In a study of 59 patients with unknown dermatitis of the foot, 42 were found to have specific allergic contact dermatitis.

Eruptions of contact dermatitis usually appear as itchy feet, generally of a chronic nature. Although many contact dermatitides appear on the dorsal aspect of the foot, they can also appear on the plantar aspect. Other diagnoses, such as tinea, psoriasis, and other papulosquamous diseases, should be ruled out. Children are often diagnosed as having "sneaker rot" or "sweaty sock" dermatitis. Secondary infection occurs frequently, especially in stasis and contact dermatitis. Treatment with antibiotics is essential in order to help clear the dermatitis that has a secondary bacterial infection. Sometimes systemic steroids, such as triamcinolone (40 mg intramuscularly) or a short course of prednisone orally, are necessary. If a specific allergic contact dermatitis is expected, the patient can be given a patch test with material from his or her own shoes. Small samples of the shoe can be cut out and tested on the patient's back. As previously mentioned, a shoe contact dermatitis kit is available from Hollister-Stier.

Infectious Eczematoid Dermatitis

With infectious eczematous dermatitis, usually there is an infection, such as otitis externa or osteomyelitis. Exudate spreads over surrounding skin and produces an eczematous dermatitis. With treatment of the underlying infection, the surrounding dermatitis resolves.

Lichen Amyloidosis

Lichen amyloidosis is usually an intensely pruritic dermatitis localized to the lateral legs just below the knee. Primary lesions are papular and tend to coalesce into large plaques. Treatment is with topical steroids under occlusion. Histology reveals amyloid deposits in the upper dermis. There is no association with plasma cell dyscrasia or multiple myeloma.

Wiskott-Aldrich Syndrome

Patients with Wiskott-Aldrich syndrome have an immune deficiency (X-linked re-

cessive trait) characterized by severe recalcitrant dermatitis, thrombocytopenia with bleeding, and recurrent pyogenic infections. Defects in cell-mediated and humoral immunity, deficient gamma M immunoglobulin (IgM) levels, and compensatory increase in gamma A immunoglobulin (IgA) and IgE levels are present.

Hyperimmunoglobulin E Syndrome

Extremely high immunoglobulin E levels, repeated cutaneous infections, and chronic dermatitis mark hyperimmunoglobulin E syndrome. Defective neutrophil chemotaxis and peripheral blood eosinophilia are present.

Intertrigo

Intertrigo is superficial inflammatory dermatitis in areas where the skin is in apposition. As a result of friction, heat, and moisture, skin becomes erythematous, macerated, and secondarily infected.

Papulosquamous Diseases

Papulosquamous diseases are characterized by scaly papules and plaques.

Psoriasis

Psoriasis is a common, chronic, recurrent, inflammatory disease characterized by rounded, circumscribed, erythematous, dry, scaly patches of various sizes appearing on extensor surfaces of the limbs, elbows, knees, and sacral region. Itching and burning may be present. On removal of the scales, bleeding points appear, known as *Auspitz' sign. Koebner's phenomenon* is present frequently. This response is the appearance of typical lesions of psoriasis at sites of injury. The mean age of onset of psoriasis is 27 years. The cause is unknown, but psoriasis represents one of the hyperproliferative disorders of keratinization. Types include seborrheic, inverse, guttate, pustular, erythrodermic, and arthritic.

The therapeutic regimen for psoriasis includes topical corticosteroids, tars, anthralin, and ultraviolet light. Specific treatments include

1. PUVA: oral psoralen and ultraviolet A radiation (UVA).

2. Ingram's method: tar bath, ultraviolet B radiation (UVB) and anthralin.

3. Goeckerman's method: tar and UVB.

4. Systemics: methotrexate and retinoids.

Lichen Planus

Lichen planus is an inflammatory dermatitis that is primarily papular in origin. Polygonal, violaceous papules appear that are highly pruritic. The presence of a consistent immunofluorescent pattern suggests an immunologic etiology. Ovoid globular deposits of IgM, gamma G immunoglobulin (IgG), IgA, complement, or a combination are present.

Koebner's phenomenon is defined as the induction of a skin lesion by physical trauma. Lesions appear on flexor surfaces of the wrists and forearms, the lumbar area, the ankles, the glans penis, the anterior aspect of the lower legs, and the dorsal surfaces of the hands. Mucous membranes are affected in more than 50% of patients. Nails are affected in about 10%. Acute lichen planus resolves in 6 to 18 months. Chronic lichen planus may persist for more than a decade. Variants of lichen planus include annular, linear, hypertrophic, atrophic, vesiculobullous, actinicus, erythematous, planopilaris, and ulcerative.

Pityriasis Rosea

Pityriasis rosea (PR) is a common, self-limited papulosquamous eruption primarily affecting children and young adults, with a lower incidence in summer. Herald, or mother, patch is a round or oval erythematous, scaly lesion that appears a few days before papulosquamous lesions erupt over the trunk, upper arms, and upper thighs. The long axis runs parallel to the ribs, producing a "Christmas tree" pattern. This pattern persists for 3 to 8 weeks and then spontaneously clears. A viral cause is suspected but is not proved. Pruritus is quite variable, and papular, vesicular, urticarial, and purpuric lesions may occur. Treatment is with topical steroids or ultraviolet light.

Pityriasis Rubra Pilaris

Pityriasis rubra pilaris (PRP) is an uncommon, chronic skin disease characterized by acuminate follicular papules, yellow-pink scaly plaques that often contain islands of normal skin, and palmoplantar keratoderma. This disorder usually occurs in either childhood or the 40s. Some cases of PRP are familial, possibly inherited as an autosomal-dominant trait. Pityriasis rubra pilaris represents a hyperproliferative disorder of keratinization. The sides and back of the neck, the trunk, and the extensor surfaces of the extremities are affected. Ectropion may occur where there is heavy, waxy scaling of the face. Lesions may become generalized resulting in an exfoliative erythroderma. The scalp is involved, and a yellow-orange keratoderma is common. The treatment for PRP is administration of oral vitamin A, synthetic retinoids, or methotrexate.

Seborrheic Dermatitis

Seborrheic dermatitis usually begins between 20 and 40 years of age and persists for life. Seborrheic dermatitis occurs in hairy areas and clinically consists of mild erythema covered with a greasy scale. The most common forms are the following:

1. Scalp seborrhea may mimic psoriasis, but it is less scaly, more diffuse, and more easily managed. In addition to the scalp, the retroauricular area and the external auditory carnal may be involved.

2. Facial seborrhea appears with a mild erythema and greasy scale in the paranasal area. Involvement of the eyebrows, eyelashes, and moustache or beard may occur. This form is more common in hospitalized patients, in whom seborrheic dermatitis is related to stress, and in patients with neurologic diseases, such as Parkinson's disease, stroke, and head injury.

3. Truncal seborrhea occurs as small circinate or petaloid patches in the central chest.

4. Flexural seborrhea occurs in the axillae, the groin, and the inframammary areas, appearing similar to the disease on the scalp.

Patients may have one or several of the forms simultaneously. The etiology is unknown, but reports of response to ketoconazole therapy support an infectious component, possibly *Pityrosporum orbiculare.* Therapy is usually simple, with keratolytic shampoos and mild topical steroids. Simple scaling of the scalp, pityriasis sicca, or dandruff, is considered a separate condition.

Lichen Nitidus

Lichen nitidus is an unusual, self-limiting disorder, affecting young persons and consisting of 1- to 2-mm shiny-topped papules. This disorder may be a variant of lichen planus but usually does not itch. Lichen nitidus does not respond to treatment.

Lichen Striatus

Lichen striatus is a self-limiting, linear dermatosis of young children, consisting of coalescing lichenoid papules. Lichen striatus is of sudden onset, forming a band 2 mm to 2 cm in width, usually running down an extremity. Resolution without scarring occurs in less than 1 year.

Parapsoriasis

Parapsoriasis is a nosologic nightmare. Parapsoriasis consists of a group of slightly scaly, slightly erythematous patches with lesions of small (benign) or large (premalignant/malignant) size.

Papulosquamous Drug Eruptions

Papulosquamous drug eruptions include lichen planus–like eruptions that occur with administration of gold, quinidine, hydrochlorothiazide, and phenothiazines. Psoriasis-like eruptions occur with beta-blockers, such as propranolol (Inderal) and practolol. Lithium and antimalarials worsen psoriasis. Gold and captopril may produce pityriasis rosea–like eruptions.

Reiter's Syndrome

Reiter's syndrome, consisting of conjunctivitis, urethritis, and arthritis, occurs predominantly in young men within 1 month of an episode of nongonococcal urethritis (Chlamydia or dysentery). The most commonly affected joints are the knee, the ankle, and the metatarsophalangeal. Although each episode lasts less than 6 months, as many as 50% of patients may have multiple episodes. Occasionally patients have severe, persistent disease. Skin lesions are clinically and histologically similar to psoriasis. Characteristic lesions, referred to as keratoderma blennorrhagica, occur on the glans penis (balanitis circinata) 20% of the time and on the soles 10%.

Infectious Diseases

Bacterial Infections

Bacterial infections of the foot are quite common and can occur with a myriad of different clinical signs and symptoms. These problems are further complicated by the fact that different bacteria can cause similar clinical syndromes, which can result in confusion concerning therapy (Table 12–11).

Infections are caused usually by *Staphylococcus, Streptococcus,* and *Pseudomonas.* Less common, although also prevalent, are infections with *Corynebacterium minutissimum.* These infections are contagious, and heat and moisture are conducive to bacterial growth. Patients who are debilitated or who have chronic diseases, such as diabetes mellitus, are

Table 12–11. BACTERIAL INFECTIONS OF THE FOOT

Staphylococcus—abscess, cellulitis, lymphangitis and lymphadenitis, paronychia, folliculitis and furunculosis (boils), impetigo and impetiginous reactions (crusting and bullous), scalded skin syndrome
Streptococcus—abscess, cellulitis, lymphangitis and lymphadenitis, paronychia, folliculitis and furunculosis (boils), impetigo and impetiginous reactions (crusting), ecthyma, erysipelas
Pseudomonas—paronychia, swamp foot (immersion foot), green nails, toe web infections, ecthyma gangrenosum
Corynebacterium minutissimum—erythrasma
Micrococcus—pitted keratolysis
Atypical mycobacteria—swimming pool granuloma (*Mycobacterium marinum*; same as *Mycobacterium balnei*), granulomatous reactions (atypical *Mycobacterium* infections other than *M. marinum*), buruli ulcer (*Mycobacterium ulcerans*)
Mycobacterium leprae—leprosy
Mycobacterium tuberculosis—tuberculosis verrucosa cutis
Actinomyces—Madura foot
Erysipelothrix rhusiopathiae—erysipeloid
Clostridium—gas gangrene
Treponema pallidum—2 syphilids, ham-colored macules

more susceptible to bacterial infections and should be treated vigorously. Early treatment can prevent severe complications. Because different bacteria can cause similar clinical syndromes, cultures are important when possible to help make an exact diagnosis. Folliculitis, furunculosis, and abscesses are clinical conditions caused by bacterial infections.

Lesions, usually caused by *Staphylococcus* or *Streptococcus,* consist of collections of pus, usually circumscribed, surrounded by erythema, and are quite tender. There is usually a central suppuration. Lesions may be pointing or draining. Cellulitis may also accompany an infected lesion. Cellulitis usually consists of tenderness and erythema, along with induration and edema. These inflammations may lead to systemic infections. Linear erythematous lesions, lymphangitis, along with swelling of the lymph nodes, lymphadenitis, are indicative usually of pyogenic infections. These lesions are tender and usually associated with a cellulitis or an abscess. Infections occurring in toe webs and around toes are usually the result of *Staphylococcus* or *Streptococcus* combined with *Pseudomonas* and *Candida albicans.* These infections are tender and sometimes may develop into an abscess.

Bacterial Paronychia

Bacterial paronychia is an inflammatory reaction involving the folds of the skin surrounding the nail. This infection can be acute or chronic, with purulent, tender, painful, and swollen tissues. These signs and symptoms are caused by an abscess in the nail fold, which may follow a simple injury or a microtrauma. Chronic paronychia results from prolonged immersion in water, exposure to irritating solutions, or vigorous manicuring. Paronychia is also an occupational disease, seen in cannery workers, bartenders, and domestic workers. The causative bacteria associated with acute paronychia are *Staphylococcus* and *Streptococcus.* Chronic infections are caused by *Pseudomonas* and *Proteus. Candida* may also be responsible for paronychia. Gram's stain and bacterial and fungal cultures are used for diagnosis. Treatment involves incision and drainage and is directed by the causative organism. Parenteral antibiotics, topical antifungals,

systemic antifungals, and drying agents are part of the armamentarium.

Toe Web Infections

Toe web infections are usually mixed infections, primarily caused by fungi or yeast, but they can also be caused by *Pseudomonas.* These infections consist of maceration, bogginess, and tenderness, usually between the fourth and fifth toes.

Erythrasma

Erythrasma is characterized by a brownish discoloration in the toe webs, usually between the fourth and fifth toes. The lesions are asymptomatic and fluoresce coral red with a Wood's light, which demonstrates the causative organism, *C. minutissimum.*

Cellulitis

Cellulitis occurs as a complication of a wound or an ulcer but may also develop in previously normal skin, especially in the presence of edema. This diffuse, brawny inflammation of the skin and subcutaneous tissues, with circumscribed indurated lesions that pit on pressure, is caused most frequently by *Streptococcus pyogenes.* The area looks dusky red and is hot and tender with borders that are poorly defined. A minor distinction between streptococcal cellulitis and erysipelas is that the latter is more superficial with sharper margins. Diagnosis is made through culturing fluid, crust, or aspirate. Treatment includes penicillin and supportive care.

Erysipelas

Erysipelas is an acute beta-hemolytic group A streptococci cellulitis, also known as St. Anthony's fire, involving the superficial dermal lymphatics. This acute infection is characterized by local redness; swelling; heat; and a highly characteristic raised, indurated border. These physical signs are usually accompanied by prodromal symptoms of malaise for several hours, with severe constitutional symptoms of chills, high fever, headache, vomiting, joint pain, and a leukocytosis of 20,000 per mm^3 or more. Predisposing factors include operative wounds and fissures in the nares, the auditory meatus, under the earlobes, and between or under the toes; abrasions; and scratches. Vesicular or crusted lesions can be diagnosed through Gram's stain or culture of fluid, crust, or aspirate. Treatment is with oral or parenteral penicillin. Erythromycin can be given to the penicillin-allergic patient.

ECTHYMA

Ecthyma is usually caused by a beta-hemolytic *Streptococcus,* which begins with a vesicle or vesicopustule that develops on an inflamed base. The lesion enlarges, becomes encrusted, and evolves into a superficial ulcer, which may heal with scar formation. The lower legs are most commonly involved. Infection usually follows minor trauma, such as insect bites or scratches. Diagnosis is made with Gram's stain and bacterial culture. Treatment includes compresses and washes, antibiotic ointments, and parenteral antibiotics.

NECROTIZING FASCIITIS (HEMOLYTIC STREPTOCOCCUS GANGRENE)

Necrotizing fasciitis is a fulminating infection of the superficial and deep fascia. Thrombosis of subcutaneous vessels occurs, with gangrene of underlying tissues. This disorder usually follows a cutaneous injury, such as needle puncture, insect bite, or laceration. Early in the course, the infected area becomes hot, edematous, and red. Pathognomonic signs develop between the second and fourth days, when the affected skin assumes a blue, dusky tinge. Blisters may also be present. The process advances to areas of frank cutaneous gangrene with eventual sloughing. Crepitation may be found on physical examination in some patients. Radiographic examination of the involved site discloses gas in most patient. Diagnosis is through radiograph, Gram's stain, and culture of fluids and blood. Treatment involves early incision and drainage, parenteral antibiotics, and vigorous supportive care.

IMPETIGO CONTAGIOSA

Impetigo contagiosa is primarily caused by streptococci. This infection is characterized by discrete, thin-walled vesicles that rapidly become pustular and then rup-

ture with formation of crusts. Impetigo contagiosa can be identified by the honey-colored crust, which appears to be "stuck on" and is tender. The crust occurs on the face, hands, neck, and extremities. Diagnosis is via Gram's stain and culture. Treatment involves topical and systemic antibiotics. Antibiotics include penicillin, erythromycin, and dicloxacillin. Topical mupirocin ointment (Bactroban) is equally as effective. Group A beta-hemolytic streptococcal skin infections are sometimes followed by acute glomerulonephritis.

BULLOUS IMPETIGO

Bullous impetigo is due to *Staphylococcus aureus.* This disorder occurs characteristically in newborns and is highly contagious. In warm climates, adults may develop bullous impetigo, most often in the axillae and the groin. Diagnosis is by Gram's stain and culture. Treatment includes administration of erythromycin and penicillinase-resistant penicillin. Topical mupirocin ointment (Bactroban) is equally as effective.

FOLLICULITIS

Folliculitis is a pyoderma that originates within a hair follicle. *Bockhart's impetigo,* or superficial pustular folliculitis, a superficial folliculitis with small, dome-shaped pustules at the orifices of the pilosebaceous glands, is most frequently caused by *Staphylococcus aureus.* Treatment includes cleansing, administration of topical antibiotics, and administration of systemic antibiotics.

Sycosis barbae is a deep type of folliculitis. This *Staphylococcus* infection, which occurs in the beard or mustache regions, is characterized by the presence of inflammatory papular pustules, with a tendency to recur and occasionally with a granulomatous response.

Furuncles and carbuncles, also a deep type folliculitis, are tender red nodules that become fluctuant and develop in relation to hair follicles. These occur on buttocks, neck, face, axillae, and areas underlying a belt. A carbuncle is merely two or more confluent furuncles with multiple heads. *Staphylococcus aureus* causes furuncles and carbuncles. Systemic disorders that lower resistance, such as cachexia, malnutrition, diabetes mellitus, obesity, and immune deficiencies, may predispose to this type of lesion. These lesions are also complications of secondarily infected dermatoses, such as pediculosis, scabies, and excoriations. One may develop recurrent furunculosis. Diagnosis is made with Gram's stain and culture. Treatment includes hot compresses and administration of penicillinase-resistant penicillins.

HIDRADENITIS SUPPURATIVA

Hidradenitis suppurativa is a disease of apocrine sweat glands that occurs in the axillae and the groin and on the buttocks. Nodules develop into abscesses with suppuration and formation of sinus tracts.

STAPHYLOCOCCAL SCALDED SKIN SYNDROME

Staphylococcal scalded skin syndrome is a febrile, rapidly evolving, generalized, integumentary infectious disease, in which localized bullous eruptions and widespread exfoliations appear on the skin. The lesions extend far beyond areas of actual staphylococcal infection by action of the epidermolytic exotoxin, exfoliatin. Other signs and symptoms include positive Nikolsky's sign, purulent conjunctivitis, otitis media or occult nasopharyngeal infection, and skin tenderness. The causative agent in most of the cases has been *S. aureus* of group 2, phage type 71, the exotoxin of which causes cleavage in the epidermal granular area. Diagnosis is made with bacterial culture of eyes, nares, and oropharynx and Gram's stain of exudate. Treatment includes fluid and electrolyte monitoring and administration of penicillinase-resistant penicillins (dicloxacillin, nafcillin) or erythromycin.

GENERAL TREATMENT CONSIDERATIONS

Therapy for different bacterial problems depends on correctly identifying the causative agent. Cultures and sensitivities for *Staphylococcus*, *Streptococcus*, and *Pseudomonas* taken from pus are usually quite helpful. Identification of *C. minutissimum* infections is usually made on a clinical basis and with use of the Wood's light. The appropriate topical or oral antibiotic should be administered for *Staphylococcus* and *Streptococcus* infections. Treatment of *Pseudomonas* infections with topical polymyxin (Neosporin) is often effective. *Corynebacterium minutissimum* infections can be treated with topical erythromycin, topical clindamycin (Cleocin), or with oral erythromycin.

Fungal Infections

DERMATOPHYTOSIS

Dermatophytosis (i.e., ringworm or tinea) is a term restricted to infections caused by a group of physiologically and morphologically related fungi, the dermatophytes. Most of the known species of dermatophytes grow in the keratinized layers of skin, hair, and nails and cause clinically well-defined lesions. The dermatophytes are classified in three genera: *Microsporum*, *Trichophyton*, and *Epidermophyton*.

Tinea pedis, also called ringworm of the feet or athlete's foot, is a dermatophyte infection involving the skin of the feet. Tinea pedis can be caused by several different organisms and can be an acute, a subacute, or a chronic dermatitis. Tinea pedis is among the most common infectious diseases known to humans and is the most common fungal disease in humans. Tinea pedis is said to be the price of civilization and the result of wearing shoes. The heat and moisture generated by footwear and socks provide an environment favorable for fungi. Hydration of the stratum corneum turns it into a culture medium for these dermatophytes.

Tinea pedis is worldwide in occurrence and appears equally in both sexes. Although tinea pedis can affect all ages, it usually occurs in adult life. Estimates for the prevalence of tinea pedis vary from 30 to 79% of the population, although many of these cases are believed to be subclinical. Infection is probably related to repeated exposure to the organism, so that individuals using common bathing facilities, as in gymnasia, are more prone to acquire the infection. Continued exposure, along with facilitating conditions, such as hot and sweaty feet, and predisposing genetic factors, such as a specific defect in one's immunity, contribute to the widespread existence of this problem.

Trichophyton mentagrophytes, Trichophyton rubrum, and *Epidermophyton floccosum* are the main causative agents in most cases of tinea pedis. The rate of occurrence for each organism varies. The relative percentage of organisms can vary greatly in different studies, although *E. floccosum* is usually less common. Clinical presentation is diverse and makes clinical classification difficult. However, itching, foul odor, and discomfort seem to be the most common symptoms. The most commonly seen types of tinea are discussed subsequently.

Tinea Pedis

Chronic Interdigital Tinea Pedis. This disorder is characterized by maceration and dermatitis commonly between the third and fourth and fourth and fifth toe webs. The skin is white and has a foul odor. The condition is exacerbated in hot weather and may become severely pruritic. Chronic interdigital tinea pedis is also very persistent.

Chronic Papulosquamous Hyperkeratotic Tinea Pedis. This form is associated with *T. rubrum* and is characterized by fine dry white scales that may be patchy or may cover the entire foot in a mocassin-like distribution. The scaling can vary in thickness and is usually bilateral. Chronic papulosquamous hyperkeratotic tinea pedis is very difficult to cure.

Vesicular or Subacute Tinea Pedis. This disorder is often associated with *T. mentagrophytes.* The lesions are characterized by tense vesicles and bullae containing a serous fluid. These lesions can be few or quite numerous and cover large areas of the foot. The acute form can resolve spontaneously but may recur in hot weather. Vesicular tinea pedis can be quite inflammatory and debilitating. This form is most often responsible for the id reaction on other parts of the body. Lymphadenitis, lymphangitis, and cellulitis may occur.

Acute Ulcerative Tinea Pedis. In this variation, there is a rapid spread of an eczematoid vesiculopustular process. Secondary bacterial infection can occur, and the vesicular fluid turns purulent. Acute ulcerative tinea pedis can involve large areas of the foot and can appear with cellulitis, lymphadenitis, and lymphangitis. The id reaction is common. In the acute form, intraepidermal vesicles, along with edema and spongiosis with an inflammatory infiltrate, are seen. These vesicles are usually subcorneal.

Diagnosis and Treatment of Tinea Pedis. The diagnosis can usually be made with a potassium hydroxide (KOH) preparation or a fungal culture in 95% of the cases. Multiple infections with mixed dermatophytes or *C. albicans* are common. Bacterial infections can also complicate the clinical picture. Erythrasma can be differentiated with a Wood's lamp showing a coral red fluorescence. *Pseudomonas, Micrococcus,* and *Acinetobacter* can mimic tinea pedis. The differential diagnosis of tinea pedis also includes contact dermatitis, psoriasis, pustular psoriasis, dyshidrosis, various causes of hyperkeratosis, secondary syphilis, and ingestion of drugs. Bacterial infections with both gram-positive and gram-negative bacteria are common in tinea pedis. Cellulitis may be superimposed on severe tinea pedis. The bacteria possibly gain access through cracking and fissuring of the skin caused by tinea pedis. The causative organism is usually *Streptococcus,* although *Staphylococcus* and in *rare* cases gram-negative organisms may be involved. Bacterial culture results are usually inconclusive even by needle aspiration technique. Signs of cellulitis include erythema, edema, and tenderness, with or without signs of swelling; tenderness of regional lymph nodes; or some combination. Fever may be present but is usually absent. The complete blood count (CBC) may show an increase in polymorphonuclear leukocytes.

Therapeutic success can vary greatly. Factors such as host resistance, chronic reexposure to the organism, a more resistant organism (*T. rubrum* is believed to be particularly difficult to eradicate), and patient compliance can affect the outcome. General rules of hygiene, such as washing and drying, wearing and washing rubber sandals instead of going barefoot, cleaning personal bathrooms, and using antifungal powder in shoes and on feet to prevent fungal infections, should be observed. Topical imidazole agents have helped in the treatment of tinea pedis. These agents, which are effective against yeasts as well as fungi, have eliminated the need for two separate medications. As a rule, application twice daily for 2 to 4 weeks should produce a cure.

Griseofulvin is available in microsized and ultramicrosized capsules, and 250 to 1000 mg/day for several weeks is required.

Although usually tolerated well, griseofulvin can cause headaches, nausea, and diarrhea. When these symptoms occur, it is best to stop the drug for 1 or 2 days and then restart at a lower dose until the patient grows tolerant of the side effects. Griseofulvin is usually quite safe, but it has been associated with red blood cell aplasia and liver problems. This agent can also interfere with the metabolism of other medications, usually by speeding up catabolism. Complete blood count and liver enzyme studies are sometimes required. Pretreatment and follow-up studies probably should be performed routinely on anyone who is taking the drug for more than a few weeks. Ketoconazole is a new oral imidazole, although it is not approved for dermatophyte infections. Ketoconazole is indicated for the treatment of patients with severe recalcitrant cutaneous dermatophyte infections who have not responded to topical therapy or oral griseofulvin or of patients who are unable to take griseofulvin.

Tinea Capitis. Most cases in the United States of tinea capitis, or scalp ringworm, are caused by *Trichophyton tonsurans.* Other causes include *Microsporum audouinii, M. canis, T. violaceum, Trichophyton verrucosum,* and *T. mentagrophytes.* The noninflammatory type is characterized by multiple scaly lesions, areas of broken hair, and minimal inflammatory response. Inflammatory tinea capitis appears with scaly, erythematous, papular eruptions with loose and broken hair and varying degrees of inflammation. Kerion celsus, a localized boggy and indurated area with pronounced swelling, exuding pus is a complication that may lead to permanent baldness. Diagnosis is made by use of a Wood's light, KOH preparation of scales and hair, and fungal culture of scales and hair. Treatment includes administration of griseofulvin or ketoconazole. Oral steroids or saturated solution of potassium iodide (SSKI) is administered for kerion.

Tinea Barbae. This form of tinea is commonly referred to as barber's itch and is most often seen in farm workers who are in contact with animals. Superficial crusted tinea barbae appears with pustular folliculitis with or without broken-off hairs and is caused by *T. rubrum* and *T. violaceum.* The deep nodular suppurative type of tinea barbae appears with nodular thick-

enings and kerion-like swellings associated with *T. verrucosum* and *T. mentagrophytes.* Diagnosis of both disorders is made through KOH preparation and culture of hair. The treatment is with griseofulvin.

Tinea Faciale. Tinea faciale is frequently misdiagnosed. *Trichophyton rubrum, T. mentagrophytes,* and *M. canis* are the offending organisms. Potassium hydroxide preparation of scales and culture of scales are usually diagnostic. Treatment includes administration of griseofulvin, topical imidazoles, or both.

Tinea Corporis. Tinea corporis is characterized by one or more circular, sharply circumscribed, slightly erythematous, dry, scaly patches with progressive central clearing. Majocchi's granuloma is caused by trichophytic granuloma and occurs with a deep, pustular, follicular type of tinea corporis. This disorder is diagnosed by a KOH preparation of the scale and culture of the scale. Treatment consists of administration of topical imidazoles, griseofulvin, or both. Ketoconazole is used for resistant infections.

Tinea Cruris. This infection, commonly known as jock itch, manifests on the upper and inner thighs. The responsible organisms include *T. rubrum, T. mentagrophytes,* and *E. floccosum.* The diagnosis is made by culture and KOH preparation of scales. Treatment includes administration of griseofulvin and topical imidazoles.

Tinea Versicolor. Tinea versicolor is characterized by finely scaling, guttate or nummular patches occurring on the upper trunk and extending onto the neck and arms. This disorder is caused by a dimorphic yeast, *Pityrosporum orbiculare.* Potassium hydroxide preparation of the scales confirms the diagnosis. Treatment includes administration of selenium sulfide, topical imidazoles, propylene glycol, ketoconazole or some combination.

Tinea Manuum. This infectious disorder is usually dry and scaly and occasionally moist, vesicular, or eczematous. The organisms responsible include *T. rubrum* and *T. mentagrophytes.* Potassium hydroxide preparation and culture of scales are diagnostic. Treatment includes administration of griseofulvin and topical imidazoles.

Tinea Nigra. This disorder is characterized by brown or black spots that resemble nevi, melanomas, or stains. Tinea nigra most frequently occurs on the palms but also occurs on the soles and elsewhere. The responsible organism, *Cladosporium werneckii*, is identified by a KOH preparation. Tinea nigra is treated with administration of keratolytic agents, debridement with a no. 10 or no. 15 blade, or both.

YEASTS

Yeasts is common vernacular for unicellular fungal organisms that reproduce by budding. In humans, the most common cause of yeast infection is *C. albicans. Candida albicans* is a normal inhabitant of the alimentary tract. The same factors that favor dermatophyte growth also favor yeasts. Heat and moisture cause the keratin to swell and become a suitable medium to support microbiologic growth. Tight footwear combined with heat, humidity, and sweat helps to make conditions favorable for yeast infections. Other pathogenic species include *Candida guilliermondi, Candida krusei, Candida pseudotropicalis, Candida tropicalis,* and *Candida stellatoidea*, with mucocutaneous surfaces the most frequent tissues involved. A chronic mucocutaneous, mild, localized, or severe generalized condition of candidiasis represents a spectrum of cellular immunodeficiencies, and further investigation is warranted.

The clinical presentation of *C. albicans* infection on the foot is either interdigital maceration, usually between the third and fourth or fourth and fifth toes, or paronychia, usually in concert with bacteria. The maceration is usually whitish and occasionally itchy or painful due to the depth of the lesion. The paronychia is usually a painful and tender erythematous swelling around the great toenail. There may be a small abscess, or the lesion may be draining pus. *Candida* can invade the nails and result in a thickened, brownish-colored nail plate. The nail plate is not friable as it is with dermatophyte infections.

The diagnosis should be suspected on clinical grounds and can be confirmed with a KOH mount. Yeasts appear somewhat differently than dermatophytes under the microscope in that the hyphae are larger, without septation, and there may be budding present. Nevertheless these infections are quite commonly mixed. The dif-

ferential diagnosis for toe web infections includes tinea pedis, psoriasis, bacterial infections, and hyperhidrosis.

Topical treatment is often successful against the yeast, but other causes must be treated simultaneously. By cooling and drying the area, much can be done to alleviate the symptoms. For interdigital infections, the newer imidazole agents, nystatin, and amphotericin B are quite effective topically. Because imidazoles are also effective against tinea, there might be a case for using them. Systemic therapy includes administration of amphotericin B and 5-fluorocytosine (Flucytosine). Paronychia infections probably require concomitant oral antibiotic therapy. Often a topical steroid cream, along with soaking the painful toe three or four times a day in warm water, helps. It is important to thoroughly dry the toe after soaking and to reapply whatever topical agent one is using, such as clotrimazole solution.

SUBCUTANEOUS AND DEEP FUNGAL INFECTIONS

Sporotrichosis. Sporotrichosis is a fungal infection of a chronic nature characterized by nodules that have a tendency to spread via the lymphatics. The causative agent is *Sporothrix schenckii*, which usually gains access through some traumatic break in the skin, such as a thorn puncture or an insect bite. The distribution of the fungus is quite widespread.

Lymphocutaneous sporotrichosis at first appears as a firm nodule at the site of a traumatic puncture within weeks or months. The nodule may ulcerate and become a sporotrichotic chancre. Over the next few months, other lesions along the lymphatic drainage appear. These lesions also may drain, and the condition can persist for many years. Uncommonly, the disease can become widespread and invade internal organs in severe forms.

The diagnosis is dependent on finding cutaneous nodules and ulcerations characteristically located at intervals ascending the limb overlying lymphatic channels. Culture of either the pus or the tissue confirms the clinical impression. The fungus is difficult to find on a biopsy specimen, however, even with the use of a special stain.

Mycetoma (Madura Foot, Maduramycosis). The term mycetoma refers to infection by a wide variety of agents, resulting in a chronic indolent condition consisting of the triad of tumefaction, draining sinuses, and grains (microcolonies of the organism). This subcutaneous fungal infection is more common in underdeveloped countries and the southeastern United States. Mycetoma is caused by a wide variety of bacteria (actinomycotic mycetoma) and fungi (eumycotic mycetoma), all of which are found in the soil and on plants and decaying matter. No matter which agent is the cause, infection begins with an initial implantation, which then may form a locally invasive indolent tumorlike mass. As the mass slowly enlarges, sinus tracts form, swelling occurs, and edema and induration on standing for long periods lead to scarring into a wooden firmness in parts of the tissue. New nodules form on the foot, and more sinus tracts develop, leading to destruction of normal soft tissue and bone. The foot eventually becomes distorted. Characteristically these chronic suppurating abscesses and their draining sinuses produce grains.

The triad of tumefaction, draning sinuses, and grains, along with the chronicity of such infections, should not make the diagnosis difficult. Microscopic examination of the grains reveals hyphae, or rays coming from the colonies. Culture should help identify the specific agent. This is important since the etiologic agent may be a bacterium or a fungus, which influences the type of therapy to be administered (Table 12–12). Early diagnosis, if possible, is important because the prognosis for complete recovery naturally decreases as the infection causes more damage. Differential diagnosis includes tumors and Kaposi's sarcoma.

Treatment of mycetoma includes surgical debridement of abscesses and removal of infected tissue, with appropriate antimicrobial therapy depending on whether the cause is bacterial or fungal. Specific therapy is dependent on the organism isolated and is best carried out in consultation with an infectious disease specialist. Chemicals such as amphotericin B are toxic and should be administered by persons experienced in their use.

Viral Infections

Viral infections of the foot are usually warts, more technically known as verrucae.

Table 12–12. SUMMARY OF FUNGAL AND YEAST INFECTIONS OF THE FOOT

Yeast

Candida albicans: paronychia, interdigital maceration, nails

Superficial Fungal Infections

Dermatophytes

Trichophyton, Epidermophyton: tinea pedis (athlete's foot)
  Trichophyton rubrum: dry mocassin type
  Trichophyton mentagrophytes: blistering variety
Piedraia hortae: black piedra
Trichosporon beigelii (Trichosporon cutaneum): white piedra

Subcutaneous Fungal Infections

Allescheria boydii: Mycetoma (most common cause in United States), Madura foot
Sporothrix schenckii: sporotrichosis
Fonsecaea: Chromomycosis

Deep Fungal Infections

Infections with herpesvirus, poxvirus and enterovirus are also encountered but to a much lesser degree. Viruses are obligatory intracellular parasites classified as either RNA or DNA, depending on their nuclear structure. Viruses can inhabit either the cytoplasm or the nucleus of the cell and are contagious.

WARTS (VERRUCA VULGARIS)

Warts are benign growths caused by papillomaviruses of the papovavirus group. Warts can occur on all areas of the skin and are quite commonly found on the foot. There are multiple serologically distinguishable strains of papillomavirus associated with warts, and the list is expanding all the time by researchers using DNA-hybridization techniques. These are slow growing DNA-containing viruses that replicate in the nucleus of cells.

Warts can appear in different sizes and shapes. Verruca vulgaris is the most common form of wart. Usually occurring in childhood, this wart is generally an elevated tumor with a characteristic verrucoid appearance. Warts can take weeks or months to grow and are usually multiple. On the foot, warts usually occur periungually but can appear on all surfaces. Verruca plantaris, or plantar wart, is so named for its appearance on the sole of the foot. Plantar warts can be located on pressure points and cause difficulty walking. Frequently these lesions fuse to form groupings, termed mosaic warts, commonly on the heel of the foot. On all warts, if they are pared down, one can find bleeding points, or grains. These points are actually blood vessels near the surface.

Microtrauma is thought to play a role in the initiation of the virus into the skin. This seems logical from the standpoint of the location of warts, but there are no good controlled studies. Immunologically warts are only slightly antigenic. Cell-mediated immune components are involved in the rejection of warts. Persons with atopic heredity have more trouble rejecting wart tissue, possibly related to IgE-blocking antibodies. Immunosuppressed individuals, such as those with lymphoma, those undergoing chemotherapy, and those with acquired immunodeficiency syndrome (AIDS), also may have rather exuberant wart infections. Usually the diagnosis is obvious. Warts can be confused with corns, but paring down a corn reveals only a clear keratin growth going down and not the characteristic grains of warts.

Treatment. An over-the-counter (OTC) preparation of 40% salicylic acid plaster is available in pad form. In our hands, 40% salicylic acid is far and away the best way to treat plantar warts. The advantages of this method are that it is painless, usually quite effective, and quite safe. The patient is instructed to cut a circle approximately the size of the wart, peel away the plastic undercoating, and apply the acid side of the pad to the wart. Tape is then applied and left on for 24 hours. When the pad is removed, the skin is white and somewhat macerated because of the destructive action of the acid. The foot is soaked in water, and the macerated material is scraped away. The patient can be given a scalpel to take home, or a nail file can be used. The patient then applies a new pad of salicylic acid, which is left on for another 24 hours. The macerated material is then scraped away again. This process is repeated for approximately 1 week, at which time a painless hole is left in place of wart tissue. The patient is then instructed to allow the lesion to heal in. If the lesion recurs, the patient can retreat it a second or even a third time. Frequent (every 2 weeks or so) office visits are recommended, especially in younger patients, to encourage compli-

ance and monitor progress. In our experience, a more destructive technique, such as liquid nitrogen freezing, hyfrecation, or laser surgery (see subsequent discussion) is often necessary to eliminate the base or root of the wart. The preparatory paring by the patient increases the efficacy and minimizes the discomfort of the subsequent destructive technique.

Acids are obtainable in commercial form, usually consisting of salicylic acid and lactic acid in some solvents, such as collodion. These solvents are applied in drop form and allowed to dry once or twice a day for several days. The area is pared down before reapplication.

Cantharidin is an extract from blister beetles and is available commercially from several suppliers. The wart can be pared down and the cantharidin is applied directly. The cantharidin is then covered with a bandage, and the patient is instructed to expect that a blister will form. This treatment is useful for plantar warts but it can create painful blisters. The painful blisters sometimes make it difficult for the patient to walk for 1 to 2 days. When using cryosurgery (liquid nitrogen freezing), a thaw time of 5 to 10 seconds is quite sufficient to destroy a lesion of moderate thickness. The patient experiences some pain, but this disappears quickly. Afterward, the patient can expect blister and crust formation and, it is hoped, a complete resolution of the process within a week. This method can be used on any type of wart.

Surgical intervention with electrodesiccation for a wart involves anesthetizing the wart. Then fine scissors, scalpel, or spatula is used to cut around the wart. At that time, a curet can be used to shell out the wart, which should come out as a whole. Then electrodesiccation is applied to the base for hemostasis and destruction of any residual virus. This method can result in permanent scarring. Carbon dioxide lasers for destruction of warts have proved to be quite effective. Pain is less than after standard surgery with electrodesiccation, but healing time is prolonged.

Podophyllin is a resin of the mandrake root and is useful for many different types of warts. For warts on the feet, podophyllin should be prepared in a 20% solution mixed with 20% linseed oil and 60% lanolin. This combination creates a brownish paste which, after a wart is pared down, can be applied and covered for 24 hours. Many times merely covering a wart with tape or moleskin and occluding it for several days result in a "smothering" of the wart. This method is painless and quite simple. Bleomycin injected intralesionally results in destruction of a wart, although this can be very painful.

HERPES INFECTIONS

Herpes Simplex. Herpes infections of the feet are not common. Herpes simplex infections with Herpesvirus hominis are similar to those herpes infections elsewhere. These viruses live in nerves and are reactivated by various trigger factors. These factors can vary from anxiety to sunlight exposure. Herpes simplex infections consist of a group of vesicles on erythematous bases, usually preceded by a burning or itching sensation. These vesicles can be recurrent.

Treatments for herpes simplex infections are myriad. Oral acyclovir is effective in aborting acute recurrences and can be taken daily to prevent further recurrences. Unfortunately no real cure has been found. Most cases recur only once or twice and are self-limiting, eventually burning themselves out.

Herpes Zoster. Herpes zoster, or shingles, is an infection with the varicella-zoster virus. Herpes zoster shows itself as grouped vesicles, usually occurring along a nerve route distribution. This infection usually appears only once and is a reactivation of chickenpox, which is caused by the same virus. The main problems with zoster infection are scarring, which is usually the result of secondary bacterial infection, and pain. There is usually some pain associated with the acute attack. A more vexing problem can be a prolonged period of residual pain or paresthesias, known as postherpetic neuralgia.

Treatment is aimed at preventing secondary bacterial infection by the use of solutions to dry the vesicles and topical antibacterial ointments. In patients with severe infections or in immunosuppressed patients, we have found the administration of oral or intravenous acyclovir quite useful. High-dose oral corticosteroids have been advocated to prevent the occurrence

of postherpetic neuralgia, but no conclusive study has been done.

MOLLUSCUM CONTAGIOSUM

Molluscum contagiosum infections are caused by poxviruses. These infections are described as dome-shaped papules and as translucent dome-shaped papules with an umbilication in the center. There are usually several papules, and they are asymptomatic. Treatment consists of either cryosurgery or curettage. It is important to alert the patient to return if new lesions appear because these can seed others.

Molluscum contagiosum commonly occurs in patients with AIDS and tend to be persistent and occur frequently in the genital and oral areas. Commonly the face and neck regions are involved. These lesions may become quite large, forming giant molluscum bodies. Recurrence is frequent, and eradication may prove difficult (Table 12–13).

Keratodermas

Keratoderma is frequently used synonymously with keratoma, hyperkeratosis, tylosis, and keratosis. These terms signify some form of thickening of the stratum corneum. Keratoses of the palms and soles are hereditary or idiopathic. Excessive scaling

Table 12–13. VIRAL INFECTIONS OF THE FOOT

Papovavirus, Papillomavirus (Warts)

Deep plantar—HPV I
Common warts, mosaic plantar warts—HPV II
Flat warts—HPV III
Common and plantar—HPV IV

Herpesvirus

Herpesvirus hominis—Herpes simplex
Varicella—Herpes zoster (shingles), chickenpox

Poxvirus

Molloscum contagiosum
Orf (sheep handler's nodules—contagious ecthyma)
Milker's nodules
Vaccina (cowpox)
Variola (Guarnieri's bodies—smallpox)

Enterovirus

Hand-foot-and-mouth disease (coxsackievirus A-16)

HPV, Human papilloma virus.

and keratin on the soles can be either acquired or congenital. Keratosis palmaris et plantaris (Unna-Thost syndrome), keratosis punctata of Hallopeau's disease, and keratosis of the palms and soles associated with Darier's disease are genetically induced disorders. Keratosis is also associated with systemic diseases, such as syphilis, diabetes mellitus, and various collagen disorders. Pathogenesis depends on etiology. Nonmechanically induced keratosis of the soles due to genetic causes or systemic disease is often misinterpreted as simple callus tissue or hyperkeratosis. Features exist that may help in the differentiation of the keratotic lesions. Pressure-induced hyperkeratotic changes are not limited to the epidermis, as seen in nonmechanically induced keratosis. The mechanically induced lesion involves the dermis and fat as well. Diagnosis depends on history and presence of hyperkeratosis and other defects elsewhere. Histologic sections taken from the keratotic lesions may be diagnostic and should be determined if clinically indicated.

Keratoderma Climactericum

Keratoderma climactericum is the most common form of acquired keratoderma. This keratoderma is also known as Haxthausen's syndrome and is seen mainly on the palms and soles of obese menopausal or postmenopausal women, who may exhibit hypertension and hyperuricemia. The hyperkeratosis leads to fissuring and pain. Estrogen replacement to treat keratoderma climactericum has been disappointing. Treatment consists of overnight urea preparations under occlusion, with administration of steroids if coexisting inflammation appears.

Keratoma Plantare Sulcatum

Keratoderma plantare sulcatum is a bacterial infection and is the other main cause of acquired keratoderma.

Keratoma Hereditarium Mutilans (Vohwinkel's Syndrome)

Keratoma hereditarium mutilans is a rare hereditary deforming dermatosis that consists of diffuse palmar and plantar hyperkeratosis, slowly progressive fibrous construction developing in the digitoplantar fold; and discrete linear and star-shaped keratosis on the dorsa of the hands, feet, elbows, and knees. The plantar aspects of both feet are usually covered with extensive diffuse hyperkeratosis, with sharp medial and lateral borders of the keratosis where plantar meets dorsal skin. A consistent finding in this disorder is constriction of the distal phalangeal joints of the third and fourth toes of the right foot. A predilection for females has been reported. The pathogenesis of the ainhumlike constrictions may be due to compression of the neurovascular nerve by the hyperkeratotic tissues that circumscribe the digit. This compression is capable of causing the distal aspect to become necrotic and necessitate amputation.

Keratosis Punctata

Keratosis punctata is dominantly inherited and appears with multiple cornlike papules on the palmar and plantar aspects of the hands and feet. Most cases develop before puberty and may be mistaken for pressure-induced corns or calluses. There is no effective treatment. Administration of vitamin A is promising, but side effects preclude its use on a long-term basis.

Purpuric Hyperkeratosis

Purpuric hyperkeratosis is a phenomenon that is commonly observed within or under plantar calluses and is associated with systemic disorders, local disorders, or both that affect the cutaneous microvasculature. These lesions are frequently seen in patients with vasculitis associated with rheumatoid arthritis and in diabetics with cutaneous angiopathy and neuropathy.

Acrokeratosis Verruciformis (Hopf's Keratosis)

Acrokeratosis verruciformis is characterized by small punctate keratotic papules located on the dorsal hands, feet, and ankles.

Precancerous, Benign, and Malignant Lesions

For practical purposes, we need to divide skin tumors into benign and malignant neoplasms. Although almost any neoplasm can grow on the lower extremity, attention here is given only to those growths that occur with some frequency on the lower extremity.

Benign Tumors

SEBORRHEIC KERATOSES

Seborrheic keratoses are common lesions that generally have a waxy brown appearance. These lesions tend to appear stuck on the surface of the skin. There is frequently a familial tendency, and the onset is late middle age. Seborrheic keratoses have essentially no malignant potential. Removal is mainly cosmetic and may be accomplished by freezing with liquid nitrogen, curettage, or shaving with a scalpel. Little depth is required because the lesions tend to grow above the dermoepidermal junction and do not invade the dermis. Biopsy is useful to rule out malignant tumors, such as melanomas and pigmented basal cell carcinomas. A variant of seborrheic keratosis called stucco keratosis has a predilection for the lower extremities, mainly around the ankles and dorsa of the feet. These lesions tend to be flesh colored to slightly pale. Morphologically these lesions resemble actinic keratosis and flat warts. A shave biopsy specimen of a representative lesion is sufficient if there is any doubt about the diagnosis. Neither seborrheic keratoses nor stucco keratoses occur on the palms or soles.

DERMATOFIBROMAS

Dermatofibromas are also very common tumors and have a predilection for the lower extremity. These are usually reddish to brown, very firm, slowly growing tumors. The skin just overlying is frequently slightly thickened. Lateral pressure on the skin with fingers characteristically causes the tumor to become slightly depressed. This is the "button" or "dimple" sign.

Dermatofibromas are usually so characteristic morphologically that biopsy is generally not necessary. Full thickness excision is necessary to remove the lesion. The resultant scar is generally more disfiguring than the original tumor. Kaposi's sarcoma (see subsequently) may resemble a dermatofibroma. Therefore punch biopsy is

indicated in a setting suggestive of Kaposi's sarcoma.

VASCULAR TUMORS

Vascular tumors can be congenital or acquired. Generally congenital tumors are more common on the legs. The flat portwine nevus or nevus flammeus is present at birth and darkens with age. This nevus can be in a linear arrangement along a dermatome. A variant is the Klippel-Trenaunay syndrome, with involvement of one limb. Arteriovenous fistulas cause hypertrophy of the soft tissues and bones of the affected extremity.

Capillary hemangiomas also occur at birth but are less likely to be found on the lower extremity. These lesions appear during the first year of life and tend to regress spontaneously by late childhood, so that 70% resolve by age 7, and 94% ultimately resolve.

Cherry angiomata develop during adulthood. These are small red papules that tend to occur on the trunk. Appearance is characteristic, and assurance is all that is necessary. If removal is desired electrodesiccation is frequently successful.

ECCRINE POROMAS

Eccrine poromas are usually flesh-colored papules or nodules with a predilection for the palms and soles. The morphology is nondescript, and a biopsy, preferably punch or elliptic subtotal excision specimen is necessary to determine the diagnosis. A malignant variant exists but is extremely uncommon.

PYOGENIC GRANULOMAS

Pyogenic granulomas frequently occur on the toes and consist of dull red pedunculated, generally solitary lesions. The surface may ulcerate and ooze and bleeds easily when traumatized. Shave biopsy with cauterization of the base generally removes the lesion and prevents recurrence.

GLOMUS TUMORS

Glomus tumors appear on the extremities as purplish, generally solitary nodules. These nodules are characteristically painful when pressure is applied. The histology is characteristic. A malignant variant exists.

LIPOMAS AND ANGIOLIPOMAS

Lipomas are common tumors and may occur as single or multiple lesions on the extremities. These are soft subcutaneous nodules. The skin moves more or less freely over the top of the lesions. Removal is usually for cosmetic purposes only. Recurrence is not uncommon. Malignant transformation is exceedingly rare.

Angiolipomas are similar to lipomas. As the name would imply, vascular cells as well as fat cells are involved. These tumors frequently occur in younger persons and can be quite tender to palpation.

Pigmented Tumors

MELANOCYTIC NEVI

Melanocytic nevi can be either benign or malignant. The vast majority are benign, but the malignant variety (malignant melanoma), unlike most other skin cancers, tends to spread rapidly and metastasize early with high mortality. Definitive diagnosis depends on histologic evaluation of biopsy or excisional specimen. Junctional nevi are flat, brown to black, and generally uniform in color. These lesions may occur anywhere, including the soles. A small number of these lesions may undergo malignant change. Intradermal nevi are more common than junctional nevi and tend to be papular, often fleshy, and lighter in color. These lesions also can appear on the soles. On the soles, nevi are frequently darker along dermatoglyphic ridges, or "fingerprint" ridges, than between the ridges, making them look somewhat zebralike. Malignant transformation of intradermal nevi is rare. Compound nevi share some characteristics of both junctional and intradermal nevi.

HALO NEVI

Halo nevi are junctional or intradermal nevi that have undergone spontaneous regression. The dark central nevus is surrounded by a hypopigmented ring or halo. Because melanomas may begin in this manner, special notice should be taken of halo nevi.

LENTIGO

A lentigo is a flat and generally uniformly light to medium brown patch. Clinically this patch resembles a large freckle. A lentigo may develop spontaneously or in areas of sun exposure.

Malignant Tumors

MALIGNANT MELANOMAS

Malignant melanomas may arise from pre-existing nevi or de novo. There are four recognized types of melanoma: superficial spreading melanoma, lentigo maligna, nodular melanoma, and acral-lentiginous melanoma.

Superficial Spreading Melanoma. The most common variety is superficial spreading malignant melanoma. This melanoma occurs in younger patients. Superficial spreading malignant melanoma may appear anywhere on the body. Sun exposure seems to be a factor by virtue of the fact that this melanoma occurs on the upper trunk in males and the lower extremities in females. As the name would imply, these lesions spread laterally before invading the dermis to any extent.

Lentigo Maligna. This lesion, also known as malignant freckle, begins as a tan macule that extends peripherally, with gradual uneven darkening over the course of several years.

Nodular Melanoma. This melanoma becomes quite thick and invades early. The typical lesion may be described as a pigmented nodule of varying size, present for a few months or even many years, which has arisen in other forms of melanoma or which has suddenly developed de novo.

Acral-Lentiginous Melanoma. This lesion is the most common melanoma in blacks and occur on palms, soles, toes, fingers, and nail beds. Acral-lentiginous melanoma is the least common type of melanoma and is very aggressive with early metastasis.

Biopsy Techniques. A few words should be said about biopsy techniques with pigmented lesions. Early melanomas may have scattered areas of malignant change, and a small punch biopsy may miss the area. Also histologic evaluation of the border of the lesion is one of the factors critical in deciding whether the lesion is malignant or not. Thickness of the lesion is a prognostic indicator of the clinical course. Therefore shave biopsy technique should be condemned if there is any question of malignancy in the lesion. A full thickness, preferably excisional biopsy is the first choice. Because a full thickness excisional biopsy is not always feasible, especially on the legs and feet, the next best technique is subtotal resection with an ellipse, making certain to get both lateral borders if possible. Further treatment and evaluation of melanomas is best left to oncologists or other persons with special expertise in melanomas.

ACTINIC KERATOSES

Actinic keratoses are early dysplastic changes believed to be secondary to solar damage. As one might expect, these lesions occur more frequently on the upper body, but they may occur on the legs, especially among women. Actinic keratoses are flesh-colored to slightly red scaling papules. The patient reports these papules continue to scale in the same place after the scale is picked off. A very low percentage of these papules, if left untreated, eventuate into squamous cell carcinoma. Fairly light freezing with liquid nitrogen is generally sufficient to remove the papules. Extensive or numerous lesions may require 5-fluorouracil topically, which has proved to be extremely effective. If the lesion does not respond, biopsy is the next step. The differential diagnosis includes squamous cell carcinoma, nodular prurigo, and basal cell carcinoma.

LEUKOPLAKIA

Leukoplakia appears as a whitish thickening of the epithelium of the mucous membranes. Lips, gums, cheeks, and edges of the tongue are the most common sites, but the lesion may arise on the anus and the genitalia. Leukoplakia is found chiefly in men over 40 years of age. Leukoplakia may result because of excessive use of tobacco, poorly fitting dentures, sharp and chipped teeth, and improper oral hygiene. Carcinoma in leukoplakia usually begins as a localized induration, often about a fissure, or as a warty excrescence or a small ulcer.

SQUAMOUS CELL CARCINOMA

Squamous cell carcinoma (SCC) occurs not only on the skin but also on the mucous membranes. Squamous cell carcinoma may begin at the site of actinic keratoses on sun-exposed areas, such as the face and back of the hands, and may appear on the legs. The lesion is superficial, discrete and hard and resembles a wart arising from an indurated, rounded, elevated base. After a period of time, the lesions become larger, deeply nodular, and ulcerated. The risk of metastases to lymph nodes is greatest in lip lesions. The principal regions involved by SCC are exposed parts, mucocutaneous junctions, lower lip, face, back of the hands, nipples, genitals, and extremities. Ultraviolet light and x-ray can be predisposing factors. Squamous cell carcinoma is very common in areas of thermal burn scars or in chronic draining sinus tracts or osteomyelitic sinus tracts. In contrast to SCC from other causes in which metastasis is a late and infrequent occurrence, SCC arising in osteomyelitic sinus tracts metastasizes in 31% of cases in some series. These lesions may be scaling or ulcerative, and they are frequently thicker than actinic keratoses.

BOWEN'S DISEASE

A variant of SCC is Bowen's disease. This disease is an intraepidermal lesion and may be accompanied by arsenical keratoses. Some workers believe that all Bowen's disease is related to arsenic exposure. As arsenic is being used less today, other predisposing factors for Bowen's disease will probably emerge. Clinically Bowen's disease can resemble SCC. Bowen's disease appears on any part of the body as an erythematous, slightly crusted, noninfiltrated patch from a few millimeters to many centimeters in diameter. The patch tends to be red with irregular but sharply defined borders. The biopsy specimen is diagnostic. The mucous membranes may also be involved.

BASAL CELL CARCINOMA

Basal cell carcinoma (BCC) is a tumor composed of none or a few small, waxy, semitranslucent nodules forming around a central depression that may or may not be ulcerated, crusted, and bleeding. The edge of larger lesions has a characteristic bold border. Telangiectases course through the lesion. Bleeding on slight injury is a common sign. Basal cell carcinoma is most frequently found on the face and especially on the nose. Any part of the body may be involved, and there are several varieties including pigmented, morphea-like, superficial, and rodent ulcer. Metastases are extremely rare. Excessive sunlight exposure, chemical carcinogens, and genetic determinants are probable causes of BCC. These lesions tend to be less keratotic than SCC and frequently have a slightly shiny, pearly border. These lesions may ulcerate early, hence the name rodent ulcer. Basal cell carcinoma tends to be slower growing than SCC. A rare variant of BCC is the basal cell nevus syndrome. This syndrome is transmitted as an autosomal-dominant trait and starts in childhood. Palmar and plantar pits are almost always present. Other abnormalities, such as ameloblastoma of the jaw and skeletal and central nervous system defects, may be present.

ARSENICAL KERATOSIS

Arsenical keratosis is characterized by keratotic, pointed, 2- to 4-mm wartlike lesions on the palms and soles and sometimes on the ears of a person with a history of arsenic ingestion. These keratoses are precancerous lesions that can evolve into SCC.

VERRUCOUS CARCINOMA

Verrucous carcinoma is a distinct, well-differentiated variety of SCC. Verrucous carcinoma is a collective term that may include such entities as Buschke-Löwenstein tumor, or giant condyloma acuminatum; epithelioma cuniculatum; and oral florid papillomatosis. These lesions must be excised completely, or they have a tendency to recur.

KAPOSI'S SARCOMA

There are three known variants of Kaposi's sarcoma: classic, African, and AIDS forms. Classic Kaposi's sarcoma tends to occur in older men, largely of Jewish or Mediterranean extraction. There is the gradual development of bluish red or dark brown papules or nodules on the legs and feet. The disease is slowly progressive. Lymph node metastasis is present in only 10% of cases even after years of the disease. The disease is believed to be multicentric in origin, with lesions developing de novo rather than from metastasis of existing lesions. Because patients are generally elderly, death occurs from diseases independent of Kaposi's sarcoma. Radiation therapy affords some control of the lesions. Other malignancies of the skin include primary lymphomas, such as mycosis fungoides, and metastatic tumors from other organs. The reader is referred to primary dermatology texts for further information on these conditions.

EXTRAMAMMARY PAGET'S DSEASE

Extramammary Paget's disease manifests as a nonhealing eczematous patch, which may persist in the anogenital or axillary region for several years. This patch is frequently mistaken for a fungus infection. Intense pruritus is common, and sometimes pain is also present, frequently associated with an underlying glandular adnexal carcinoma.

MYCOSIS FUNGOIDES (CUTANEOUS T-CELL LYMPHOMA)

Mycosis fungoides is a T-cell lymphoma that initially and primarily involves skin. Mycosis fungoides can also involve lymph nodes and viscera. Clinically there is an erythematous pretumor stage that progresses to thickened, indurated, plaque-like lesions. Ultimately tumor results. Extracutaneous dissemination of mycosis fungoides is no longer considered uncommon. Visceral involvement is noted in two thirds of cases at autopsy. Staging for prognosis will have impetus as treatment protocols are developed.

METASTATIC CARCINOMA

Cutaneous metastases may occur from almost any malignant growth. The metastatic nodules are usually located in the dermis. The most frequent lesion is a nodule, which may occur as an uncharacteristic single lesion. Also there may be multiple, hard, infiltrative nodules. In women, the most common source of cutaneous metastases is mammary carcinoma. In males, the most common source of cutaneous metastases is lung carcinoma.

Dermatologic Presentations in Sexually Transmitted Diseases

Sexually transmitted diseases (STDs) are a common but changing spectrum of diseases transmitted by sexual contact. Clinically STDs are usually manifested in one of three forms: ulcers (ulcerations or erosions), drips (discharge or dysuria), and bumps (papules). The acquisition of multiple infections simultaneously is common (Table 12–14).

Table 12–14. DERMATOLOGIC LESIONS IN SEXUALLY TRANSMITTED DISEASES*

Ulcers

Herpes Simplex Virus

Primary infection: widespread blistering eruption with autoinoculation
Recurrence: majority, often with a prodrome of tingling and itching, followed by grouped blisters in the genital area (most common cause of genital ulcers in United States)
Diagnosis: Tzanck's smear or culture
Contagious: blisters or erosions present; viral shedding from cervix can occur
Prevention/treatment: Condoms, acyclovir

Chancroid

Causes a painful, dirty, soft ulceration at the site of inoculation; associated inguinal adenopathy (bubo) is often present
Treatment: Erythromycin, trimethoprim/sulfamethoxazole, or ceftriaxone

Candida Albicans

Erosive or ulcerative balanitis, especially in the circumcised male
Female: diagnosis is suspected in partner with candidal vaginitis confirmed by KOH test
Treatment: imidazole (a fixed drug eruption may look very similar)

Drips (Penile Discharge)

Gonococcal Urethritis

Diagnosis: Urethral culture and Gram's stain
Treatment: ceftriaxone, penicillin, or amoxicillin/ampicillin (uncomplicated gonorrhea); treat for concomitant Chlamydia infection

Disseminated Gonococcal Infection

Skin lesions: few (<10) acrally located violaceous macules that evolve into hemorrhagic pustules
Joint involvement (Dermatoarthritis): knee most common; monoarticular acute arthritis in the young adult is gonococcal arthritis until proven otherwise; most common cause of septic arthritis in this age group

Table 12–14. (continued)

Nongonococcal Urethritis

Most frequently due to Chlamydia, ⅓ by other organisms
Diagnosis: fluorescent antibody tests
Treatment of choice: erythromycin, empiric course if other than Chlamydia

Bumps (Papules)

Genital Warts

Caused by human papillomavirus
Lesions: occur on the skin or mucosal surfaces; appear elevated, velvety, rough surfaced papules
Treatment: destructive
Recurrence: common

Molluscum Contagiosum

In adults is spread venereally
Lesion: multiple pearly umbilicated papules in genital area; if extensive, work-up for immune suppression, such as AIDS

Scabies

Lesions in the axilla and groin
Lesion: pruritic erythematous superficially eroded papulonodules, glans penis common site for scabetic nodules
Treatment: Topical tar, steroids, or both

* Contact tracing and treatment of contact is of critical importance in sexually transmitted diseases.
AIDS, Acquired immunodeficiency syndrome; KOH, potassium hydroxide.

Syphilis

Syphilis is an infectious disease caused by *Treponema pallidum* and acquired principally through sexual exposure. Dermatologic manifestations include chancre at the site of inoculation in the primary stage. The chancre begins as a papule and then ulcerates. The secondary stage appears with influenza-like systemic symptoms; generalized adenopathy; and generalized nonpruritic macular, papular rash. *Condyloma latum* is a papular lesion, relatively broad and flat, located on folds of moist skin, especially about the anus and the genitals. Occasionally pustular mucous patches are seen. The latent stage demonstrates a reactive serologic test result only and a nonreactive spinal fluid reagin test result. Tertiary, or late-stage, syphilis has not only mucocutaneous involvement but also osseous, visceral, cardiac, and neurologic involvement. Skin lesions may be nodular, noduloulcerative, or gummatous (granulomatous ulcer). Treatment includes administration of penicillin, tetracycline, erythromycin, doxycycline, and cephaloridine.

Acquired Immune Deficiency Syndrome

A variant of Kaposi's sarcoma related to AIDS has been reported in the United States and other developed countries, primarily involving homosexual males and intravenous drug users. This variant attacks younger persons and is rapidly progressive, with an average life expectancy after diagnosis of less than 3 years. This Kaposi's sarcoma may be associated with lymphadenopathy, weight loss, fevers, and night sweats. Unusual opportunistic infections may be present, such as pneumocystic pneumonia, cryptococcal meningitis, atypical mycobacterial infection, and intestinal cryptosporidiosis. Lymphomas may also be associated.

In 1981, the first cases of AIDS were discovered in the United States. The ensuing years have seen the disease emerge as a major epidemic that has had an unprecedented adverse effect on the health and social structure of society. Acquired immune deficiency syndrome is a preventable disease. The causative agent is the human immunodeficiency virus (HIV), a retrovirus. Human immunodeficiency virus is transmitted in the population through risk behaviors. The virus is spread through blood and body fluids. All health care providers have among their patients individuals who either have already been infected by HIV, which is indicated by the presence of HIV antibodies, or who are at risk of infection. Therefore it is essential that all health care providers become expert in the approaches to counseling patients about the specific steps they should take to prevent the spread of infection.

The oral and cutaneous manifestations of AIDS develop as helper cell function deteriorates. Patients develop a variety of cutaneous manifestations, reflecting deteriorating immune function. Most disorders appear when helper-cell numbers fall below 100 cells-mm^3. Multiple cutaneous disorders frequently exist in a single patient. The oral and cutaneous manifestations can be divided into distinct categories.

Infections

Viral infections include herpes simplex, molluscum contagiosum, herpes zoster, Epstein-Barr virus (EBV), and papillomavirus. *Herpes simplex* infections are consistently present in patients with AIDS. Recurrent herpes attacks are often quite severe, disfiguring, and persistent. These lesions may develop secondary bacterial infections, which may disguise the true nature of the condition. *Molluscum contagiosum* occurs commonly and frequently in the genital and oral areas, face, and neck. These lesions may become quite large, forming giant molluscum bodies. Recurrence is frequent, and eradication may prove difficult. Patients with AIDS appear to be extremely susceptible to *varicella zoster*, and infection is explosive and more extensive than in nonimmunocompromised patients. Numerous lesions may be associated with varicella pneumonia. Patients may also develop severe shingles, resulting in deep scarring with persistent, intractable herpetic pain. Oral hairy leukoplakia is associated with the development of AIDS and contains *EBV*. Hairy leukoplakia is an epithelial hyperplasia of the oral mucosa and may contain papillomavirus in addition to EBV. Patients with AIDS may have extensive *papillomavirus* warts on their hands and feet, face, and anogenital region.

The most common clinical presentation of *fungal* infection is oral *candidiasis*. This infection often precedes the onset of other opportunistic infections. Tinea versicolor may be extensive and is commonly refractory to topical management. Patients have been described with tinea cruris, lesions resembling keratoderma blennorrhagicum of the palms and soles, and onychomycoses. These *dermatophytoses* are frequently due to *T. rubrum*.

Bacterial infections of the skin are quite common in patients with AIDS. Intravenous drug abusers are particularly susceptible. Intravenous drug abusers frequently have numerous track marks as manifestations of scars and infections at injection sites. These infections can be caused by *S. aureus, group A, C, G streptococci,* and ulcerated lesions containing *Pseudomonas.* Other bacteria responsible for clinical infections include *Haemophilus influenzae,* and *Rhodococcus equi.* In spite of their state of immunosuppression, these patients usually respond well to appropriate antibiotic therapy. Other infections include *syphilis,* particularly in homosexuals. Secondary syphilis may not have a classic presentation. It is appropriate to evaluate the serologic status of individuals with a variety of dermatologic manifestations of AIDS. Arthropod, protozoan, and mycobacterial infections have also been seen.

BENIGN VASCULAR LESIONS

A variety of vascular lesions have been reported, including *multiple cutaneous angiomas, multiple splinter hemorrhages* in the nail beds, *telangiectases* of the shins, *petechiae*, thrombophlebitis of the leg, and palpable *purpura* representing *vasculitis*. These lesions are associated with systemic signs and symptoms, such as fever, liver abnormalities, and chronic venous obstruction.

EPIDERMAL HYPERPROLIFERATIVE CONDITIONS

Seborrheic dermatitis occurs in about 83% of patients with AIDS. Severity correlates with the degree of clinical deterioration. The dermatitis is usually severe, with thick scales that may appear on the trunk, groin, and extremities, or the skin may actually develop a generalized *erythroderma*. Active psoriasis may develop after a diagnosis of AIDS. *Acquired ichthyosis* has been reported, with an associated keratoderma of the palms and soles. The oral and cutaneous manifestations of AIDS are numerous. It is important for the physician who first treats a patient with possible HIV infection to recognize these early lesions.

Cutaneous Drug Reactions

Statistics show that 5% of all drug administrations cause some adverse effect. The ordinary patient in the hospital receives, on the average, nine drugs. As many as 30% of these patients have adverse drug reactions. The most common reactions in order of frequency include nausea, drowsiness, diarrhea, vomiting, skin rash, arrhythmia, and itching. Skin rash develops in 2 to 3% of medical inpatients following drug administration (Table 12–15). Some drugs that produce a low rate of skin reactions are prescribed often, and the reactions from them are seen quite frequently. Consequently, if a person develops a skin rash, it is wise to suspect all

Table 12–15. DRUGS ASSOCIATED WITH SKIN ERUPTIONS

Drug	Rate (%)
Sulfamethoxazole-trimethoprim	5.9
Ampicillin	5.2
Semisynthetic penicillins	3.6
Penicillin G	1.6
Gentamicin sulfate	1.6
Cephalosporins	1.3
Quinidine	1.2
Barbiturates	0.5
Digoxin	<0.3
Meperidine	<0.3
Acetaminophen	<0.3
Aspirin	<0.3
Codeine	<0.3
Prednisone	<0.3
Allopurinol*	<0.3
Diphenhydramine	<0.3

* Except in patients with borderline renal functions.

drugs being taken. Most skin rashes develop within 2 weeks of beginning therapy. Therefore it is logical to consider drugs the patient has been taking most recently. Some drugs are more likely than others to cause a particular type of skin eruption (Table 12–16). If one can distinguish these different eruptions and a suspect drug is being used a diagnosis of drug-induced reaction is usually simple to make. Difficulties arise, however, if a common type of reaction is encountered in a patient taking multiple drugs. In such a case, knowledge of the incidence of reactions for a given drug helps identify the most likely culprit.

Exanthem

Exanthem is the most common form of drug eruption and is the maculopapular or morbilliform type. Exanthem first appears on the upper body in pressure spots and then spreads widely to become confluent. There may be variable, usually mild involvement of mucous membranes and purpura. Exanthem occurs in dependent areas. Pruritus, sometimes intense, is a frequent feature. Patients may have slight fever and eosinophilia. Eruptions usually begin within 8 days of the first dose of the provoking drug, but they can begin 1 to 2 weeks after the drug has been stopped. Drugs that cause this type of reaction may be used again in a life-threatening situation. Ampicillin and sulfamethoxazole-trimethoprim are responsible for this type of rash in about 5% of patients. In patients

Table 12–16. COMMON FORMS OF DRUG ERUPTIONS WITH PARTIAL LIST OF
RESPONSIBLE DRUGS

Exanthems (Morbilliform, Maculopapular)

Penicillins, nitrofurantoin, chlorpromazine, isoniazid, tetracycline, gold salts, pyrazolones, sulfonamides, phenytoin, benzodiazepines, streptomycin, phenacetin, salicylates, ampicillin, barbiturates, chloramphenicol, thiazides, amitriptyline, furosemide, lincomycin, sulfamethoxazole-trimethoprim, phenylbutazone, erythromycin, carbamazepine, allopurinol, quinine, sulfones

Urticaria (Nonimmunologic)

Opiates, polymyxin B, ASA, contrast media, indomethacin, other NSAIDs, benzoates

Urticaria (Immunologic)

Penicillin, chloramphenicol, sulfonamides, tetracycline, barbiturates

Vasculitis

Sulfonamides, iodides, gold salts, phenothiazines, thiazides, tetracycline, other metals, hydantoins, aspirin, penicillin, horse serum, thiouracil, phenacetin, vaccines, allopurinol

Erythema Multiforme (Stevens–Johnson Syndrome, Toxic Epidermal Necrolysis)

Sulfonamides, tetracycline, griseofulvin, salicylates, allopurinol, gold salts, penicillin, phenytoin, trimethadione, chloramphenicol, tolbutamide, quinine, ampicillin, phenolphthalein, phenylbutazone, chlorpropamide, phenothiazines, sulfones, hydralazine, barbiturates, antipyrine, vaccines, tetanus antitoxin, nitrofurantoin

Fixed Drug Eruptions

Barbiturates, phenolphthalein, phenacetin, tetracycline, pyrazolone, sulfonamides, meprobamate, phenylbutazone, chlordiazepoxide, oral contraceptives, laxatives, food coloring

Erythema Nodosum

Sulfonamides, codeine, iodides, streptomycin, salicylates, sulfones, penicillin, oral contraceptives

Lichenoid Eruptions

Quinidine, tetracycline, bromides, gold salts, thiazides, iodides, quinine, methyldopa, sulfonamides, chloroquine, dapsone, arsenicals

Exfoliative Dermatitis

Sulfonamides, phenylbutazone, gold salts, phenothiazines, quinidine, antimalarials, phenytoin, heavy metals, codeine, tetracycline, penicillin, mephenytoin, iodides, actinomycin D, vitamin A, allopurinol, trimethadione, ASA, barbiturates, isoniazid

Acneiform Eruptions

Iodides, ACTH, trimethadione, bromides, hydantoins, lithium, isoniazid, phenobarbital, oral contraceptives, corticosteroids, androgenic hormones, vitamin B_{12}

Drug-Induced Systemic Lupus Erythematosus

Procainamide, phenytoin, phenothiazines, quinidine, hydralazine, primidone, sulfonamides, penicillin, isoniazid, griseofulvin, propylthiouracil, PAS, barbiturates, oral contraceptives, tetracycline

Photosensitive Eruptions

Tetracyclines, chlorpromazine, disinfectants, quinethazone, thiazides, protriptyline, phenothiazine, chlorothiazide, sulfonamides, griseofulvin, dyes, nalidixic acid, coal tar, psoralens, essential oils

ACTH, Adrenocorticotropic hormone; ASA, Acetylsalicylic acid; NSAIDs, nonsteroidal anti-inflammatory drugs; PAS, para-aminosalicylic acid.

with infectious mononucleosis, cytomegalovirus, and lymphocytic leukemia, the incidence of exanthems as a result of ampicillin administration is much higher. Treatment consists of discontinuing the medication and giving antihistamines, topical steroids, or for severe cases a short course of systemic steroids. In making the differential diagnosis, consider viral exanthems, although the findings of pruritus and eosinophilia favor drug-induced eruption.

Urticaria

Clinically urticaria, which is also common, appears as evanescent, well-circumscribed, pruritic, migratory plaques. The individual lesions are red and plateaulike. If one observes the lesions over a period of time one finds that the edges of the lesions move and the plaques clear up in one site only to appear in another. If the swelling involves subcutaneous tissue and the plaques are less well defined the lesions are called angioedema. No true urticarial lesions last more than 24 hours. Drug-induced urticarial reactions often favor pressure points, such as under a waistband or bra strap. There are several different mechanisms, nonimmunologic and immunologic, that may cause these drug-induced eruptions. In any patient with urticaria, any OTC drug as well as prescribed drug must be considered as the possible culprit. Other causes of angioedema and urticaria must also be considered. These causes include physical stimuli, such as heat, cold, pressure, and light; heredity (e.g., atopy, hereditary angioedema); food; pollens; and parasites. The possibility of these other physical causes makes careful history taking an important step in therapy. Besides stopping the offending drug or exposure to the offending agent, therapy consists of administration of antihistamines and occasionally systemic steroids.

Vasculitis

Clinically the lesions of drug-induced vasculitis may appear as palpable purpura, which distinguishes them from other forms of purpura. Drugs, such as gold and quinidine, can cause nonpalpable purpura by inducing thrombocytopenia. Usually vasculitic eruptions begin as erythematous macules that progress to palpable lesions, which may ulcerate. Characteristically the lesions occur in crops on the lower legs and ankles, but they may progress elsewhere. Livedo reticularis (reddish blue, netlike mottling of the skin) may be seen. The patient may also have fever, arthritis, arthralgia, and neuropathy. Other organs may be involved, such as the kidneys. Eosinophilia occurs in 10 to 20% of patients. This vasculitis is identical to that in subacute bacterial endocarditis, in meningococcemia, in rickettsial disease, in hepatitis B, in connective tissue disease, and following common streptococcal infections. The drugs implicated most frequently include the sulfonamides, thiazides, and those listed in Table 12–16. Treatment involves stopping administration of the incriminated agent and if necessary giving steroids, and rarely antimetabolites parenterally.

Erythema Multiforme

Erythema multiforme is an acute eruption of the skin and mucous membrane characterized by a distinctive target lesion. The prodrome is nonspecific. As the severity of the disease increases, the patient may become very ill. The forms of lesions may be target-type, urticarial plaques; bullae or vesicles arising on pre-existing macules; or a combination of both in a distribution similar to target lesions. In 25% of the cases, erythema multiforme lesions are limited to the oral cavity; these cases form a link between erythema multiforme and the more severe Stevens-Johnson syndrome. Erythema multiforme is a self-limiting disorder and is most often treated with antihistamines and topical steroids. Although many drugs have been implicated, other causes include herpes simplex and mycoplasma infections, deep x-ray, and internal malignancy.

Stevens-Johnson Syndrome (Erythema Multiforme Major)

Stevens-Johnson syndrome usually follows a 1- to 14-day prodrome of fever, malaise, cough, sore throat, arthralgia, and myalgia. Many inflammatory bullous lesions suddenly appear on the mucous membranes, especially the bulbar conjunctiva and the lips, which are characteristically covered by hemorrhagic crusts. Bilateral purulent conjunctivitis appears. The nares, pharynx, larynx, esophagus, and lower respiratory tract may be involved. Balanitis or vulvovaginitis may occur. Skin involvement varies from urticarial to target or bullous lesions.

Patients require careful monitoring and aggressive therapy if a systemic complication, such as renal failure or severe pneumonia, develops. Large doses of systemic steroid are usually given. The mortality for patients with Stevens-Johnson syndrome who are not treated is 5 to 15%. Complications include blindness, scarring of the skin, nail loss, and genital scarring.

Toxic Epidermal Necrolysis

Toxic epidermal necrolysis (TEN) is a rare, severe reaction characterized by widespread erythema and detachment of the epidermis resembling scalding. Sulfonamides, phenylbutazone, and hydantoins are the most frequently associated drugs. The onset of TEN is acute, with burning of the eyes, skin tenderness, fever, malaise, and arthralgia. Within hours to 1 to 2 days, a maculopapular rash appears, mostly on the face and extremities, and rapidly becomes confluent. Target lesions and blisters may develop. The vesicles coalesce, and sheets of epidermis detach from the dermis. There may be extensive mucosal involvement in the oral cavity and in the respiratory, gastrointestinal, and genitourinary tracts. The nails are shed. Patients with TEN are very ill with high fever, leukocytosis, abnormal liver function, albuminuria, and similar symptoms. Overall patients resemble those with extensive burns. Treatment requires superb nursing care and careful medical management, with large doses of steroids (120 to 180 mg of prednisone or equivalent per day). The outlook for TEN is guarded. Relapses may occur, and mortality is about 30%. It is important to differentiate this reaction from staphylococcal scalded skin syndrome, which involves separation of the uppermost portion of the epidermis, induced by circulating toxin. Other causes of TEN include measles, varicella zoster, herpes simplex, *Escherichia coli* sepsis, vaccines, lymphomas, leukemias, and carbon monoxide poisoning.

Fixed Drug Eruptions

Fixed drug eruptions appear as solitary or multiple oval erythematous plaques with or without vesicles and may show central clearing, as in target lesions. Lesions recur at the same site with each administration of the provocative drug. New sites may appear with each episode, but all the old lesions also are reactivated. The favored sites are the lip, the glans penis, the palms, and the soles, but any area of the skin may be involved. The dusky red plaques fade within 7 days, leaving hyperpigmentation that may last for years. Treatment of the eruption consists of eliminating the offending agent.

Erythema Nodosum

Erythema nodosum is an eruption of inflammatory cutaneous nodules, usually limited to the anterior aspects of the limbs, particularly the lower legs. The eruption may be ushered in by fever, arthralgia, pain, and occasionally gastrointestinal upset. Multiple bilateral subcutaneous nodules appear over the shins and occasionally on the thighs, forearms, and soles. Initially the lesions are red, slightly elevated, and 1 to 5 cm in diameter with diffuse borders. Nodules evolve through the color changes of a bruise, from red to blue to yellow with a greenish tint. These nodules may last between 1 and 2 weeks. Many infectious and inflammatory diseases can cause erythema nodosum, but responsible drugs include oral contraceptives and sulfonamides. Steroids are not particularly effective for treating patients with erythema nodosum, and they are contraindicated in cases resulting from infectious diseases. Salicylates and other nonsteroidal anti-inflammatory agents, however, may be given. Potassium iodide is most effective in clearing erythema nodosum. The starting dose is usually 5 to 15 drops, depending on weight, three times a day. The dose is increased 1 drop per administration per day until symptoms clear. The results are usually dramatic.

Exfoliative Dermatitis

Exfoliative dermatitis is a generalized induration with redness and scaling of the skin. This disorder occurs more frequently in men, beginning as erythema of the genital area, trunk, or head. Within days or weeks, the erythema spreads to cover the entire body, including the palms and soles. Mucous membranes, however, are spared. Exfoliation, or shedding of scales, follows the erythema and is accompanied by nail dystrophy and alopecia. The skin feels thick and usually very dry. Systemic signs include increased or decreased temperature found in 40 to 80% of patients, hepatomegaly in about 20 to 50%, and lymphadenopathy in 60%. Splenomegaly is common in exfoliative dermatitis in general but uncommon in that induced by drugs. Anemia is seen in 65% of patients and eosinophilia in 30%. Allopurinol may cause a particularly severe dermatitis if given to patients with borderline renal function who are receiving thiazides. In these cases, renal function is worsened, liver enzyme levels are elevated, and many of the patients die. Withdrawal of the provocative drug from allergic patients may not reverse the condition for as long as a year. Treatment includes not only discontinuation of the drug but also careful management of fluid and electrolytes and temperature and use of topical steroids, lubrication agents, occasionally systemic steroids, and in severe cases antimetabolites. The prognosis is guarded, with an overall mortality of 30%.

Lichenoid Eruptions

Lichenoid or lichen planus–like eruptions occur with a variety of medications, especially quinidine, gold salts, antimalarials, tetracyclines, and thiazides. The lesions appear as pruritic red to violet polygonal papules that coalesce or expand to form plaques. Scaling is a minor feature. The differential diagnosis includes lichen planus, systemic lupus erythematosus (SLE), and secondary syphilis. Skin biopsy specimens are helpful for differentiating these entities. Discontinuing the offending drug and using topical steroids lead to resolution.

Drug-Induced Systemic Lupus Erythematosus

Cutaneous lesions are uncommon (fewer than 20% of cases) in drug-induced SLE. Serosal and joint symptoms are generally more significant. Patients regularly have positive antinuclear antibody (ANA) test results. The drugs that most commonly induce SLE-type lesions are procainamide, hydralazine, and isoniazid, all of which are acetylated in the liver. Discontinuing the drug leads to clearing of symptoms, but ANA test results may remain positive for months. Steroids can induce a more rapid resolution.

Acneiform Drug Eruptions

Acneiform drug eruptions consist of follicular, inflammatory lesions, usually erythematous papules and pustules. The reactions start 2 to 5 weeks after the patient begins taking provocative drugs. Lesions may be outside of normal acne areas, in persons outside of the acne age group, and accompanied by other symptoms of drug toxicity. Initially comedones are absent, although they may appear late in the course of drug therapy (not early, as in acne vulgaris). Cysts are rare, and scarring is uncommon. Females receiving androgens for bone marrow stimulation may develop classic acne with comedones, papules, and cysts. Halogens, systemic and topical corticosteroids, and anticonvulsants may exacerbate pre-existing acne vulgaris. Treatment includes discontinuation of the inciting agent and topical therapy with benzoyl peroxide, isotretinoin, or both.

Photosensitive Eruptions

Photosensitive eruptions may be either phototoxic or photoallergic. Phototoxic eruptions appear as an exaggerated sunburn and may occur in any patient who takes the appropriate drug in large enough doses even for the first time and who receives enough ultraviolet light exposure. Common photosensitizing agents are tetracyclines, thiazides, and sulfonylureas. All photosensitizing agents can induce photoallergic responses with a maculopapular, eczematous, or lichenoid appearance. These responses are much less common than phototoxic reactions and are probably immune mediated. Therapy includes withdrawal of the drug and use of topical steroids, anti-inflammatory agents, and in rare cases systemic steroids. Sun screens may be of limited benefit for some photosensitive eruptions. Some patients become persistently reactive to light and continue to develop lesions for years after the offending medication has been discontinued. Differential diagnosis includes SLE and polymorphous light eruption.

Vasculitis

Vasculitis is a process characterized by inflammation and necrosis of blood vessels. Vasculitis may affect any size or type of vessel in any organ system. The basic cause is an abnormal immune response. Pathogenesis involves antigen exposure, formation of circulating soluble antigen-antibody complexes, deposition in vessel walls rendered permeable by platelet-derived vasoactive amines, and activation of complement components. Attraction of polymorphonuclear leukocytes, which infiltrate the vessel wall and release collagenase and elastase, to other lysomal enzymes occurs, causing necrosis of the wall followed by hemorrhage, thrombosis, occlusion, and surrounding ischemic necrosis of tissue. Cell-mediated immune reactivity may also be involved in the pathogenesis of vasculitis.

Polyarteritis Nodosa

Polyarteritis nodosa is characterized by necrotizing vasculitis, affecting the small- and medium-sized muscular arteries of such caliber as the hepatic and coronary vessels and arteries in the subcutaneous tissue and sometimes adjacent veins. Painful, tender nodules occur in about 25% of patients. These nodules may ulcerate. Common sites are the lower extremities, especially below the knee. Internal manifestations are hypertension, tachycardia, edema, and weight loss. Arthralgia, myocardial and intestinal infarctions, glomerulosclerosis, and peripheral neuritis may also develop. The lungs and spleen are rarely involved. Polyarteritis nodosa frequently develops after an acute infection. The disease may follow the use of certain drugs or may be a manifestation of bacterial allergy. Corticosteroids are most helpful in treating this serious disease.

Allergic Granulomatosis (Churg-Strauss Syndrome)

Allergic granulomatosis is characterized by the highly distinctive initial manifestation of asthma. Diffuse angitis, involving the heart, liver, spleen, kidney, intestines, and pancreas, subsequently develops. A fatal outcome is likely in about 50% of cases. Skin lesions are not always present, but nodules may appear on the extensor surfaces of the extremities and on the scalp.

Hypersensitivity Vasculitis

Hypersensitivity vasculitis is also known as leukocytoclastic angitis and anaphylactoid purpura (Henoch-Schönlein syndrome), serum sickness and vasculitis incidental to cryoglobulinemia, malignancy, or other diseases. Anaphylactoid purpura occurs most frequently in the 3- to 10-year-old age group, although it may occur at any age. Infections are most likely the triggering event. Skin lesions usually involve the lower legs and start with palpable purpura. Hemorrhagic vesicles and bullae may develop. Nodules with arthralgia may occur. Systemic features include fever, malaise, and myalgia. Kidney manifestation is usually glomerulonephritis. Gastrointestinal involvement may be noted with the presence of hematemesis, bloody stools, ulcerations in the esophagus and stomach, anorexia, vomiting, nausea, and diarrhea. Pneumonitis may also be present. Hypersensitivity vasculitis is most frequently attributable to drugs. Infections are also implicated. Treatment with corticosteroids is helpful.

URTICARIAL VASCULITIS

Urticarial and erythema multiforme—like rashes may predominate or may be the only cutaneous manifestation of leukocytoclastic vasculitis. Other features may include arthralgia or arthritis, angioedema, and mild glomerulonephritis.

Wegener's Granulomatosis

Wegener's granulomatosis is a syndrome of necrotizing granuloma of the respiratory tract, generalized necrotizing angitis affecting medium-sized blood vessels, and focal necrotizing glomerulitis. Skin nodules may appear in crops, along the extensor surfaces of the extremities. These nodules may ulcerate to form necrotic centers.

Lymphomatoid Granulomatosis

Lymphomatoid granulomatosis, a severe systemic disease, has as its main component a necrotizing pulmonary angitis. Skin lesions are present in about 40% of cases. Usually these lesions are subcutaneous or dermal nodules, but macular erythema, papules, ulcers, alopecia, annular lesions, vesicles, and acquired ichthyosis have been reported. Systemic complaints of fever, malaise, weight loss, and myalgia are common.

Giant Cell Arteritis

Giant cell arteritis is characterized by an unusual necrotizing panarteritis with granulomas and giant cells, which produce unilateral headache and exquisite tenderness in the scalp over the temporal or occipital arteries. Fever, anemia, and a high sedimentation rate are usually present.

Malignant Atrophic Papulosis (Degos's Disease)

Malignant atrophic papulosis is a fatal cutaneointestinal obliterative arteritis syndrome. This syndrome is usually characterized by pale rose, rounded, edematous papules mostly on the trunk. The center of the papule becomes porcelain-white. Infarcts involve the intestine to produce acute abdominal symptoms. Death is due to fulminating peritonitis.

Thromboangiitis Obliterans

Thromboangiitis obliterans is an obliterative vascular disease affecting the medium- and small-sized arteries, especially those of the feet and hands. This disease is most often seen in men between the ages of 20 and 40 who smoke heavily. Pain is a constant symptom. The skin supplied by affected arterioles tends to break down, with central necrosis and ulceration and eventual gangrene.

Nodular Vasculitis

Nodular vasculitis is characterized by recurrent tender nodules located chiefly below the knees, especially the calves, in women past their 30s. Nodules often ulcerate. The cause is mostly unknown.

Mondor's Disease

Mondor's disease occurs three times as frequently in women as in men and mostly in the age range of 30 to 60. The disease is characterized by the sudden appearance of a cordlike thrombosed vein, which is at first red and tender and subsequently changes into a painless, tough fibrous band. There are no systemic symptoms. The cause is unknown.

Granulomatous Diseases

Sarcoidosis

Sarcoidosis is a systemic granulomatous disease of undetermined etiology. Cutaneous lesions are encountered in about one third of patients. The most common type of cutaneous lesion consists of brownish red or purplish papules and plaques. When the papules and plaques are situated on the nose, cheeks, and ears, the term lupus pernio is applied. Very rare manifestations are erythrodermic, ichthyosiform, and ulcerating lesions.

Cheilitis Granulomatosa

Cheilitis granulomatosa is characterized by a chronic, often somewhat fluctuating swelling, usually of one lip but occasionally of both lips. Associated with this swelling may be recurrent facial paresis and lingua plicata.

Granuloma Annulare

Granuloma annulare is characterized by small, firm, asymptomatic nodules that are flesh colored or pale red and are often grouped in a ringlike, or circinate, fashion. The lesions may be many, or there may be just one. The lesions are found most commonly on the hands and feet.

Necrobiosis Lipoidica Diabeticorum

Necrobiosis lipoidica diabeticorum is characterized by one or several sharply but irregularly demarcated patches, usually on the shins. These patches appear yellowish in the center and violaceous at the periphery. About three fourths of patients with necrobiosis lipoidica diabeticorum are female, and approximately two thirds have diabetes mellitus.

Tuberculosis

Tuberculosis may be divided into the localized forms and the exanthematous or hematogenous forms. The localized forms are primary inoculation complex, lupus vulgaris, tuberculosis verrucosa cutis, scrofuloderma, and tuberculosis cutis orificialis. The hematogenous forms are miliary tuberculosis, lupus miliaris disseminatus faciei, papulonecrotic tuberculid, lichen scrofulosorum, and erythema induratum.

Atypical Mycobacteriosis

Several atypical acid-fast bacilli (*Mycobacterium marinum, M. fortuitum, M. chelonei, M. szulgai*) may cause skin infections that are referred to as atypical mycobacteriosis. A particular form of this condition causes nodular and ulcerative lesions in the skin and is termed swimming pool or fish tank granuloma.

Leprosy

Leprosy is a chronic, systemic infectious disease of humans caused by *Mycobacterium leprae*. Leprosy manifests itself in the development of specific granulomatous or neurotrophic lesions in the skin, mucous membranes, nerves, bones, and viscera. The predominant types of leprosy are tuberculoid leprosy and lepromatous leprosy.

Diseases of Appendages

Nails

Frequently conditions affecting the skin of the body also produce changes in the nails (Table 12–17). Whole texts are available on nail disorders alone. It is beyond the scope of this chapter to discuss less

Table 12–17. NAIL DISORDERS

Psoriasis—subungual keratosis, nail pitting, onycholysis, discoloration (oil spots)
Lichen planus—longitudinal grooving and ridging, shedding of nail plate and atrophy of nail bed, pterygium formation, subungual hyperpigmentation
Darier's disease—longitudinal subungual red and white streaks, distal wedge-shaped subungual keratoses
Alopecia areata—pitted (stripped) nails
Onycholysis—separation of nail plate from nail bed; causes include psoriasis, hypothyroidism, hyperthyroidism, pregnancy, manicuring, moniliasis, nail hardeners, artificial nails, photo-onycholysis, and administration of tetracyclines
Clubbing—biliary cirrhosis, chronic respiratory illnesses, congenital heart defects, familial
Spoon nails (koilonychia)—faulty iron metabolism, familial, inflammatory skin diseases, idiopathic
Onychogryphosis—hypertrophy and curvature; trauma or circulatory disorder
Anonychia—Stevens–Johnson syndrome, epidermolysis bullosa; absence of nails
Beau's lines—transverse furrows; systemic illness, trauma
Onychoschizia—splitting of distal nail plate into layers, dehydration of nail plate
Half and half nails—proximal white, distal red; renal disease
Muehrcke's lines—narrow, white, transverse bands occurring in pairs; hypoalbuminemia
Mee's lines—white transverse lines, single or multiple; arsenic poisoning
Onychorrhexis—brightness with breakage of nails
Terry's syndrome—distal 1–2 mm normal pink color, proximal end has white appearance; cirrhosis
Racquet nails—inherited disorder
Median nail dystrophy—inverted fir tree; trauma

common medically related nail problems or to discuss the more surgical or mechanical problems, such as traumatic onycholysis and ingrown nails. Nails, even more so than skin, have limited ways to demonstrate disease morphologically. Therefore different conditions may look identical, and frequently further diagnostic procedures are necessary.

ONYCHOMYCOSIS

Onychomycosis is perhaps the most common disorder encountered on toenails. Approximately 22% of the United States population have onychomycosis. There are four different presentations of onychomycosis: (1) distal subungual; (2) white superficial; (3) proximal subungual; and (4) candidal, involving the whole nail plate. The most common organisms are *T. rubrum, T. mentagrophytes*, and *C. albicans*. Other organisms include *Cephalosporium, Aspergillus*, and *Fusarium*.

Diagnosis is made by KOH preparation of scrapings from the nail plate or subungual debris either immediately if shavings are thin enough or after overnight digestion in KOH solution. Fungal cultures from shavings inoculated onto dermatophyte test medium (DTM) or other similar culture media have the advantage of being more sensitive tests that enable the differentiation between pathogenic and saprophytic fungi. Differential diagnosis of other conditions causing dystrophic thickening of the nails should be considered, such as psoriasis, lichen planus, and congenital nail conditions.

Prior to the introduction of systemic antifungals, surgical avulsions and debridement combined with topical solutions was only partially effective in treatment. Best results are achieved with systemic antifungals, such as griseofulvin and ketoconazole, for fingernails. Toenails show a poor clinical response. After 2 weeks of therapy, surgical or chemical nail avulsions increase the chance of cure by removing infected tissue and by stimulating faster growth of the new nail. Systemic antifungals should be continued until all of the infected nail has been removed and the new nail has grown in fully. This takes about 12 to 18 months. Blood tests to check for drug toxicity should be obtained prior to treatment, at 3 to 4 weeks into treatment, and every 4 months thereafter. Tests of renal, hepatic, and bone marrow function are recommended. *Candida* may be treated by topical imidazoles (clotrimazole, ketoconazole, miconazole, oxiconazole, sulconazole). A topical drying agent, such as thymol 4% in chloroform or absolute alcohol, is useful. Patients should be advised to keep their feet dry as much as possible.

PSORIASIS

Some skin conditions frequently involve the nails and produce characteristic changes. Nails are involved in psoriasis between 10 and 50% of the time, depending on criteria. Pitting of the nail is the most common finding. Pitting is not specific and may be caused by a variety of other conditions, such as alopecia areata and eczema. Onycholysis, especially lateral onycholysis, is also a common finding. Dystrophic thickening of the nails, clini-

cally indistinguishable from onychomycosis mentioned previously, also occurs. A KOH or fungal culture is necessary to distinguish between funal and psoriatic involvement. Psoriatic arthritis is said to be more common in patients with psoriatic involvement of the nails. Treatment with local steroid injections may be helpful. Methotrexate is effective in controlling nail involvement, but the risk of using such a drug seems unjustified for what is essentially a cosmetic deformity.

Table 12–18. DISORDERS OF THE HAIR

Alopecia areata—rapid and complete hair loss in round or oval patches, usually on the scalp, bearded area, eyebrows, eyelashes, rarely hairy body parts

Alopecia totalis—total loss of scalp hair

Alopecia universalis—hair loss over the entire body, including scalp, associated with several autoimmune diseases including thyroiditis, pernicious anemia, Addison's disease, vitiligo, several connective tissue diseases, and atopy

Telogen effluvium—early, excessive loss of normal club hairs, related to tight braids, winding too tight on curlers, seen in pregnancy, after febrile illness, certain drugs, crash dieting, and various chronic systemic diseases

Anagen effluvium—anagen hair loss, occurs 1–2 wks after administration of cancer chemotherapeutic agents; thallium and boron may also produce this type of hair loss

Male pattern alopecia—shows itself during the late 20s or early 30s by gradual loss of hair especially at the vertex and frontotemporal regions; inherited familial factors and testosterone metabolism in hair follicles predisposes to this type of baldness

Androgenetic alopecia in women—hair loss mainly at the vertex, slightly at temporal margin, may have a diffuse pattern; cause is believed to be excessive androgen response; serum testostrone levels usually not elevated

Trichotillomania—neurotic practice of plucking or breaking hair from the scalp or eyelashes

Pressure alopecia—occurs frequently on the occipital areas in babies lying on their backs; in adults, seen most often after prolonged pressure on the scalp, such as long general anesthesia

Syphilitic alopecia—has a typical moth-eaten appearance

Tinea capitis—is usually manifested by one or several patches of alopecia with scaling

Endocrinologic alopecia—may occur in various endocrinologic disorders, including hypothyroidism, hyperthyroidism, and diabetes mellitus, and in the use of oral contraceptives

Trichorrhexis nodosa—hair shafts have small white nodes and breaks occur at these nodes; usually due to trauma to the hair shafts

Pseudofolliculitis barbae—hairs that, after appearing at the surface, curve back and pierce the skin as ingrowing hairs

Hirsutism—an increase in growth of facial and body hair in women with a masculine distribution on the beard, chest, and abdominal areas; the most common type is found on the upper lip only

BACTERIAL INFECTIONS

Green Nail Syndrome. Green nail syndrome is characterized by lifting of the nailplate from the nail bed (onycholysis) and usually a striking greenish discoloration in the separated area. This syndrome results from growth of *Pseudomonas aeruginosa* under the nail.

Pitted Keratolysis. This infection consists of asymptomatic discrete round pits, 1 to 3 mm in diameter, which may become confluent, usually on weight bearing areas such as the heel. Pitted keratolysis is common in people with sweaty feet and is often malodorous. This infection is caused primarily by *Micrococcus* species.

Hair

Anagen hairs are growing hairs. Catagen hairs are those undergoing transition from growing to the resting stage. Telogen hairs are resting hairs. Approximately 90% of human hairs are in the anagen stage, and the remaining 10% are composed of catagen or telogen hairs. The normal scalp contains approximately 100,000 hairs, with a growth rate of approximately 1 cm/month. Human hair is designated as lanugo, vellus, and terminal. Lanugo hair is the fine hair present on the body of the fetus. Vellus hairs are fine, usually light-colored fuzz and are characteristically seen on children's arms and faces. Terminal hairs are coarse, thick, and dark except in blonds. Table 12–18 describes several different disorders of the hair.

Bibliography

Bailin PL (ed): Lasers in dermatology. Cleve Clin J Med 50:53, 1983.

Dolen J, Varma SK, South MA: Chronic mucocutaneous candidiasis: Endocrinopathies. Cutis 28:592, 1981.

Fauci AS, et al.: The acquired immunodeficiency syndrome: An update. (NIH conference) Ann Intern Med 102:800, 1985.

Rees RB: The treatment of warts. Clin Dermatol 3:179, 1985.

Robertson MH, et al.: Ketoconazole in griseofulvin-resistant dermatophytosis. J Am Acad Dermatol 6:224, 1982.

Tkach JR, Rinaldi MG: Severe hepatitis associated with ketoconazole therapy for chronic mucocutaneous candidiasis. Cutis 29:482, 1982.

PART **II**

SPECIAL TOPICS IN GENERAL MEDICINE AND IN GENERAL MEDICAL CARE OF THE SURGICAL PATIENT

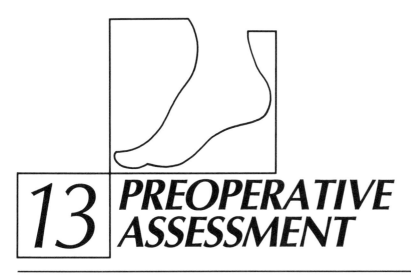

13 PREOPERATIVE ASSESSMENT

BENNETT G. ZIER

OVERVIEW

Clinical podiatric practice has tended toward a greater emphasis on surgical correction of foot pathology. Undergraduate as well as graduate teaching in podiatry settings has emphasized the need for assessing the patient's general medical status before a patient is brought to surgery. A number of states have passed laws allowing podiatrists to admit their surgical patients without consulting a co-admitting medical physician. The sum total of these and other forces has made it imperative that podiatrists learn to assess patients preoperatively from a general medical viewpoint.

The science of preoperative medical evaluation has grown. There are a number textbooks that deal specifically with this subject. The purpose of this chapter is to give the podiatrist an organized method of gathering pertinent medical information from the preoperative patient. To this end, this chapter has been organized into sections on the preoperative history and physical examination, laboratory and physiologic data, and preoperative assessment of the patient with specific medical problems by a systems approach. The goal of this chapter is to allow the podiatrist to accept the responsibility of submitting the sole preoperative history and physical examination and admitting the patient without a co-admitting physician. Also, the podiatrist should be aware of what constitutes a thorough preoperative evaluation and should be able to draw up a perioperative care plan that is dictated by that evaluation. Such a plan allows excellent communication with consulting physicians, which should only serve to improve the medical care of the surgical patient. Besides the systemic implications of a good preoperative evaluation, the podiatrist should be better able to detect problems that could lead to local morbidity of the operative site, such as aspirin abuse that could lead to a hematoma. The podiatrist who is knowledgeable in preoperative assessment should be able to more correctly and efficiently order preoperative tests.

The ability to define surgical risk is extremely useful for assessing the medical status of a preoperative patient. Anesthesiologists use a rating scale to correlate a patient's clinical status with a classification of surgical risk (Table 13–1). Surgical risk is defined as the probability of morbidity or mortality resulting from a procedure. There are five classes of surgical risk, as determined by the American Society of Anesthesiologists (ASA), ranging from class 1 (least risk) to class 5 (most risk). The mortality risk from the same operation obviously jumps considerably when comparing a patient with a class 1 risk with that of a patient with a class 5 risk. Most patients who have elective surgery should qualify for a class 1 or a class 2 risk. If the risk group is class 3 or worse there must be extremely extenuating circumstances that warrant any consideration for elective surgery.

DATA COLLECTION

History

Obtaining the patient's medical history is an essential part of preoperative evaluation. Just as some clinicians believe that 95% of diagnoses can be made through obtaining a careful history, so too can an excellent assessment of the patient's preoperative risk be made through obtaining a careful history. A preoperative history is specific for surgical risk assessment and need not be as extensive as the type of historical data obtained in an internist's comprehensive medical assessment of a new patient. The essential elements of a preoperative history are delineated in Table 13–2. One of the most productive areas of this questionnaire has to do with past medical history. It is essential that the interviewer obtain all information about previous operations. Specific questions regarding medical, surgical, and psychologic complications from previous surgeries may be very rewarding in terms of preparing the patient for the planned surgery. It is important to gather information about any medications the patient may be taking. Special emphasis should be given to in-

Table 13–1. THE AMERICAN SOCIETY OF ANESTHESIOLOGISTS PHYSICAL STATUS MEASURE

Class 1	*Normal and healthy.* No physiologic, biochemical, or psychiatric disturbance; pathologic process for which operation is to be performed is localized and not conducive to systemic disturbances; example—a fit patient with a heel spur
Class 2	*Mild systemic disease.* Mild to moderate systemic disturbance caused either by the condition to be treated surgically or by other pathophysiologic processes; examples—presence of mild diabetes mellitus, essential hypertension
Class 3	*Severe systemic disease that is not incapacitating.* Rather severe systemic disturbance or pathology from whatever cause, even though it may not be possible to define the degree of disability with finality; examples—severe diabetes mellitus with vascular complications, moderate to severe degrees of pulmonary insufficiency
Class 4	*Incapacitating systemic disease that is a threat to life.* Indicative of a patient with a severe systemic disorder already life threatening and not always correctable by the operative procedure; examples—advanced degrees of cardiac, pulmonary, renal, hepatic, and endocrine insufficiency
Class 5	*Moribund patient who is not expected to live with or without surgery.* This category defines the patient who has little chance of survival but is submitted to operation in desperation; example—massive pulmonary embolus.
Emergency Operation (E)	Any patient in one of the classes listed above who is operated on as an emergency is considered to be in somewhat poorer physical condition; the letter E is placed beside the numerical classification

Table 13–2. PREOPERATIVE HISTORY

Introductory Statement

Name, age, sex, referring physician, planned procedure, primary care physician

Patient Profile

Geographic living situation, support system (husband, wife, significant others, children), line of employment

Present Medical History

Narrative description of events leading up to decision to undergo planned surgical procedure

Past Medical History

Previous Operations and Complications
Medications:
    Prescribed, OTC, recreational drugs, alcohol, nicotine
Allergies
Nonsurgical Hospitalizations
Immunization Status
    (e.g., hepatitis, tetanus)
Pertinent Review of Systems:
    Head: history of headache, head trauma
    Eyes: vision, glasses, contact lenses, glaucoma
    Ears: hearing, history of vertigo/dizziness, infection
    Nose: nasal stuffiness or obstruction, nose bleeds
    Mouth: condition of teeth, bleeding gums, any oral lesions
    Respiratory: cough, sputum production, hemoptysis, asthma, COPD, history of pneumonia, TB screening, last CXR,
      recent URI, history of pulmonary function screening
    Cardiac: history of SOB, dyspnea, orthopnea, paroxysmal nocturnal dyspnea, chest pain (angina), history of MI, PND,
      edema, chest pain, palpitations, hypertension, rheumatic fever, heart murmurs, pacemaker, last ECG
    Peripheral vascular: intermittent claudication, history of thrombophlebitis, lower-extremity ulcers
    Gastrointestinal: heartburn, hematemesis, melena, rectal bleeding, constipation, diarrhea, hepatitis, abdominal pain,
      jaundice, history of liver disease, diet and nutritional status
    Genitourinary/renal: polyuria, nocturia, dysuria, hematuria, incontinence, urinary tract infection, history of renal dis-
      ease; male: hernia, discharge from or sores on penis; female: last menstrual period, possibility of pregnancy
    Musculoskeletal: joint pains, arthritis, backache, gout
    Neurologic: seizures, fainting, blackouts, paralysis, memory, cognition, burning in feet, dementia, delerium, past or
      present history of psychiatric problems
    Hematology: anemia, easy bruising or bleeding, past blood transfusions, history of thrombocytopenia, history of post-
      operative bleeding
    Endocrine: thyroid disease, diabetes mellitus, history of osteoporosis, history of recent use of steroids, history of
      hyperparathyroidism
    Infectious disease: history of AIDS risk factors, history of sexually transmitted diseases

Family History

Occurrence within the family of any signficant medical condition, including diabetes mellitus, TB, heart disease, hy-
    pertension, stroke, kidney disease, cancer, arthritis, anemia, complications of surgery

---

AIDS, Acquired immunodeficiency syndrome; COPD, chronic obstructive pulmonary disease; CXR, chest x-ray; ECG, electrocardiogram; MI, myocardial infarction; OTC, over the counter; PND, paroxysmal nocturnal dyspnea; TB, tuberculosis; URI, upper respiratory infection.

formation about over-the-counter medications (e.g., aspirin and nonsteroidal anti-inflammatory medications), recreational drugs, caffeine intake, and nicotine use.

Allergies are of primary importance. It is necessary to document the specific type of allergic response, such as respiratory, dermatologic, syncopal, and so forth. In addition, careful identification of the alleged offending drug must be accomplished via review of previous medical records, communication with other physicians who have cared for the patient, or both. It is important also to ask about nonsurgical hospitalizations. Very often patients identify previous hospitalizations only by the surgeries that they have had and fail to mention those that were necessitated by medical problems.

Perhaps the most vital part of the past medical history is the review of systems. This section is a comprehensive analysis of organ systems in a serial fashion. These series of questions are designed to uncover any possible historical data that may have a bearing on the patient's surgical risk. The review of systems is the physician's checklist of historical data that may directly affect surgical morbidity or mortality. Table 13–2 includes a carefully designed section on review of systems.

The last part of the preoperative history is that of family history. Of most concern are any obvious diseases, such as hemophilia, or anesthesia reactions that may have a specific impact on the patient in consideration for surgery.

Physical Examination

The physical examination of the preoperative patient mainly emphasizes the cardiopulmonary systems because it is these organ systems that contribute most toward perioperative morbidity and mortality. Table 13–3 describes the physical examination data that are necessary to evaluate a podiatric surgical patient from a general medical standpoint.

Vital signs are the most important part of the physical examination and should not be obtained by anyone other than the admitting physician. Hypertension, hypotension, tachycardia, bradycardia, irregular pulse, fever, tachypnea, obesity, and malnutrition are all readily discernible by performing vital signs. Because hypertension is often newly discovered on routine preoperative examinations, careful blood pressure recording is an essential task.

Eye examination may reveal evidence of hypertensive or diabetic retinopathy. Podiatrists should be familiar enough with funduscopic examination to recognize

---

Table 13–3. PREOPERATIVE PHYSICAL EXAMINATION

Introduction, General Survey	**Chest/Lung**
Succinct paragraph describing patient's general physical appearance	Presence of rales, wheezes, rhonchi, or pleural rub
Vital Signs	**Heart**
Height, weight, temperature, blood pressure, pulse, respiratory rate	Rate, regularity, presence or absence of heart murmur
	Abdomen
Head	Scars, presence of bowel sounds, splenomegaly, hepatomegaly, tenderness, masses
Size, shape, trauma	
	Extremities
Eyes	Presence of clubbing, cyanosis, edema, pulses in all extremities, podiatric pathology
PERLA, EOM	
Sclera color, ophthalmoscopic examination (fundi)	**Skin, Nails, Hair**
Ears	Erythema, eruptive lesions, rashes
Patency of canals, appearance of drum, light reflex	Texture, configuration
	Texture, distribution
Nose	**Musculoskeletal**
Patency of choanae, septal deviation	Joints and ROM, symmetry, tone, deformities
Mouth	**Nervous System**
Buccal mucosa, state of health of oral structures; teeth, gum, palate, tongue, appearance of pigmentary spots or petechiae	Mental status (orientation), cranial nerves, sensory, cerebellar
	Motor, reflexes, gait
Throat	**Lymphatic System**
Presence of obstruction, gag reflex, presence of exudate or erythema	Presence of adenopathy in cervical, axillary, epitrochlear, or inguinal area
Neck	
Neck vein distention, tracheal deviation, presence of carotid bruits	
Presence of goiter, adenopathy, ROM	

EOM, Extraocular movement; PERLA, pupils equal, react to light and accommodation; ROM, range of motion.

these entities. Nasal examination should carefully note any obstruction because this is important information for consideration for intubating patients for general anesthesia. Examination of the neck should denote any presence of carotid bruits; goiter, which may have implications in terms of thyroid disease; and elevated neck veins, which may indicate right-sided congestive heart failure. It is important for a patient who is to undergo endotracheal intubation to have excellent range of motion of the neck.

Chest and lung examination is extremely important for detecting findings that may indicate congestive heart failure (rales), emphysema (barrel chest, hyper-resonant percussion), bronchitis (rhonchi), and asthma (wheezing). Examination of the heart may reveal a heart murmur, fast or slow apical pulse, or an irregular heart rate. The presence of a heart murmur may indicate underlying valvular heart disease, whereas a slow, fast, or irregular heart rate may indicate a cardiac rhythm or conduction disturbance. Abdominal examination must be performed to rule out liver enlargement (acute hepatitis or cancer), splenic enlargement (viral infection, lymphoma, or portal hypertension), and abnormal abdominal masses or pulsations (aortic aneurysm). The presence of bowel sounds must be noted both preoperatively and postoperatively, as this indicates active bowel function.

Examination of the lower extremities is of obvious importance in podiatry. From a medical view, the podiatrist is most concerned about an intact vascular and neurologic system that would promote excellent wound healing. The musculoskeletal system must be examined because it is very helpful in determining the presence of any type of arthritis as well as the existence of any muscular weakness, which may indicate an underlying myopathy. The neurologic examination is of importance in terms of ruling out any involuntary movement disorders, focal deficits, and cognitive problems that may indicate underlying neurologic disease. The lymphatic system should be examined for the presence of lymphadenopathy, which may represent a myriad of disorders ranging from AIDS-related complex (ARC) to lymphoma to cellulitis.

Genitalia, rectal, and breast examinations are not routinely suggested unless the patient specifically requests that these be done or there is some need uncovered in the history or other parts of the physical examination that would necessitate doing these.

Laboratory Data

Most textbooks of surgery and anesthesia recommend certain specific laboratory tests for preoperative evaluation. These recommendations often call for a standard complete blood count (CBC), chest radiograph, electrocardiogram (ECG) on any patient over 45 years of age, specific blood chemistries, and tests of hemostasis. However, there is little scientific justification for performing these tests. No prospective and few retrospective trials have been carried out to evaluate the necessity of these or any other laboratory tests in the routine presurgical evaluation of otherwise healthy patients. Studies of the value of preoperative chest radiographs and partial thromboplastin time (PTT) tests in healthy individuals show that no significant clinical abnormalities are detected that would not have been apparent from the history or physical examination alone. Suffice it to say that most abnormalities found from laboratory and physiologic data may be predicted from obtaining a careful history and physical examination.

A minimal number of specific laboratory examinations should be carried out on any individual being considered for surgery. Obviously all individuals must have a preoperative history and physical examination. Any individual who is found to have a significant abnormality through history and physical examination can no longer be considered an ASA class 1 risk and should therefore be evaluated for the specific condition. The following procedures are recommended tests for otherwise healthy preoperative patients. These tests are the most common ones utilized in preoperative assessment of the podiatric patient.

Complete Blood Count

A CBC includes basic data on red and white blood cells, such as red blood cell (RBC) count, hemoglobin concentration, hematocrit measurement, white blood cell (WBC) count, and WBC differential. In addition, the laboratory comments on the morphology of the red or white blood cells if either appears abnormal.

Blood Hemoglobin Concentration. Blood hemoglobin concentration is reduced in all forms of anemia, and its reduction is a measurement of the severity of the disease because it reflects the oxygen-transporting capacity of the blood. Hemoglobin concentration is increased in polycythemia.

Hematocrit Measurement. The hematocrit measurement, or packed cell volume, is a measurement of the combined volume of the RBCs in a sample of blood. This measurement is expressed as the percentage of total blood volume that consists of erythrocytes packed by centrifuge in a given volume of anticoagulated blood. Packed cell volume is reduced in all types of anemia. It is important to detect anemia. Most workers would agree that a hematocrit measurement of less than 30% is probably detrimental to the patient's undergoing surgery.

Red Blood Cell Morphology

Anisocytosis. Anisocytosis is excessive variation in the size of RBCs, as seen in megaloblastic anemias, thalassemia major, and spherocytosis.

Poikilocytosis. Poikilocytosis is excessive variation in the shape of RBCs, as seen in sickle cell anemia, pernicious anemia, and spherocytosis.

Red Blood Cell Indices. Red blood cell indices are arithmetic ratios from the RBC count, the hematocrit measurement, and the hemoglobin concentration that are helpful in the diagnosis of anemias. The most useful of these ratios is the mean corpuscular volume (MCV), which is a measurement of hematocrit divided by the RBC count. The importance of the MCV is that it is low, that is less than 82 U, with microcytic anemia and greater than 100 U with megaloblastic anemia.

White Blood Cell Count. The WBC count can be either decreased, as in leukopenia, or increased, as in leukocytosis. Leukopenia can result from overwhelming infection, such as septicemia; viral infection; ingestion of certain drugs, especially antineoplastics; and radiation. Leukocytosis can result from acute bacterial infection, leukemia, acute hemorrhage, and tissue necrosis.

Differential White Blood Cell Count. The differential WBC count is a reflection of 100 WBCs that are morphologically examined in a peripheral smear. The numbers of different types of WBCs are expressed as a percentage of the whole. In the differential WBC count, neutrophils, which may increase in acute systemic or localized infections; lymphocytes, which may increase in infectious mononucleosis or lymphocytic leukemia; monocytes, which may increase in monocytic leukemia and protozoan infections; and eosinophils, which may increase in allergic reactions and parasitic infections, are seen. A left shift denotes an increase in neutrophils; an increase in nonsegmented neutrophils (band forms), which is a sign of increased turnover or demand for WBCs; or both. This left shift is seen most commonly in acute bacterial infections.

Reticulocyte Count

The reticulocyte count includes those early forms of RBCs with inclusions that are fragments of endoplasmic reticulum, which are known as reticulocytes. Increased numbers of reticulocytes reflect increased formation of RBCs, resulting from hemolysis, hemorrhage, or successful treatment of anemia. The reticulocyte count is considered an excellent measurement of bone marrow function.

Blood Tests for Hemostasis

Blood tests for hemostasis include the platelet count, the prothrombin time, and the PTT. Some hemostatic screens include a bleeding time.

Platelet Count. This count provides quantification of thrombocytopenia but gives no indication of platelet function. The normal range of platelets is 150,000 to 300,000. However, the platelet count must be very low (< 25,000) before spontaneous bleeding occurs. In the absence of any symptoms suggestive of thrombocytopenia, routine platelet counts are usually not recommended.

Prothrombin Time. This test provides a laboratory measurement of the extrinsic blood coagulation pathway and of the factors common to both the extrinsic and intrinsic pathways. Prothrombin time is prolonged by deficiencies in fibrinogen; prothrombin; and factors V, VII, and X.

This test measures several coagulation defects and is commonly used to monitor patients taking anticoagulant drugs, such as warfarin (Coumadin). Prothrombin time is increased under conditions such as vitamin K deficiency; impaired fat absorption, causing malabsorption of vitamin K; severe liver disease; and ingestion of warfarin-type drugs. Normal values are reported as a percentage of the control value, which is approximately 11 to 13 seconds. Prothrombin time remains normal in patients with hemophilia A and B and patients with platelet deficiencies.

Partial Thromboplastin Time. This test provides a laboratory measurement of the intrinsic blood coagulation pathway and of the factors common to both the intrinsic and extrinsic pathways. This measurement is the best single screening test for disorders of coagulation. Partial thromboplastin time is prolonged by deficiencies in fibrinogen; prothrombin, and factors V, VIII, IX, X, XI, and XII. Partial thromboplastin time is increased in patients with hemophilia A or B and patients with prothrombin complex disorders. Normal values are 24 to 36 seconds. Values remain normal in patients with platelet deficiencies and in patients with a defect in factors VII and XIII.

Bleeding Time. This is a standard in vivo assay that measures the effectiveness of platelet plug formation. Bleeding time is increased if platelet function is abnormal. Bleeding time remains normal, however, if the hemorrhagic disorder is confined to the coagulation system. This test is usually performed in patients who are suspected of having a qualitative platelet disorder, such as patients who have recently taken anti-inflammatory medications, such as aspirin, and patients who have von Willebrand's disease.

Blood Chemistries

Sequential Multiple Analyzer (SMA 12). This is an automated battery of serum chemistry assays that usually includes 12 tests. The battery of tests may vary from one laboratory to another. The SMA 12 is commonly used as a relatively inexpensive screening examination to measure hepatic, renal, cardiac, metabolic, and endocrine functions. The individual assays in the SMA 12 may be grouped according to the

organ system or disease being considered (Table 13–4). The following section lists only the more common causes of quantitative changes in each of the tests in the SMA 12 battery.

Calcium. Calcium ion concentration is closely controlled by a complex hemostatic mechanism, making its measurement a sensitive indicator of several pathologic conditions. Calcium level is increased in patients with hyperparathyroidism, hypervitaminosis D, bone tumors, milk-alkali syndrome, and some metastatic bone carcinomas and in patients who are immobilized. Calcium level is decreased in patients with hypoparathyroidism; malabsorption; hypoalbuminemia; and osteomalacia, or hypovitaminosis D.

Phosphorus. Phosphorus level is usually determined in the phosphate form and is correlated with calcium level. In patients with parathyroid or renal disease, phosphorus levels tend to vary inversely to calcium levels. Phosphorus level is elevated in patients with renal failure, owing to the inability of the kidneys to excrete phosphorus. Phosphorus level, similar to potassium level, is inversely related to

---

Table 13–4. SERUM CHEMISTRY ASSAYS INCLUDED IN THE SEQUENTIAL MULTIPLE ANALYZER (SMA 12/60)*

Tests

Calcium, phosphorus, chloride, albumin, creatinine, SGOT, CPK, sodium, total protein, glucose, cholesterol, LDH, BUN, carbon dioxide, uric acid, alkaline phosphatase, total biluribin

Disease Being Considered

Renal

Uric acid, creatinine, BUN

Cardiac

CPK, SGOT, LDH

Hepatic

Total bilirubin, alkaline phosphatase, SGOT, LDH

Bone and Parathyroid

Calcium, phosphorus, alkaline phosphatase

Metabolic

Total protein, albumin, calcium, phosphorus, cholesterol, uric acid, glucose

---

* Content may vary from laboratory to laboratory.

BUN, blood urea nitrogen; CPK, creatine phosphokinase; LDH, lactate dehydrogenase; SGOT, serum glutamic-oxaloacetic transaminase.

blood pH. Therefore in patients with metabolic acidosis due to renal failure, serum phosphorus level is increased. Serum phosphorus level is also elevated in patients with renal insufficiency, hypoparathyroidism, hypervitaminosis D, and bone disease. Serum phosphorus levels are decreased in patients with hyperparathyroidism, vitamin D deficiencies of rickets and osteomalacia, malabsorption, and uncontrolled diabetes mellitus.

Alkaline Phosphatase. The two main sources of this enzyme are liver and bone. Alkaline phosphatase mediates some of the complex reactions of bone formation and is involved in osteoblastic activity. When the osteoblasts are actively depositing bone matrix, they secrete large quantities of alkaline phosphatase.

Elevations of alkaline phosphatase levels are seen in patients with hyperparathyroid disease, Paget's disease, bone-forming neoplasms, and healing fractures. Alkaline phosphatase levels are also elevated in patients with obstructive liver disease, as in hepatitis, cirrhosis, and hepatic neoplasm. This enzyme is usually increased during normal growth periods in children, when expanded osteoblastic activity deposits calcium in bone. Alkaline phosphatase levels decrease uncommonly in patients with hypovitaminosis D, milk-alkali syndrome, scurvy, and malnutrition.

Glucose. The utilization of glucose by the body cells is intimately related to insulin. Mild hyperglycemia is observed in patients with diabetes mellitus, exogenous or endogenous hypercortisolism, hyperthyroidism and in patients who are taking thiazide diuretics. Hypoglycemia is seen in patients with pancreatic neoplasm, Addison's disease, hypothyroidism, pituitary hypofunction, severe liver disease, and reactive hypoglycemia.

In the individual who is asymptomatic, it is unlikely that one would undertake any preoperative management of diabetes mellitus, even if the patient were to have mild hyperglycemia. Therefore it is not necessary to do a screening test for diabetes mellitus, including serum glucose and postprandial glucose levels, in asymptomatic patients.

Cholesterol. An increase or decrease of cholesterol level may be found in many metabolic and hormonal diseases. Cholesterol level is elevated in patients with obstructed biliary flow, hereditary hypercholesterolemia, untreated diabetes mellitus, and chronic pancreatitis. Hypercholesterolemia has been associated with increased risk for arteriosclerosis. Hypercholesterolemia is a much publicized risk factor for coronary artery disease.

Total Bilirubin. An elevation of total bilirubin level may be due to increased unconjugated (prehepatic) or conjugated (hepatic or posthepatic) bilirubin. The total bilirubin measurement does not differentiate between increased unconjugated and conjugated bilirubin. Significant elevation of total bilirubin level occurs in patients in the obstructive phase of hepatitis and in patients with hepatic cellular damage, cholangiolitis, lower biliary tract obstruction by stone or carcinoma, and hemolytic disease.

Uric Acid. This substance is an end product of purine (nucleoprotein) metabolism. If many cells die suddenly the concentration of uric acid in the serum increases. Levels show great variation in the same individual. Uric acid level is elevated in patients with gout; renal failure; and myeloproliferative diseases, such as leukemia, multiple myeloma, and polycythemia. Uric acid level is decreased in patients who are taking adrenocorticotropic hormone (ACTH).

Albumin. The liver manufactures all the serum albumin and most of the globulins. A decrease in total protein level and reversal of the usual 2 to 1 albumin-to-globulin ratio are often indicators of liver disease. Albumin level is decreased in patients who are suffering from chronic liver disease, starvation, nephrosis, malabsorption, and myeloproliferative disease and in patients who are in the second and third trimesters of pregnancy. Albumin level is increased in patients who are suffering from dehydration.

Total Protein. If values for total protein level are abnormal serum protein electrophoresis determines which class of plasma protein is involved. Total protein level is increased in patients who are suffering from dehydration and diseases that feature increased gamma globulin levels. Total protein level is decreased in patients who are suffering from hypogammaglobulinemia, liver disease, starvation, and malabsorption.

Lactate Dehydrogenase. This serum enzyme is normally found in numerous tissues, with the highest concentrations in liver, erythrocytes, cardiac muscle, and skeletal muscle. An increased concentration of lactate dehydrogenase (LDH) is neither sensitive nor specific. Diseases involving inflammation or necrosis are often associated with a release of LDH from the pathologically involved cells. Lactate dehydrogenase level is increased in patients with myocardial infarction, pulmonary infarction, liver disease, hemolytic anemias, and muscle trauma and in patients who have undergone surgery. Lactate dehydrogenase can be separated electrophoretically into five isoenzymes. Levels of LD_1 and LD_2 are important in the diagnosis of myocardial infarction. In acute myocardial infarction, LD_1 exceeds LD_2. The isoenzyme LD_5 is associated with liver cell injury. Isoenzyme determination is useful in the differential diagnosis of total LDH elevations.

Serum Glutamic-Oxaloacetic Transaminase. This enzyme is also called aspartate aminotransferase (AST) and is found in most tissues, with highest concentrations in liver, cardiac muscle, and skeletal muscle. Under normal conditions, only a small amount of serum glutamic-oxaloacetic transaminase (SGOT) is present in the serum. Whenever cellular necrosis occurs, serum SGOT level rises. Increases of SGOT levels are seen in patients with myocardial infarction, liver disease, muscle trauma, and hemolytic anemias.

Creatine Phosphokinase. This enzyme is ubiquitous, similar to LDH and SGOT. Isoenzyme studies of creatine phosphokinase (CPK), similar to those of LDH, are helpful in the diagnosis of cardiac disease. The creatine phosphokinase-MB isoenzyme (also known as CK_2) is specific for myocardial cells. Therefore total creatine phosphokinase elevations with more than 3 or 4% MB isoenzyme generally indicate an acute myocardial infarction. Creatine phosphokinase levels may also be increased with muscle trauma, inflammatory muscle diseases, and brain infarction (cerebrovascular accident), in patients who are receiving intramuscular injections, and in patients in postpartum status.

Sequential Multiple Analyzer (SMA 6/60). This automated battery of serum chemistry assays includes the following: creatinine, urea nitrogen, sodium, potassium, chloride, and carbon dioxide. These tests are not usually performed as part of a screening examination but are useful in the diagnosis or monitoring of many metabolic, renal, and fluid and electrolyte abnormalities. The following section lists only the more common causes of quantitative changes in each of the tests in the SMA batteries.

Blood Urea Nitrogen. Urea and creatinine are two substances in the serum that are uniquely dependent on the kidney for excretion. Because of this dependence, measurement of urea and creatinine provides an index of renal function. Urea is an end product of protein metabolism, is synthesized in the liver, and is the principal nitrogenous constituent of the urine. In various pathologic conditions, primarily those impairing renal function, urea is not adequately excreted, and its concentration in the serum rises proportionately. Azotemia is defined as increased nitrogenous substances in the blood and is characterized by a blood urea nitrogen (BUN) level greater than 20 mg/100 ml in an asymptomatic patient. The BUN level alone as an estimate of renal function is not reliable because it is influenced by many extrarenal factors. The serum creatinine level depends on the relative rates of creatinine production and excretion, which is affected by age, gender, and lean body mass. The BUN-to-creatinine ratio is 10 to 1 in normal individuals. In patients with acute renal failure, both BUN and creatinine levels rise, and the ratio may be unchanged. Care must be taken when evaluating this ratio. Blood urea nitrogen level alone is increased in patients with renal disease, gastrointestinal bleeding, and increased protein metabolism. Blood urea nitrogen level is decreased in patients with severe cirrhosis and inadequate protein intake and in patients who are pregnant.

Creatinine. The concentration of creatinine in the serum has a linear relationship to glomerular filtration, making its determination a more sensitive indicator of renal disease than BUN concentration. Creatinine level rises in patients with renal disease, gigantism, acromegaly, and increased dietary intake of creatinine from roasted meats. If the patient is going to be treated with medications known to be metabolized through the kidney one may wish to evaluate renal function. If this is not the case a BUN or creatinine determination does not necessarily have to be ordered.

Sodium. The level of the principal cation of the extracellular fluid is increased in patients with dehydration, primary aldosteronism, and Cushing's syndrome and in the use of some diuretic drugs. Sodium level is decreased in fluid retention, as seen in patients with congestive heart failure and ascites. Sodium depletion also occurs in patients through loss of body fluids without replacement, such as in vomiting, diarrhea, and excessive sweating, and in patients with Addison's disease.

Potassium. This is the principal cation of the intracellular fluid. Potassium level may be increased (> 5.5 mEq/L) in patients with renal failure, mineralocorticoid deficiency, acidosis, massive tissue necrosis, and hemolysis and in patients who are receiving exogenous potassium supplement, massive blood transfusions, and high-dose penicillin. Hypokalemia (serum potassium level < 3.5 mEq/L) may occur in patients with chronic diarrhea, primary or secondary aldosteronism, and Cushing's syndrome and in patients who are receiving diuretic drugs.

Chloride. This is the principal anion in the blood. Concentration of chloride tends to decrease along with sodium to maintain electrical charge equilibrium. Therefore chloride level is decreased in the same conditions in which sodium level is decreased. Chloride is increased in patients who are suffering from dehydration and renal failure.

Carbon Dioxide. The measurement of carbon dioxide provides a way to approach the differential diagnosis of a change in blood pH, or acidosis or alkalosis. Carbon dioxide level is higher in respiratory alkalosis, as seen in patients with pulmonary emboli, asthma, and liver disease. Carbon dioxide level also rises in patients with metabolic acidosis, as seen in increased formation of acid, such as in diabetic ketoacidosis; in patients with decreased excretion of hydrogen ions, such as in renal failure; and in patients with increased loss of alkaline fluids, as in chronic diarrhea.

Arterial Blood Gas Studies

Another blood test commonly used in clinical podiatry is the arterial blood gas test. This test is the best single determination of lung function. Arterial blood gas level refers to the determination of arterial oxygen and carbon dioxide tensions plus the pH. Indications for blood gas studies include assessment of preoperative lung function; documentation of pulmonary disease; continuing assessment of critically ill patients with a variety of cardiopulmonary diseases; and diagnosis of acute pulmonary insults, such as pulmonary embolism.

Urinalysis

Because surgery may result in the administration of renal-excreted medications and at times may involve catheterization of the urinary tract, renal function and presence of pre-existing urinary tract infections should be assessed. Urinalysis is the most useful reasonable screening test because of its sensitivity and low cost.

Pregnancy Test

Women who could possibly be pregnant should have a screening test for pregnancy. Even though surgical morbidity has not been shown to be increased during pregnancy, it is clearly in the best interests of the patient and the fetus to be aware of this condition prior to surgery. Potential legal issues arising from doing nonemergency surgery on a woman who is unknowingly pregnant make it imperative that pregnancy tests be carried out on all women of child-bearing age who are scheduled for any type of surgery. A recent menstrual period argues against pregnancy but by no means rules it out.

Physiologic Data

Electrocardiogram

It is commonly recommended that any patient over the age of 40 have a preoperative resting ECG. However, the ECG is a very poor predictor of ischemic heart disease. In asymptomatic patients, the ECG is not a very useful predictor of perioperative cardiac morbidity or mortality. An accurate physical examination demonstrates the absence or presence of significant cardiac arrhythmias. If an arrhythmia is present an ECG is indicated. The podiatrist should correlate the electrocardiographic interpretations with the patient's clinical status. Any ECG that shows evidence of acute or chronic ischemia, electrolyte imbalance, or ventricular arrhythmia needs to be promptly investigated before any elective surgery may be undertaken. For any patient who has an ECG interpretation of myocardial infarction of indeterminate age, elective surgery must be delayed at least 6 months, unless it can be proved from a prior ECG or other historical data that the myocardial infarction did occur prior to 6 months ago.

Chest Radiograph

The standard chest radiograph complements the history and physical examination as a starting point for the diagnosis of suspected pulmonary disorders. By far the most important chest radiograph for the podiatrist to be able to interpret is that of congestive heart failure. Other abnormalities that may be derived from chest radiographic data include pulmonary masses; pleural effusions; and acute parenchymal infections diseases, such as pneumonia. A chest film is not a reliable indicator for operative risk. In fact, a patient with severe obstructive disease may have a normal chest film. An abnormal chest film, however, does not necessarily indicate high surgical risk. Careful studies have shown that there is no value in obtaining routine preoperative chest radiographs. No significant clinical abnormalities are detected that would not be apparent from the history and physical examination alone.

Pulmonary Function Evaluation

Spirometry is an excellent standard for documenting pulmonary function. Pulmonary spirometry along with arterial blood gas determinations should be considered for every patient with a positive systems review for pulmonary disease, including history of smoking, shortness of breath, dyspnea, hemoptysis, chronic sputum production, wheezing, abnormal chest film, history of tuberculosis, and so forth. Positive pulmonary physical examination findings should also highlight the need for objective documentation of pulmonary function with blood gas determinations and spirometry.

SPECIFIC PERIOPERATIVE ASSESSMENT

General Considerations

The operative mortality for a healthy patient (ASA class 1) having an elective procedure is approximately 1 in 10,000. This risk is minimized by attention to three specific areas: coagulation disorders, drug history, and previous anesthetic complications. It is important to obtain a careful history about any previous episodes of postoperative or postpartum bleeding, spontaneous bleeding, family record of coagulation disorders, and recent ingestion of aspirin or nonsteroidal anti-inflammatory drugs (NSAIDs). If these questions do not elicit a positive response it is not necessary to obtain a hemostatic screen. Many drugs interact with anesthetic agents and a history of recent administration of such drugs may affect choice or dosage of anesthetic agents. Succinylcholine chloride is potentiated by antibiotics, particularly aminoglycosides and clindamycin, lithium, quinidine, cyclophosphamide, other antineoplastic drugs, and diethylstilbestrol.

Patients should also be asked about an immediate family history of anesthetic complications. Attention should be given to a history of postoperative jaundice. Records should be obtained if possible and reviewed to ascertain whether jaundice was associated with halothane administration. Halothane should not be readministered to a patient with a history of halothane-associated hepatitis.

Malignant Hyperthermia. Malignant hyperthermia, or hyperpyrexia, is a catastrophic reaction to general anesthesia. Malignant hyperthermia is a disorder of skeletal and myocardial muscle metabolism. In some families, this disorder is inherited as an autosomal-dominant trait. In most cases, however, the event is sporadic, and it is likely that there is more than one kind of susceptibility. Malignant hyperthermia has an incidence of about 1 in 20,000 patients. Preoperatively these patients are generally asymptomatic, although some may have evidence of myopathy, such as muscle hypertrophy, lumbar lordosis, and mild hip weakness. On exposure to anesthetic agents, usually halothane and succinylcholine, the patient exhibits fasciculations and increased muscle tone, particularly of the masseter muscle. Jaw clenching during the induction of anesthesia is a typical early sign. The body muscles become rigid, and excessive body heat is produced. Marked lactic acidosis develops. The anesthesia must be discontinued, and the patient should be cooled. Intravenous dantrolene sodium has a therapeutic effect. In any patient with a family history of anesthetic-induced hyperthermia or unexplained sudden death during induction of anesthesia, a CPK test should be done. The CPK level is elevated in approximately 79% of patients with malignant hyperthermia. A positive family history and an elevated enzyme level are sufficient evidence to consider a patient susceptible. All immediate relatives of patients who have had attacks should be reported to the anesthesiologist before elective surgery.

Other Preoperative Considerations. Two further preoperative considerations that apply to all patients are nutritional assessment and psychologic preparation for the operation. Malnutrition is prevalent in certain groups of patients, such as alcoholics, elderly individuals, and those admitted to the hospital for medical disease. Several tests can assess nutrition, namely serum albumin level, serum transferrin level, hematocrit measurement, and total lymphocyte count. It is important for the surgeon as well as the primary care physician to play a role in the psychologic preparation of patients for surgery. Providing patients with information about what to expect and discussing coping techniques for the postoperative period has been shown to reduce pain-medication requirements and to shorten hospital stays.

Cardiac Disease

The presence of cardiac disease is a predictor of operative morbidity and mortality and is responsible for approximately one third of operative deaths. As noted in Chapter 1, Goldman and coworkers published a prospective study of approximately 1000 patients evaluated for cardiac risk factors. These factors affecting risk, along with their relative importance, have been carefully delineated. At highest risk were patients with uncompensated congestive heart failure and patients with a myocardial infarction within the last 6 months. Additional risk factors were signs of aortic stenosis, age older than 70 years, ventricular arrhythmias, and several laboratory values indicating organ system disease.

Stable angina is not a contraindication to an operation. Therapy with beta-blockers and nitrates should be continued preoperatively and resumed postoperatively. If a history of myocardial infarction is obtained an elective surgical procedure should be postponed until 6 months following infarction. If evidence of an old infarction is found on ECG without a history of chest pain a previous ECG should be obtained. If an old ECG is not available it is prudent to delay surgery for 6 months. Patients with permanent pacemakers require monitoring at surgery, especially while cauterizing units are in use.

Ventricular and atrial premature contractions may be an index of underlying cardiac disease. Patients with these abnormalities should be carefully monitored and given antiarrhythmic medications if more complex arrhythmias or hemodynamic compromise occurs. Prophylactic therapy is not recommended. Echocardiography should be considered in any patient who has criteria for pathologic heart murmurs. Endocarditis prophylaxis should be given for patients with acquired valvular heart disease, congenital valvular heart disease, and prosthetic valves, depending on the duration of surgery, the invasiveness of the particular surgery, and whether or not the surgery is contaminated. Patients with prosthetic valves who are receiving anticoagulant medications require careful management. Anticoagulant therapy may be briefly discontinued 2 days prior to surgery and then immediately restarted postoperatively.

Hypertension alone is not a risk for cardiac complications for a surgical procedure, but it is often associated with coexisting cardiovascular disease. Surgical risk in patients with mild diastolic hypertension (a diastolic blood pressure of less than 110 mm Hg) was not increased in prospective studies. Surgical procedures in patients with higher elevations in blood pressure should be postponed until blood pressure is lowered. All patients who are receiving antihypertensive agents require careful intraoperative and postoperative blood pressure management. In general, antihypertensive medications should be continued before and after an operation.

Potassium levels in all patients taking diuretics should be preoperatively measured and if necessary be adequately replaced before a surgical procedure to prevent hypokalemia-associated cardiac arrhythmias. A serum potassium level of 3 mEq/L or less is an indication of total body potassium deficit and requires adequate replacement stores preoperatively.

Pulmonary Disease

Pulmonary disease is a major contributor to perioperative morbidity and mortality. Anesthesia, medications, chest wall bandages, and immobilization in the supine position all adversely affect respiratory function. The major postsurgical complications are atelectasis and infection. Besides pulmonary disease, other factors that predict increased pulmonary risk include smoking, obesity, and age older than 60 years old. Several preoperative measures can minimize preoperative risk. Education in the use of incentive spirometers and deep-breathing exercises increases compliance in postoperative respiratory maneuvers. Patients should be advised to discontinue smoking before an operation. Pre-existing reversible bronchial obstruction and respiratory tract infection should be treated before an operation.

Subcutaneously administered mini-dose heparin is provided in selected situations for prophylaxis of venous thromboembolic disease. In general, mini-dose heparin therapy is indicated in certain situations for any patient more than 40 years old with no history of bleeding disorders, normal coagulation studies, and no aspirin ingested for 10 days. Selected situations in which mini-dose heparin therapy may be considered are those in which a patient has a previous history of idiopathic thrombophlebitis, a patient who has congestive heart failure, and a patient who has other diseases in which venous stasis may occur

(massive obesity, cancer) and that patient is bedridden postoperatively.

Endocrinology

Management of diabetes mellitus and thyroid disease and prior steroid therapy are the most common preoperative endocrine considerations. Diabetic management in diabetics undergoing a surgical procedure is discussed in Chapter 5. In addition to diabetes mellitus, uncorrected hypothyroidism is a contraindication to surgical procedures. Hypothyroidism is associated with postoperative hypotension, prolonged sedation, hypoventilation, and hyponatremia. Patients may have hypothyroidism diagnosed with a careful history, physical examination with special attention to the thyroid gland, and thyroid function studies. Patients with adrenal suppression require exogenous steroid therapy during the perioperative period. Any patient who undergoes more than 2 weeks of continuous high-dose steroid therapy any time during the 12 months just prior to surgery should also receive perioperative steroids.

Gastrointestinal Disease

The importance of a history of postoperative jaundice has been noted in Chapter 6. Additionally patients with a history of jaundice or abnormal liver function values should have the hepatitis B surface antigen status determined. Because morbidity, mortality, prognosis, and prophylaxis vary with the type of hepatitis virus, it is essential to understand the serologic markers for viral hepatitis and their interpretation. Universal precautions for all body fluids and needles or any contaminated sharp objects, as outlined in a hospital infection-control manual, are essential for all patients not just those with positive serology values. Any patient with active bleeding from the gastrointestinal tract, as noted from the history (hematemesis, melena, and hematochezia) or physical examination (bright red blood in the rectum and positive stool-guaiac examination), must have this investigated before any elective surgery is allowed to proceed.

Renal Disease

Because many medications given during the perioperative period are metabolized through the kidney, it is very important to assess a patient's renal function preoperatively. In an asymptomatic patient, renal function can be assessed most easily by urinalysis, which reveals any evidence of protein in the urine and any presence of urinary tract infection through bacteria or WBCs in the urine. If a urinalysis is abnormal more specific tests of renal function, such as BUN and creatinine measurements, may be obtained.

Fluid balance is another important consideration in the perioperative period. It is imperative that the surgeon be aware of the patient's preoperative weight as well as fluid intake and fluid output so as to prevent iatrogenic fluid overload, which may result in congestive heart failure. Dehydration is another common postoperative problem that can be avoided with careful fluid monitoring.

Hematology

Asymptomatic patients do not require a hemostatic screen. However, any patient who has a history of prolonged oozing or bleeding after surgery does need preoperative prothrombin time, PTT, platelet count, and bleeding time measurements. Diseases, such as von Willebrand's disease, may be uncovered via bleeding time. A preoperative CBC should be done on every patient for any type of surgery whether it be elective or nonelective. Any anemic patient should be investigated for the cause of anemia before any elective procedure is undertaken.

Rheumatology

Rheumatic diseases are among the most common medical conditions treated by physicians. An understanding of the disease process, complications, and problems that may arise as a result of drug therapy in treatment is imperative. The effects of corticosteroids, NSAIDs, penicillamine, immunosuppressive drugs, and cytotoxic drugs on wound healing and blood coagulation need to be understood. Some of these drugs may also cause problems in the postoperative period.

Postoperatively functional capacity can deteriorate rapidly in patients who are confined to bed. Active polyarthritis and deformities may cause difficulties in postoperative rehabilitation. Patients who are undergoing elective surgery should have a preoperative evaluation of the extent of joint disease and particularly the functional capacity of the ability to walk with or without assistance, to move around in bed unaided, and to stand from a sitting position. An evaluation of musculoskeletal problems also helps in the correct positioning of deformed joints in an operating room to avoid unnecessary stress and forceful manipulation. A physical therapy consultation may be helpful in developing a suitable program for postoperative rehabilitation and maintenance of joint function.

Infectious Disease

Clearly any patients who are at risk for hepatitis or acquired immunodeficiency syndrome (AIDS) need to be identified before elective surgery is attempted. It is also necessary to identify the cause of an unexplained fever in a patient before elective surgery is undertaken. Patients with self-limiting infectious problems, such as upper respiratory infection and urinary tract infection, generally should have the illnesses resolved before any surgery occurs.

Neurology

Patients with underlying seizure disorders must be identified. If these patients are on anticonvulsant medications these medications should be continued throughout the perioperative period, even if the medications need to be given parenterally during the perioperative period. Demented patients should also be identified, and any possible cause of pseudodementia, such as hypothyroidism or nutritional deficiency, should be investigated.

Geriatric Patients

The perioperative care of geriatric patients is particularly demanding. Elderly patients may have pre-existing problems that complicate the primary disease process for which surgery is indicated. Drug metabolism and excretion by the hepatic and renal systems are often reduced. The stress of surgery, added to pre-existing disease, increases morbidity and mortality in the aged.

Pediatric Patients

The perioperative management of the infant and child offers a special challenge and requires specific understanding of the infant and child as patients. Children cannot be thought of as merely small adults. There may be many unfamiliar experiences to deal with, including the surgical process, immobilization, pain, separation from loved ones, and hospital environment. The podiatrist must be aware of normal growth and development, variations in drug metabolism and excretion, anesthetic considerations, and unique perioperative needs of the patient and parents.

Bibliography

Barnett PA, et al.: The frequency and prognostic significance of electrocardiographic abnormalities in clinically normal individuals. Prog Cardiovasc Dis 23:299, 1981.

Bor DH, Himmelstein DU: Endocarditis prophylaxis in patients with mitral valve prolapse. Am J Med 76:711, 1984.

Breslin DJ, Swinton NW, Jr: Elective surgery in hypertensive patients: Preoperative considerations. Surg Clin North Am 50:585, 1970.

Caranasos GJ: Drug reactions and interactions in the patient undergoing surgery. Med Clin North Am 63:1245, 1979.

Caselli MA: Considerations in the use of medications in the pediatric patient. J Am Podiat Med Assoc 71:54, 1981.

Gohil P, Forman WM: Malignant hyperthermia: Description and case report. J Foot Surg 21:7, 1982.

Goldmann DR, et al. (eds): Medical Care of the Surgical Patient: A Problem-Oriented Approach to Management. Philadelphia: JB Lippincott Co, 1982.

Hurst J (ed): Medicine for the Practicing Physician. Boston: Butterworth Publishers, 1983.

Loder RE: Routine preoperative chest radiography. Anaesthesia 33:972, 1978.

Molitch ME: Management of Medical Problems in the Surgical Patient. Philadelphia: FA Davis CO, 1982.

Polk HC: Principles of preoperative preparation of the surgical patient. In Sabiston DC (ed): Textbook of Surgery, 11th ed. Philadelphia: WB Saunders Co, 1977.

Robbins JA, Mushlin AL: Preoperative evaluation of the healthy patient. Med Clin North Am 63:1145, 1979.

Rubenstein E, Federman DD (eds): Scientific American Medicine. New York: Scientific American, Inc, 1987.

Wyngaarden JB, Smith LH (eds): Cecil Textbook of Medicine. Philadelphia. WB Saunders Co, 1985.

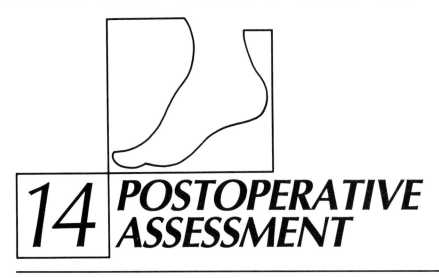

14 POSTOPERATIVE ASSESSMENT

STEPHEN BECKER

OVERVIEW

Postoperative care may be the most challenging aspect of treatment in many podiatric patients. The prevalence of coexisting medical problems and the advanced age of many patients set the stage for numerous complications. The number and severity of these problems can be reduced by careful preoperative screening and preparation. Certain postoperative complications can be anticipated, and every effort to prevent or minimize these problems should be made. Once a complication has developed, a directed and systematic approach is necessary to arrive at the correct diagnosis in a timely and cost-effective fashion. Early consultation with an internist often facilitates this process.

The aim of this chapter is to discuss postoperative complications and treatments.

The number of potential postoperative problems is large; however, several are found to occur more frequently. Fever, altered mental status, fluid and electrolyte disturbances, renal failure, chest pain, shortness of breath, and hypertension are discussed. I have selected a problem-oriented approach to aid the clinician in diagnosis and treatment of these problems.

The importance of a thorough preoperative evaluation cannot be overemphasized. A patient with reactive airway disease who is not properly prepared for surgery is likely to develop intraoperative or postoperative complications. Diabetic patients, especially those treated with insulin, should whenever possible be scheduled for surgery in the morning. This scheduling reduces the metabolic disturbances of the fasting preoperative state and permits better postoperative glycemic control. Patients with chronic pulmonary disease are often at their worst in the morning, and a later surgery time may be beneficial.

Several types of anesthesia are commonly employed in podiatric surgery. The risks and complications of surgery under general anesthesia are clearly different from those of a procedure done under local anesthesia. A hospitalized patient who develops cough and fever and has an abnormal chest radiograph after prolonged general anesthesia and a patient with the same findings following a procedure done under local anesthesia must be viewed differently. Whereas both may have pneumonia, the risk of aspiration pneumonitis is clearly higher in the patient who has undergone general anesthesia.

One must approach postoperative problems in a systematic fashion. Not all disorders have the same probability of occurrence. The general state of health of the patient, underlying medical conditions, medications, age, type of anesthesia, and type of surgery all influence the potential for developing postoperative problems. The effective clinician is able to establish the likelihood of an event in a given clinical context. The clinician is then able to confirm or exclude the likely possibilities in an efficient and a timely fashion in order to arrive at the correct diagnosis.

ASSESSMENT OF POSTOPERATIVE PROBLEMS

Fever

Fever is probably the most common postoperative problem and as such is often expected in the postoperative period (Table 14–1). Postoperative fevers may be

Table 14–1. COMMON CAUSES OF POSTOPERATIVE FEVER

Atelectasis*
Aspiration pneumonitis*
Drug reaction*
Wound infection†
IV-site phlebitis
Deep venous thrombosis
Urinary tract infection

---

* Usually apparent within 20 hrs of surgery.
† Group A streptococcus infection may occur early in the postoperative course.

divided into three groups, including (1) those due to a specific operative procedure, (2) those specific to any postoperative patient, and (3) those unrelated to surgery. The time of occurrence of fever is a useful clinical guide.

Causes

Fever that occurs within 24 hours of surgery is the most common. Causes include atelectasis from hypoventilation, aspiration of gastric or oral contents, and drug reactions. In patients who have received blood or blood products, transfusion reactions should be considered. Drug fever is not uncommon, and all drugs, including those used on a long-term basis, should be suspected. Virtually every drug has been reported to cause fever. Cardiac drugs quinidine and procainamide, antihypertensive agents methyldopa (Aldomet) and hydralazine (Apresoline), and antibiotics are the most frequently implicated. One clue to the diagnosis of drug fever is that the patient often appears less ill than the fever would suggest.

Fever that occurs later than the 24-hour period following surgery has many causes. Pulmonary complications, such as atelectasis and aspiration, may certainly become manifest in this period. Other causes include wound infections, intravenous-site phlebitis, urinary tract infection, deep venous thrombosis (DVT), and hepatitis. Causes related to the surgery itself may also be apparent. Wound infections classically begin 3 to 7 days following surgery. Tissue reaction, such as erythema, warmth, swelling, and tenderness, out of proportion to that expected by the surgical procedure itself should prompt consideration of wound infection. The wound should be carefully inspected and any exudate expressed. Properly obtained anaerobic and aerobic cultures are necessary as are blood cultures if the patient appears to have sepsis. An important exception to the 3- to 7-day rule is infection by group A streptococci, which may occur earlier in the postoperative period.

Phlebitis at the site of the intravenous lines should be considered in any patient with a fever. The duration of use and the type of catheter are factors in the development of phlebitis. Plastic catheters are more likely to become infected and do so sooner than metal catheters. Evidence of inflammation is usually present, although the absence of signs of local infection does not preclude the diagnosis. Any intravenous device in place longer than 48 hours is suspect. In a febrile patient without an obvious source of fever, all intravenous lines and intravenous solution bags should be changed.

The urinary tract may be a source of fever and infection, especially when there is an indwelling Foley's catheter. Bladder irrigation, once thought to suppress bacterial growth, does not decrease the incidence of urinary tract infection. Diabetics, females of all ages, and elderly males are at highest risk for the development of urinary tract infections. A properly obtained urine sample should be examined for evidence of infection.

Deep venous thrombosis frequently occurs in the postoperative period. Lower-extremity surgery, especially combined with use of blood pressure cuffs for hemostatic control, and immobilization are major predisposing factors. The clinical diagnosis of DVT is difficult at best and may be further complicated by the normal post-surgical inflammatory processes. A high index of suspicion is necessary, and the development of fever in the postoperative period should prompt consideration of DVT.

Evaluation

Whether fever occurs within the first 24 hours or later in the postoperative period, this problem requires a detailed and systematic approach. A data base, including history, physical examination, and laboratory evaluation, is required. Several points merit special attention. First, it should be ascertained whether a fever existed preoperatively. Secondly, it should be determined whether an episode of vomiting or regurgitation with aspiration has occurred. This occurrence suggests aspiration pneumonitis as the cause of fever. The patient should be questioned about chills, especially shaking chills; cough, with or without sputum production; chest pain, abdominal pain, dysuria, and incisional pain, all of which give an indication of ongoing processes that may be responsible for fever.

Physical examination should begin with a general assessment of the patient. Vital signs, state of hydration, and signs of toxicity or jaundice should be determined. Attention should be directed to any site suggested by the history. In addition, careful chest, cardiac, abdominal, and extremity examinations should be done. Special attention should be given to the wound, and all intravenous sites should be examined for evidence of phlebitis.

Laboratory evaluation is directed by findings from both the history and the physical examination. Laboratory evaluation should include complete blood count (CBC), urinalysis, and chest radiograph as initial studies. Failure to diagnose the cause of fever after a careful history, physical examination, and laboratory assessment should prompt consultation.

As a general rule, a fever should not be treated until its cause has been determined. The exceptions to this rule are extreme patient discomfort, dehydration, delirium or convulsions, and precipitation or exacerbation of heart failure. Antipyretics, either aspirin or acetominophen, should be administered on an every-3-to-4-hours basis until the underlying disease process has been controlled.

Altered Mental Status

Alteration of mental state may occur in a variety of postoperative settings. Underlying medical problems, stress of surgery, complications, and unfamiliar surroundings of the hospital may all contribute to changes in mental status. Often these changes are obvious, with agitation and dilirium at one extreme and obtundation and coma at the other. However, most patients with alteration of mental status present in a more subtle fashion. Often it is the family or nursing staff who note the less obvious clues. "He's not himself" or similar expressions by those familiar with a patient's baseline mental state should not be dismissed. Whereas many instances of altered mental status do not have a clear etiology and are self-limiting, some instances may be the first indication of serious, even life-threatening illness. It is incumbent on the physician to exclude a number of treatable causes of observed or reported changes in mental status.

The most common alteration in mental status is confusion. The patient's attention is disturbed, with either inattention or undue attention to unimportant details. The patient is unable to sustain normal conversation or thought patterns. Judgment is impaired. The patient commonly exhibits disorientation. As mentioned, the patient may be agitated or obtunded but most often is withdrawn or sluggish

Causes

Knowledge of a patient's baseline mental state, underlying medical and psychiatric problems, use of medications, and details of the recent operative procedure provide the context that permits the clinician to detect alteration of function and predict potential treatable causes. Table 14–2 lists some of the frequent causes of altered mental status in the postoperative patient. Regardless of cause, alteration in mental status occurs most often in the elderly, although clearly all ages are at risk.

Metabolic disorders are common and are readily correctable. Hyponatremia is an important cause of altered mental status, frequently occurring in patients with cardiac, renal, or hepatic dysfunction. The de-

Table 14–2. CAUSES OF ACUTE ALTERATION OF MENTAL STATUS IN THE POSTOPERATIVE PATIENT

Metabolic
Dehydration
Hyperglycemia
Hypercalcemia or hypocalcemia (rare)
Hyponatremia or hypernatremia (rare)
Hypoglycemia
Acidosis (includes shock, sepsis, diabetic ketoacidosis, renal failure, respiratory failure)

Fever

Sepsis

Cardiac
Acute myocardial infarction
Arrhythmia with cerebral hypoperfusion

Pulmonary
Hypoxia
Hypercarbia

Neurologic
Ischemia
Seizures (including postictal state)

Drug Toxicity
Analgesics
Alcohol (including withdrawal)
Sedatives
Others: digoxin, theophylline, antihypertensive agents

Idiopathic

gree of hyponatemia and the rate of decline of serum sodium level determine the severity of symptoms. Confusion, lethargy, and anorexia result when serum sodium concentrations fall to 120 to 125 mEq/L. Seizures and coma may occur with serum sodium levels less than 115 mEq/L.

The prevalence of diabetes mellitus among the general population and especially among podiatric patients makes disorders of glucose metabolism a common and important cause of altered mental status. The signs of altered mental status may be produced by either hyperglycemia or hypoglycemia. Any diabetic being treated with hypoglycemic agents (insulin or oral agents) who manifests altered mental status should be assumed to be hypoglycemic. Blood for serum glucose determination should be drawn and the patient treated immediately with intravenous dextrose. An oral route is acceptable if the clinical condition permits. In most cases, the derangement is due to hypoglycemia, and the administered dextrose produces a prompt resolution of symptoms. If the altered mental status has been the result of hyperglycemia the additional dextrose causes no harm.

Glucose-related disorders occur frequently in hospitalized patients. The stress of surgery, infection, or both and alterations of the usual outpatient dietary and and exercise regimen contribute to these changes. Infection and surgery are well-known precipitants of diabetic ketoacidosis as well as of a nonketotic hyperosmolar state. Ketoacidosis occurs most often in insulin-dependent (type 1) diabetics, although it can occur in those with type II diabetes mellitus during periods of stress. The nonketotic hyperosmolar state usually appears in elderly, type II diabetics. These patients have sufficient endogenous insulin to prevent ketosis and present with elevated serum glucose level (usually greater than 700 mg/dl) and altered mental status, including confusion, lethargy, and coma.

Acid-base disturbances, notably acidosis, can produce alteration of mental status. The acidosis can be either respiratory or metabolic. Sepsis, shock (i.e., hypovolemic, cardiogenic, or anaphylactic), diabetic ketoacidosis, and renal failure are frequent causes in the postoperative patient.

Fever and sepsis, particularly in the elderly, may appear with altered mental status. Pneumonia, urinary tract infection, wound infection, and infected intravenous sites are the most common sources in the hospitalized patient. Cardiopulmonary causes include myocardial infarction, with or without chest pain; arrhythmias, with cerebral hypoperfusion; and acute hypercarbia or hypoxia of whatever etiology. Careful assessment of cardiac and respiratory function is necessary in any patient with altered mental status.

Primary neurologic processes are usually readily identifiable. Cerebrovascular events are usually accompanied by focal neurologic signs. Seizures may be another cause of altered mental status and are often witnessed in the hospitalized patient.

Drugs are an important cause of altered mental status and should be considered early in the evaluation, especially in the elderly. Sedative hypnotics and analgesics are the prime offenders, particularly when given in combination. Toxicity may manifest as confusion in the elderly. Multiple drugs and drug interaction in the hospitalized patient may cause toxicity even when a stable dosage has not been changed.

In a significant number of patients, no apparent cause for altered mental status can be found even after careful evaluation. Common to this group of patients is older age, multiple underlying problems, and prolonged or emergency surgery.

Evaluation

The evaluation of a patient with altered mental status should include current medical and psychiatric problems, history of medications and drugs, and careful examination of all current medications. Determination of vital signs detects shock states and cardiac arrhythmias. An increased respiratory rate may suggest hypoxia or metabolic acidosis, whereas a low rate may suggest carbon dioxide narcosis. A rectal temperature should be obtained. Physical examination should include a general inspection of the patient for cyanosis or signs of fever or toxicity. The neck should be examined for signs of meningeal irritation. The heart and lungs as well as surgical wounds and intravenous sites should be examined. Mental status examination that reveals disorientation to time and place is a nonspecific finding. Disorientation to person is significant, however, in a patient with an altered mental status. Laboratory investigation depends somewhat on the findings from the history and physical examination. An assessment of electrolytes, glucose, and renal function is indicated in most cases. Arterial blood gas determination, CBC, chest radiograph, electrocardiogram (ECG), and specific drug serum level determination may be necessary when suggested by the clinical findings.

Fluid and Electrolyte Disturbances

Disturbances of fluid and electrolyte balance are common postoperative problems. These disturbances occur most frequently in those patients with impaired renal concentrating mechanisms and in those with cardiac and hepatic disease. Fluid and electrolyte abnormalities may be manifested preoperatively, as in a patient receiving diuretics, or may develop in the postoperative period, as a result of improper fluid replacement; increased bodily loss, through vomiting, diarrhea, or fever; medications, and stress. Dehydration, hyponatremia, and hypokalemia are the most commonly encountered abnormalities.

Hydration

The minimum daily water requirement can be calculated as insensible, or evaporative, loss and urine output necessary to excrete solute load, (i.e., water produced from endogenous metabolism). In the average adult, insensible losses are 800 to 1000 ml/day, urine output necessary to excrete daily solute load is approximately 500 ml/day, and water produced is approximately 300 ml/day. Thus the administration of 2000 to 3000 ml/day to maintain a urine output of 1000 to 1500 ml/day is desired in most circumstances. Certain common clinical conditions in the postoperative period may alter fluid requirements. Fever and increased respiratory rate, for example, increase insensible loss. For each degree of fever above 37°C (98.6°F), insensible water loss is increased by 100 to 150 ml/day. Sensible losses, such as sweat, may vary tremendously depending on ambient and body temperatures and physical exertion. The kidneys' ability to excrete the daily solute load may vary as a result of age, renal dysfunction, and diuretic therapy.

The state of hydration can be best assessed by certain clinical parameters, including blood pressure, pulse rate, skin turgor, weight, and recorded volumes of intake and output. Dehydration is manifested as poor skin turgor (best tested on the forehead and sternum), dry oral mucous membranes, sunken eyes, and tachycardia. Orthostatic hypotension may be present as well if the fluid deficit is marked. Excess fluid volume is most reliably detected by weight gain. Edema is not usually apparent until 2 to 3 kg of fluid is retained. Edema manifestes initially in the most dependent portions of the body. In the bedridden patient, edema is noted in the sacral and presacral regions.

There are no specific laboratory tests that accurately reflect volume status. The serum sodium measurement indicates the relationship of total body water and sodium and is therefore not a useful guide to volume status. Serum and urine osmolality, blood urea nitrogen (BUN) to creatinine ratio, and urine sodium excretion may provide additional evidence. However, the state of hydration is largely a clinical determination.

Sodium Disorders

Disorders of sodium, particularly hyponatremia, are common. Once a decreased level of serum sodium is noted, it is important to determine the patient's volume status. Postoperative hyponatremia may occur with volume excess, volume depletion, and normovolemia. Hyponatremia with volume expansion is frequent in the elderly and in those with congestive heart failure and renal disease. Frequently these patients have received hypotonic intravenous solutions. Because the disturbance is the result of impaired water excretion, treatment includes water restriction, often in conjunction with diuretics. Hyponatremia with volume depletion exists when sodium losses are disproportionally greater than water losses, which may result from renal or nonrenal causes. Renal causes include diuretic therapy, osmotic diuresis (e.g., uncontrolled diabetes mellitus), and various nephropathies. Extrarenal causes include vomiting; diarrhea; and third-

space sequestration, such as ascites. Treatment is volume expansion with isotonic saline. Hyponatremia with normovolemia appears in two settings: water intoxication and the syndrome of inappropriate antidiuretic hormone (SIADH) secretion. Water intoxication may be the result of water or hypotonic intravenous solutions administered to patients with impairment of renal diluting mechanisms. Patients with renal and cardiac disease are at particular risk, as are all patients who have undergone operative procedures under general anesthesia.

The SIADH secretion in postoperative patients is believed to be the result of surgical stress, anesthetic agents, or both. As the name implies, there is an excessive secretion of antidiuretic hormone in the absence of physiologic need. The result is excretion of a small volume of highly concentrated urine. Because most patients continue to ingest water normally, there is water retention and dilutional hyponatremia. Increased renal excretion of sodium follows, further lowering the serum sodium level. The clinical picture is characterized by (1) hyponatremia; (2) normal volume status; (3) serum hypo-osmolality; (4) inappropriately high urine osmolality; (5) high urinary sodium level; (6) normal renal, adrenal, and thyroid function; and (7) absence of diuretic therapy. Syndrome of inappropriate antidiuretic hormone is a diagnosis of exclusion and depends on a very careful assessment of volume. Serum uric acid level is frequently low in SIADH and may be a useful clue to the diagnosis. Although it is rarely severe or prolonged, SIADH is a common postoperative problem. Diseases of the chest and central nervous system are frequently associated with the syndrome. Numerous drugs, some common to podiatry, are also associated with SIADH (Table 14–3). Treatment of SIADH in the usual postoperative patient is fluid restriction. Symptomatic or se-

Table 14–3. DRUGS ASSOCIATED WITH SYNDROME OF INAPPROPRIATE ANTIDIURETIC HORMONE

Chlorpropamide (Diabinese)
Clofibrate
Analgesics (especially morphine)
Sedatives (especially amitriptyline [Elavil])
Psychotropics

verely hyponatremic patients (serum sodium <115 mEq/L) require aggressive therapy with saline and diuretics.

A spurious hyponatremia may exist with hyperglycemia, severe hyperlipidemia, and hyperproteinemia. In hyperglycemia, osmotic diuresis results in the obligatory loss of abnormally large amounts of sodium and water. Hyperglycemia is the most common cause, and a simple formula allows correction of the serum sodium level. Each 100-mg/dl rise in serum glucose leads to a 1.6 mEq/L decrement in serum sodium. Treatment is correction of the underlying abnormality.

Potassium Disorders

Potassium disorders are frequent problems in the postoperative period. Although most disorders are mild, severe hypokalemia or hyperkalemia may be life threatening. Potassium is the primary intracellular cation; only 2% is found in the extracellular fluid. Therefore serum potassium level is only a general indicator of total body potassium stores. Several common clinical states may cause a shift in potassium distribution, with or without a change in total body stores. These states include acid-base disorders, increased serum osmolality, and insulin deficiency.

Hypokalemia occurs most often in patients who are receiving diuretics. Other common causes include vomiting; diarrhea; osmotic diuresis; certain antibiotics, including amphotericin B and antipseudomonal penicillins; and high doses of glucocorticoids. Symptoms usually do not appear until serum levels fall below 2.5 mEq/L. A rapid rate of all, however, may induce symptoms at higher levels. Weakness, fatigue, and paralysis are the usual symptoms. Cardiac abnormalities, including arrhythmias, orthostatic hypotension, and ECG changes, may be evident. Of special concern is the development of hypokalemia in patients who are receiving digoxin. Hypokalemia may precipitate or worsen digitalis toxicity, a potentially life-threatening condition. Electrocardiographic changes of hypokalemia include flattening of T waves, presence of U waves, and ST segment depression. Therapy is the replacement of potassium with potassium chloride. Oral supplementation is adequate in mild hypokalemia, with serum levels greater than 3.0 mEq/L. In those patients with severe hypokalemia, those with ECG abnormalities, and those unable to take oral supplements, intravenous administration is necessary. The rate of replacement is dependent on the degree of depletion but in general should not exceed 10 to 20 mEq/hour in concentrations of 30 to 50 mEq/L. Repeated tests of serum potassium level are necessary to prevent excess replacement and hyperkalemia.

Hyperkalemia is much less common than hypokalemia but a far more lethal abnormality. Neuromuscular manifestations, including weakness, paresthesias, and paralysis, occur with potassium levels greater than 6.5 mEq/L. Cardiac manifestations, including bradycardia, ventricular fibrillation, and cardiac standstill, occur when the serum potassium level exceeds 7.5 to 8.0 mEq/L. Hyperkalemia rarely exists in healthy individuals. Renal failure; metabolic acidosis; exogenous sources of potassium, such as supplements; increased tissue breakdown, as seen with hemolysis; crush injuries; and rhabdomyolysis are the major causes of significant hyperkalemia. A spurious hyperkalemia may be seen when potassium is released from cells in thrombocytosis, marked leukocytosis, and blood-sample hemolysis. Therapy for hyperkalemia is determined by the serum level of potassium and the presence of ECG changes. Potassium serum levels of 7.0 mEq/L or greater require immediate treatment. A useful approach to treatment involves the following:

1. Protecting the cardiac cell from the effect of potassium on myoelectric activity. This is accomplished by the administration of calcium chloride.

2. Shifting potassium from the extracellular to the intracellular space. Sodium bicarbonate, glucose, and insulin infusions effect this shift.

3. Reducing the total body potassium load. Cation exchange resins (sodium polystyrene sulfonate [Kayexalate]) and in rare instances dialysis are used for this purpose.

Acute Renal Failure and Oliguria

Acute renal failure (ARF) is a feared postoperative complication. The result of a diminished glomerular filtration rate,

ARF may be oliguric, with urine output less than 500 ml/day, or nonoliguric, with urine output more than 500 ml/day. Anuria occurs infrequently and usually suggests bladder outlet obstruction. The causes of ARF may be categorized by the site of abnormality as prerenal, intrarenal, and postrenal. Many prerenal and postrenal causes are reversible and should be the focus of the clinician's attention.

Causes

Prerenal oliguria is the result of inadequate renal blood flow. Dehydration, hemorrhage, and hypotension are the most frequent causes. If recognized early these causes are amenable to prompt therapy and return of normal renal function. The most important cause of postrenal failure in the postoperative patient is bladder outlet obstruction. This obstruction is often the result of drugs given in the perioperative period, notably meperidine (Demerol). The combination of bed rest, prostatic hypertrophy, and analgesic use is often the cause of postrenal failure in elderly males. Bladder catheterization permits ready diagnosis and treatment.

There are many intrarenal causes of oliguria, but ischemic insults and nephrotoxic drugs are the most common in the postoperative period. Ischemia secondary to an episode of intraoperative hypotension frequently leads to the development of renal failure. Hypovolemia; administration of anesthetic agents, particularly methoxyflurane; sepsis; and heart failure should be considered as causes of the hypotensive insult. Correction of the hypotension and treatment of its underlying cause should be initiated promptly. Nephrotoxic drugs, especially aminoglycoside antibiotics, may result in ARF. Contributing factors include advanced age, pre-existing renal dysfunction, and excessive dosages of the drugs.

Evaluation

The approach to a patient with ARF includes obtaining a history of antecedent renal dysfunction, measuring urine volumes, and determining medication use. The state of hydration and cardiovascular status should be assessed. If postrenal obstruction is considered a possibility bladder catheterization is indicated. Laboratory evaluation includes examination of a fresh urine sample. Prerenal and postrenal azotemia yields a benign urine sediment, whereas ischemic ARF reveals a brownish sediment with numerous casts. Additional laboratory studies include serum and urine sodium levels, creatinine level, osmolality, and BUN level. There are several specific tests that assess the kidneys' abilities to concentrate and to reabsorb sodium. These tests are extremely useful in differentiating prerenal azotemia from intrarenal disease. An underperfused but otherwise normal kidney is capable of conserving both salt and water. A kidney damaged by ischemia loses its ability to retain salt and concentrate maximally. The renal failure index (RFI) and calculation of the fractional excretion of sodium (FE_{NA}) are sensitive means of differentiating prerenal from intrarenal causes of azotemia. These measurements require only a determination of urinary and plasma sodium levels and creatinine concentrations. The formulas to calculate these values as well as other tests in the evaluation of renal failure are summarized in Table 14–4. A summary of the

Table 14–4. LABORATORY STUDIES IN THE EVALUATION OF OLIGURIC RENAL DYSFUNCTION

	BUN-Creatinine Ratio	Urine Sodium	Renal Failure Index*	Fractional Excretion of Sodium†
Prerenal Azotemia	>15	<20	<1	<1
Acute Renal Failure	<15	>40	>1	>2

$$\text{Renal failure index} = \frac{\text{urine sodium}}{\text{urine-plasma ratio of creatinine}}.$$

$$\text{Fractional excretion of sodium} = \frac{\text{urine-plasma ratio of sodium}}{\text{urine-plasma ratio of creatinine}} \times 100.$$

BUN, Blood urea nitrogen.

diagnostic approach to postoperative renal failure is found in Table 14–5.

Treatment is directed toward correction of underlying causes. When no reversible cause is discovered, treatment consists of careful fluid, electrolyte, and dietary management in consultation with an internist. Treatment of renal failure is discussed in greater detail in Chapter 8.

Chest Pain and Shortness of Breath

There are several common and serious causes of chest pain and shortness of breath (SOB) in the postoperative period. Myocardial infarction, pulmonary embolus, and pneumonia are the usual diagnoses of concern. Perioperative infarction has a substantially higher mortality rate, up to 70%, than infarction unrelated to surgery. Procedures done utilizing general anesthesia are more likely to precipitate infarction than those done under local anesthesia or a balanced regimen. Podiatric patients are at particular risk because they generally are of advanced age and have a high prevalence of diabetes mellitus, hypertension, and atherosclerotic disease.

Myocardial Infarction

The diagnosis of myocardial infarction is discussed in the Chapter 1; however, several points are of particular importance in the postoperative patient. Silent ischemia, that is, the absence of typical chest pain, occurs often in the postoperative patient. General anesthesia, sedation, and analgesia may obscure the usual symptoms. Acute infarction may therefore appear as unexplained hypotension, SOB, nausea with or without vomiting, or syncope. The clinician should have a high index of suspicion

Table 14–5. DIAGNOSTIC APPROACH FOR OLIGURIA AND ACUTE RENAL FAILURE

1. Assess volume and cardiovascular status
2. Rule out postrenal obstruction: bladder catheterization
3. Discontinue nephrotoxic drugs
4. Test serum electrolytes: BUN, creatinine and osmolality
5. Spot test urine sodium and creatinine
6. Calculate fractional excretion of sodium or renal failure index

with the occurrence of any of these signs or symptoms. An ECG is mandatory and may reveal changes consistent with infarction. In a patient with typical chest pain, however, a normal ECG does not exclude the diagnosis of infarction. The clinician must carefully consider the patient's history and clinical context in making a decision for critical care treatment.

Pulmonary Embolus

Thromboembolic disease is a major cause of morbidity and mortality in the surgical patient. The exact incidence of DVT with pulmonary embolism is unknown, but some estimate it to be approximately 500,000 cases per year. Surgery of the lower extremity, bed rest, and older age increase the risk. Previous DVT and congestive heart failure add further to a patient's risk. The diagnosis is often difficult to make. Massive emboli may occur as sudden death, hypotension, acute right-sided heart failure, or syncope. Smaller emboli usually appear as dyspnea with or without chest pain. Hemoptysis occurs if there has been pulmonary infarction. Acute agitation or confusion, either alone or certainly when accompanied by SOB, should prompt consideration of the diagnosis.

Physical examination is rarely helpful, and even findings of phlebitis (present in one third of patients) are not specific for DVT. The ECG and chest radiograph are usually abnormal but are not specific for pulmonary embolus. The value of the ECG is largely the exclusion of acute myocardial infarction. The chest radiograph may vary from completely normal to the wedge-shaped peripheral infiltrate and associated pleural effusion of pulmonary infarction. The usual finding is atelectasis, which is of little help because it is common in postoperative patients. Arterial blood gas determinations are important. Hypoxia and hypocarbia are invariably present, though at times only transiently. The greatest difficulty in the interpretation of arterial blood measurements is the determination of the departure from the norm for a given patient. A pO_2 of 76 mm Hg may be distinctly abnormal in a young patient without coexisting pulmonary disease, whereas it may be the norm for a patient with chronic obstructive pulmonary disease (COPD). Interpretation is further complicated by factors that normally lower the pO_2, such as lying in the supine position, obesity, and older age. In general, the clinician is often required to make a judgment as to whether relative hypoxia exists. The constellation of signs and symptoms and the clinical context must be taken into consideration, together with the ECG, chest radiograph, and arterial blood gas determinations, to establish a probability of diagnosis. If the likelihood is high further diagnostic studies are required.

The ventilation-perfusion radionuclide lung scan is an extremely useful and safe test. The sensitivity of the scan is sufficiently high that negative findings essentially rule out the diagnosis of pulmonary embolus. The lung scan, however, lacks specificity, and findings may be positive in other acute pulmonary disorders. The combination of ventilation and perfusion scanning with the plain chest radiograph allows a determination of probability of significant embolic disease. For example, perfusion defects that correspond to an area of normal lung parenchyma on chest radiograph would be considered high probability for pulmonary emboli. Lung scans are therefore considered to be normal or with a graded probability, high, low, and intermediate, of pulmonary embolus. The approach to the patient thought to have a pulmonary embolus is outlined in Chapter 3. If the diagnosis remains in doubt after lung scanning pulmonary angiography should be obtained. Angiography is the most sensitive and specific test for pulmonary embolism. Angiography is also the most invasive test.

The treatment of pulmonary embolism is intended to prevent further propagation of existing blood clots. Many drugs commonly employed in postsurgical patients interact with the anticoagulants heparin and warfarin. The concomitant use of antibiotics, aspirin and other anti-inflammatory agents, oral agents to control diabetes mellitus, and agents to control epilepsy must be carefully monitored, preferably in collaboration with a clinical pharmacist.

Other causes of dyspnea in the postoperative period include anxiety, which is often the result of pain; atelectasis, aspiration; and congestive heart failure. The onset of symptoms, including associated chest pain, cough, sputum production, and fever or chills, is an important factor in the diagnosis. Physical examination should include a careful evaluation of the cardiorespiratory system. Of particular importance are signs of localized pulmonary processes and evidence of consolidation, such as egophony and increased fremitus.

Pneumonia

A distinction between aspiration pneumonitis and aspiration pneumonia should be made. Although both are frequent postoperative problems, aspiration pneumonitis and aspiration pneumonia represent different syndromes with distinct etiologies, pathophysiologies, courses, and treatments. Aspiration pneumonitis results from the aspiration of sterile, acidic gastric contents. This aspiration causes chemical pneumonitis usually without bacterial infection. Aspiration pneumonia occurs when polymicrobial oral secretions of physiologic pH are introduced into the pulmonary tree. Bacterial pneumonia is the usual result.

Aspiration pneumonitis follows an episode of vomiting or regurgitation. Dyspnea; bronchospasm; and production of thin, frothy sputum appear within several hours of the event. Hypoxia may be marked. Aspiration pneumonitis carries a significant mortality rate. The chest radiograph may be useful in diagnosis because aspiration has predilection for certain lung segments, depending on gravity and position of the patient. The right upper and lower lobes and the left lower lobe are most commonly involved. Treatment is mainly supportive. Corticosteroids and prophylactic antibiotics are of no proven value. Antibiotics are indicated only if signs of secondary pneumonia develop. Measures to prevent aspiration include airway protection during the induction stage of general anesthesia and proper placement of patients with altered mental status in a lateral decubitus, head-down position.

Aspiration pneumonia occurs when oropharyngeal contents are introduced into the lung. Those individuals with impaired upper airway defenses are at highest risk, such as recently anesthetized patients, alcoholics, epileptics, drug addicts, and persons with disorders of swallowing. The episode of aspiration is rarely observed, and the clinical course is gradual. Cough, productive of purulent sputum; fever, and an infiltrate on chest radiograph are the usual signs. The microbiology of aspiration pneumonia is complex, and its occurrence in a hospitalized patient further complicates matters. The orpharynx contains numerous aerobic and anerobic bacteria (10^8 to 10^{11}; bacteria per ml of saliva). Aspiration pneumonia is therefore almost always polymicrobial in nature. Hospitalized patients and especially those with COPD have a more complex oral flora. Gram-negative organisms and *Staphylococcus aureus* are frequently isolated from these individuals. Treatment is therefore different, depending on the anticipated microbiology at the time of aspiration.

Community-acquired infections can be treated effectively with penicillin (2 to 5 million μ/day), whereas hospital-acquired infections require an antibiotic combination that provides additional coverage against most gram-negative organisms and *S. aureus*. An aminoglycoside plus penicillin, or a semisynthetic penicillin, or a cephalosporin are usually selected for treatment.

Postoperative Hypertension

Postoperative hypertension is a frequent problem. Postoperative hypertension is defined as a sustained blood pressure greater than 190/100 mm Hg. Several studies suggest an incidence of postoperative hypertension of approximately 4%. Postoperative hypertension usually arises in those patients with an antecedent history of hypertension, particularly among those with evident end-organ damage. Most cases arise in the first hour after the completion of surgery and the majority of those within the first 30 minutes.

Causes and Treatments

Most cases of postoperative hypertension are associated with pain and anxiety as anesthesia dissipates. In these instances, analgesia and sedation when appropriate are usually sufficient treatment. Other causes to be considered are hypoxia and hypercarbia, hypothermia, and volume overload.

Overdistention of the urinary bladder is known to be a cause of hypertension, with significant elevation of both systolic and diastolic pressures. Treatment in these situations is directed toward the underlying cause. Another cause of postoperative hypertension is acute preoperative discontinuation of certain antihypertensive drugs. The central-acting sympatholytic agents clonidine (Catapres), guanabenz (Wytensin) and methyldopa (Aldomet) are most likely to cause this reaction. Reinstitution of therapy usually restores a normal blood pressure. Because of this reaction and the well-known tendency for rebound angina following abrupt discontinuation of beta-blocking agents, it is suggested that antihypertensive agents be continued up to the time of surgery and resumed as soon as possible postoperatively.

If the treatment of pain, anxiety, and other secondary causes does not lower blood pressure, treatment with oral or parenteral antihypertensive agents may be warranted. The decision to treat elevated blood pressure is based on several factors, including the absolute blood pressure itself; the presence of symptoms, including central nervous system and cardiac manifestations; the history of hypertension; and the previous treatment. Numerous oral and parenteral antihypertensive agents are available. Treatment choice is dependent on the urgency of the situation. Most hypertensive emergencies require the podiatric physician to seek consultation.

Bibliography

Aduan RP, Fauci AS, Dale DC, Herzberg JH, Wolff SM: Factitious fever and self-induced infections. Ann Intern Med 90:230, 1979.

Barlett JG: Aspiration pneumonia. Clin Notes Respir Dis 18:3, 1980.

Bergofsky EH: Respiratory failure in disorders of the thoracic cage. Am Rev Respir Dis 119:643, 1979.

Biello DR, Mattar AG, McKnight RC, Siegel BA: Ventilation-perfusion studies in suspected pulmonary embolism. Am J Roentgenol 133:1033, 1979.

Coon WW: Epidemiology of venous thromboembolism. Ann Surg 186:194, 1977.

Curtis AM, Knowles GD, Putman CE, et al.: The three syndromes of fat embolism: Pulmonary manifestations. Yale J Biol Med 52:149, 1979.

Dalen JE, Albert JS: Natural history of pulmonary embolism. Prog Cardiovasc Dis 17:259, 1975.

Dinarello CA, Wolff SM: Approach to the patient with fever of unknown origin. In Mandell G, Bennett JE, Douglas RG (eds): Principles and Practices of Infectious Diseases, Vol 1. New York: John Wiley & Sons, 1979.

Fairbairn JF II, Juergens JL: Principles of medical treatment. In Juergens JL, Spittell JA, Jr, Fairbairn JF, II (eds): Peripheral Vascular Diseases, 5th ed. Philadelphia: WB Saunders Co., 1980.

Fichman VP, Vorherr H, Kleeman CR, Telfer N: Diuretic-induced hyponatremia. Ann Intern Med 75:853, 1971.

Fratantoni J, Wessler S: Prophylactic therapy of deep vein thrombosis and pulmonary embolism. DHEW Publication No. (NIH) 76-866, 1975.

Gold W: Dyspnea. In Blacklow RS (ed): Signs and Symptoms: Applied Pathologic Physiology and Clinical Interpretation, 5th ed. Philadelphia: JB Lippincott Co, 1979.

Goldmann DR, et al. (eds): Medical Care of the Surgical Patient: Problem-Oriented Approach to Management. Philadelphia: JB Lippincott Co, 1982.

Grieco MH (ed): Infections in the Abnormal Host. New York: Yorke Medical Books, 1980.

Hinshaw HC, Murray JF: Diseases of the Chest, 4th ed. Philadelphia: WB Saunders Co, 1980.

Hinton RC, Kistler JP, Fallon JT, Friedlich AL, Fisher CM: Influence of etiology of atrial fibrillation on incidence of systemic embolism. Am J Cardiol 40:509, 1977.

Hurst, JW (ed): Medicine for the Practicing Physician. Boston: Butterworth Publishers, 1983.

Irwin RS, Rosen MJ, Branan SS: Cough: A comprehensive review. Arch Intern Med 137:1186, 1977.

Kakker VV, Corrigan TP, Fossard DP: Prevention of fatal postoperative pulmonary embolism by low doses of heparin: An international multicenter trial. Lancet 1:45, 1975.

Kempczinski RF: Lower extremity arterial emboli from ulcerating atherosclerotic plaques. JAMA 241:807, 1979.

Levy M: The pathophysiology of sodium balance. Hosp Practice 13:105, 1978.

Light RW: Pleural effusions. Med Clin North Am 61:1339, 1977.

Martin L: Respiratory failure. Med Clin North Am 61:1369, 1977.

Martinez-Maldonaldo M: Inappropriate antidiuretic hormone secretion of unknown origin. Kidney Int 17:554, 1980.

Neward SR, Dluhy RG: Hyperkalemia and hypokalemia. JAMA 231:631, 1975.

Rubenstein E, Federman DD (eds): Scientific American Medicine. New York: Scientific American, Inc, 1987.

Salzman EW, Davies GC: Prophylaxis of venous thromboembolism. Ann Surg 191:207, 1980.

Schwartz AB: Potassium-related cardiac arrhythmias and their treatment. Angiology 29:194, 1978.

Wyngaarden JB, Smith LH (eds): Cecil Textbook of Medicine. Philadelphia: WB Saunders Co, 1985.

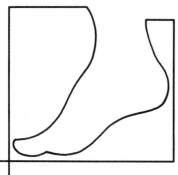

15 PEDIATRICS

LEON SMITH

OVERVIEW

Podiatric Relevance to General Pediatrics

Many childhood problems related to the lower extremity, foot, and gait are seen by the podiatrist. These problems may be associated with genetic disorders or systemic disease or may be specific, localized foot problems. It is not the main purpose of this chapter to review specific foot problems because the podiatrist is well versed in them. Those problems involving the foot in a medical, biomechanical way may be related to other systemic problems not yet being treated or recognized by the child's pediatrician. The podiatrist should be aware of the many disorders that may appear as lower-extremity problems but are manifestations of more widespread systemic disease.

Appropriate referrals should be made when the podiatrist recognizes manifestations of systemic disease. Diagnosed problems must also be considered by the podiatrist when medically and surgically managing the pediatric patient. Consultation should be sought when indicated to ensure the best possible care for the pediatric patient.

General Pediatrics

Pediatrics, as defined by the American Academy of Pediatrics, spans birth to age 21 years. Numerous podiatric problems occur within this age group, and statistics indicate that many pediatric patients are seen by podiatrists for lower-extremity problems. To properly evaluate these patients, podiatrists need a broad general pediatric background. Infants, children, and adolescents differ significantly from adults and from each other. Adult standards for physical findings, laboratory data, drug dosages, and pharmacologic and psychologic responses are not necessarily valid in the pediatric patient.

Pediatric evaluation and appropriate plan of care must take into account not only the presenting problem, but the family history; pregnancy, birth, and developmental history; patterns of growth; immunization status; history of bleeding problems; and allergies, especially to medications. In the adolescent, a history of drug use, sexual activity, and known pregnancy may influence diagnosis, laboratory studies, and therapeutic approaches.

To treat the pediatric patient either medically or surgically, special knowledge is necessary regarding medication, anatomic

PLEASE ANSWER THOSE QUESTIONS APPLICABLE TO YOUR CHILD

FIRST VISIT DATE _____

CHILD'S NAME _____ BIRTH DATE _____

CHIEF COMPLAINT (reason for the visit) _____

P.I. (history of present illness)
I. Family History   <u>Name</u>   <u>Age</u>   <u>Blood Type</u>   <u>Rh</u>
Mother _____
Father _____
Brothers & Sisters _____
_____
_____

Please circle any disease present in the child's immediate family (parents, siblings, grandparents, uncles and aunts):
Allergy   Asthma   Hayfever   Eczema   Sinus Trouble   Bronchitis
Drug Reactions   Anemia   Bleeding   Diabetes   Cancer   Leukemia
Tuberculosis   Epilepsy   Convulsive Disease   Emotional Problems
Inherited Disease
Please explain above: _____
_____

II. Past History
1. Birth History: Birth Date _____ Date Due _____ Weight _____
                Length _____
During pregnancy, did the mother have any of the following? (please circle)
Anemia   Bleeding   Infections   Surgery   Weight Gain over 20 lbs
Edema   Injuries   Convulsions   High Blood Pressure
Vomiting   Weight Loss   Other Illness (please explain):
_____
_____
What medications or vitamins were taken by mother? _____
_____

Labor: 1. Onset: spontaneous or induced _____
        2. Length of Labor _____ hrs.
        3. Type: breach, vertex (head first) or c. section _____
        4. Type of anesthesia _____
        5. Forceps used? _____
Baby: Required Resuscitation? _____ Oxygen? _____ Incubator? _____
Any problems in the nursery: (please circle)
Jaundice (yellow)   Bleeding   Breathing Difficulties   Rash   Seizures
Blue Spells (cyanosis)   Vomiting   Infection
III. Early Developmental History: (indicate the age at which child)
Rolled Over _____ Sat Without Support _____ Crawled _____
Walked Alone _____ Talked in Sentences _____ Toilet Trained _____
IV. Immunizations: (check off those received)
DPT _____ Oral Polio _____ Measles (10 day) _____ Mumps _____
Rubella (German Measles) _____ Hib _____ Others _____
Tuberculin Testing: Date _____ Results _____
V. Later Developmental History and School History:
Present Grade _____ School Name _____
Estimate Achievement: Slow   Average   High
Problems with speech? Concentrating on a single project? Distractibility? Hyperactivity? _____
_____ Any Testing? _____

Figure 15–1. Patient history form.

VI. Behaviors: (circle if present)
Bedwetting   Nail Biting   Constipation   Nightmares   Nervousness
Speech Problems   Toilet Problems   Hyperactivity
Does your child get along well with children? _____   Adults? _____
At school? _____
Any concerns regarding eating habits or nutrition? _____

VII. Illnesses: (circle if child has had)
Measles   Mumps   Chickenpox   Roseola   Whooping Cough   Scarlet Fever
Pneumonia   Bronchitis   Croup   Other _____
Any severe illnesses? _____
Any injuries? _____
Hospitalizations? _____
Surgery? _____

VIII. General Survey: (circle if present)
1. Central Nervous System: Frequent Headaches   Seizures   Dizziness
Head Injury   Black Out Spells
2. Ear Problems   Eye Problems   Nose Problems   Throat Problems
3. Chest Problems   Lung Problems
4. Heart Problems: Murmur   Palpation   Congenital Heart Defect
5. Infections: Gastrointestinal   Kidney   Bladder
6. Muscles and Coordination: Problems with Gait or Walking   Speech
Coordination   Weak Muscles   Joint Swelling   Joint Pain   Fractures
Braces   Special Shoes
7. Skin: Any Chronic Rashes or Other Skin Problems
8. Allergies: Frequent Colds   Bronchitis   Pneumonia   Asthma   Hayfever
Sinus Trouble   Eczema   Hives   Drug Reactions
9. Blood: Anemia   Bleeding Problems
10. Episodes of Fever with Known Cause: _____
11. Habits: Diet _____
Drug Use—smoking, alcohol, other _____
Sexual Activity _____
Exercise _____
Sleep _____
Medications _____
Toxic Exposures _____
Social Activities, Friends _____
Jobs _____
Hobbies _____
Religious Affiliations _____

Figure 15–1 *continued.*

variations, preoperative and postoperative management, and fluid and electrolyte problems. In addition to the history, physical findings, developmental and growth patterns, and personality, one needs to remember that every pediatric patient is part of a family, and knowledge of that family, the family's lifestyles, and the family's capacity to cope with illness is important in caring for the child. Adolescent relationships to peers, school, and community may also have an important bearing.

The ability of the physician to empathize with both the patient and the family is of great importance. Parents and children like to be called by name. The physician should ask for preferences; not all Williams want to be called Billy or Bill. If one likes children they generally return the feelings and warmth spontaneously.

History forms, which the parent or adolescent fills out to give a broad, general history, are useful. The present illness must be reviewed in detail, with the physician asking all questions deemed important to establishing a diagnosis. The parent and patient must be allowed to ask anything of concern to them. The physician should lis-

General Appearance:

Pulse _____ Resp _____ BP _____ Temp _____ Ht _____ Wt _____

Head _____

Head: Symmetry:
　　　Fontanelle:

Skin:

Nodes:

Eyes: Cover Test:
　　　Pupils:
　　　EOM:
　　　Fundi:
　　　Conjunctiva:

Ears: External:
　　　Drums:
　　　Hearing Screen:
　　　Weber, Rinne:

Mouth: Teeth:
　　　　Tonsils:
　　　　Pharynx:

Nose:

Neck: Thyroid:
　　　Masses:

Chest: Cage Abn.:
　　　Lungs: Excursion
　　　　　　Fremitus
　　　　　　Percussion
　　　　　　Auscultation

Heart: Rate:
　　　Rhythm:
　　　Murmurs:
　　　Size:

Abdomen: Liver:
　　　　　Spleen:
　　　　　Kidney:
　　　　　Masses:

Back: CVA:
　　　Spine:
　　　Forward Bend:

Pulses: Pedal:
　　　　Radial (Compared):

Neurological: Mental Status:
　　　　　　　Cranial Nerves:
　　　　　　　Motor Function:
　　　　　　　Sensory:
　　　　　　　Reflexes:

Extremities: (also see Podiatry Exam Sheet)
　　　　　　　Hips:

Gait:

Developmental Screen:

Impression:

1. Major Problems:
   a. Acute
   b. Chronic
2. Minor Problems
   a. Acute
   b. Chronic
3. Emotional Concerns
4. Social Concerns

Labs:

Figure 15–2. Physical examination form.

Plan:

1. Acute Treatment
2. Chronic Treatment
3. Health Maintenance
4. Follow-Up

Signed _____ DPM

Figure 15–2 *continued.*

In order to assist us in making your initial visit as productive as possible, please fill in the following information and bring this with you at the time of your visit.

Child's Name _____

First Visit Date _____

Age _____ Date of Birth _____

Reason for Visit _____
_____

Child's Physician _____

Please check or circle each of the following, where appropriate.

1. Disease present in child's immediate family (parent's, siblings, grandparents, aunts and uncles):

Allergy	Asthma	Hay Fever	Eczema
Sinus	Bronchitis	Drug Reaction	Anemia
Diabetes	Cancer	Leukemia	Bleeding Disorder
Tuberculosis	Epilepsy	Convulsive Disease	

2. Pregnancy:
   Drugs taken during pregnancy _____
   Illness during pregnancy _____

3. Birth History:
   Due Date _____ Weight _____ Length _____ Head Circumference_____

   Labor:
   1. Onset: Spontaneous _____ Induced _____
   2. Length of Labor _____
   3. Type of Delivery: Breach _____ Vertex (head first) _____
      Cesarean Section _____
   4. Type of Anesthesia _____
      Drugs During Labor _____
   5. Forceps Utilized _____

   Baby:
   Required Resuscitation _____ Oxygen _____
   Apgar Score (if known) 1 Minute _____ 5 Minutes _____
   Incubator Requires? _____

Figure 15–3. Pediatric information sheet. (Revised from Ronald Valmassy, DPM.)

Illustration continued on following page.

Any Problems in the Nursery: (circle where appropriate)

Jaundice	Bleeding	Blue Spells	Breathing Difficulties
Rash	Vomiting	Seizures	Infection

4. Development History:
   Indicate Age At Which Child:
   Sat without Support _____ Crawled _____
   Stood with Support _____ Walked Alone _____
   Talked in Sentences _____ Toilet Trained _____

   While Walking or Running My Child Is:
   Coordinated _____ Often off Balance _____
   Clumsy _____ Always Tripping _____
   My Child:
   Likes to Walk _____ Likes to Run _____
   Does Not Walk for Long Distances _____
   Tires Easily _____ Asks to Be Carried _____
   Complains of Foot/Leg Pain or Cramping _____
   Awakens During the Night Complaining of Foot/Calf Pain or Cramping _____
   My Child's Shoes Are Generally Replaced Because They Have Become
   Too Small _____ Have Worn Out _____
   Previous Treatment for Leg Problems _____

5. Immunizations (yes or no)
   DPT _____ Oral Polio _____ Measles _____ Mumps _____ Rubella _____
   Hib _____ TB Skin Test _____

6. Illness (yes or no)
   Severe Illness _____
   Injury _____
   Hospitalizations _____
   Surgery _____

If you have an infant, please bring a bottle of milk or juice to be used during the examination. Please bring a pair of worn shoes, if possible.

Thank you for taking the time to fill out this form.

Figure 15–3. continued.

ten carefully to understand and respond to all questions. Many standard history forms are available and can be sent to the parents prior to the appointment (Figs. 15–1, 15–2, and 15–3). The form can be filled out and brought at the time of the appointment. The physician can provide his or her own form if it is more appropriate to needs or style. When development is a consideration in evaluating the problem, the physician should compare the child's development with established standards, such as the Denver Developmental Screening Test (Figs. 15–4 and 15–5). This test in- volves observing the child performing stated tasks.

PATHOPHYSIOLOGY

Embryology

The podiatrist should have some awareness of embryologic development of the lower extremities. This background is important to the podiatrist in understanding some of the foot problems that occur in

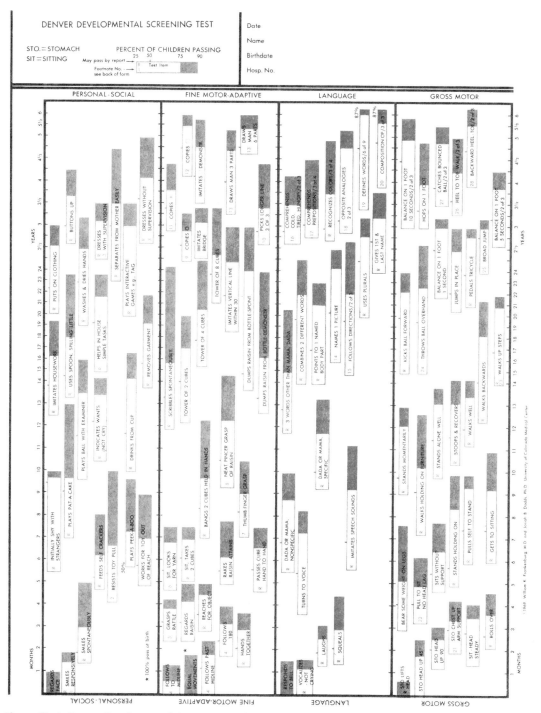

Figure 15–4. Denver Developmental Screening Test form, part 1. (From William K. Frankenburg, MD, and Josiah B. Dodds, PhD, University of Colorado Medical Center, 1969. Courtesy of Mead Johnson Laboratories.)

DATE _____

NAME _____

BIRTHDATE _____

HOSP. NO. _____

DIRECTIONS
1. Try to get child to smile by smiling, talking or waving to him. Do not touch him.
2. When child is playing with toy, pull it away from him. Pass if he resists.
3. Child does not have to be able to tie shoes or button in the back.
4. Move yarn slowly in an arc from one side to the other, about 6″ above child's face. Pass if eyes follow 90° to midline. (Past midline; 180°)
5. Pass if child grasps rattle when it is touched to the backs or tips of fingers.
6. Pass if child continues to look where yarn disappeared or tries to see where it went. Yarn should be dropped quickly from sight from tester's hand without arm movement.
7. Pass if child picks up raisin with any part of thumb and a finger.
8. Pass if child picks up raisin with the ends of thumb and index finger using an over hand approach.

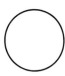 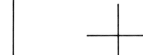

9. Pass any enclosed form. Fail continuous round motions.
10. Which line is longer? (Not bigger.) Turn paper upside down and repeat. (3/3 or 5/6)
11. Pass any crossing lines.
12. Have child copy first. If failed, demonstrate

When giving items 9, 11 and 12, do not name the forms. Do not demonstrate 9 and 11.

13. When scoring, each pair (2 arms, 2 legs, etc.) counts as one part.
14. Point to picture and have child name it. (No credit is given for sounds only.)

 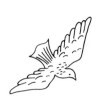 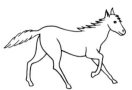 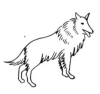 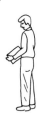

15. Tell child to: Give block to Mommie; put block on table; put block on floor. Pass 2 of 3. (Do not help child by pointing, moving head or eyes.)
16. Ask child: What do you do when you are cold? . . . hungry? . . . tired? Pass 2 of 3.
17. Tell child to: Put block on table; under table; in front of chair, behind chair. Pass 3 of 4. (Do not help child by pointing, moving head or eyes.)
18. Ask child: If fire is hot, ice is ?; Mother is a woman, Dad is a ?; a horse is big, a mouse is ?. Pass 2 of 3.
19. Ask child: What is a ball? . . . lake? . . . desk? . . . house? . . . banana? . . .

Figure 15–5. Denver Developmental Screening Test form, part 2. (From William K. Frankenburg, MD, and Josiah B. Dodds, PhD, University of Colorado Medical Center, 1969. Courtesy of Mead Johnson Laboratories.)

curtain? . . . ceiling? . . . hedge? . . . pavement? Pass if defined in terms of use, shape, what it is made of or general category (such as banana is fruit, not just yellow). Pass 6 of 9.

20. Ask child: What is a spoon made of? . . . a shoe made of? . . . a door made of? (No other objects may be substituted.) Pass 3 of 3.
21. When placed on stomach, child lifts chest off table with support of forearms and/or hands.
22. When child is on back, grasp his hands and pull him to sitting. Pass if head does not hang back.
23. Child may use wall or rail only, not person. May not crawl.
24. Child must throw ball overhand 3 feet to within arm's reach of tester.
25. Child must perform standing broad jump over width of test sheet. (8½ inches)
26. Tell child to walk forward, ◖▬◗◖▬◗◖▬◗◖▬◗→ heel within 1 inch of toe. Tester may demonstrate. Child must walk 4 consecutive steps, 2 out of 3 trials.
27. Bounce ball to child, who should stand 3 feet away from tester. Child must catch ball with hands, not arms, 2 out of 3 trials.
28. Tell child to walk backward, ←◖▬◗◖▬◗◖▬◗◖▬◗ toe within 1 inch of heel. Tester may demonstrate. Child must walk 4 consecutive steps, 2 out of 3 trials.

DATE AND BEHAVIORAL OBSERVATIONS (how child feels at time of test, relation to tester, attention span, verbal behavior, self-confidence, etc.):

Figure 15–5 *continued.*

newborns and infants. The development of the individual from embryo to fetus repeats evolutionary development to a great extent, and this is evident in studies of the lower extremities. The 5-week-old embryo develops paired limb buds, parallel to the long axis of the body.

The prehuman foot is very flexible and has loosely connected bones, large digits, and a large heel, with a mobile great toe and a flat longitudinal arch. The evolution of bipedal gait necessitated changes in foot structure, which is evident in embryology. At 7 weeks of age, the embryonic extremities of the human extend at right angles to the body, the foot in line with the leg (equinus) in marked supination, with the plantar surfaces facing each other and with forefoot adduction. With further development, the lower limb rotates inward at about 8 weeks' gestation. By 16 weeks, the foot has everted and dorsiflexed, beginning to prepare for plantar weight bearing and ankle joint articulation.

The human plantigrade foot is less conducive to speed. Predecessors of humans were arboreal and used an opposable hallux to move through the trees. As these predecessors moved to the ground and became terrestrial, the foot became more rigid with an unopposable hallux. Humans became orthograde, and the foot adapted for ambulation. The rear foot became larger and stronger, and the axis of function shifted toward the second toe. Ligamentous and osseous structures became the major support rather than muscle. Longitudinal and transverse arches developed, and the great toe became larger to enhance balance in the upright posture. Increasing ankle flexion brought the heel to the ground, giving a functional increase in length and better balance.

Pregnancy, Labor, Delivery, and the Newborn

Just as the lower extremity undergoes remarkable change as it forms, so too does every part of the developing embryo. In the majority of pregnancies, the end result is a normal baby with no significant abnormalities. The fetus is generally well protected against problems that may threaten the health of the mother. However, exposures or insults that seem to have little effect on the mother, such as drug therapies necessary for the well-being of the mother (e.g., phenytoin [Dilantin]), may have deleterious effects on the fetus (Table 15–1). Unnecessary drugs willingly taken by the mother, such as alcohol, heroine, cocaine, antimetabolites, and nicotine from cigarettes, may seriously affect embryogenesis, or development of the fetus. German measles, acquired immunodeficiency syndrome (AIDS), cytomegalovirus (CMV), and other infectious diseases severely affect the development and general health of the fetus. X-ray was the first proven external source to malform an embryo. The best-known malforming substance is thalidomide, a sleeping medication formerly used in Europe, which caused many cases of limb defects, such as amelia and phocomelia. Poor nutrition may also affect embryogenesis. In late pregnancy, optimum nutrition and adequate placental function are critical, particularly to protect the developing brain.

If fetal well-being is in question invading the uterine cavity may be advisable.

Table 15–1. DRUGS WITH SIGNIFICANT ADVERSE EFFECTS ON THE FETUS

Drug	Trimester	Effect
Aminopterin	1st	Multiple gross anomalies
Barbiturates	All	Neonatal dependence with chronic use
Chloramphenicol	3rd	Increased risk: gray baby syndrome
Chlorpropamide	All	Neonatal hypoglycemia
Cortisone	1st	Increased risk: cleft palate
Diazepam	All	Neonatal dependence with chronic use
Diethylstilbestrol	All	Vaginal adenocarcinoma
Ethanol	All	Fetal alcohol syndrome (high risk)
Heroin	All	Neonatal dependence with chronic use
Iodide	All	Congenital goiter, hypothyroidism
Methadone	All	Neonatal dependence with chronic use
Methylthiouracil	All	Hypothyroidism
Phenytoin	All	Cleft lip and palate
Tetracycline	All	Discoloration of teeth
Thalidomide	1st	Phocomelia
Trimethadione	All	Multiple congenital anomalies
Warfarin	1st, 3rd	1st: Chondrodysplasia, hypoplastic nasal bridge; 3rd: risk of bleeding

Amniocentesis is done by inserting a needle in the amniotic space and withdrawing fluid for cellular and biochemical analysis. (The first amniocentesis was done in 1882.) Amniocentesis has made it possible to diagnose a significant number of inherited disorders prenatally, early enough in pregnancy to consider abortion. The most frequent use of this technique has been in the woman over 35 years of age to detect Down's syndrome, the most common chromosomal abnormality (Fig. 15–6). In late pregnancy, fetal blood incompatibility (Rhesus [Rh] factor) can be evaluated by bilirubin measurement, and Coombs's test can be done on amniotic fluid. Appropriate management can then be planned. The ratio of lecithin to sphingomyelin in amniotic fluid, determined in late pregnancy, gives an index of lung maturity to guide obstetric and pediatric management. Elevated alpha-fetoprotein in amniotic fluid is found in association with fetal brain and spinal cord malformations. With the use of fetoscopy, the fetus can be viewed directly and fetal blood samples collected to diagnose thalassemia, Duchenne's muscular dystrophy, and severe hemophilia. Blood transfusions are possible in the fetus, and fetal surgery has been performed for urinary tract defects. Exciting new possibilities for fetal surgery have been opened. Another prenatal diagnostic technique is evaluation of aspirated chorionic fetal villi, which can be done very early in pregnancy and is used for chromosome, enzyme, and DNA analyses (Fig. 15–7).

When pregnancy nears its end, the normal fetus still has to undergo the stress of labor and delivery, and at that point it is the concern of the obstetric team to protect the baby against serious asphyxia. Even full-term infants may suffer asphyxia sufficient to affect development. The goal of fetal monitoring is to prevent hypoxia. The primary measurement is the fetal heart rate, but fetal pH, fetal pO_2, and base excess or deficit measurements may be made on fetal scalp blood after rupture of the membranes.

Fetal heart rate ranges from 120 to 160 beats/minute. With uterine contractions, the heart beat decelerates. Early in labor, deceleration associated with pressure on the fetal head parallels the uterine contraction. Variable deceleration occurs with decreased fetal circulation, as with cord

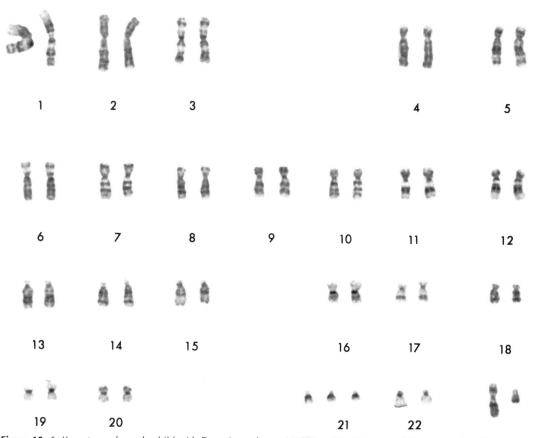

Figure 15–6. Karyotype of a male child with Down's syndrome (47 XY + 21). (Courtesy of University of California, San Francisco, Cytogenic Laboratory.)

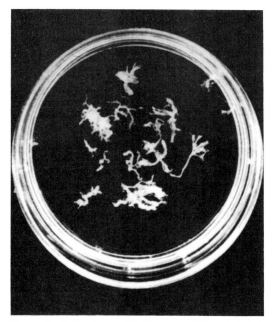

Figure 15–7. Chorionic villi. (Courtesy of Dr. Mitchell S. Golbus, MD, University of California, San Francisco, School of Medicine.)

compression at the time of contraction. Late decelerations occur with myocardial hypoxia, owing to poor placental blood flow. A long, difficult labor may also result in myocardial glycogen depletion.

Even in normal labor, there is progressive acidosis, hence the great potential for insult to the neonatal brain. The standard for evaluating the infant's status in assessing perinatal asphyxia is based on 1-minute and 5-minute Apgar scores (Table 15–2). Scores of 0, 1, and 2 indicate severe asphyxia; scores of 3 and 4 indicate moderate asphyxia; and scores of 5, 6, 7, and 8 indicate mild asphyxia. Scores of 9 and 10 are considered normal. A 1-minute Apgar score mandates delivery room action. A 5-minute score better predicts long-term outcome. A 5-minute score of 6 or less indicates asphyxia of significance and requires ongoing intensive care. Low Apgar scores are a stimulus to action and not an absolute indication of outcome. A combination of many biologic and chemical factors dic-

Table 15–2. APGAR SCORING CHART

Sign	0	1	2
Heart rate	Absent	Slow (<100 beats/min)	>100 beats/min
Respiratory effort	Absent	Weak cry, hypoventilation, irregular	Good, strong cry
Muscle tone	Limp	Some flexion of extremities	Well-flexed extremities, active motion
Reflex irritability	No response	Some motion, grimace	Cry
Color	Blue, pale	Body pink, extremities blue	Completely pink

tates the significance of the effect of hypoxia on the infant's brain. Infants may appear well oxygenated at birth, with good Apgar scores. However, within a few minutes, because of suppressive influences, such as maternal medications, chilling, and so forth, infants may become increasingly asphyxic and cyanotic, with poor perfusion, hypotonia, and falling heart rate, as glycogen stores are lost. These infants need active resuscitation, which includes suction, oxygen, artificial inhalation, and temperature control.

The perinatal health and labor and delivery history is meaningful, pertinent information to the podiatrist. This history may be an important source of information when evaluating gait abnormalities in childhood and determining etiology and influencing factors. Birth asphyxia may have significant long-term effects on neuromotor function. However, the majority of infants who have brain hypoxia at birth are subsequently normal. In addition, normal term infants may later show evidence of cerebral injury.

Genetics

Genetics is an important aspect of human disease and of great significance to the podiatrist as well as the pediatrician. Approximately 2.5% of newborn infants have some sort of genetic disorder, and 10 to 30% of pediatric hospitalizations are the result of genetic disease. It is estimated that 25% of developmental defects are primarily genetic or chromosomal; 10% are caused by known environmental factors, such as alcohol, cigarettes, methyl mercury, lead, selenium, plastics, and so forth; and 65% are of unknown cause but may be related to exposure during pregnancy.

Genetic inheritance is referred to as ge-notype. There are three basic types of genetic defects: single-gene, chromosomal, and multifactorial. In dealing with these disorders, it is necessary to recognize the child's problem as genetic, to establish the patterns of inheritance, to deal with clinical manifestations, and to provide genetic counseling to reduce future incidence.

Single-Gene Disorders

Single-gene disorders have an approximate 1% incidence. The gene's DNA, a series of nucleotides, determines the synthesis of one polypeptide. DNA determines the amino-acid sequence of polypeptides and proteins. Over 1200 genes of a possible 50,000 or more have been identified. Disorders follow one of four patterns: autosomal recessive, autosomal dominant, X-linked recessive, and X-linked dominant.

Autosomal-Dominant Gene Abnormalities. Hundreds of disorders are transmitted through autosomal-dominant abnormalities, though overall they are rare as a cause of human disease. The disease may be manifest or expressed in variable severity, so that one person may be much more severely affected than another. A father who is only mildly afflicted (forme fruste) may transmit Marfan's syndrome to his child, who may be severely afflicted. Sometimes the condition in a parent might not be diagnosed until the child's problems are clarified. These disorders tend to produce visible abnormal structural changes. Single-gene–dominant disorders not infrequently occur in children of normal parents, the result of mutation. Achondroplasia is a classic example of this phenomenon, in which more than four fifths of cases occur as mutations. Parent age also may influence the risk of genetic disorders, with an older parent increasing the risk.

Autosomal-Recessive Gene Abnormalities. There are over 500 autosomal-recessive abnormalities known. The risk of disease when both parents are carriers is one in four. In contrast to the autosomal-dominant type, with obvious physical abnormality, the autosomal-recessive type is characterized by chemical abnormalities. The heterozygous carrier, although clinically normal, may have evidence of mild abnormal biochemical function. This fact has been the basis of screening programs to detect risk, as with mild hexosaminidase-A deficiency in carriers of Tay-Sachs disease in the Ashkenazi Jewish population.

Sex-Chromosome Gene Abnormalities. Nearly 200 loci on the X chromosome and 2 on the Y have been identified in sex-chromosome abnormalities. Characteristically in a typically normal female with two X chromosomes who is carrying a defective gene on one of them, 50% of her offspring carry the gene, but only the male with an abnormal X chromosome is afflicted. The two most common disorders are hemophilia A and Duchenne's muscular dystrophy. Chromosomal sex-linked dominant disorders are very rare. Vitamin D–resistant rickets is an example.

Chromosome Disorders

In 1956, human chromosome numbers were correctly confirmed. In 1959, Down's syndrome was linked to a chromosome abnormality. Down's syndrome is a multiple-gene disorder that carries a visible chromosome change. Chromosome abnormalities occur in less than 1% of newborns but account for 10% of congenital defects. About half are autosomal abnormalities, and half are associated with sex chromosomes.

To determine a person's karyotype, peripheral whole blood cells are collected; stimulated to divide; and then fixed, stained, and photographed. The divided chromosomes are then paired according to size and structural characteristics. In each somatic cell, there are 46 chromosomes, 22 matching pairs called autosomes and 2 additional sex chromosomes, known in the female as XX and in the male as XY. Somatic cells contain 46 chromosomes; gametes contain only 23 as the result of meiosis, which is a halving process. Therefore the combination of sperm and ova each containing 23 chromosomes restores the original 46, half from each parent. Chromosome disorders are the result of (1) alterations of numbers of chromosomes, which may involve either autosomes or sex chromosomes; (2) loss of part of a chromosome; and (3) interchanges of genetic material from one chromosome to another, known as translocation.

Autosomal Disorders
Down's Syndrome (Trisomy 21). Down's syndrome is the most common chromosome abnormality for which people request genetic counseling. Advancing maternal or paternal age seems to predispose to the disorder. Down's syndrome occurs once in about 650 live births; 30% of cases occur in women over age 35 years. The risk of a second affected progeny is less than 2%, regardless of the mother's age. Most cases occur as a result of nondisjunction. However, if either parent has a 21-21 translocation the risk is 100%. Children with Down's syndrome have classic characteristics, and most cases can be diagnosed soon after birth. Those without obvious characteristics may not be diagnosed for months. There is also a significant variation in intelligence. Clinically children with Down's syndrome classically have an oval face with mongoloid appearance, reverse epicanthal folds, flat occiput, Brushfield's spots in the iris, hypotonia, retardation, wide spaces between the great and second toes, simian lines on the palms, and abnormal dermatoglyphics (Fig. 15–8). Congenital heart disease is also frequently associated with Down's syndrome.

Other Trisomies. Other trisomies are rare, with trisomy 18 (Edwards's syndrome) being the next best known. Findings with trisomy 18 include mental retardation; craniofacial anomalies; congenital heart disease; and limb abnormalities, including rocker-bottom foot.

Sex-Chromosome Disorders
Turner's Syndrome (Gonadal Dysgenesis) (XO). Loss of an autosome is fatal, but survival is possible with loss of an X chromosome. This loss most often results in spontaneous abortion. However, Turner's syndrome (XO chromosome pattern) may

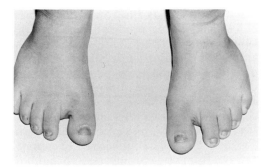

Figure 15–8. Classic Down's syndrome presentation in foot. Note the wide space between great and second toe.

also result. Diagnostic characteristics of Turner's syndrome include short stature; webbed neck; small, downturned mouth; lymphedema; cubitus valgus; shield chest with wide-spaced nipples; short metatarsals; increased incidence of congenital heart disease, especially coarctation; and ovarian dysgenesis with inability to conceive. Buccal mucosal smears are negative, with no Barr bodies, and of course, chromosomal analysis reveals only a single X chromosome.

Klinefelter's Syndrome (XXY) Klinefelter's syndrome occurs with a frequency of approximately 1 in 1000 births. Male characteristics are present, but these boys are slight, slender, and tall, with gynecomastia and small testicles with impaired spermatogenesis. Affected boys have increased gonadotrophins and low testosterone levels. There is an increased incidence of retardation.

Structural Chromosome Changes. Part of a chromosome may be translocated to another chromosome. If this does not affect genetic function the individual is phenotypically normal. However, the individual may pass along this translocation during meiosis in the gametes, creating an ovum (in the case of the woman) that, once fertilized, causes a congenital abnormality. This translocation accounts for some Down's syndrome cases. More than one fourth of early spontaneous abortions are the result of such chromosomal anomalies.

Polygenic Disorders

Polygenic, or multifactorial, disorders occur in about 10% of infants, accounting for nearly 60% of all genetic disorders. The inheritance pattern cannot be explained by mendelian theory or demonstrated by visible chromosome abnormality and would appear to be the result of more than one gene alteration as well as environmental influences. Many disorders fall into this classification. The incidence in subsequent offspring is around 4 to 5%, if the parents are not affected, ranging from 2 to 10% but with much higher frequency in identical twins. Examples of polygenic inheritance include clubfoot, cleft lip and palate, congenital hip dislocation, diabetes mellitus, schizophrenia, Hirschsprung's disease, and ankylosing spondylitis.

Congenital defects are not necessarily inherited, and inherited defects are not necessarily congenital. Congenital defects may be due to extrinsic causes, such as radiation, infection (e.g., rubella), and drugs (e.g., thalidomide).

Genetic Counseling

Genetic counseling is advisable in any patient with a genetic disorder, both to plan care and anticipate needs in the patient and to discuss risk in future pregnancies and availability of prenatal diagnostic techniques. Chromosome analysis is available for chromosome disorders. The most frequent use of this technique has been to diagnose Down's syndrome in the fetus of a woman over 35 years of age. Neural tube disorders are diagnosed with about 95% accuracy by the measurement of fetus-specific globulin, alpha-fetoprotein. There are over 50 biochemical inherited disorders, that can be detected by amniocentesis. Fetal chorionic villi aspiration analysis gives an earlier answer than amniocentesis. Fetal chorionic villi aspiration analysis is still being studied but appears to be an equally safe fetal diagnostic procedure. These diagnostic procedures carry very little adverse effects for the mother or fetus. However, one should realize that abortion of a known defective fetus is of great emotional impact on the family and may result in significant maternal emotional problems and subsequently a higher rate of divorce.

Growth and Development

Growth

In general, an outstanding characteristic of children is that they are constantly changing, physically and functionally. This changing is the major factor that sets children apart from adults. Therefore knowledge of normal growth and development is essential to podiatric physicians when they are caring for infants and children who present with lower-extremity problems. Growth is defined as physical maturation and development as functional maturation (Figs. 15–9 to 15–16). Children develop in a specific sequence. The acquisition of skills occurs not only in a sequence but also tends to be fairly specific within a rather narrow age range for achievement. Normally growth and development are closely related, proceeding in such a manner that the infant or child matures in all aspects, mental, physical, emotional, and social. Growth and development may vary widely in infants and children yet still fit normal patterns.

An important consideration in medical supervision of infants and children is whether the individual is maturing normally. Evaluation of growth and development should be a part of each examination performed on the pediatric patient. This evaluation must be done if one is to diagnose abnormalities as well as advise and guide parents concerning proper management of the child. Four well-defined periods of growth occur in all normal individuals after birth:

1. Relatively rapid growth during infancy.
2. Slow and uniform growth lasting until puberty.
3. Pubertal growth spurt.
4. Gradual decrease in growth rate until it ceases.

Progress is from a reclining, nonspeaking infant with poor fine motor and gross motor function, with variable response, to a walking, talking sociable child with considerable fine and gross motor skills. It is important to have a knowledge of these developmental milestones in order to properly interpret a child's development and not to interpret a late normal development of a given milestone as pathologic (Table 15–3).

A number of factors may influence the acquisition of skills and development. These factors include inherited disorders and prenatal factors, such as maternal disease, including diabetes mellitus, rubella in the first trimester, syphilis, toxoplas-

Table 15–3. EARLY DEVELOPMENTAL MILESTONES

Age (Months)	Milestone
1	Smiles
2	Follows objects with eyes
3	Holds head up when prone
4	Turns self from prone to supine
5–6	Cuts first tooth
6	Sits with support
7–9	Sits without support
8	Crawls
9	Pulls up
10	Feeds self with spoon
10–12	Walks holding on
12–15	Walks alone
15–18	Uses words
18–21	Combines words
21–24	Uses sentences
24–30	Toilet training (females)
30–36	Tolet training (males)

mosis and other infections, diseases, and insults that can affect the fetus. Recurrent or chronic infection, trauma, hypoxia, hypoglycemia, hyperbilirubinemia, malnutrition, social deprivation, and isoimmunization due to Rh or ABO blood type incompatibility may also influence development. Premature infants have a higher incidence of congenital malformations, anemia, infections, feeding problems, and cerebral damage. If a child's activity is markedly impaired because of illness motor development may be hindered. Motor activity begins in utero by about 9 weeks' gestation as the neuromotor apparatus develops. The mother is usually aware of fetal movement early in the second trimester. This movement is reflexic and is dependent on function of the sensory system to initiate reflex motor activity.

After birth, the infant continues to develop progressively in a general cephalic to caudal pattern, first with head control, then rolling, crawling, sitting, pulling up, standing, walking, climbing, and on to complex movements. As stated, fine motor, language, and social responses are developing concomitantly. This head-to-toe progression is more complex than generally presented. The use of the lower extremities to facilitate upper body function comes into play in the first months of development. Gait development is particularly important to the podiatrist in analyzing a child's gait. At first, children "cruise," that is, walk while holding onto something for

Text continued on page 488

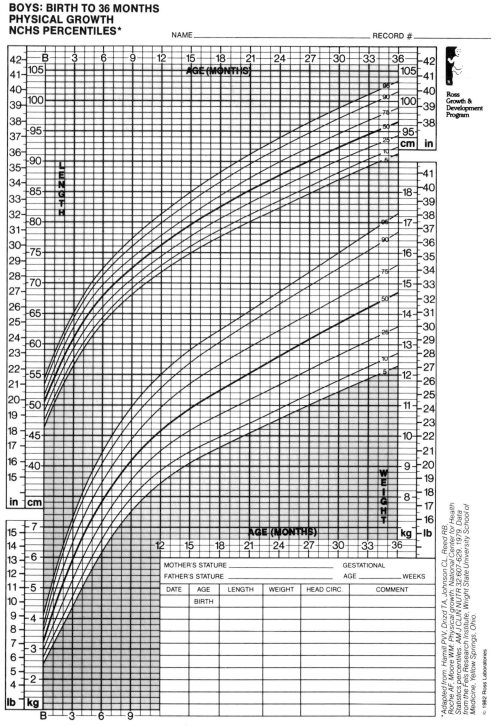

BOYS: BIRTH TO 36 MONTHS
PHYSICAL GROWTH
NCHS PERCENTILES*

Figure 15–9. Normal growth and development chart for boys, birth to 36 months. (Adapted from Hamill PVV, Drizd TA, Johnson CL, Reed RB, Roche AF, Moore WM: Physical growth: National Center for Health Statistics percentiles. Am J Clin Nutr 32:607–629, 1979. Data from the Fels Research Institute, Wright State University School of Medicine, Yellow Springs, Ohio. Used with permission.)

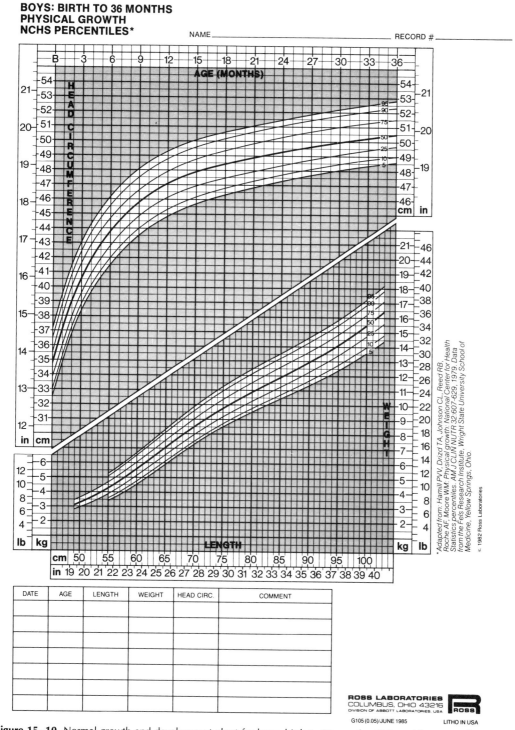

BOYS: BIRTH TO 36 MONTHS
PHYSICAL GROWTH
NCHS PERCENTILES*

NAME_____ RECORD #_____

Figure 15–10. Normal growth and development chart for boys, birth to 36 months. (Adapted from Hamill PVV, Drizd TA, Johnson CL, Reed RB, Roche AF, Moore WM: Physical growth: National Center for Health Statistics percentiles. Am J Clin Nutr 32:607–629, 1979. Data from the Fels Research Institute, Wright State University School of Medicine, Yellow Springs, Ohio. Used with permission.)

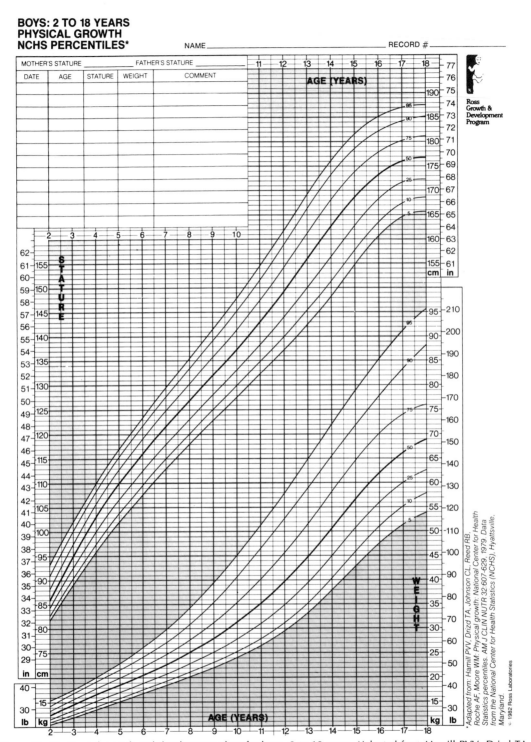

Figure 15–11. Normal growth and development chart for boys, 2 to 18 years. (Adapted from Hamill PVV, Drizd TA, Johnson CL, Reed RB, Roche AF, Moore WM: Physical growth: National Center for Health Statistics percentiles. Am J Clin Nutr 32:607–629, 1979. Data from the Fels Research Institute, Wright State University School of Medicine, Yellow Springs, Ohio. Used with permission.)

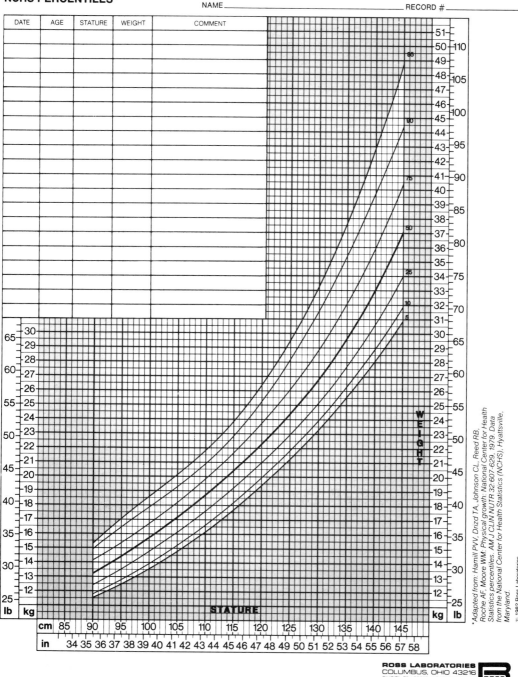

BOYS: PREPUBESCENT PHYSICAL GROWTH NCHS PERCENTILES*

Figure 15–12. Normal growth and development chart for prepubescent boys. (Adapted from Hamill PVV, Drizd TA, Johnson CL, Reed RB, Roche AF, Moore WM: Physical growth: National Center for Health Statistics percentiles. Am J Clin Nutr 32:607–629, 1979. Data from the Fels Research Institute, Wright State University School of Medicine, Yellow Springs, Ohio. Used with permission.)

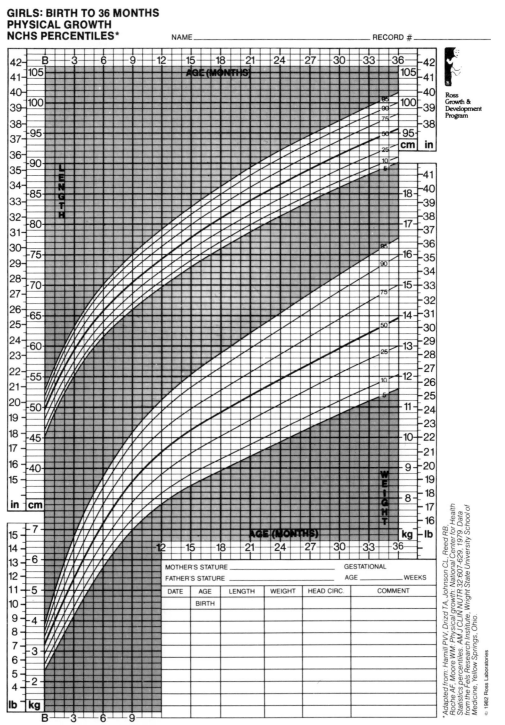

Figure 15–13. Normal growth and development chart for girls, birth to 36 months. (Adapted from Hamill PVV, Drizd TA, Johnson CL, Reed RB, Roche AF, Moore WM: Physical growth: National Center for Health Statistics percentiles. Am J Clin Nutr 32:607–629, 1979. Data from the Fels Research Institute, Wright State University School of Medicine, Yellow Springs, Ohio. Used with permission.)

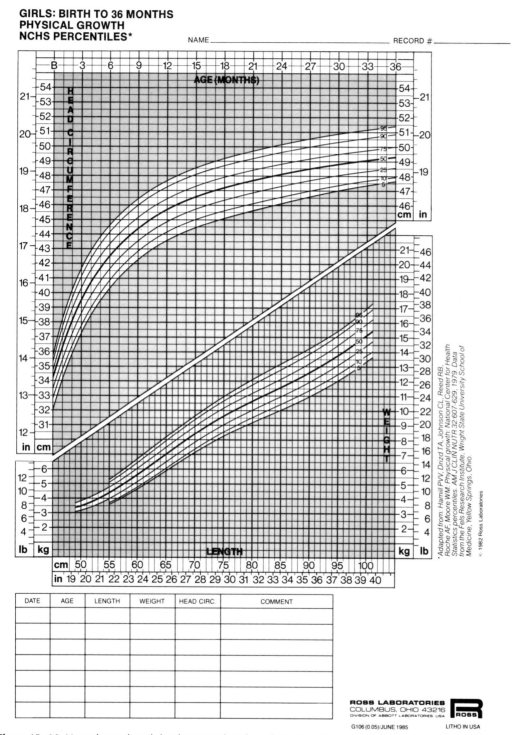

GIRLS: BIRTH TO 36 MONTHS
PHYSICAL GROWTH
NCHS PERCENTILES*

NAME_____ RECORD #_____

ROSS LABORATORIES
COLUMBUS, OHIO 43216
DIVISION OF ABBOTT LABORATORIES, USA

G106 (0.05)/JUNE 1985   LITHO IN USA

Figure 15–14. Normal growth and development chart for girls, birth to 36 months. (Adapted from Hamill PVV, Drizd TA, Johnson CL, Reed RB, Roche AF, Moore WM: Physical growth: National Center for Health Statistics percentiles. Am J Clin Nutr 32:607–629, 1979. Data from the Fels Research Institute, Wright State University School of Medicine, Yellow Springs, Ohio. Used with permission.)

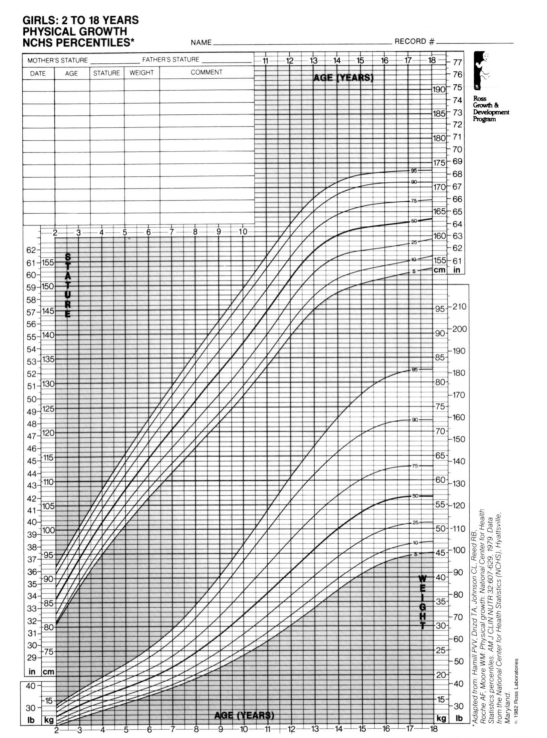

Figure 15–15. Normal growth and development chart for girls, 2 to 18 years. (Adapted from Hamill PVV, Drizd TA, Johnson CL, Reed RB, Roche AF, Moore WM: Physical growth: National Center for Health Statistics percentiles. Am J Clin Nutr 32:607–629, 1979. Data from the Fels Research Institute, Wright State University School of Medicine, Yellow Springs, Ohio. Used with permission.)

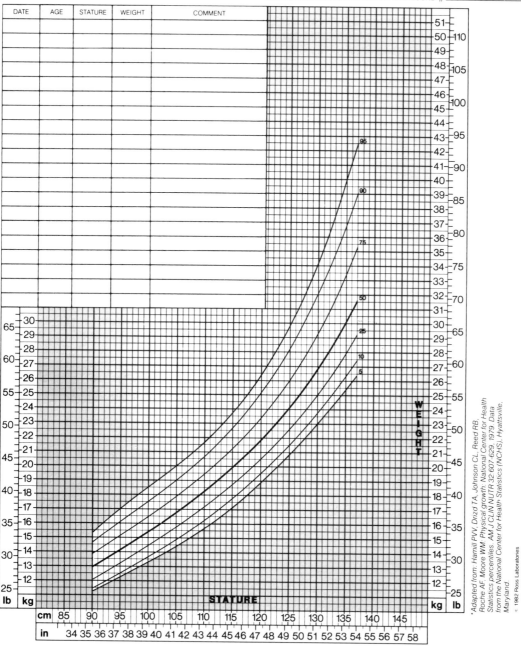

GIRLS: PREPUBESCENT PHYSICAL GROWTH NCHS PERCENTILES*

Figure 15–16. Normal growth and development chart for prepubescent girls. (Adapted from Hamill PVV, Drizd TA, Johnson CL, Reed RB, Roche AF, Moore WM: Physical growth: National Center for Health Statistics percentiles. Am J Clin Nutr 32:607–629, 1979. Data from the Fels Research Institute, Wright State University School of Medicine, Yellow Springs, Ohio. Used with permission.)

support. Cruising occurs at about 9 to 12 months of age and is followed by walking without support. Initially this unsupported gait occurs by keeping the legs abducted and externally rotated, providing a wide base, flexed at knees and hips, which lowers the pelvis and brings the center of gravity closer to the ground. The arms are also abducted and flexed, aiding in balance. With ambulation, the foot strikes toe first or flat, with typical heel-toe gait occurring at age 3 years or later. If screening developmental history suggests a delay more extensive evaluation should be done.

Physical growth is appraised by measurement of height; weight; and head, chest, and abdominal circumference. An osseous dental evaluation is also included. A podiatric physician who cares for children must know factors that affect their development, the role illness may play, and how to identify common emotional problems, so that appropriate referrals can be made when warranted.

Short Stature. Short stature is defined as height below the third percentile. Particular attention must be paid to children who are severely short, with a height less than 3.5 standard deviations, whose parents' heights suggest the child should be above the third percentile, and those whose serial measurements show progressive deviation from normal. Short stature may be caused by polygenic inheritance factors, preterm or small-for-gestational-age birth, congenital infection, maternal drug use, certain syndromes, endocrine dysfunction, chromosomal abnormalities, cystic fibrosis, chronic renal failure, Fallot's tetralogy, and juvenile rheumatoid arthritis (JRA). Organic short stature may also be associated with mental handicap. Investigation of short stature reveals that a majority of children have a history of genetic or social basis for their problem, and a more detailed investigation is appropriate. A few children are short because of abnormalities, such as thyroid deficiency, growth hormone deficiency, disorders of bone growth, malnutrition, metabolic disorders, chronic infections, prolonged steroid therapy, and congenital malformations. Those cases of definite abnormal growth lacking such an explanation require accurate arthropometry. In addition to height, trunk versus leg length allows recognition of disproportionate short stature.

Tall Stature. The majority of children with excessive height come from tall families and are accepted as normal. Pathologic causes of excessive height include endocrine disorders, such as eosinophilic adenoma of the pituitary gland, thyrotoxicosis, and early stages of precocious puberty. Other disorders associated with excessive height are cerebral gigantism (Sotos's syndrome), Marfan's syndrome, Klinefelter's syndrome, neurofibromatosis, adrenogenital syndrome, and homocystinuria. The most important factor in tall stature is genetic potential. Extrinsic and intrinsic factors affect the individual's chances of meeting that potential.

Foot Growth. The foot increases in length by about 75% in the first year and over the first 3 years averages $2\frac{1}{2}$ shoe sizes, or about $\frac{7}{8}$ inch/year. For the next 2 years, feet grow an average of 2 shoe sizes, or $\frac{2}{3}$ inches/year. Between 5 and 10 years, growth slows to $1\frac{1}{2}$ shoe sizes, or $\frac{1}{2}$ inch/year. From 10 years to 16 years, growth accelerates again. At about $2\frac{1}{2}$ years, the foot has reached about half its adult length. Similar to other body parts, feet are generally larger than in past generations. A man's average shoe size in 1776 was $6\frac{1}{2}$, and today it is $9\frac{1}{2}$. These changes are primarily attributed to improved nutrition.

Lower-Extremity Dysmorphia. About 6% of children have structural abnormalities that are discovered at birth or later. It is necessary to make a proper diagnosis in order to make a prognosis and establish preventive measures. Specific lower-extremity dysmorphologies are listed in Table 15–4. The podiatrist should refer the patient for further medical evaluation.

Behavior Variations

Many childhood illnesses are associated with a behavior problem. Children in conflict with themselves, their family, or environment may present with symptoms that mimic organic disease. Recognizing and understanding behavioral disturbances is an important part of the physician's knowledge base. These disorders include diseases that interfere with cerebral homeostasis and perception, mental retardation, and autism. These behavioral disturbances are addressed in pediatric texts.

Child Abuse and Neglect. The battered child syndrome was first described in 1962. Since then, all states have passed

Table 15–4. LOWER-EXTREMITY DYSMORPHOLOGIES

Arthrogryposis Multiplex Congenita
Caused by anything that decreases intrauterine movement of joints causing congenital contractures; types include myopathies, abnormal nerve function or innervation, connective tissue disorders, and mechanical limitations

Amniotic Bands (Streeter's Horizons)
Partial or complete ringlike constrictions, which encircle fetal parts and restrict growth or deform

Malformation of Feet
May be clues to serious problem, asymmetric length of toes, clinodactyly of 2nd toe with overlapping; short first metatarsal with dorsiflexion of hallux; syndactyly, cutaneous or osseous, of the 2nd–3rd toes most common; hypoplasia of nails; short, broad toenail; deep crease between hallux and 2nd toe; wide gap between hallux and 2nd toe

Trisomy 21 (Down's Syndrome)
Hypotonia with protruding tongue, joint hyperflexibility, wide gap between 1st and 2nd toe; plantar crease between 1st and 2nd toe, abnormal dermatoglyphics, simian crease (45%)

Ehlers-Danlos Syndrome
Hyperflexibility of joints and skin, poor wound healing, clubfeet, overlapping toes, often premature

Apert's Syndrome
Syndactyly, polydactyly, distal hallux broad and malformed, mental retardation variable, tower skull, maxillary hypoplasia, flat facies, antimongoloid slant

Fetal Hydantoin
Hypoplasia and irregular ossification of distal phalanges, producing short, narrow, misshapen fingers and toes; nail dysplasia; borderline IQ; most have additional deformities

lems; difficult-to-rear child (premature, handicapped, or blemished); other family stress (financial or legal); and lack of support system or relief. About one third of cases of abuse occur under 1 year of age, one third from 1 year to 6 years of age, and one third over 6 years of age. About 4000 children per year die as a result.

Child abuse must be reported when one acquires knowledge of or has a reasonable suspicion that a child has been a victim of abuse. A report must be made as soon as possible by phone. A written report must be forwarded within 36 hours of receiving the information regarding the incident. Correct forms can be requested from local child protective agencies, police or sheriff's departments, and county probation or welfare departments. Professionals legally required to report suspected child abuse have immunity from criminal or civil liability for reporting. The primary intent of the reporting law is to protect the child. It is equally important to provide help for the parents. Parents may be unable to ask for help directly, and child abuse may be their way of calling attention to family problems. Certain abuses must be reported by all legally mandated reporters when a victim is a child (under age 18) and the perpetrator is any person, including another child (Table 15–5).

Suicide. There is an increasing inci-

laws requiring that suspected child abuse or neglect be reported to a child protective agency.

Deviant behavior by adults may be manifested through injurious acts toward children. Every child has the right to develop to his or her full potential. Child abuse is any action or omission by an adult responsible for that child that either temporarily or permanently interferes with development. Murder, cruelty, neglect, abuse, molestation, and child pornography all fall into this category. Patterns of abuse vary, but about 25% of cases are sexual, 70% are physical, and 5% are nutritional deprivation.

Child abuse occurs in families from all walks of life but is most common in underprivileged families and in families that are more demonstrative than verbal. Common elements in the child abuse setting include parents who had a troubled, deprived, or abused childhood; marital prob-

Table 15–5. TYPES OF CHILD ABUSE THAT MUST BE REPORTED

Physical Injury
Inflicted by other than accidental means on a child

Sexual Abuse, Including Sexual Assault and Sexual Exploitation
Includes sex acts with children and child molestation, and does not require force or lack of consent; sexual exploitation includes child pornography and child prostitution

Willful Cruelty or Unjustifiable Punishment
Including inflicting or permitting unjustifiable physical pain or mental suffering or the endangerment of the child's person or health

Corporal Punishment or Injury
Willfully inflicted, resulting in a traumatic condition

Neglect of a Child, Whether Severe or General
Must also be reported if the perpetrator is a person responsible for the child's welfare; includes acts of omission and harming or threatening to harm the child's health or welfare

Any of Above Abuses Occurring During Out-of-Home Care

dence of adolescent suicide attempts. Suicide is the third most common cause of death in adolescents. Threats of suicide should be taken seriously. Individuals who attempt suicide may do so in reaction to an overwhelming number of life changes within a relatively brief period of time.

With each patient visit, the physician should give the patient or parent an opportunity to talk about problems or concerns other than the chief complaint. Time should be allotted for an adequate interview with the parents and teenager, allowing them to talk first about their concerns and then going back into the family history. Talking through problems is important. To make an evaluation of emotional problems in children, it is helpful to have a format. One way to approach the evaluation is to begin with present symptom, onset, details surrounding the symptom, reaction of each family member to it, and methods of dealing with it. The physician should proceed to other symptoms associated with the problem and complete the family history. The physician should ask about illnesses, serious injuries, separations, marital discords, births of siblings, and changes in environment. Counseling should be recommended and help sought for any depressed child or adolescent.

As children grow older, they mask their feelings, and in uncertain situations they are more likely to demonstrate actions rather than words.

A relaxed, friendly atmosphere is essential for the success of the interview. The physician should be sensitive when making the first introduction. The physician should always know the child's name and what he or she would like to be called. The physician should not refer to a baby as "it." The physician should confirm the relationship of the adult who is accompanying the child. The ability and willingness of the child to describe his or her own symptoms vary widely. An important question to ask the child is why the child thinks he or she has been brought to see the physician. As Dr. John Dower has pointed out in lectures, "The child is not always the real patient. The identified problem may not be the real problem." The physician obtains clues to the child's motor skills, mental abilities, attention span, interests, and personality by observing his or her play. The interplay between the child and parents and the child and physician gives some indication on how best to examine the child. If a child stays on the parent's lap performing at least the preliminary examination on the parent's lap is probably wisest.

PEDIATRIC HISTORY AND EXAMINATION

The medical history is a method of gathering data to aid in diagnosis and counseling of patients, in order to maintain health, to cure illness, or to improve health. The pediatric history provides the opportunity to interview both the child and the parent in order to gather information about the child's health, development, relationships with others, and general care. The interview provides the opportunity for the child to become acquainted with the practitioner before being examined. The informant for the history may be a parent, a relative, a caretaker, or the child. The interviewer must identify the source and degree of reliability in the history. The information gained from the child must be indicated as such in the history. First impressions are important. Even the very young sense an atmosphere and the parent's reaction to it.

History

The pediatric history is an adaptation of the model used for an adult history. It incorporates areas uniquely pertinent to the child. A history should be taken as noted before, carefully documenting the chief complaint and present illness. If there are a number of complaints an open problem list may help. Each problem and associated signs and symptoms can be expounded on.

Chief Complaint and Present Illness. The chief complaint statement gives the reason for the visit and may be recorded in the words of the adult or the child. The history of the present illness incorporates the same categories of information obtained in the adult health history. This information should be carefully detailed, including a description of the chronology of the illness; onset; character; duration; frequency; time of day; progression; aggravating or relieving factors; prior treatment and results; and patient's perception, major concern regarding the problem, and expectation of outcome with treatment. Pertinent organ systems that relate to the illness should be reviewed. This information should not be repeated in the past history. A statement about usual health, any relevant family history, negative information, and disability assessment should be included.

Past History. Background information is essential. It is important to collect information about the child's own life. In any child with a possible developmental deficiency, the following information should always be included. The physician should ask about the health of the mother during pregnancy, the mother's feelings about pregnancy, the amount and type of prenatal care, and history of any complications, such as excessive weight gain or loss, hypertension, vaginal bleeding, infection, and use of drugs or alcohol. The birth history, including length of gestation, mother's parity, nature and duration of labor and delivery, use of medications and anesthesia, birth weight, status of infant at birth, and use of special procedures, is important. The physician should ask: How was the baby during the first few days of life? Was the child bottle- or breast-fed, and when was he or she weaned? The physician should inquire about the main stages of development. Older children should be asked about their progress in school. A history of common childhood communicable diseases, noting age, severity, and complications; hospitalizations (for what, where, when); serious illnesses; and injuries, all with dates, treatment, and complications, should be obtained. The immunization history should document a properly completed series with dates, including boosters. Medications given to the child with dose, frequency, route, duration, and purpose should be noted. Allergies to food and drugs, with description of reaction and treatment, if needed, and any history of hay fever, asthma, and eczema should be noted. An compulsive inquiry about all the bodily functions is usually not necessary and interrupts the flow of the interview.

Nutritional History. The nutritional assessment includes data that reflect caloric intake, liquid and solid intake, and pattern of output. The physician should ask the mother of an infant whether she is breast-feeding or using a formula. If the mother is breast-feeding her use of medications and daily dietary intake should be explored. The nature and amount of any supplement or plans to introduce new foods or weaning should be determined. If the infant is formula-fed the use of an iron-fortified formula, the frequency and amount of feedings, and the intake of solid food should be documented. The physician should ask whether the child is taking any vitamin or mineral supplements. The assessment should be summarized with the mother's interpretation of her child's growth, weight gain, and appetite and comparison of the child to other siblings at the same age for insight into family patterns and parental expectations.

Family History. The family history should include questions about family illnesses; hereditary disorders; anomalies; health and age of grandparents and parents; and age, sex, and health of siblings. The cause of and age at death of members of the family are also included.

Habits. A description of habits includes eating patterns, sleeping behaviors (e.g., disturbances, restlessness, and nightmares), play interests, amount of exercise, urinary and bowel continence, development of independence and control, and conduct problems (e.g., bed wetting, temper tantrums, fighting, biting). Any use of drugs, alcohol, forms of tobacco, and forms of caffeine should be noted.

Social History. The social history includes information about the child's pattern of health care, place of birth in family, placement and progress in school, relationships with family members, relationships with peers and important people outside the home, socioeconomic status of family, and marital status of parents.

Review of Systems. The review of systems is essentially the same as that of the adult history except for age-appropriate modifications.

Physical Examination

The diagnostic clues obtained from the physical examination can become extremely valuable, especially when the child is unable to communicate or when the parents are poor historians. Performance of the examination varies according to age, development, and behavior of the child. A fine appreciation of the physical differences and developmental milestones according to age helps guide an examination and results in a successful examination. Each health care visit is a learning experience for the child and parents. The experience may result in an increased confidence in themselves and others or may result in a feeling of failure and distrust. Separation of the child from the parent may provoke anxiety and increase fear and distrust.

If a child is fearful or fatigued the practitioner may choose a selective examination. If a complete examination is needed the practitioner must be quick and efficient. The parents can help with the examination by holding or distracting the child, unless the child is developing independence and needs to have some control. The child's independence must be respected. Children vary in their responses individually and at different ages. A child may be passive, accepting, or curious; cautiously resistant; or angrily and actively opposed to examination. The physician should proceed in a calm, slow manner, explaining at a level the child understands what he or she is doing. The physician should always be truthful and should prepare parent and child for any new or painful techniques or procedures.

The physical examination of the child needs to be organized and systematic. Distressing parts of the examination are performed at the end (e.g., ear, nose, and throat). The order of the examination may be altered to accommodate behavior, such as listening to the heart and lungs first before crying starts or becomes vigorous. The examination of a child should start with a body part that is least likely to interfere with his or her sense of trust and confidence, such as the hands and feet.

From the ages 1 to 3 or 4, children are normally negative to a request of "Will you please . . . ," responding with an emphatic "No." Rephrasing to "Please take off your shoes" may result in compliance. If there is resistance at any point in the examination the physician should proceed to another part and come back to the more difficult parts later. If the child is totally uncooperative and the problem is not urgent it is best to defer to another day. The parents should be instructed on how to better prepare the child for a visit to the doctor by reading the child a book written specifically for this experience. It is often helpful to schedule an appointment early in the day or after nap time when the child is well rested.

An older child or adolescent may be modest about undressing even partially. One needs to be sensitive to the child's feelings. A significant degree of evaluation can be done without touching the child, including noting skin for pallor, cyanosis, and dermatologic lesions; body proportion; gait; symmetry; tremors; spasticity; balance; speech; breathing patterns; cardiac impulse; and protruding abdomen.

The physician can essentially proceed the same as with an adult except for deferring uncomfortable procedures until the latter part of the examination. The podiatric examination of a child should always include general observation; evaluation of the upper and lower extremities; basic neurologic evaluation; and evaluation of the spine, including full range of motion. After the examination, any questions the parent and child may have should be answered.

COMMON PEDIATRIC PROBLEMS

Dermatologic Disorders

Scabies

For treatment of scabies, lindane (Kwell) is the medication of choice. Lindane should be applied and left on for 4 hours and removed by showering. A single application is adequate. The patient should not shower before lindane is applied. This agent should not be left on overnight. The absorption of this toxic substance is greatly enhanced by these unnecessary practices. Bed partners should be simultaneously treated, and bed clothing should be washed. Itching may persist for some time after treatment until the broken-down products of the organism have been completely absorbed. This persistent itching is not an indication for repetitive treatment. Pyrethrins or piperonyl butoxide (RID or A-200) is a second choice of medication if lindane has been used recently.

Flea Bites

For treatment of flea bites, administration of vitamin B$_1$ (thiamine) (25 to 50 mg/day in two doses) may be helpful. The physician should also provide local treatment for itching. Treatment of pet contacts with flea powders instead of impregnated collars is most effective to prevent recurrence.

Infections

The prevalence of dermatologic problems indicates infection as the most common problem in podiatric patients. Viral and fungal infections predominate.

FUNGAL INFECTIONS

Fungal infections are rare on the feet of children and require confirmation by culture specimen. When fungal infection does occur, as it does in the older child and adolescent, treatment is with an antifungal, such as clotrimazole (Lotrimin cream or lotion).

VIRAL INFECTIONS

Viral infections, such as verrucae, herpes zoster, herpes simplex, varicella, molluscum contagiosum, and viral exanthem, are mostly treated expectantly with local or symptomatic therapy.

BACTERIAL INFECTIONS

Periungual infections, impetigo, cellulitis, lymphangitis, boils, abscesses, and locally infected wounds are frequently seen in children. These bacterial infections are most commonly due to beta-hemolytic streptococci and *Staphylococcus aureus*. Mixed infections with both organisms occur, in which *S. aureus* is considered an opportunistic invader. Lesions form pustules and boils, which encrust, and frequently occur over pre-existing conditions, such as eczema and bites. Local treatment with compresses soaked in aluminum acetate solution (Burow's solution) (1 tablet per quart of water) is helpful in relieving the crust. Most patients require systemic treatment. Patients generally respond well to penicillin and erythromycin. Local antibiotic ointment is helpful in preventing spread of the infection initially. Lesions

caused by *S. aureus* may require treatment with synthetic penicillins. In addition to drainage of boils and abcesses, heat and elevation are important adjunctive treatments. Deep infections of soft tissue, muscle, joints, and bone are rare but serious.

Although *S. aureus* causes most of these infections, one must be alert for other organisms, such as *Clostridium, Haemophilus influenzae, Mycobacterium tuberculosis,* and *Neisseria gonorrhoeae.* Infections caused by these organisms often require vigorous treatment locally and systemically. Management of wound infection necessitates tetanus immunization when indicated. Preoperative planning, even for minor procedures, should include appropriate tetanus immunization. If past immunization has been given reimmunization every 10 years for superficial wounds and every 5 years for penetrating wounds is indicated. If the patient requires tetanus immunization he or she should also be given diphtheria immunization. The combination of adult-type tetanus and diphtheria toxoids (Td) should be given ($\frac{1}{2}$ mm^3 intramuscularly). For children who have never received tetanus immunization, human tetanus immune globulin should be given intramuscularly in a dose of 250 to 500 U. Tetanus toxoid should be given at the same time.

Erysipelas, Impetigo, and Cellulitis. Group A streptococci and penicillin-sensitive *Staphylococcus* are the common offending organisms with erysipelas, impetigo, and cellulitis. If the patient is to undergo elective surgery these disorders should be treated prior to the procedure. Treatment is with penicillin V potassium (125 to 500 mg by mouth four times a day [q.i.d.] for 7 to 10 days). If a surgical procedure cannot be delayed antibiotic therapy should be started prior to surgery and continued for 10 days. The hospital patient may be given initial penicillin intravenously (10 mg/kg every 6 hours). For the penicillin-allergic adolescent patient, erythromycin (250 mg by mouth every 6 hours for 7 to 10 days or 400 mg twice a day [b.i.d.]) can be administered. In the child, a total of 40 mg/kg/day of erythromycin in four divided doses should be used.

Furuncles with surrounding cellulitis may be treated with any of the following agents. When the offending organism is a pencillin-resistant *Staphylococcus*, dicloxacillin (7.5 mg/kg, up to 25 mg/kg every 6 hours, given 1 hour after meals for 10 days) may be employed. Cephalosporins are also used; however, 5 to 10% of penicillin-allergic patients are sensitive to cephalosporins. Erythromycin (10 mg/kg every 6 hours for 10 days) is used in patients with a history of penicllin allergy. Vancomycin (20 to 40 mg/kg/day in divided doses) is administered to patients with an infection resistant to pencillins who are allergic to both penicillin and cephalosporins. If the offending organism is *Pseudomonas* gentamicin (Garamycin) (6.0 to 7.5 mg/kg/day divided into three doses) is effective. Infant doses of gentamicin are smaller. Doses of this medication must be adjusted for renal impairment. Blood levels can and should be measured. Acylureido penicillins, mezlocillin, piperacillin, and azlocillin, which are available in intravenous preparations only, and ceftriaxone (Rocephin) can also be used.

Allergic Disorders

At some time in their growing years, 15% of children have an allergic disorder. An allergy is a state of altered tissue reactivity to an allergen (antigen). The allergic response may result in immunity or a clinical hypersensitivity disease. Allergens are usually proteins that may be ingested, inhaled, or brought into contact with the skin. Symptoms depend in part on inheritance; nature of allergen; and degree, duration, and nature of exposure. Two basic types of reactions include immediate and delayed (Table 15–6). Treatment principles include eliminating the cause, decreasing immunologic reactivity (immunotherapy), and managing symptoms.

Anaphylaxis

Anaphylaxis may be acute and life threatening. Initial management may be required in the office (Table 15–7). Symptoms may appear in seconds or minutes. The quicker the symptoms appear, usually the more serious the reaction.

Contact Dermatitis

A variety of chemicals, such as dyes, soaps, rubber, and nickel, and locally ap-

Table 15–6. COOMBS'S CLASSIFICATION OF ALLERGIC DISORDERS

Immediate

Type 1
Reagin-dependent anaphylaxis

Type 2
Cytotoxic (e.g., hemolytic disease of the newborn)

Type 3
Arthus reactions; antigens reacting with antibody in tissue spaces (serum sickness)

Delayed

Type 4
Mediated by allergized lymphocytes going to the site of antigen (e.g., tuberculosis skin test)

plied medications, such as polymyxin B and Neosporin, commonly cause local sensitivity rashes. Treatment of contact dermatitis consists of withdrawal of the contactant and application of local compresses and local steroid cream or ointment. If the contact dermatitis is severe and no contraindication exists, systemic treatment with prednisone (initial dosage of 1 to 2 mg/kg/day) is advised. With improvement, prednisone can be reduced to alternate-day dosage and tapered to zero over a total of 10 to 20 days. Prednisone should not be used in a child with immune deficiency or a child with tuberculin conversion.

Asthma

Asthma is the most common chronic respiratory disease of childhood. Asthma is characterized by hyper-reactivity of the

Table 15–7. IMMEDIATE TREATMENT OF ANAPHYLAXIS

Injection or Insect Sting the Cause
1. Place tourniquet immediately above injection site if possible
2. Inject 0.01 ml/kg up to 0.35 ml of 1:1000 epinephrine into injection site
3. Give hydrocortisone 4–5 mg/kg or equivalent IV and hook up IV fluid
4. If dyspnea and wheezing are present give aminophylline IV very slowly 6–7 mg/kg
5. Antihistamine may be helpful later if angioneurotic edema appears (e.g., chlorpheniramine [Chlor-Trimeton] 10 mg q 6 h)
6. Hospitalize for follow-up observation; if acute reaction is controlled prognosis is excellent. If insect sting is the cause desensitization should be done later by an allergist

airways leading to paroxysmal attacks of airway obstruction that produce coughing, respiratory distress, and wheezing. The paroxysmal dyspnea is caused by a spasm of the bronchi, by swelling of the mucous membranes with secretions, or both. There is a wide spectrum of disease, ranging from an isolated mild wheezing episode to continuous wheezing with an occasional severe exacerbation. Asthma in children is usually graded as mild, with an occasional attack often precipitated by infection; intermediate, with severe or recurrent episodes; and severe, with attacks varying in severity but never without symptoms.

Asthma attacks are influenced by secondary factors, including exercise, cold, and emotions. Acute attacks may be relieved by a number of drugs, such as epinephrine, ephedrine, terbutaline, albuterol, and aminophylline. Steroids may also be necessary to control status asthmaticus. Steroids should be used only as long as necessary because of serious side effects. Sedatives, expectorants, and antibiotics for infection are also used. Basic treatment of acute asthma includes epinephrine (1:1000 in a dose of 0.01 ml/kg subcutaneously every 15 minutes for three times, if necessary, up to maximum of 0.3 ml) and isoetharine (Bronkosol) 0.25% by nebulizer aerosol (0.5 ml in 4.5 ml saline). If the patient has a poor response to epinephrine and isoetharine administration of corticosteroids should be considered. Causative factors must be controlled. Cromolyn sodium is used for prophylaxis and is not of value for treatment of an attack.

Hay Fever (Allergic Rhinitis)

Hay fever, a classic type I reaction, is the most common allergic manifestation in children. Hay fever is seldom due to hay and is infrequently associated with fever. Seasonal symptoms are usually due to pollens of trees, grasses, and weeds. In perennial rhinitis, the offenders may be pollens, house dust, animal dander, mold spores, and mites. The conjunctiva may be inflamed, and the nasal mucous membrane may be pale, boggy, bluish, and edematous-looking, with thin, watery discharge. The child frequently rubs the nose. Peripheral white blood cell (WBC) count may show an increase in eosinophils, and nasal secretions may have many eosinophils.

Treatment of hay fever includes avoidance of antigen; hyposensitization; and administration of antihistamines, corticosteroids, and nasal cromolyn.

Hematologic Disorders

Anemias

Growth increases demand for blood, and so during childhood, various anemias may have dramatic manifestations. Children present with tiredness, lethargy, pallor, and occasionally pica. Anemia is often discovered only during investigation for other conditions, such as infection and poor weight gain.

Iron Deficiency Anemia

Most anemia is due to dietary iron deficiency. Overt gastrointestinal bleeding is rare in children, but it is important to exclude this possibility and any other underlying disease. A hypochromic, microcytic blood smear is usually sufficient evidence to justify a trial of oral iron therapy. Children who fail to respond to iron therapy warrant a more detailed investigation.

Aquired Aplastic Anemia

Acquired aplastic anemia occurs at any age and may follow infection; drug therapy, such as with chloramphenicol; and chemical exposure, such as to benzene. Those patients who have severe pancytopenia respond poorly to treatment with androgens and corticosteroids. Transplantation with human leukocyte antigen (HLA)–compatible marrow is the treatment of choice.

Hemolytic Anemia

Hemolytic anemia is basically due to a shortened survival time of red blood cells (RBCs) and may be either congenital or acquired. The majority of hemolytic anemias encountered in childhood are due to RBC disorders. These disorders are characterized by anemia, increased reticulocyte count, unconjugated hyperbilirubinemia, and skeletal changes secondary to compensatory marrow hyperplasia. Causes include spherocytosis, RBC enzyme deficiencies, glucose-6-phosphate dehydrogenase deficiency, and pyruvate kinase deficiency. Splenectomy produces improvement but increases the risk for pneumococcal sepsis. Pneumococcal vaccine should be given.

Hemoglobin Synthesis Disorders

Hemoglobin synthesis disorders fall into two categories, those with an amino-acid substitution in the globin portion of the molecule, such as sickle cell anemia, and those with failure of globin chain synthesis, such as thalassemia.

Sickle Cell Anemia. The homozygous condition is referred to as sickle-cell disease and the heterozygous as sickle cell trait. Sickle-cell disease is a serious condition with many complications in addition to anemia. Painful swelling of the hands and feet is a common early presentation. Repeated infarctions in the spleen may produce an autosplenectomy. Crises are usually precipitated by infection and may be complicated by dehydration, poor tissue perfusion, hypoxia, and acidosis. Treatment is largely symptomatic, with administration of fluids being primary. Pain medication should be given liberally. Any underlying infection should be treated with appropriate antibiotics.

Thalassemia. This inherited anemia is common in Italians, Asians, and Greeks and is subdivided into alpha-thalassemia and beta-thalassemia, depending on the hemoglobin polypeptide chain affected by synthetic failure. Beta-thalassemia is more common and results in severe hemolytic anemia with hypochromic, microcytic cells. The compensatory bone marrow hyperplasia produces a characteristic overgrowth of the facial and skull bones as well as fragile limb bones. Death may be delayed by repeated transfusion. The problem of chronic iron overload results in progressive organ failure.

Bleeding Disorders

A variety of disorders may lead to excessive bleeding in children. Past history is important in distinguishing congenital from acquired problems. Family history of excessive bleeding after circumcision or dental extraction may help give clues to etiology.

Von Willebrand's Disease

Von Willebrand's disease is a clotting disorder that should be considered in a girl who bleeds easily, has frequent nosebleeds, or experiences menorrhagia. Skin and mucous-membrane bleeding is common. The characteristics of von Willebrand's disease include a prolonged bleeding time, low factor VIII, and reduced platelet adhesiveness.

Hemophilia

Male babies with hemophilia may have a history of prolonged bleeding associated with circumcision.

The more severe hemophilias become evident in the first year of life ($< 1\%$ factor VIII). Joint hemorrhage is most likely due to hemophilia if it relates to a bleeding disorder. Petechiae are associated with platelet deficiencies and capillary wall leaks. Clotting defects do not produce petechiae, adenopathy, or hepatosplenomegaly. The character of the bleeding problem and four basic coagulation tests—platelet count, bleeding time, prothrombin time, and partial thromboplastin time (PTT)—determine that a bleeding disorder is present.

Purpuras

Purpuras are the result of skin hemorrhage, either ecchymosis or petechiae.

Thrombocytopenia. A platelet count below 40,000 is associated with a variety of disease states, including aplastic anemia, leukemia, drug-induced disease, and autoimmune disease. Idiopathic thrombocytopenic purpura is the most common form of thrombocytopenia and is thought to have an immunologic basis mediated by antiplatelet antibodies. This disorder often follows a viral infection. Idiopathic thrombocytopenic purpura usually has an acute self-limiting course, with spontaneous recovery by 6 months. Splenectomy is considered for refractory cases. Immunosuppressive drugs are used if splenectomy fails. Aspirin should be avoided.

Drug-Induced Purpura. Although this disorder is unusual in children, it is becoming increasingly recognized. Aspirin is the most commonly associated drug in children.

Purpura Associated with Blood Vessel Defect. Small blood vessel defects also cause purpura and are seen in Henoch-Schönlein purpura (anaphylactoid purpura), scurvy, disease associated with some toxins, meningococcal infection, trauma, and chronic disease.

Defective Platelets. Defective platelets result in petechiae or ecchymosis. Defective platelets are related to aspirin ingestion, uremia, and von Willebrand's disease.

Cardiac Disorders

Although increasing in incidence again, rheumatic fever is rare, and congenital abnormalities are the main causes of heart disease in children.

Heart Murmurs

Murmurs may be (1) organic, caused by structural heart abnormalities; (2) secondary, associated with increased cardiac output by a normal heart; and (3) innocent, occurring with normal output and a normal heart. Innocent murmurs are systolic but not holosystolic. Murmurs are well localized and vibratory, measuring a grade III or less and without a thrill. Loud murmurs (grades IV through VI) are those with a thrill, those that radiate, and those that are holosystolic or diastolic. Loud murmurs must be considered organic. In addition to murmurs, widely split second heart sounds that persist with inspiration and expiration and fourth heart sounds (gallop) are also indicative of organic heart disease.

INNOCENT MURMURS

Innocent murmurs can be characterized as follows:

	Characteristic	Grade
Systolic	I Still's musical	II/VI
	II Basal blowing	II/VI
	III Carotid blowing	II/VI
	IV Physiologic peripheral pulmonic stenosis	II/VI
Continuous	V Mammary souffle (whisper)	II/VI or <
	VI Venous hum	II/VI or >

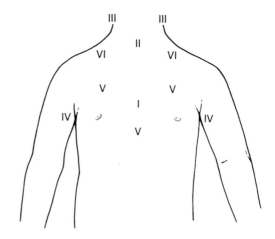

With exercise, fever, and reclining, all these murmurs get louder except venous hum, which may decrease.

Bicuspid aortic valve (one large and one small cusp) occurs in 2% of children and gives a basal murmur, usually harsh with an ejection click.

Venous hum is a blowing, continuous murmur heard at the base of the heart, often just below the clavicles. The hum varies with respiration and position of the head and disappears when the child lies down. Venous hum is related to blood flow through the superior vena cava. Venous hum is the most common murmur heard. The so-called Still's murmur ("twangy string" murmur) is almost as common as the venous hum. Still's murmur is a grade III or less systolic murmur, localized along the left sternal border.

Congenital Heart Disease

Congenital heart disease may be cyanotic or acyanotic. The child usually presents in one of three ways, with heart murmur, heart failure, or central cyanosis. Heart murmur is the most common presentation and is usually detected in the first year of life. A baby who presents with cyanosis ("blue baby") has a right-to-left shunt. Long-standing cyanosis results in clubbing of the fingers and toes and secondary polycythemia. Most children now survive these defects because of skillful cardiac surgery. Cyanosis in the infant is most likely associated with transposition, tetralogy of Fallot, tricuspid atresia, and truncus arteriosus.

Suggestive symptoms of congenital heart

disease in the infant are sighing spells with pallor, respiratory difficulties, stridor, hyperextension of the neck, poor weight gain, and feeding difficulties.

ACYANOTIC CONGENITAL HEART DISEASE

Patent Ductus Arteriosus. A murmur may be absent early in patent ductus arteriosus (PDA). The systolic component may be present alone before the classical "machinery-like" combined systolic-diastolic murmur becomes apparent in the second and third left intercostal spaces. The high aortic pressure shunts blood into the pulmonary artery. The left ventricular output is increased, and pulse pressure is wide. Radiographs show enlargement of the left ventricle with increased pulmonary vascular markings. The "hilar dance" of the enlarged pulmonary artery may be visualized on fluoroscopy. The electrocardiogram (ECG) may show left ventricular hypertrophy. Subacute bacterial endocarditis or congestive failure is a risk. (Indomethacin is a drug that may cause closure of a PDA, thereby avoiding surgery.) Surgical division and ligation is recommended in infants with large PDA who show failure to improve with indomethacin.

Coarctation of the Aorta
Infantile (Preductal) Type Coarctation. Constriction between the subclavian artery and the ductus arteriosus causes infantile type coarctation of the aorta. This disorder results in death if the ductus closes. Treatment is surgical.

Adult (Postductal) Type Coarctation. Adult type coarctation is often asymptomatic in early childhood. This coarctation is associated with Turner's syndrome and Noonan's syndrome. A systolic murmur may be heard at the base or in the back. Strong radial pulses and pulsations at the sternal notch with weak femoral pulses are typical. *To evaluate, arm and leg pulses must be compared simultaneously.* The systolic blood pressure in the arms is considerably higher than in the legs, whereas the diastolic is nearly the same. In most cases, left ventricular hypertrophy is evident clinically by ECG and by radiograph, unless there is associated patent ductus or septal defect. Notching of the ribs is not usually apparent before age 5. The hypoplastic aorta may be demonstrated by barium swallow. Treatment is surgical.

Septal Defects
Interatrial Septal Defects. The three types of interatrial septal defects are as follows:
1. Ostium primum defect, which is low in the septum and often associated with a defect in the mitral or tricuspid valve.
2. Ostium secundum, which is high in the septum and is rarely troublesome.
3. Lutembacher's syndrome, which is an atrial septal defect associated with congenital or acquired mitral stenosis.

All types of defects have murmurs. In the uncomplicated primum type, the murmur is generally not loud (grades II to III), heard in systole in the left second intercostal space. The heart is globular, with enlargement of the right side. Pulmonary vessels are enlarged, whereas the aorta is small.

Electrocardiogram shows right ventricular hypertrophy and bundle-branch block. Infants are rarely symptomatic. Shunt is left-to-right. With catheterization, it is usually easy to enter the left atrium through the defect. Color Doppler effect is replacing catheterization to a great extent. There is increased oxygen content in the right atrium. Early opacification of the right atrium occurs on selective right atrial angiocardiography. Associated subacute bacterial endocarditis is rare.

Surgery ensures complete cure in uncomplicated atrial septal defects. The treatment varies and must be based on the cardiologist's evaluation.

Endocardial Cushion Defects. Endocardial cushion defects occur in about 50% of children with Down's syndrome.

CYANOTIC CONGENITAL HEART DISEASE (OUTFLOW TRACT DEFECTS)

Tetralogy of Fallot (right ventricular outflow defect) is *the most common cause of cyanotic congenital heart disease.* Patients with this defect may survive for a long period. There is pulmonary stenosis or atresia with intraventricular septal defect, right ventricular hypertrophy, and dextroposition of the aorta. Physiologically tetralogy of Fallot is a pulmonary stenosis with right-to-left shunt.

Antibiotic Prophylaxis for the Child With Congenital Heart Disease Undergoing Surgery. Antibiotic prophylaxis may be necessary for podiatric surgery in patients with prosthetic heart valve or mitral prolapse with regurgitation or congenital heart lesions. For patients who are undergoing clean surgery, no prophylaxis is needed. For patients who are undergoing infected surgery, penicillin (2 g by mouth 1 hour prior to surgery and 1 g 6 hours following surgery) is recommended. In the infant and young child, 1 g should be given by mouth prior to surgery and 500 mg should be given 6 hours following surgery. Each case should be reviewed with the patient's physician prior to surgery.

Rheumatic Heart Disease

Rheumatic heart disease is immunologically related to infection with group A beta-hemolytic streptococci. The streptococcal infection usually precedes the rheumatic state by 1 to 3 weeks. This disease had decreased dramatically in incidence but is increasing again. Rheumatic heart disease can cause serious illness in children and permanent valvular damage in adults. The decline was attributed to antibiotics, diminished virulence of beta-hemolytic streptococci, and improved social conditions. There is no specific diagnostic test. Diagnosis is confirmed by Jones's criteria, the presence of two major signs or one major and two minor signs. Major signs include migratory polyarthritis, acute carditis, erythema marginatum or annulare, subcutaneous nodules, and Sydenham's chorea. Minor signs include arthralgia, previous history of rheumatic fever, group A beta-hemolytic streptococcal infection, ECG-prolonged P-R interval, mild anemia, elevated sedimentation rate, elevated C-reactive protein levels, elevated gamma globulin level, and elevated antistreptolysin-O (ASO) titer: (33 U borderline; 500 U indicate recent infection). The arthritis is reversible, but the cardiac involvement may progress to serious sequelae. Other symptoms include chest and abdominal pain, dyspnea, purpura, epistaxis, and pneumonitis with or without pleural effusion. Treatment includes penicillin (1.2 mU/day for 10 days [penicillin G or penicillin V potassium orally or procaine penicillin 1 mU]) followed by penicillin G benzathine (Bicillin) (1.2 mU intramuscularly monthly) or, if the patient is allergic to penicillin, sulfadiazine 0.5 g daily for children less than 30 kg and 1.0 g for those over 30 kg. Other treatment includes rest; high-protein diet; administration of acetylsalicylic acid (ASA); and for severe carditis, administration of steroids.

Arrhythmias

BRADYCARDIA

Bradycardia is a slow pulse rate at rest of less than 80 in infants and less than 60 in older children. Bradycardia may be familial and may occur in the active person or the athlete. This disorder sometimes occurs during convalescence from acute infections, such as hepatitis and typhoid, and in association with increased intracranial pressure. Bradycardia may also be associated with heart block.

HEART BLOCK

The conductive system may be blocked anywhere along its pathway (sinoatrial node, atrial muscle, atrioventricular node, bundle of His, left and right branches, and Purkinje's network). First degree block is usually associated with myocarditis. P-R interval is prolonged. Wenckebach's phenomenon is progressive prolongation of P-R interval until a ventricular beat is skipped (second degree block). Complete block is a rate of 40 to 60/minute, probably caused by a congenital defect in the main stem of the bundle of His. Auricles and ventricles beat independently. Because of increased stroke volume, systolic pressure is elevated, and a water-hammer–type pulse is present. There may be associated murmur. Prognosis is good, though syncope may occur at times and occasionally may require a pacemaker implant.

PAROXYSMAL TACHYCARDIA

Paroxysmal tachycardia is usually idiopathic and is more common in men than in women. There are two types, supraventricular and ventricular. This disorder may be accompanied by Wolff-Parkinson-White syndrome (short P-R interval and prolonged QRS complex). Paroxysmal tachycardia most commonly originates in an atrial ectopic focus. Attacks start and stop abruptly, lasting from a few seconds to a few days but rarely longer. The heart rate ranges from 150 to 250.

Symptoms of paroxysmal tachycardia are ashen color; sometimes mild cyanosis; sweating; restlessness; vomiting; fever; "toxic" look; and tachypnea, particularly if heart failure is supervening. Signs of this disorder are rapid pulse rate, steady in supraventricular type, variable in ventricular type; possibly enlarged heart with variable murmurs; and signs of heart failure with prolonged attack. Electrocardiogram demonstrates no P waves and normal QRS complex in the supraventricular type, P waves present but not related to QRS complex in the ventricular type, and shortened P-R interval with prolonged QRS complex in Wolff-Parkinson-White syndrome.

Treatment is urgent. Oxygen must be administered. Vagal stimulation by *unilateral* pressure on the eyeball or carotic sinus, or by gagging, is potentially hazardous but may abort the attack. Digitalis in full digitalizing doses (or verapamil, 0.1 mg/kg i.v.) is administered to patients who have supraventricular paroxysmal tachycardia. Quinidine sulfate (15 to 30 mg orally) is administered to patients who have ventricular paroxysmal tachycardia. If tolerated, quinidine sulfate should be given in doses of 6 mg/kg orally every 2 hours. The prognosis for this disorder is good, with attacks usually disappearing with increasing age. Digitalis should be given for several months and then withdrawn under observation.

Childhood Hypertension

Approximately 1.9% of children aged 4 to 15 years have persistent hypertension. Unfortunately blood pressure measurement is often overlooked in children. In children over 10 years old, a persistent systolic pressure measurement over 140 mm Hg or a diastolic pressure measurement over 90 mm Hg is abnormal. For children under 10 years old, see published standards for age. These measurements must be confirmed on several occasions before a child can be regarded as having an abnormal blood pressure. The majority of children with mild, asymptomatic hypertension fall into the primary or essential category. Nonessential hypertension is most commonly related to renal parenchymal disease. Hypertension may be manifested as persistent headache, dizziness, disturbed vision, irritability, and convulsions. Other neurologic signs may also be present. Paroxysmal episodes of palpitation and sweating raise the possibility of a pheochromocytoma. Early detection and control of an underlying problem reduces morbidity and mortality.

Ear, Nose, and Throat and Pulmonary Disorders

Epistaxis

Nose bleeds are more frequent on hot summer days or with change in altitude. Causes include trauma; infection, such as viruses and purulent rhinitis; allergy; foreign body; tumor; and rheumatic fever. Occasionally epistaxis is associated with the onset of menstruation. Swallowed blood may give coffee-ground vomitus and dark to tarry stools. Treatment includes correcting any underlying cause and putting the patient in semi-sitting position, applying pressure to the nose at least 10 minutes, with an ice pack at the back of the neck. A cotton pledget soaked in 0.25% phenylephrine (Neo-Synephrine) held in the nostril or a Gelfoam pack left in place is helpful for anterior nose bleed. Posterior nose bleed requires consultation with an ear, nose, and throat specialist.

Tonsillitis and Pharyngitis

The peak incidence for tonsillitis and pharyngitis is in the fourth to seventh years, with the majority of the cases being viral. Group A beta-hemolytic streptococci are the only bacteria significantly involved. *Mycoplasma* may account for a few cases. Exudate may be seen in the throat. Viral disease should be suspected if coryza, cough, or hoarseness occurs. Complications include scarlet fever, adenitis, peritonsillar abscess, otitis media, and pneumonia. Rheumatic fever and glomerulonephritis are occasional complications of beta-hemolytic streptococcal infection. Hematogenous spread could result in meningitis, septic arthritis, and osteomyelitis.

Otitis

Otitis media is one of the most common infections, with viruses being the most common etiologic agents. Bacterial pathogens include *Streptococcus*, pneumococci, *Staphylococcus*, *Haemophilus influenzae*, and *Branhamella catarrhalis*. *Streptococcus pneumoniae* is the most common cause. *Haemophilus influenzae* infections are common in children under 5 years old. In chronic otitis media, drums may be scarred or perforated, with some conductive hearing loss. Mastoids may be tender. Cholesteatoma may develop, leading to destruction of ossicles. Mastoiditis is usually related to chronic otitis media or recurrent otitis. Consultation with an ear, nose, and throat specialist is indicated. External otitis is related to trauma, eczema, foreign bodies, and irritants. Swimming may also result in external otitis.

Croup (Acute Laryngotracheobronchitis)

The larynx, trachea, and bronchi are all involved in the inflammatory process of acute laryngotracheobronchitis. Croup tends to occur in epidemics, particularly in autumn and early spring. This disease is characterized by difficult breathing. The five main classifications are viral, spasmodic, foreign body, acute epiglottitis caused by *H. influenzae*, and diphtheritic croup. The child presents with a barking cough and stridulous breathing, especially on inspiration, with anxiety exacerbating the natural tendency for the airway to collapse on inspiration. Treatment is symptomatic for viral croup. Epiglottitis is a life-threatening emergency. The incidence of epiglottitis should be reduced with *Hemophilus influenzae* type B (HIB) immunization.

Airway Obstruction

When normal patency of the respiratory tract is reduced, use of accessory muscles of respiration is necessary. Hoarseness, aphonia, stridor, and wheezing may occur. Symptoms of airway obstruction caused by a foreign body include choking, gagging, coughing, stridor, and cyanosis. If a bronchial foreign body is present for more than a few days, local infection begins with subsequent abscess formation.

Bronchitis

ACUTE BRONCHITIS

Both viral and bacterial acute bronchitis tend to occur with a paroxysmal cough, which worsens at night, with mild or no fever. Chest findings include tachypnea, rhonchi, and rales. White blood cell count generally reveals relative neutropenia in viral disease and leukocytosis in bacterial disease. Most cases of acute bronchitis are probably viral or associated with pertussis, measles, influenza, scarlet fever, and *Mycoplasma* infection. Treatment includes administration of antibiotics if indicated, fluids, mist, expectorants, chest percussion, and postural drainage.

CHRONIC BRONCHITIS

In children, chronic bronchitis is usually associated with allergy or chronic infection of the sinuses or nasopharynx. Bronchiectasis, cystic fibrosis, immunodeficiency, and esophageal reflux may predispose to these symptoms. The child should be evaluated for possible cause.

Pneumonias

Influenzal pneumonia and mycoplasma pneumonia are the most common forms of this illness. Children so affected do not usually appear very ill. White blood cell counts are variable but often are normal or low, with predominant lymphocytes. Cold agglutinin is often positive in mycoplasma pneumonia but is not specific. The drug of choice for mycoplasma pneumonia is erythromycin (20 mg/kg/day divided into four doses). Tetracycline is also satisfactory, but it is not used in young children because of its propensity to stain teeth. Penicillin-sensitive organisms constitute the majority of other bacterial pneumonias in children. The work-up in the seriously ill child includes sputum culture and sensitivity, blood cultures, and chest radiograph.

Lobar pneumonia occurs with acute toxicity, chills, fever, cough, dyspnea, tachycardia, and rusty sputum. White blood cell count is elevated, with predominance of polymorphonuclear neutrophils (PMNs) in blood and sputum. Sedimentation rate is high, and pneumococci are present in the sputum smear and culture specimens. There is an increasing incidence of gram-negative pneumonias. Blood culture is an important part of diagnostic evaluation. Treatment should be initiated with a broad-spectrum antibiotic, such as ampicillin, erythromycin, or cephalosporin, and then changed to the drug of choice as soon as the organism is identified. Amphotericin B is indicated for fungal infection. General therapy includes bed rest; use of a saline gargle; use of lozenges; use of a humidifier; administration of an antipyretic; administration of an agent for mild sedation, such as phenobarbital; administration of codeine or dextromethorphan for a severe cough; and administration of oxygen if the patient is dyspneic or cyanotic. Abscess or empyema may require surgical drainage.

Cystic Fibrosis

Cystic fibrosis involves the exocrine glands, especially those secreting mucus. This disease results in duct obstruction, which leads to pancreatic insufficiency; chronic suppurative lung disease; abnormally high sweat electrolyte levels; male infertility; and in some cases, biliary cirrhosis. Incomplete forms of the disease lead to variations in the manifestations. Ciliary mechanism defect leads to recurrent infection. Although prognosis is poor, with the advent of effective antibiotics, the life span of patients with cystic fibrosis has been prolonged. Respiratory physical therapy; inhalation mist therapy; addition of pancreatic enzymes; and a diet low in fat and high in calories and proteins, with vitamins, are all helpful but not curative. The defective gene has been identified.

Tuberculosis

The pattern and incidence of tuberculosis has changed markedly in the last 50 years. In 1920, nearly 80% of 20-year-old individuals were tuberculin positive. Today, less than 5% are tuberculin positive. After initial contact and spread into the lymphatic system, normal immune mechanisms cause regression of lesions and dormancy of tubercle bacilli. With a breakdown of body defenses even years later, active disease may occur. Cases tend to be sporadic and insidious, with vague symptoms of malaise, tiredness, unexplained fever, decreased appetite, and weight loss. Cough in children is uncommon except in infants. Older adults are the most likely contact. Children seldom transmit the disease. Diagnosis of tuberculosis is most often made by routine tuberculin skin testing. The primary complex, Ghon complex, is a lesion in the periphery, with enlargement of regional nodes. Progression of disease is through local extension and via endobronchial, lymphatic, and hematogenous routes to both lungs and other parts of the body.

In children, physical findings are usually normal or minimal. Even in miliary tuberculosis, the chest examination may be negative. The patient may be toxic. Splenomegaly is often present. Complications include miliary tuberculosis; meningitis; and bone, joint, kidney, and bowel involvement. Treatment includes evaluation of contacts, administration of bacille Calmette-Guérin (BCG) vaccine to newborns of mothers with tuberculosis, and normal diet with vitamin supplement if indicated. Asymptomatic patients have no restrictions in activity. Symptomatic patients should reduce their activity or rest in bed if needed and return to normal activity as soon as possible. Protection from other infections is imperative. Mainstay drugs include isoniazid (INH); para-aminosalicylic acid (PAS); streptomycin; rifampin; ethambutol; pyrazinamide; and in specific circumstances, prednisone.

Gastrointestinal Disorders

Anorexia

Anorexia may be physiologic and part of normal development or accompany illness. Anorexia nervosa is an extreme form of self-starvation, usually seen in adolescent girls. Hospitalization is often necessary for proper nutritional observation and intensive psychotherapy. Administration of cyproheptadine (Periactin) has been reported as a useful adjunct in treatment.

Failure to Thrive

Failue to thrive is a descriptive diagnostic term to indicate an infant or child who fails to gain weight or grow without a readily discernible explanation. Failure to thrive may be due to physical or psychologic deprivation or may be organic in nature, relating most likely to central nervous system disease, chronic urinary tract infection, renal failure, congenital heart disease, and malabsorption syndromes. Appropriate evaluations should be made.

Vomiting and Diarrhea

Vomiting and diarrhea are common symptoms but may represent serious disease. If symptoms are prolonged or severe or associated with significant pain the child should be examined. A baseline weight at the onset may be very helpful later. General examination is important. Appendicitis and other surgical abdominal disease or acute nonsurgical abdominal disease should not be overlooked, particularly when "intestinal flu" is in the community.

One general treatment method is dietary restriction. Vomiting can usually be controlled with a short period of no or reduced intake, slowly increasing volume beginning with clear fluids. Commonly used drugs include dimenhydrinate (Dramamine), phosphorated carbohydrate solution (Emetrol), and promethazine (Phenergan). Prochlorperazine (Compazine) can cause central nervous system reactions. A variety of juices should be given to avoid excessive salt intake. Water alone may cause hyponatremia. Boiled skim milk may cause hypernatremia. Strained orange juice and bananas are good sources of potassium. Small, frequent feedings (2 to 4 ounces every 2 to 4 hours) should be given, using dilute fruit juices, tea, water, bouillon, gelatin, sherbet, crushed Popsicles, rice cereal, apple sauce, and bananas. Increased amounts may be given to older children, along with carbonated beverages. Soups, crackers, lean meats, and toast may be tolerated. Pedialyte and Lytren are commercial rehydration fluids available for infants and children. In patients with severe hydration (10% acute weight loss), intravenous fluid therapy may be necessary.

Diet control is an important part of treatment for diarrhea. Kaolin (Kaopectate) (2 to 4 tsp every 4 to 6 hours) may be useful. Preparations of diphenoxylate and atropine (Lomotil) are contraindicated in chil-

dren. Bismuth and paregoric (0.4 mg morphine/ml) should be used with caution and only if the patient has been examined. Some workers think *Lactobacillus* (given three times a day [t.i.d.]) may be useful. Donnagel (opium, hyoscyamine, atropine, and scopolamine with kaolin and pectin) given every 6 to 8 hours may help to relieve severe cramping. However, some workers believe these drugs may aggravate or prolong the infection. Differential diagnoses include enteric infections, acute gastroenteritis, postantibiotic diarrhea, fungal infections, and parasites.

Reye's Syndrome

The prodrome of Reye's syndrome suggests a mild virus infection followed by vomiting, stupor, convulsion, and coma. The characteristic liver lesion shows diffuse small droplets, fatty infiltration of hepatocytes, and absent glycogen. Some workers believe the liver changes and the encephalopathy are due to hyperammonemia, not to the viral infection, and the basis may be a genetic metabolic defect. Reye's syndrome is particularly associated with influenza virus infections and chicken pox. In persons with genetic predispositions, aspirin appears to be an added trigger. For this reason, aspirin is generally not used in children or young adolescents. Reye's syndrome is rare after age 16. Treatment is symptomatic, aimed at controlling cerebral edema and ammonemia.

Inflammatory Bowel Diseases

CROHN'S DISEASE

Crohn's disease is characterized by segmental transmural ulcerations most commonly involving the ileum and colon. Crohn's disease manifests with fever, poor appetite, weight loss, growth failure, crampy abdominal pain, diarrhea, and joint symptoms. The cause is unknown. Treatment is palliative or surgical.

ULCERATIVE COLITIS

Ulcerative colitis predominantly affects teenagers. Onset begins with mild recurrent bouts of diarrhea associated with cramping. Subsequently blood appears in the stool. Ulcerative colitis is associated with anorexia, weakness, weight loss, anemia, and arthritis. Perirectal ulceration and abscesses may occur. The rectum and distal colon are most frequently involved. Pyoderma gangrenosum of the skin may also occur. The chronic stooling and anorexia may lead to hypoproteinemia. Stool culture specimen and ova and parasite studies are negative. Arthritis is seen in 10 to 20% of patients, with the knee and ankle being especially affected. The differential diagnoses include allergy, irritable bowel syndrome, amebic colitis, bacillary dysentery, ischemic colitis, antibiotic colitis, and Crohn's disease. Treatment consists of adequate rest and diet high in protein and iron with no laxative foods, milk, or alcohol. Psychologic support and administration of anticholinergics and antispasmodics may help control mild diarrhea. Opiates and corticosteroids can be administered in severe cases. Blood transfusions may be necessary with severe anemia. About 20% of patients ultimately require surgery, either ileostomy or colectomy. About 50% of patients recover completely or improve significantly. With prolonged disease, carcinoma of the colon may develop.

Constipation

With constipation, stools are hard, dry, and small with variable frequency. Constipation may be related to underlying disease, such as hypothyroidism, congenital megacolon, and anemia; diet; faulty toilet habits; rectal fissures; rectal stenosis; and mechanical obstruction. Ingestion of certain drugs may also be associated. Treatment includes administration of mineral oil, diet therapy, administration of Maltsupex, administration of docusate (Colace), ingestion of fluids, and management of underlying disorder.

Celiac Syndrome

Celiac syndrome is a malabsorptive disorder that may manifest in a variety of ways. Presentation includes malodorous, bulky, fatty, frothy stools; abdominal distention; and malnutrition, including vitamin deficiencies. This syndrome is seen with absence of pancreatic lipase, as in cystic fibrosis, protein deficiency, and hypoplasia of exocrine pancreas. Biliary atresia and hepatitis both lead to bile deficiency with impaired fat digestion and appear as described. Other causes of celiac syndrome include milk allergy, celiac disease (gluten-induced enteropathy), disaccharidase deficiencies, and idiopathic steatorrhea. Screening tests include serum carotene level, serum sweat level, iodized oil (Lipiodol) absorption, oral glucose tolerance test, vitamin A tolerance test, stool pH, stool for reducing substance, and if indicated small bowel biopsy. The most reliable test is chemical determination of fecal fat by balance studies, but this is difficult to perform. Management depends on etiology.

Surgical Problems of the Abdomen

Gastrointestinal Bleeding

The site of bleeding, its duration and severity, age of the child, and associated symptoms and findings are all critical in determining the cause and significance and hence treatment of gastrointestinal bleeding.

Vomiting of blood (hematemesis) is usually associated with swallowed blood following epistaxis, surgical procedures, and repeated vomiting due to gastritis. Elevated fever and WBC count may be associated with blood in the gastrointestinal tract. Anal fissures are the most common cause of rectal bleeding. Ulcers, volvulus, intussusception, gastrointestinal infection, ulcerative colitis, amebiasis, polyps, and milk allergy are also associated. Other bleeding sites in the body may suggest anaphylactoid purpura, thrombocytopenia, hypoprothrombinemia, and leukemia.

Management of children with gastrointestinal bleeding includes administration of intravenous fluids, blood type and crossmatch, restoration of fluid volume, and restoration of blood volume, if loss is severe. The source of bleeding must be found and the basic cause treated.

Intussusception

Intussusception is a telescoping of one part of the intestine into a distal portion, most commonly the ileum into the colon, cutting off blood supply and causing local necrosis. Most intussusceptions have no known cause but may relate to a polyp, a

Meckel's diverticulum, or a viral infection. Symptoms include acute onset of severe colicky, paroxysmal pain, usually in an infant under 1 year of age. A mass may be felt in the right midabdomen. A "currant jelly" blood clot in the stool may appear with incarceration. Barium enema may demonstrate an inverted cap. In two thirds of cases the intussusception may be reduced by a skilled radiologist; otherwise surgery is indicated. Older children should undergo surgical exploration to determine cause of occurrence.

APPENDICITIS

The most common childhood condition that requires intestinal surgery is appendicitis. The cause is most commonly a fecalith but may be associated with measles, other viral infections, and pinworms. Appendicitis often presents a difficult diagnostic dilemma. Typically pain is periumbilical at onset, gradually shifting to the right lower quadrant. Vomiting, diarrhea, or both may occur, and urinary symptoms may be associated. The child usually looks acutely ill, lies doubled up, or if upright walks bent over holding the right side. Examination of the abdomen reveals variable peristalsis; guarding; tenderness, particularly over the appendix; referred pain from other areas; and rebound tenderness. White blood cell count is usually elevated. Differential diagnoses include mesenteric adenitis, pyelonephritis, gastroenteritis, pneumonia, constipation, pinworms, peritonitis, and diverticulitis.

CONGENITAL MEGACOLON
(HIRSCHSPRUNG'S DISEASE)

Congenital megacolon is seen mostly in males and is usually evident from the first day of birth. The disorder is related to lack of Meissner's or Auerbach's plexus developing in the small bowel. Main signs are constipation, abdominal distention, and vomiting. The anus is tight and elongated on examination, which may reveal the "glove finger" sign (as if the examining finger were inserted into a glove). Barium enema may show the spastic segment, especially on the lateral view, and the distention of bowel above. Confirmation depends on a rectal biopsy specimen that shows absence of ganglion cells. Treat-

ment is a temporary colostomy with resection of the aganglionic segment and reanastomosis later.

Genitourinary Tract Disorders

Urinary tract disorders in the infant and child should always be considered as a cause of illness. Failure to grow, bouts of unexplained fever, vague abdominal pain, and any change in urinary habits may indicate primary genitourinary disease. Specific symptoms include urinary changes, such as frequency, urgency, dysuria, incontinence, and enuresis; fever; chills; costovertebral angle (CVA) pain; anemia; elevated blood pressure; and edema. Laboratory findings may include fixed specific gravity of urine, pyuria, proteinuria, cellular abnormalities, and casts and crystals in urine. Culture specimens obtained by midstream showing more than 100,000 colonies suggest infection. Chemical studies may reveal decreased serum protein levels, elevated blood urea nitrogen levels, low calcium levels, elevated phosphorus levels, and elevated creatinine levels or decreased creatinine clearance. Proteinuria is usually absent in urinary tract infection. Pyuria does not necessarily correlate with bacteriuria.

Orthostatic Albuminuria

Orthostatic albuminuria is generally a benign finding. Significant protein spilling usually occurs in the upright position but not in the recumbent position. Orthostatic albuminuria may be an early sign of glomerulonephritis. Several examinations of urine collected in both recumbent and upright positions should be performed. Several urine specimens should be examined for cellular elements. Renal function tests should be done.

Urinary Tract Infection

Urinary tract infection is more common in girls. This infection is most frequent in the first 2 years. Urinary tract infection most often involves only the urethra and bladder but may involve the kidneys (pyelonephritis). In girls, pinworms and poor toilet habits may be triggering factors. Obstructions are important factors. *Esche-*

richia coli is the most common infecting organism, and spread is generally ascending and not hematogenous. Most infections involve one organism only. Because chronic undiagnosed urinary tract infection in childhood may lead to serious morbidity and mortality in adulthood, it is critical to evaluate, diagnose, and treat in childhood. A single infection in a boy is an indication for a sonogram and possibly a urogram. An intravenous pyelogram (IVP) and a voiding cystourethrogram may also be indicated. With girls, some workers believe studies are necessary only after a recurrent infection. In either case, after the initial infection is treated, urine should be examined and cultured every 3 months for 2 years. With recurrent infection, sonograms, urograms, and voiding cystourethrograms are indicated to demonstrate reflux.

Acute cystitis appears with frequency, urgency, dysuria, suprapubic pain, tenderness, and usually a low-grade fever. Causative organisms include *E. coli* (80%), *Klebsiella* (15%), enterococci, *Streptococcus viridans*, *Staphylococcus*, *Proteus*, and *Pseudomonas*. Children with diabetes mellitus and obstruction are predisposed to acute cystitis.

Acute Pyelonephritis

In patients with acute pyelonephritis, high fever, chills, back and abdominal pain, nausea and vomiting, CVA and abdominal tenderness, and symptoms of cystitis may be present. Differential diagnoses include appendicitis, surgical abdomen, perinephric abscess, and acute glomerulonephritis. Treatment is with fluids and chemotherapy. Drugs used for a first infection are sulfisoxazole (150 mg/kg/day in 4 doses), nitrofurantoin (5 to 7 mg/kg/day in 4 doses) (not effective against *Pseudomonas*), and ampicillin (100 mg/kg/day in 4 doses) up to 250 mg/dose. Ampicillin has 20 to 30% resistance; maximum 2 g/day or high single doses of 3 to 4 g in an adult should be given. Nalidixic acid (55 mg/kg/day in 4 doses) and methenamine mandelate (Mandelamine) (50 mg/kg/24 hours to maximum of 250 mg/dose for children under 5; 500 mg q.i.d. for children aged 6 to 12) are recommended for recurrent infections. Other drugs are sulfamethoxazole-trimethoprim (Bactrim, Septra), car-

benicillin for *Pseudomonas* and *Proteus*, and cephalexin (Keflex) for children, 25 to 100 mg/kg/24 hours, divided in 4 doses. Acute pyelonephritis should be treated for 6 months if recurrent. Follow-up screening tests can be done at home using the nitrites test with confirmatory culture in the laboratory, plus routine culture for 2 years.

Acute Glomerulonephritis (Bright's Disease)

Acute glomerulonephritis is a hypersensitivity reaction to beta-hemolytic streptococcal infection. This disease occurs predominantly in children. Signs are smoky urine, edema, hypertension, abdominal pain, headache, vomiting, chills, coma, and convulsions. Diagnosis is based on urine findings, including RBC casts and proteinuria, with reduced renal function. Complete recovery occurs in about 90% of cases but may take more than a year. Even though the patient is asymptomatic and kidney function normal, hematuria and proteinuria may persist for years. Treatment is bed rest; high-carbohydrate, low-protein, low-sodium diet; and restricted fluids. Control of hypertension and seizures and treatment of streptococcal infection are essential.

Chronic Glomerulonephritis

Chronic glomerulonephritis may follow acue glomerulonephritis. Often this disorder has no apparent cause. Chronic glomerulonephritis may be triggered by poisoning, syphilis, systemic lupus erythematosis (SLE), anaphylactoid purpura, and renal vein thrombosis. A congenital familial form is associated with deafness (Alport's syndrome).

Nephrosis (Nephrotic Syndrome, Minimal Change Disease)

The etiology of nephrosis is unknown, though it may be associated with syphilis, SLE, chronic glomerulonephritis, poison oak contact, bee sting, and nephrotoxic drugs. Clinically the child presents with generalized edema, severe proteinuria, hypoproteinemia, and hypercholesterolemia. Hematuria, hypertension, and azotemia may be present. Average age at onset is $2\frac{1}{2}$ to 3 years. Annual incidence is 2 cases per 100,000 live births. Edema is the usual onset symptom, with increased pallor, lassitude, and decreased appetite. Malnutrition may become severe because of bowel wall edema and malabsorption. These so-affected children are particularly prone to infection. Proteinuria of 2 to 10 g/day occurs. Hyaline granular and cellular casts are abundant and may contain lipid bodies. Serum albumin is decreased, frequently below 1 g/100 ml serum. Serum cholesterol level rises sharply, above 300 mg/100 ml. Complement activity is usually normal, with a markedly elevated sedimentation rate. Treatment includes restriction of sodium, administration of steroids, and administration of diuretics.

Musculoskeletal Disorders

Arthritides

Inflammatory joint disease is manifested by swelling, pain, stiffness, loss of motion, inflammation, and warmth of the involved joint. Pain alone is termed arthralgia. Swelling is the most reliable confirmatory sign of arthritis. Swelling is due to synovial fluid, synovial thickening, and periarticular edema. If the joint structures are damaged joints are permanently affected. Bone, nerve, and muscle pain may be confused with joint pain. Arthritis in childhood or diseases that mimic arthritis can be categorized into rheumatic diseases of childhood, infectious arthritides, noninflammatory conditions, and malignancies.

JUVENILE RHEUMATOID ARTHRITIS

Juvenile rheumatoid arthritis (JRA) is a chronic synovitis that is subdivided into polyarticular and pauciarticular types.

Polyarticular Arthritis. Three subgroups in polyarticular JRA include systemic-onset disease, typified by spiking fever, rash, hepatosplenomegaly, lymphadenopathy, polyserositis, myalgia, arthralgia, leukocytosis, and anemia; seronegative polyarticular arthritis; and seropositive polyarticular arthritis. *Systemic-onset disease* involves large and small joints and tends to be symmetric. Average age at onset is 5 years, with equal sex predilection. Serologic tests are negative. There is severe joint destruction in about 25% of patients. Arthritis may be chronic. *Seronegative (rheumatoid factor–neg-*

ative) polyarticular arthritis is more frequent in girls, with a median onset age of 3 years. Of patients, 25% have positive antinuclear antibody (ANA) test results. Patients are HLA-B27 negative, with mild systemic manifestations. The disease generally burns out, with 35 to 90% recovery.

Seropositive (rheumatoid factor–positive) polyarticular arthritis has a median age at onset of 12 years and equal sex predilection. Of patients, 75% have positive ANA test results. Patients are HLA-B27 negative. Subcutaneous and rheumatoid nodules are common. Seropositive polyarticular arthritis tends to be a chronic destructive joint disease.

Pauciarticular Arthritis. Only a few joints are involved in pauciarticular arthritis. This disease tends to affect large joints and is often asymmetric. There are two types. Type 1 has a median age at onset of 2 years, with equal sex predilection. The rheumatoid factor is negative. Of patients, 50% have positive ANA test results. Patients are HLA-B27 negative. Iridocyclitis is chronic and the major cause of morbidity. Permanent joint damage is rare. Type 2 has a median age at onset of 10 years and a male predominance with a familial pattern. Patients have negative rheumatoid factor and ANA test results. Patients are HLA-B27 positive. Iridocyclitis is acute. Ankylosing spondylitis is the main joint residue.

Treatment. The basic objective of therapy for any of the types of JRA is to relieve pain and to maintain joint motion. However, therapy varies somewhat with type of JRA. The primary drug therapy is with salicylates (approximately 100 mg/kg/day to 3600 mg total). Tolmetin is considered the drug of choice by some experts. Gold is considered if salicylates fail. Antimalarials are occasionally helpful but still experimental. Steroids do not prevent joint destruction and are indicated only for severe pericarditis or iridocyclitis that is not controlled by topical steroids.

Physiotherapy is an integral part of treatment and perhaps more important than medication. Warm baths, range of motion exercises, and active stretching are indicated. Night splints may be helpful. Maintaining hip function and preventing flexion contracture are most important. In severe destructive disease, joint replacement may eventually be necessary.

In ankylosing spondylitis, aspirin may be helpful but steroids and gold salts are not effective. Indomethacin and tolmetin may be helpful. Stretching of paraspinous muscles, a firm bed for sleeping, and good posture are important.

INFECTIOUS ARTHRITIS

Infective bacteria may cause joint infection directly or may cause synovitis without the presence of organisms. Direct infection or septic arthritis is usually secondary to sepsis and organisms that directly involve the joint. Occasionally the organism is from a penetrating wound. The synovium swells and involves the articular cartilage. The joint is painful, swollen, hot, and inflamed. The products of infection are destructive to articular cartilage. If the infection is left untreated for only a few days permanent damage may occur. Aspirate of joint effusion contains WBCs usually in excess of 50,000, predominantly PMNs. Organisms may be seen on smear. Synovial fluid glucose levels are usually low.

The patient generally is systemically ill, with fever, chills, and malaise. More than one joint may be involved, especially in gonococcal arthritis. In tuberculous arthritis, systemic symptoms are often lacking, and a single joint is usually involved. In general, joint cultures are positive about 70% of the time and blood cultures about 15%.

Joint space aspiration and blood cultures are indicated to differentiate septic from nonseptic arthritis. If gonococcal arthritis is suspected genital, rectal, and oral cultures should be done. Chest radiograph and skin tests are indicated if mycobacteria are suspected. If septic arthritis is thought to be present appropriate antibiotics should be started intravenously and continued for 2 to 4 weeks if confirmed. Oral therapy with newer antibiotics is being studied. In infants, gram-negative bacteria may be the cause. In children under age 4 years, *S. aureus* and *H. influenzae* are the most common causes. In children over age 4 years, *S. aureus* is the most common cause. Patients with sickle cell anemia are more prone to salmonella osteomyelitis. Septic arthritis is rapidly destructive, and early treatment is critical. Patients with rheumatoid arthritis are prone to septic arthritis as are intravenous drug users and patients with pneumonia or other infections. Joint effusions may accompany adjacent osteomyelitis. The fluid has low cell counts and is sterile.

Direct synovial infection has been demonstrated in patients with rubella. Immune-complex disease occurs with detectable Australia antigen titers preceding clinical hepatitis. Chicken pox, mumps, adenovirus infection, hepatitis, and Epstein-Barr virus infection have also been associated with arthritis.

A common cause of aseptic arthritis and limp in children is so-called transient synovitis of the hip. Pain is usually mild and is exaggerated by abduction and internal rotation, which is therefore limited. Radiographs, blood count, and sedimentation rate are usually normal. If bone age is delayed Legg-Calvé-Perthes disease should be considered. Rarely neuroblastoma may appear in a similar fashion. Sickle cell anemia and salmonella osteomyelitis should be considered in black patients. With fever and elevated sedimentation rate, joint fluid should be obtained. Technetium scan may be helpful in Legg-Calvé-Perthes disease, osteoid osteoma, and osteomyelitis. An occasional child with transient synovitis develops Legg-Calvé-Perthes disease.

ARTHRITIS ASSOCIATED WITH
SYSTEMIC DISORDERS

Musculoskeletal pain about a joint suggestive of arthritis has been associated with leukemia, neuroblastoma, Hodgkin's disease, histiocytosis, and rhabdomyosarcoma. The joint may be warm and swollen. Pain is usually severe and not responsive to aspirin. Radiographs are often normal at onset. Adenopathy and hepatosplenomegaly may be present. Anemia is often associated. The sedimentation rate is frequently elevated. Ulcerative colitis and regional enteritis may appear with transient arthritis and ankylosing spondylitis. Arthritis may precede the bowel symptoms by years.

Osteomyelitis

Osteomyelitis is a pyogenic infection in bone usually hematogenous in origin, which affects the metaphysis of the long bone and is often due to *S. aureus*. *Haemophilus influenzae* and *Streptococcus pyogenes* are less common isolates. *Salmonella* is more common in the patient with sickle cell anemia. The epiphyseal plate of growing bone usually prevents its spread to the adjacent joint space. The infected limb is painful and immobile. Osteomyelitis is more frequent in boys, which presumably relates to activity and trauma. Although any bone may be affected, the distal femur, proximal tibia, distal radius, distal humerus, and calcaneus are the most common sites. Determining the responsible organism and thus the most effective antibiotic is done through direct aspiration. Radiographs are not usually diagnostic until several days after onset, with subperiosteal new bone formation and spotty rarefaction being the first radiologic signs. Bone scans show abnormality at a much earlier stage. White blood cell count is typically elevated with a left shift. The elevated sedimentation rate can serve as an index of severity.

Prompt, effective antibiotic therapy is essential for a successful outcome. Therapy includes 1 to 2 weeks of an intravenous, high-dose regimen followed by oral therapy until there is clinical response and evidence of healing. No response in the first 48 hours warrants consideration of surgical exploration and drainage. Patients with neglected osteomyelitis may develop irreversible bone necrosis, draining sinuses, and limb deformity.

Dysplasia

Dysplasia is abnormal skeletal growth that results in disproportionate short stature or deformity. Dysostoses are malformations of individual bone or bones. Clinically short stature can be classified as disproportionate, associated with skeletal dysplasias or dysostoses, or proportionate, associated with maturational, nutritional, endocrine, and chronic disease problems. If a child's height is three standard deviations below or above the mean the possibility of a dysplasia should be considered. Family history and prenatal, natal, and postnatal growth history are important. Other defects, such as renal, immunologic, cardiovascular, ophthalmic, and hearing disorders, may be the first suggestion of a dysplasia. Management is dependent on exact diagnosis and includes appropriate orthopedic care, recognition of skeletal

and nonskeletal complications, rehabilitation, genetic counseling, and psychosocial support for parents and patients. Little People of America is a lay group helpful in providing support.

EPIPHYSEAL DYSPLASIA

The characteristic abnormality in epiphyseal dysplasia is poorly developed epiphyses with delayed, irregular, or multiple centers of ossification and associated arthritis. There is a tendency to generalized ligamentous laxity resulting in genu varum or valgum, pronated feet, pes planus, and higher incidence of joint dislocations and scoliosis. The basic defect involves collagen and therefore affects soft tissue as well as bone.

Multiple Epiphyseal Dysplasia. Multiple epiphyseal dysplasia is a milder form that appears with stippling in the large globular epiphyseal cartilages. Stippling at the ankle is especially marked and characteristic. There is a defect in the primitive vascular mesenchyme that affects the development of the primary ossification center. These so-affected children resemble achondroplastic dwarfs at birth, but later vascularization corrects some of the longitudinal growth. General improvement over time is apparent. Congenital cataracts are seen in these children about 50% of the time, which is typical in mucopolysaccharide (MPS) disorders.

Spondyloepiphyseal Dysplasia. Spondyloepiphyseal dysplasia (SED) is a more severe form that is typified by Morquio's disease, or osteochondrodystrophy. Soft tissue abnormalities occur as well as bone abnormalities. Corneal clouding is common, as it is in all MPS disorders. The diagnostic feature in Morquio's disease is keratosulfate spill in urine. Clinically the face and skull appear normal, but the neck and trunk are short, and the chest is typically pigeon type. Severe genu valgum is common. Muscle tone is poor. Lower-extremity spasticity and coxa vara deformity are common. Children with SED usually appear normal at birth, with changes becoming apparent in the first few years of life.

PHYSEAL DYSPLASIAS

The basic defect in physeal dysplasias is in the proliferating cartilage of the physis.

The classic prototype is achondroplastic dwarfism. The epiphyses are normal. Hydrocephaly and vertebral stenosis with paraplegia are occasional complications. The bones of the extremities are shortened. The metaphyses are flared because the subperiosteal bone at the metaphyses develops normally. Because of lack of growth at the physis, the epiphysis tends to invaginate into the flared metaphysis. The physeal dysplasias include achondroplastic dwarfism, Marfan's syndrome (hyperchondroplasia), multiple enchondromatosis (Ollier's disease or dyschondroplasia), MPS I (Hunter's syndrome), and MPS II (Hurler's syndrome).

DIAPHYSEAL DEFECTS

Few dysplasias affect the diaphysis alone. Such dysplasias include osteogenesis imperfecta congenita and osteogenesis imperfecta tarda, which represent a basic collagen defect. Other syndromes that reflect defects in the connective tissue include Marfan's syndrome, homocystinuria, and Ehlers-Danlos syndrome.

MISCELLANEOUS DYSPLASTIC SYNDROMES

Talipes Equinovarus (Clubfoot). Fixed clubfoot is one of the most complex deformities facing podiatric surgeons. Clubfoot represents a disruption of complicated interrelationships among bone, ligament, and muscle. The incidence is 1.2/1000 live births, rising by 20-fold when there is an affected first-degree relative. Males are more at risk, with a ratio of 3 to 1. Of cases, 50% are bilateral. Clubfoot may be congenital or acquired, flexible or rigid. The rigid (intrinsic) type is more common, and its prognosis for conservative correction is poor. The flexible (extrinsic) type is a mild reducible deformity. The rigid type usually requires surgery for complete correction. Congenital forms may also be associated with spina bifida, arthrogryposis, and congenital bone anomaly. Clubfoot may be acquired secondary to a neuromuscular disorder or after trauma. Treatment should begin in infancy and includes manipulation, casting, and subsequent surgery when indicated.

Congenital Rocker-Bottom Foot. Congenital rocker-bottom foot is usually as isolated deformity but can be seen with a number of autosomal abnormalities. The forefoot is dorsiflexed, while the rearfoot is markedly plantarflexed, causing a severe subluxation at the midtarsal joints. The axis of the talus is nearly at right angle to the axis of the calcaneus. In a clubfoot, the axes of the two bones are nearly parallel. A rocker-bottom foot may follow improper casting for a clubfoot. Early treatment is necessary for success in restoring normal function to the foot. Surgery is usually necessary.

Tarsal Coalition. During the first 4 weeks of embryonic life, the tarsal bones form. Failure of segmentation in a given area results in a tarsal coalition. The foot is flat and pronated and, in the adult or teenager, may be held rigidly by the peroneals and cannot be passively inverted, hence the term peroneal spastic flatfoot. The foot may be painful. The coalition may be osseous or cartilaginous. Decreased subtalar joint motion is compensated for by hypermobility of the talonavicular joint. Radiographs show early spurring or fusion of the subtalar joint in the area of the sustentaculum. Surgery is necessary.

Apert's Syndrome (Acrocephalosyndactyly). Apert's syndrome is associated with polydactyly and syndactyly of the digits in both upper and lower extremities. Double hallux deformity is commonly seen. Typically these so-affected patients have a high forehead, prominent eyes, and mental retardation. "Mitten" hand and foot (syndactyly) are common. Cases are sporadic in nature.

Klippel-Feil Syndrome. In patients with Klippel-Feil syndrome, the scapulae are undescended bilaterally, and a failure of segmentation of the cervical spine is present, causing a shortening of the neck and pterygium colli. There may be an associated scoliosis or kyphosis and occasionally a neurologic deficit.

Arthrogryposis Multiplex Congenita (Amyoplasia Congenita). In patients with arthrogryposis multiplex congenita, subluxation of joints is common with associated hypoplasia of muscle. There is characteristic webbing across the antecubital space. On radiograph, the bone is frail and resembles osteogenesis imperfecta tarda. Clubhands are common. The hips are flexed and rotated internally. Joint motion is restricted, secondary to primary abnormal muscle development or anterior horn cell defect.

Down's Syndrome. A dysplasia occurs related to an autosomal abnormality, trisomy 21. Facial features classically include an epicanthal fold, thick lips, large tongue with deep furrows, and small nose with broad bridge. The neck is short and broad. The hand shows clinodactyly of the fifth finger. The middle phalanx is hypoplastic. Syndactyly and polydactyly are not infrequent. Classically there is a single transverse palmar crease (simian line). Joints are hypermobile. There is wide spacing between the first and second toes. Snowflakelike spots appear on the periphery of the iris (Brushfield's spots). There are many associated skeletal anomalies, such as lateral flare of the periphery of the ilium, decreased acetabular angle, dysplastic pelvis, dislocated hips, and pectus excavatum. Congenital heart defects are also common, and leukemia occurs more frequently.

Diseases of the Spine

Problems in the spine in children may be primary or part of a generalized skeletal abnormality. Diseases of the spine are usually manifested by deformity, pain, or both. Congenital anomalies produce deformity that usually progresses with growth.

SCOLIOSIS

Scoliosis is a lateral deviation of the spine that can be divided into structural, nonstructural, and idiopathic types.

The *nonstructural type* is secondary to underlying pathology, such as leg-length discrepancy, dislocated hip, and polio. Vertebral anatomy is not altered, and there is no rotation of the spine.

Structural scoliosis is the most common spine deformity, occurring in about 6 in 1000 individuals, with 85% of cases idiopathic. Congenital defects, neuromuscular disease, and unilateral muscle disease may be causes. Structural scoliosis may also be associated with neurofibromatosis, fractures, radiation, and rib excision. Diagnostic features are elevation of the shoulder on the convex side, fullness of the waist suggesting protruding hip, and rib humping with forward bending. Patients with a progressive structural curve greater than 20° need treatment. The rate of progression varies greatly, and treatment is based on the rate. Early diagnosis and treatment is very important because one cannot make

the curve better, but one can prevent progression with appropriate bracing. Once growth centers have fused, the curve rarely progresses.

Approximately 90% of cases of idiopathic scoliosis affect females with a familial history. Thoracic curve is apparent with apex to the right. In patients with both lordosis and scoliosis, early fusion may be indicated because bracing is ineffective.

Kyphoscoliosis is a combination that occurs in patients with congenital defects, neuromuscular disease, and neurofibromatosis. Progression is rapid, and early treatment is important.

SPINA BIFIDA

Spina bifida is characterized by defects in the fusion of the lamina of the neural arches that usually occur in the lumbosacral or cervical region. There may be protrusion of spinal membranes or cord tissue (myelomeningocele). In spina bifida occulta, a hairy patch may be found over the defect. Associated defects of the spine are common.

Trauma: Growth Plate and Epiphyseal Injuries

EPIPHYSEAL FRACTURES

Salter and Harris describe five types of epiphyseal injury with prognosis relating to type. Types I and II have a generally good prognosis and fortunately are the most common. Type I is a separation of the epiphysis from the metaphysis by a shearing force through the degenerative zone of the growth plate. Type II is essentially a type I fracture with a fracture of a portion of the metaphysis. The most common sites are the distal radius, distal tibia, and distal fibula.

OSTEOCHONDROSIS

All bones may be affected in osteochondrosis. Etiology appears to be primarily related to trauma or vascular disturbance. Primary osteochondrosis involves the primary center of ossification, and secondary osteochondrosis involves the secondary center of ossification. Pathology demonstrates three stages: edema of the intra-articular and periarticular soft tissue; impaired blood flow; and bone necrosis, repair, and healing. Patients present with similar symptoms regardless of area involved, including pain, limp, and joint derangement or deformity.

Legg-Calvé-Perthes Disease (Coxa Plana). Legg-Calvé-Perthes disease involves avascular necrosis of the capital femoral epiphysis. This disease is more common in boys. Of cases, 10% are bilateral. Patients may present with groin, thigh, and knee pain. Limp is antalgic in type, with abductor lurch and flexion deformity. Limitation of internal rotation and abduction is apparent. Treatment involves relieving muscle spasm to allow internal rotation and abduction, which keeps the femoral head covered in the acetabulum, followed by early weight bearing.

Osgood-Schlatter Disease. Osgood-Schlatter disease, or osteochondrosis of the tibial tubercle, is a tendonitis of the distal patellar tendon. Osgood-Schlatter disease is usually found in adolescence and affects boys more often than girls. Main symptoms are pain, on local pressure and after exercise, involving the quadriceps tendon. Radiographs show irregular ossification of the tibial tubercle and poor definition of the patellar tendon. Treatment is immobilization for 6 to 8 weeks and gradual resumption of full activity over another 6 to 8 weeks. Untreated, this tendonitis frequently heals, but occasionally avulsion of the patellar tendon may occur. The hypertrophic cartilage may ossify to form a large mass. Some workers believe the primary defect is the result of calcification in patellar tendonitis. Genu recurvatum and upriding patella are rare complications.

Sever's Disease. Sever's disease involves the posterior apophysis of the calcaneus and results in local pain on walking or on tension of the triceps surae. This disorder is common in the prepubescent boy. The child walks with an equinus gait. Radiograph shows a widening of the space between the apophysis and calcaneus. An internal padded heel lift ($\frac{1}{2}$- to $\frac{3}{4}$-inch) is usually adequate treatment. In severe cases, a walking cast for 4 to 6 weeks with the foot in slight equinus may be necessary.

Köhler's Bone Disease. Köhler's bone disease is osteochondrosis of the tarsal navicular. This disease is most common in 3- to 6-year-olds. Local pain, swelling, tenderness, and limp are present in the acute phase. Pain is aggravated by putting the posterior tibial tendon on stretch. Radiographs show proximal-distal narrowing of the bone. A soft arch support and an $\frac{1}{8}$-inch inner heel wedge may be adequate. In severe cases a short leg cast may be necessary.

Freiberg's Disease. Freiberg's disease is osteochondrosis of the head of the second metatarsal. This disease is most common in adolescence. There is localized tenderness and pain and pain on movement of the metatarsophalangeal joint. A $\frac{3}{8}$-inch metatarsal arch pad may be adequate. Occasionally resection of the metatarsal head is necessary.

Neuromuscular Disorders

The majority of neurologic disorders of childhood are nonprogressive, but they become increasingly evident as the rest of the central nervous system develops or as they affect related structures or cause complications, such as hydrocephalus. The multiplicity of anatomic defects in the brain and spinal cord are beyond the scope of this text. A pediatric or neurology text should be referred to for this information.

Cerebral Palsy

Cerebral palsy is a nonspecific term that describes a group of disorders. The disorders are secondary to a static, nonprogressive brain lesion and are manifested by spasticity and abnormal movement. Associated nonmotor disabilities include:

1. Speech defects (75%)
2. Retardation (50%)
3. Perception difficulties and behavior problems
4. Seizures (30%)
5. Heart impairment (25%)
6. Visual defects (50%)

The incidence of cerebral palsy is approximately 1 case in every 1000 live births. Cerebral palsy is usually congenital or perinatal in onset. Small-for-gestational-age babies are at higher risk, but most cases occur in full-term infants. It is not clear whether modern intensive neonatal care has significantly changed the incidence.

Periventricular damage from hypoxia or hemorrhage produces a spastic diplegia, predominantly affecting the lower extremities. Kernicterus due to hyperbilirubinemia is a decreasing cause of cerebral palsy. The primary involvement in kernicterus is the basal ganglia, resulting in an athetoid dystonic disorder. Cerebellar malformation, of unknown cause, results in an ataxic cerebral palsy.

Spastic cerebral palsy is the most common type. Diagnosis prior to 1 year of age may be difficult. Hypotonia can be assessed by measuring the degree of abduction of the hips with the knees extended. Bilateral abduction to a total of 160° or unilateral abduction to 80° is unusual and suggests hypotonia. Two helpful reflex evaluations include an asymmetric tonic neck reflex and a persistent crossed extensor reflex persisting beyond 4 months. The reflex is elicited by irritating one foot with the leg extended. The contralateral foot withdraws and then extends, abducts, and adducts. Sustained clonus is abnormal. Abnormalities in tone, primitive reflexes, and deep tendon reflexes should arouse suspicion. In establishing diagnosis, it is necessary to rule out a progressive disorder, which should be suspected if there are sensory abnormalities; absent or decreased deep tendon reflexes; skin abnormalities, such as café au lait spots; eye abnormalities, such as cataracts and optic atrophy; abnormally enlarging head; hepatosplenomegaly; and any other evidence of systemic disease. Persistent toe walking may also be an early sign of muscular dystrophy.

As soon as the diagnosis of cerebral palsy is established, the child should be referred to a cerebral palsy center for coordinated treatment. The goal is to attain the best function possible with the least possible treatment. As Dr. Eugene Bleck, children's orthopedist, Stanford University, has pointed out, "All too often children with cerebral palsy have been overmedicated and overtreated. They have a lifetime of treatment rather than a life. The goal is to help establish a person not a permanent patient."

Examining a spastic child for motor development should clarify what the child can do, how he or she does it, and what he or she cannot do. Treatment is based on the child's motor abilities. Motor training follows a normal developmental sequence. The next skill should be aided while the preceding one is being developed. Methods should be adapted to the individual child and should include nonmotor skills and consider social and emotional development. The main aspect in preventing deformities is appropriate physiotherapy and daytime management. Carrying a spastic child may aid or inhibit progress but should be discouraged if a child can walk at all. Deformities of the feet may be helped with below-the-knee supports. Back straps prevent plantar flexion, and T straps prevent pronation or supination. A child with cerebral palsy may progress remarkably if given appropriate therapy.

Muscular Dystrophies

Muscular dystrophies are characterized by progressive degeneration of certain groups of skeletal muscles and are frequently hereditary. A number of different forms have been distinguished on clinical and genetic grounds. Muscular dystrophy is the commonest cause of muscle disease in childhood.

DUCHENNE'S MUSCULAR DYSTROPHY

Duchenne's muscular dystrophy, a so-called childhood type of dystrophy, occurs in about 1 in 7500 children. Duchenne's muscular dystrophy essentially occurs only in boys. The disorder is X-linked in 50% of patients and represents a new mutation in the other 50%. These so-affected children appear to be normal in the early years, with clinical suggestion usually evident in the preschool or early school years. Duchenne's muscular dystrophy manifests as difficulty climbing stairs and a waddling gait. The calves appear large but are weak secondary to fatty infiltration. Contracture of calf muscles and weak anterior leg muscles lead to toe walking. Weakness of pelvic muscles causes the waddling gait and difficulty arising from a reclining position (Gower's sign).

Although the child may have been thought to be normal for several years, careful developmental history usually reveals delayed motor development from infancy. With progression, delayed upper limb girdle development also becomes evident. Cardiomyopathy develops in the majority of patients. Most affected children die around age 20.

Diagnosis is dependent on the clinical

picture confirmed by measurement of creatine phosphokinase (CPK) level, which is markedly elevated in early disease and may be evident even in utero. The carrier mother may also have elevated CPK level. Electromyography shows decreased amplitude and duration of motor unit potentials. Biopsy specimen reveals degeneration of muscle fibers and replacement by fat and connective tissue. There is no effective treatment. Ambulation should be encouraged as long as possible.

Becker's Muscular Dystrophy

Becker's muscular dystrophy is a milder form of sex-linked recessive muscular dystrophy.

Limb Girdle Dystrophy

Limb girdle dystrophy appears in later childhood or in early adult life. The pelvic girdle muscles are most affected. This disorder has autosomal-recessive inheritance.

Myotonic Dystrophy

Myotonic dystrophy was previously considered to be a disease of adult life, but it is now realized that onset in childhood is not uncommon. This disorder differs from the other muscular dystrophies not only in the presence of myotonia but also in the widespread involvement of other tissues. Both males and females are affected, with autosomal-dominant inheritance. The face and neck muscles are characteristically involved. Distal limb weakness may also be present. Other features include cardiac involvement, cataracts, testicular atrophy, and adrenal dysfunction.

Neurocutaneous Syndromes

The ectodermal dysplasias are often not evident at birth. Lesions involve both the skin and the central nervous system, plus a variety of other organs.

Neurofibromatosis (Von Recklinghausen's Disease)

In patients with neurofibromatosis, café au lait spots, neurofibroma, osteofibrosa cystica, and multiple central nervous system lesions occur. Sarcomatous degener-

ation may occur in the neurofibromas. Neurofibromas may need to be excised to relieve pressure. Longevity relates to malignant degeneration or expanding intracranial lesions.

Tuberous Sclerosis

Fibroadenomas of sebaceous glands, café au lait spots, depigmented spots, hemangiomas in viscera, bone cysts, nodules, and calcifications in the brain are typical in patients with tuberous sclerosis. Mental retardation and seizures are common.

Sturge-Weber Syndrome

Sturge-Weber syndrome is characterized by a trigeminal-distribution port-wine stain involving skin, skull, and meninges. Mental retardation is common. Focal seizures may occur.

Ataxia-Telangiectasia

In patients with ataxia-telangiectasia, gamma A immunoglobulin (IgA) deficiency is associated with frequent infections. Mild retardation and ataxia are typical.

Brain Tumors

Over three fourths of brain tumors affecting children are gliomas, and most are in the posterior fossa. Headache, head enlargement, and papilledema constitute the most common triad. Headache occurs freqently in the morning at onset. Ataxia, nausea, and vomiting may be associated. These findings may also be associated with venous sinus thrombosis, central nervous system infections, subdural hemorrhage, and brain abscess.

Neuromuscular Junction Disorders

Myasthenia Gravis

Myasthenia gravis is more common in girls and can develop at any age. The onset is usually gradual, with ptosis, strabismus, difficulty in chewing, loss of facial expression, and arm weakness being common manifestations. Tight heel cords are present in severe cases. Usually there is no atrophy. The weakness is variable and characteristically induced by fatigue. The diagnosis is confirmed by showing prompt improvement after an intravenous injection of edrophonium. Treatment involves the use of long-acting anticholinesterase drugs, such as neostigmine.

MYOTONIA CONGENITA (THOMSEN'S DISEASE)

Myotonia congenita is characterized by persistent muscular contraction after voluntary stimulation ceases. Atrophy develops with time (myotonia atrophica). Cataracts, baldness, and generalized atrophy of endocrine glands are also present. Quinine may relieve symptoms, but they increase with exposure to cold. Local contraction occurs with percussion. There are no sensory abnormalities, and the persistent contraction is not evident on passive movement.

FAMILIAL PERIODIC PARALYSIS

Familial periodic paralysis is characterized by recurrent episodes of transient weakness of muscles of the trunk and extremities that lasts about 24 hours. Reflexes are absent. Potassium and carbon dioxide combining power is lowered at the time of the attack. An attack usually follows the ingestion of large amounts of carbohydrates and is relieved by administration of potassium.

MISCELLANEOUS CAUSES OF NEUROMUSCULAR JUNCTION DISORDERS

Myoneural junction dystrophy also occurs in botulism and in magnesium and manganese poisoning; with some snake venoms; and from eel toxins.

Floppy Child Syndrome

Floppy child syndrome is a term used to describe children who have marked hypotonia. These children are floppy but not weak. A useful test is to hold the baby or child in ventral suspension. Paralytic causes include neuromuscular disorders, spinal cord lesions, and birth trauma. Nonparalytic causes include brain disorders, such as cerebral palsy, degenerative central nervous system disease, and Prader-Willi syndrome; chromosomal disorders, such as Down's syndrome; systemic dis-

orders, such as malnutrition, congenital heart disease, hypothyroidism, rickets, and hypercalcemia; connective tissue disorders, such as osteogenesis imperfecta; and benign hypotonia.

Limping

Limp is described as an exaggeration or deficiency in one or more of the components of normal gait. Abnormal gait may be further described as painful (antalgic) or painless (Table 15–8). A limp is an imperfect action of a limb through injury or defect.

Evaluating gait involes separate and combined examination of the lower extremities, pelvis, and trunk during locomotion. Normal gait can be altered in different ways through pain, neuromuscular paralysis, spasticity, ataxia, limb-length discrepancy, loss of supporting structures, and contractures (Table 15–9). Limp should always be considered to reflect serious disease until proven otherwise.

The history is essential. Birth history, development, past medical history, trauma, family history, recent immunizations, and thorough history of present illness should be included. The physical examination should begin with a routine evaluation prior to extremity and gait evaluation. The type of limp gives significant clues to etiology, and further likelihood is suggested by the patient's age. In evaluating, one may approach the limp from the standpoint of underlying presentation and evaluate for the disease process that fits that pattern.

Infectious Diseases

Viral Infection

MEASLES (RUBEOLA)

Measles is a common viral disease, with about a 10-day incubation period followed by a prodromal illness with fever, coryza, conjunctivitis, and cough. Generalized lymphadenopathy may be found with Koplik's spots on the buccal mucosa. After 3 or 4 days, a typical maculopapular skin eruption appears, spreading downward from the head to cover the whole body. High fever is common. Treatment includes

Table 15–8. THE CHILD WHO LIMPS

Etiologies	Gait
Pain (antalgic)	*Hip:* tries to avoid weight bearing, shortens stance phase, plantarflexes foot, externally rotates, avoids propulsion *Knee:* ankle plantarflexes, knee in flexion with no extension during push off, short stance phase, no lurch *Ankle:* foot planted flat, everted, externally rotated, short stance phase, no push off *Subtalar/Forefoot:* short stance phase, no propulsion, heel walks or walks flatfooted, supinates
Neuromuscular (paralytic)	*Gluteus Maximus:* loss of truncal stability, falls forward; forces patient to try to keep center of gravity behind hip *Gluteus Medius:* Trendelenburg gait; chief abductor, cannot feel contracting muscle *Quadriceps:* extends knee, noticeable limp; hand on thigh at heel strike, push backward to lock knee in extension; external rotation, prevents knee flexion, tilt forward *Hamstring:* genu recurvatum without significant limp *Achilles Tendon:* weak; *calcaneous gait,* external rotation, pronation in propulsion, rise of pelvis on affected side, to clear foot in swing; *dropfoot gait* from dorsiflexion loss in foot and ankle; raise leg higher in swing; toes strike, then midfoot and heel (steppage gait)
Upper motor neuron lesion	Hypertonicity, with taking over by stronger muscle groups; usually see adduction, internal rotation, hip flexion, slight knee flexion, ankle and foot in equinus
Limb-length discrepancy	Pelvis tilts down to affected side; if less than 3.5 cm normal leg, foot pronates, short leg foot supinates; if greater than 3.5 cm, walks with foot in equinus on affected side; flex hip and knee
Flexion contractures	At hip, knee, or both, in effect shortens extremity; if hip, cannot extend, results in abnormal anterior pelvic tilt in swing, posterior tilt in stance; if knee, does not fully extend at propulsion

keeping the patient well nourished and hydrated and isolated in a darkened room if photophobia is present. Symptomatic treatment is also required. Complications include measles, encephalitis, and secondary infection (otitis media, bronchopneumonia, corneal ulcers, stomatitis, gastroenteritis, and appendicitis). Measles vaccine is widely used in First World countries, where the disease is now rarely seen.

RUBELLA, OR GERMAN MEASLES (THREE-DAY MEASLES)

Rubella is an acute infectious disease that resembles both scarlet fever and measles, but it differs in its short course, slight fever, and lack of sequelae. Incubation is 14 to 21 days, with eruption of a maculopapular rash that vanishes in 2 to 3 days. The prodrome is slight or absent and includes drowsiness, slight fever, sore throat, and eruption on day 1 or 2. Treatment is nonspecific, with use of a local antipruritic for itching, rest, liquid diet, and sponging with tepid water. The importance of this disease lies in the devastating effect on the developing fetus in the pregnant woman, especially in the first and second trimesters. Immunization against rubella has markedly reduced this problem.

CHICKEN POX (VARICELLA)

Chicken pox is a mild, highly contagious disease marked by an eruption of vesicles on skin and mucous membrane and caused by the same virus that produces herpes zoster. The characteristic eruption makes its appearance in successive crops, passing through stages of macules, papules, vesicles, and crusts. Chicken pox may occur at any age but is less common in the adult. Three fourths of children have had chicken pox by age 15. Average incubation is 17 days, with a slight elevation of temperature at onset, followed by appearance of skin eruptions within 24 hours.

Complications are uncommon in healthy children. Encephalitis is rare and is usually cerebellar. The child presents with ataxia 3 to 8 days after the onset of the rash. At least 80% of patients make a complete recovery. Other complications include secondary infection, erysipelas, septicemia, and pneumonia. Children with immune deficiency, especially those being treated for leukemia or those receiving steroids, may develop a very severe form of the illness. Prognosis is favorable except in the very severe type of varicella gangrenosa.

Treatment consists of keeping the patient isolated for 7 days after first crop of vesicles, controlling scratching, keeping

Table 15–9. SUMMARY OF TYPES OF LIMP

Age (Yr)	Antalgic	Paralytic	Short Leg	Contracture	Loss of Support
Birth–4	Trauma, infection	Cerebral palsy, spinal muscular atrophy, spina bifida, hemiatrophy	Congenital, coxa vara, CHD, infection	Spina bifida, cerebral palsy, CHD, infection	CHD, trauma, coxa vara, spina bifida
5–10	Trauma, infection, rheumatoid arthritis, Legg-Calvé-Perthes disease, hemophilia, transient synovitis	Cerebral palsy, spina bifida, muscular dystrophy, polio	Spina bifida, trauma, CHD, infection, rheumatoid arthritis	Trauma, CHD, Legg-Calvé-Perthes disease, infection, rheumatoid arthritis	Trauma, polio, infection, muscular dystrophy
11–14	Trauma, synovitis, slipped capital femoral epiphysis, infection, Osgood-Schlatter disease	Muscular dystrophy, polio, peripheral nerve trauma, CNS neoplasm, ischemic contracture	Infection, trauma, slipped capital femoral epiphysis, neoplasm	Infection, trauma, Legg-Calvé-Perthes disease, slipped capital femoral epiphysis	Trauma, slipped capital femoral epiphysis, inadequate treatment, CHD

CHD, Congenital heart disease.

fingernails short and clean, administering calamine lotion locally, and administering trimeprazine (Temaril) orally for severe itching. A vaccine is being tested and should soon be released. Aspirin should not be given to a child with chicken pox because of the association of varicella, aspirin, and Reye's syndrome.

HERPES

The term herpes indicates a vesicular eruption caused by a virus, herpes simplex or herpes zoster.

Herpes Simplex. Herpes simplex is an infectious disease caused by herpes simplex virus and characterized by thin-walled vesicles that tend to recur in the same area of the skin, usually at a site where the mucous membrane joins the skin. In newborn infants, meningoencephalitis or a panvisceral infection may occur. Infants become infected during pregnancy or delivery by a maternal genital herpes infection (type 2) or less commonly by a type 1 virus in the postnatal period. Mortality is about 70%, with a high morbidity rate among the survivors. Cesarean section must be considered in the mother with active vaginal herpes at the time of delivery. Less than 10% of children with primary infection become clinically ill. Close personal contact is required for transmission of the disease. Primary infection may affect the mouth, skin, and eyes. Infection is characterized by high fever; swelling and bleeding of the gums; and extensive ulceration of the buccal mucosa, tongue, and palate, with cervical lymphadenopathy. The illness lasts about 10 to 14 days. Eating and drinking is painful. Keratoconjunctivitis is inflammation of the cornea and conjunctiva with ulcers of the cornea that may lead to scarring and loss of vision. Primary infections tend to develop in older children with eczematous skin and at trauma sites. Recurrence of lesions is variable and is associated with respiratory infections and nonspecific factors, such as exposure to sunshine, menstruation, and emotional stress. Herpes simplex virus may cause generalized infection in malnourished children or immunodeficiency. Herpes simplex is a relatively common cause of meningoencephalitis in normal children, with a high mortality rate. The electroencephalogram and brain scan demonstrate a "space-occupying lesion." A rising titer of antibody in the blood or cerebrospinal fluid confirms the diagnosis.

CYTOMEGALOVIRUS INFECTION

Cytomegalovirus produces a mild disease in adults. The disease is widespread in the community, with many pregnant women carrying the antibodies to CMV. Infection in the early part of pregnancy can cause abortion or a spectrum of malformations, including growth failure, microcephaly, cerebral calcifications, cataracts, cardiac lesions, deafness, epilepsy, and mental disability. Infection in late pregnancy may result in systemic illness, with purpura, hepatosplenomegaly, pneumonia, and encephalitis. The infection in the mother often goes undetected. The presence of virus in the urine of the newborn and rising CMV-specific immunoglobulin M (IgM) antibody confirm the diagnosis.

Bacterial Infection

SCARLET FEVER

Scarlet fever is an acute contagious disease characterized by sore throat, strawberry tongue, fever, and punctiform scarlet rash. Scarlet fever results from an erythrogenic toxin produced by group A streptococci. After an incubation period of 1 to 4 days, the child develops tonsillitis, fever (38.3° to 40.5°C [101° to 105°F]), headache, and malaise, with the rash appearing within 12 hours of onset and rapidly becoming generalized. The face is spared, but the cheeks are flushed and indeed scarlet. Convulsions may occur in the very young. The tongue has a thick white coating through which inflamed papillae project. This is known as the white strawberry tongue, which peels by day 4 or 5, leaving a red strawberry tongue. The rash disappears in a few days, sooner if penicillin is given. Scarlet fever may follow tonsillitis, burns, and infection of wounds. The treatment of choice is administration of penicillin, which leads to a rapid recovery. A 10-day course is necessary to eradicate the streptococci. Management should include isolation from time of diagnosis to 1 day after beginning antibiotic therapy, with bed rest during the acute phase. Complications include rheumatic fever and acute glomerulonephritis.

Mycoplasma Pneumonia

Several bacteria of the *Mycoplasma* genus, which are found in the human and have been called pleuropneumonia-like organisms (PPLOs), have been proved to be the cause of primary atypical pneumonia. This pneumonia affects older children, particularly those between 5 and 15 years of age, and produces a wide range of respiratory tract infections. The patient presents with generalized malaise, anorexia, headache, fever, and sore throat, followed by a cough producing mucoid sputum that may be blood tinged. The chest radiograph shows diffuse pneumonia. Treatment in children is administration of erythromycin.

Chlamydia Trachomatis Infection

Chlamydia trachomatis results in a common sexually transmitted disease. This pathogen causes vaginitis, cervicitis, and pelvic inflammatory disease and may be a major cause of infertility. A more virulent strain causes lymphogranuloma venereum. From 7 to 12 days after exposure, a vesicle similar to the herpetic lesion appears, usually on the genitals. The vesicle ruptures and heals, with regional lymphadenopathy appearing in 1 to 8 weeks. The enlarged, tender, sometimes suppurative glands are called buboes. The buboes heal and leave scars, sometimes scarring and obstructing lymph channels. Diagnosis is usually by clinical findings. Of cases of nonspecific urethritis, 50% have been found to be associated with this bacteria-like organism. Treatment is with tetracycline. Sex partners should also be treated.

COMMON PODOPEDIATRIC PROBLEMS

Neonatal Lower-Extremity Problems

Lower-extremity problems occur in about 5% of newborns. These problems can generally be divided into those resulting from abnormally formed tissue (malformation), usually of genetic or teratologic etiology, and those resulting from normal tissue that has been altered by external forces, such as uterine constraint, to produce an abnormal structure (deformation). The most common lower-extremity deformations include hip dislocation, bowing of the leg, knee dislocation, metatarsus adductus, overriding toes, calcaneovalgus, and talipes equinovarus. Constraint occurs late in gestation as the fetus occupies much of the uterine cavity. Constraint is more common with first-borns, large babies, multiple fetuses, breech position, and lack of amniotic fluid. Dr. Dennis Browne described fetal constraint as a cause of birth defects and alluded to their amelioration by conservative methods. It is not the purpose of this chapter to further describe these conditions, their diagnoses, and managements, which can be found in numerous pediatric, podiatric, and orthopedic texts.

Congenital Hip Dislocation

Early detection of congenital hip dislocation is essential to ensure a simple course of treatment and excellent outcome. Genetic influences and familial joint laxity make girls more susceptible than boys. Unilateral cases are more common than bilateral, with infants born by breech more at risk. Ortolani's sign, a palpable clunk produced when the hips are slowly abducted with knees flexed and externally rotated through a 90° arc, is used as a screening test. The dislocated hip slips back into the acetabulum during external rotation and abduction. A variety of splints are used to retain the femoral head in the acetabulum until normal relationship has developed. The Pavlik harness is the splint most commonly used.

Talipes Equinovarus (Clubfoot)

See discussion of clubfoot previously in this chapter.

Developmental Flexible Flatfoot

Developmental flexible flatfoot is the most common flatfoot in children. The significance of this finding is argued by orthopedists and podiatrists, with orthopedists minimizing its importance. In classic flexible flatfoot, no serious structural defects are present. Laxity of joint capsules and plantar ligaments is the probable etiologic factor. Weight bearing causes medioplantar flexion of the head and neck of the talus, calcaneal eversion, and forefoot abduction. Most children with flexible flatfoot are asymptomatic and remain so. Restriction of motion, pain, and calcaneal eversion exceeding 10° justify further evaluation. A long list of diagnostic possibilities includes calcaneovalgus; vertical talus; tarsal coalitions; neuromuscular disorders such as cerebral palsy; syndromes, such as Ehlers-Danlos syndrome, Marfan's syndrome, and Morquio's disease; transverse plane abnormalities; limb-length discrepancy; equinus; and forefoot varus. Severe deformity may lead to early degenerative arthritis. Appropriate diagnosis is necessary. Shoe gear is a satisfactory approach in flatfoot with calcaneal eversion exceeding 10°. Surgery is indicated only rarely.

Torsional Problems

Tibial torsion is the most common cause of in-toeing gait. In 1979, the subcommittee on Torsional Deformity of the Pediatric Orthopedic Society recommended a classification system that addressed the problem of defining torsional and angular problems. Comparable definitions had been defined previously by Thomas Sgarloto, DPM, in 1971.

Orthopedists define version as the normal angular difference between the transverse axis of each end of a long bone and torsion as abnormal version. Podiatrists define torsion as abnormal twist in bone and version as deviation of the extremity on the transverse plane related to soft tissue rather than bone. Measurement methods for the various levels of torsional deformity are outlined in most orthopedic or podiatric texts. A variety of treatment devices have been employed, including twister cables, rotation bars, derotation casts, torque heels, and shoe wedges. Medial rotations usually correct spontaneously. The indications for use of these treatment devices are debatable.

Sleeping posture may sustain a torsional abnormality. For deformities persisting beyond 18 months, a night splint is reasonably indicated. If treatment is delayed until the patient is 3 years old significant correction is unlikely. Similar deformity in a parent is an added indication for early treatment. Pediatric orthopedists believe femoral antetorsion can be treated only surgically. Pediatric podiatrists feel derotational casting is effective.

Metatarsus Adductus

Metatarsus adductus is the most common of the major foot deformities, occurring in 1 in 1000 births with no sex distinction. Causes include abnormal in utero position, short or absent medial cuneiform, heredity, spastic or tight abductor hallucis muscle, and abnormal medial insertion of the tibialis anterior or abductor hallucis muscle into the first metatarsal. Clinically the foot is C shaped, with a concave medial border and a convex lateral border. The prominent styloid process of the fifth metatarsal may become irritated and inflamed by shoes. Metatarsus primus varus, a widened first interdigital space, may or may not be present. Mild metatarsus adductus is treated with passive stretching and shoe therapy. If metatarsus adductus is rigid or associated with tibial torsion, serial casting may be indicated followed by a night brace with straight-last shoes. Shoe modifications have generally not been proved effective in treating these torsional conditions, but they prevent excessive pronation while spontaneous resolution occurs.

Angular Deformities

Angular deformities include coxa vara, genu valgum (knock-knee), and genu varum (bowleg). Bowlegs and knock-knees, unless excessive, represent normal development, and most resolve spontaneously. Genu varum is normal in the first 2 years, followed by a stage of genu valgum up to about 7 years of age. A mild valgum occurs again during the adolescent growth spurt. A varus deformity persisting beyond 2 years with a tibiofemoral angle on radiograph of 20° or greater or a valgus deformity with a tibiofemoral angle of 15° or greater beyond age 7 is abnormal. Such deformity may be associated with congenital deformity, trauma, infection, endocrine or metabolic diseases, and tumors, and appropriate studies should be made. Unilateral or asymmetric involvement suggests a pathologic defect.

Blount's Disease (Osteochondrosis Deformans Tibiae)

Blount's disease results in severe genu varum. Cause is uncertain, but Blount's disease probably represents medial tibial epiphyseal deformity due to early, excessive weight bearing in a child with marked physiologic tibial bowing. Osteotomy may be necessary if bracing prior to age 2 years is unsuccessful.

Genu Valgum

Genu valgum is normal between 3 and 5 years of age. Genu valgum may persist or become excessive (>15° tibiofemoral angle) because of abnormal forces across the knee secondary to obesity, pronated feet, laxity of the medial collateral ligaments of the knee, and abnormal development of the lateral femoral condyle. Pathologic genu valgum does not usually improve with bracing or shoe modifications. If genu valgum presents a cosmetic problem medial femoral epiphyseal arrest or osteotomy is indicated.

Leg Aches

Aching pain in the lower extremities is a common childhood complaint. Aches vary from mild to severe and are commonly referred to as "growing pains." This is a misnomer but an accepted term because it has been in common use for so many years. There are many causes of lower-extremity pain in childhood and one must not overlook serious disease while passing off the symptoms as "growing pains." Lower-limb pain can be classified etiologically as shown in Table 15–10.

PREOPERATIVE AND INTRAOPERATIVE MANAGEMENT OF THE PEDIATRIC PATIENT

History

History and physical examination are the most important parts of the preoperative evaluation. A history should be taken as noted previously, carefully documenting the chief complaint and present illness, but in addition, particular attention should be paid to family history; family and patient histories of allergies; drug sensitivities; recent drug therapy, such as with steroids or antibiotics; and medications currently taken. Prolonged use of steroids, for instance, may interfere with healing, and withdrawal before surgery can cause adrenal collapse.

Family history or personal history of bleeding problems, arrhythmias, and prolapsing mitral valve should be noted. Meperidine (Demerol) given as a pain medication or sedative may trigger paroxysmal

Table 15–10. LOWER-LIMB PAIN: ETIOLOGIC CLASSIFICATION

Traumatic: fractures (stress, pathologic), dislocation, subluxation, sprain, joint strain, contusions, hemorrhage, myositis, periostitis, synovitis, cysts, hemarthrosis
Infection: osteomyelitis, septic arthritis, soft tissue abscess, cellulitis, lymphadenitis
Avascular necrosis of bone
Vascular
Congenital
Developmental
Tumors
Collagen disease
Growing pains

---

tachycardia in those patients who are susceptible. It should also be noted whether there have been any anesthetic reactions in the family. For example, acetylcholinesterase breaks down succinylcholine, which is a muscle relaxant. A deficiency in this enzyme allows for build-up, causing apnea. This genetic defect occurs in 1 in 3000 patients and is a serious operative problem. Family history of malignant hyperthermia should be noted, and the anesthesiologist should be notified. Constant temperature monitoring is done on the patient during surgery. A muscle biopsy may be helpful in diagnosis prior to surgery.

One should note recent exposure to respiratory illnesses, particularly contact with croup, influenza, and colds. A history of asthma, asthmatic bronchitis, or wheezing in the child, with the most recent episode and treatment rendered noted, is an essential part of the preoperative history.

Other infectious disease exposure may be significant enough to delay surgery. An example is chicken pox, which can have disastrous results if it occurs following the surgical insult of anesthesia. Considerably more pox may occur in surgical lesions, so one should delay elective surgery in a child who has had chicken pox contact until the incubation period has passed. The incubation period averages 17 days, but one should allow a minimum of 21 days following contact. A patient's immunization status should be clarified, and immunizations should be brought up to standard if they are not current (Table 15–11).

The dietary history or any history of a recent weight loss or gain should be noted. No elective surgery should be performed on a patient who is in poor nutritional status. In children, teeth should be examined for dental caries and missing, loose, and capped teeth, and the anesthesiologist should be informed.

For patients with gait problems, a more extensive history is indicated. If history or general observation suggests the possibility of genetic or systemic disorders a more extensive history is also indicated.

Clinical Evaluation

After an adequate history is obtained, the physician can proceed with clinical evaluation. The podiatric examinations on pediatric patients involve the lower extrem-

Table 15–11. PEDIATRIC IMMUNIZATIONS

Immunization	Recommended Age
DPT*, polio†	2 mo/yr
DPT, polio	4 mo/yr
DPT	6 mo/yr
Booster (DPT and polio)	18 mos and 5 yr
Hib‡	18 mo/yr
MMR†,§	15 mo/yr
Td (adult)‖	15 yr and every 10 yr thereafter

 * Diphtheria, pertussis, tetanus. Pertussis is not given with history of convulsions, neurologic damage, or close family history of epilepsy.
 † Should not be given to children with immune-deficiency states or children receiving steroids or cytotoxic drugs.
 ‡ *Haemophilus influenzae* type B.
 § Measles, mumps, rubella.
 ‖ Tetanus and diphtheria toxoid.

ities, with particular attention to the foot and ankle, including evaluating pulses, screening neurologic examination, observation of the spine in both standing and forward-bending positions, and gait evaluation. In patients undergoing hospitalization for surgery with general or local anesthesia, a complete physical examination should be done by the podiatrist even though a consultation examination for surgical clearance is done by the patient's general physician. Children under 1 year of age are generally happy and easy to examine. Children between 1 and 4 years may reject strangers, although most are still cooperative. From age 4 on, most children are curious and cooperative. With a child who is fearful, a reasonable examination can usually be done on the mother's lap, where the child is more secure. As the patient approaches puberty, respecting modesty is important, and appropriate clothing or covering is necessary. For infants and young children, appointments should be timed so that the child arrives after being fed and not due for a nap. Appointments should be scheduled so that prolonged waiting is unnecessary. Clothing should be appropriate so that gait can be observed with extremities and spine visible and the child is not embarrassed to walk down a hallway. For example, a sunsuit for girls and gym shorts or a swimsuit for boys is appropriate.

A general physical examination of the pediatric patient is not significantly different from that of the adult, but the sequence may be altered. In the apprehensive child, one should listen to the heart and the lungs, feel the abdomen, and observe gait before proceeding to other parts. The approach to preoperative examination is discussed more extensively previously under Pediatric History and Examination.

Physical Examination

A general physical examination should be done in children just as in adults, with particular attention paid to vital signs, including temperature, blood pressure, pulse, and respiration. The skin should be meticulously examined for any sign suggesting systemic disorders. Any signs of upper respiratory infection or asthma that might preclude surgery should be noted. In children, teeth should be carefully examined to note any evidence of loose teeth, and the anesthesiologist should be alerted.

One should look for evidence of congenital anomalies, which may be associated with aberrant anatomy elsewhere. One should therefore review variations in anatomy in the site in which one is planning to operate. Cardiac evaluation should include rate, rhythm, any evidence of murmurs or abnormal second sounds, and the suggestion of a mitral prolapse syndrome. If any abnormality is suspected, cardiac consultation should be obtained prior to surgery.

Abdominal examination should begin with observation, noting whether the abdomen is scaphoid (sunken) in nature, suggesting cachexia, or distended, as may occur with obesity, intestinal distention, and intra-abdominal masses. The bowel should then be auscultated, noting the absence of peristalsis or the presence of high-pitched hyperperistalsis. The abdomen should be gently palpated, starting in the left lower abdomen and proceeding to the left mid and upper areas and then to the right upper, mid, and lower sections. Any evidence of organ enlargement, masses, and tenderness should be noted, and guarding or rebound should be observed. Hepatomegaly, if evident, should be evaluated by liver function testing. Children in the first several years may normally have a palpable liver edge, which is sharp and nontender. The spleen tip may also be palpable in infancy and early childhood. If the spleen tip is felt careful palpation for gen-eralized lymph node enlargement should be done, the blood count carefully noted, and the blood smear evaluated for the presence of adequate platelets.

Peripheral pulses should be palpated, comparing the upper-extremity pulses with lower-extremity pulses and noting blood pressure to detect any suggestion of coarctation. Genitalia should be examined externally to note any deviation from normal. All four extremities should be examined to note symmetry, muscle mass, ranges of motion of joints, and strength of major muscle groups. The back should be examined in the standing and bending-forward positions to exclude scoliosis.

Cranial nerves should be tested, including funduscopic examination. Deep tendon reflexes for major muscle groups should be elicited. Sensations should be noted for touch, temperature, pain, and vibration. Cerebellar tests should include finger to nose, heel to shin, and stance on one leg. Heel walking, toe walking, hopping on one foot, and regular gait should be noted.

Any other examination or testing indicated by findings on the aforementioned observations should then be done, and appropriate consultation should be requested.

Laboratory and Diagnostic Studies

Generally in children, preoperative laboratory studies need only include a standard CBC and urinalysis. Any underlying medical disorder or physical findings, however, may indicate the need for additional studies. In children, normal laboratory figures are often significantly different from those in adults and should therefore be compared with childhood standards (Table 15–12).

Complete Blood Count

Increased hemoglobin or hematocrit (polycythemia) is usually secondary in children and is uncommon except in the newborn infant, in whom it is physiologic. Anemia is usually related to chronic blood loss (normocytic, normochromic) or iron deficiency (microcytic, hypochromic). Once the diagnosis of iron deficiency ane-

Table 15-12. PEDIATRIC VALUES FOR LABORATORY STUDIES

	Infants	Adolescents	
		Male	**Female**
Erythrocytes	4 million/mm^3	4.2–5.4 million/mm^3	
Hemoglobin*	>11.5	>13	>12.5
Hematocrit	>34	>40	>38
Leukocytes	8000–12,000/mm^3	5000–10,000/mm^3	

	Birth	**3 Months**	**6 Months**	**1 Year**	**15 Years**
Hemoglobin	16	9.5	10.5	11	12.5 + –14 +
Mean Cell Volume	95–115	80–90	70–85	75–90	80–100

Hemoglobin: Grams per 100 ml blood; hematocrit usually equals 3 times the hemoglobin. In children, the normal value varies with age.

Hematocrit: The volume of packed cells per 100 ml of blood; varies with age.

If these evaluations are made at an altitude greater than 6000 feet one can add 1 g of hemoglobin to the figures for each 6000 feet of additional altitude.

mia is established, anemia should be treated with 3 mg/kg/day of elemental iron for a period of 3 months. Macrocytic anemia is rare in children. An elevated WBC count in children (>12,000) (leukocytosis) is associated with infection, hemorrhage, trauma, mild proliferative disease, leukemia, poisoning, stress, and exercise. An elevated WBC count also occurs following epinephrine injection.

Increased band forms with leukocytosis (shift to left) implies infection. Leukocytosis is more suggestive of bacterial infection. Lymphocytosis in younger children, less than 5, may occur in bacterial disease, whereas in viral disease, counts above 15,000 have been noted.

Leukopenia (WBC count below 5000) occurs in viral infections; in overwhelming bacterial infections; in association with drugs, such as chloramphenicol (Chloromycetin); in aplastic anemia; and in bone marrow depression. Leukopenia with counts below 4000 and lymphocytes predominating may also occur in overwhelming bacterial disease. A so-affected child usually looks seriously ill.

Urinalysis

Urinalysis should include measurements of protein, glucose, pH, blood, nitrites, bilirubin, and WBCs by dip stick or microscopy and culture when indicated. An excess of protein (1+ = 30 mg/dl; 2+ = 100 mg/dl) in an afternoon specimen with no other abnormality is compatible with orthostatic albuminuria. Red blood cells always appear abnormal until further evaluated and explained. White blood cells in the first 10 mm^3 of urine in a male suggest urethritis even if the patient is asymptomatic.

Sedimentation Rate

Sedimentation rate demonstrates increases in gamma globulin. A normal range for sedimentation rate is 10 to 20 mm/hour (0 to 10 mm/hour in the child and man and 0 to 20 mm/hour in the menstruating woman). Elevation above normal is an indicator of disease and is related most commonly to infection, collagen vascular disease, and malignancies. Normal sedimentation rate, however, does not always rule out serious disease.

Electrolyte and Liver and Renal Function Panels

Electrolyte and liver and renal function tests are done to evaluate liver and renal functions and are not routinely indicated. Alkaline phosphatase is normally elevated in children compared with adults and is particularly high during the adolescent growth spurts. The electrolyte panel is done to evaluate potassium levels only when indicated. Metabolic acidosis is an indicator of inadequate perfusion.

Tests for Hemostasis

Hemostasis can be evaluated when indicated by the family or personal history by one of the following:

1. Rumpel-Leede test, which determines vessel wall integrity.
2. Platelet count.
3. Prothrombin time, which screens for bleeding secondary to liver disease in the extrinsic pathway.
4. Partial thromboplastin time, which tests for factors V, VIII, X, XI, XII, and XIII in the intrinsic pathway.
5. Bleeding time.

Tuberculin Skin Test

A tuberculin skin test is done prior to elective surgery if history or physical findings are suspicious. In any patient with suspected tuberculosis infection, diagnostic skin testing is essential as well as other appropriate tests, such as chest radiograph and sedimentation rate. The tine test is easy to store and apply.

Chest Radiograph

A chest radiograph is not indicated routinely and should be done only if indicated by history (asthma, cystic fibrosis, pneumonitis, chronic cardiac disease, or pulmonary disease) or physical findings.

If history or physical examination suggests any organic disease appropriate laboratory tests should be done. For example testing for sickle cell in black children should be done.

Fluid Balance

Fluid balance is a sensitive problem in infants and children. Oral fluids can be given up to 4 hours before surgery in infants and 6 hours before surgery in children up to 5 years of age. Adequate hydration is critical to stable anesthesia. For children over age 5, the usual withholding of fluids after midnight is acceptable. No milk or solids, however, should be given less than 12 hours prior to anesthesia. Any dehydration or acidosis should be corrected prior to anesthesia and significant blood loss replaced before surgery. Most podiatric surgery is elective, and children should be in optimum condition prior to it. Before and during anesthesia, fluids can be maintained in almost all pediatric patients via peripheral or scalp veins, and except in emergency situations, cutdown is not nec-

essary. In infants and children, blood volumes are small, approximately 80 mm^3/kg. Significant blood loss may be measured in ounces. For example, a 1-year-old, 10-kg child suffers a 10% decrease in circulating volume with only 80 mm^3 of blood loss. Pediatric patients should be operated on only in places where blood is readily available.

Medications

Drug safety and effectiveness in children are major problems. It is difficult to test drugs in children. Animal testing is not reliable, as the thalidomide experience points out. Studies in adults cannot be relied on to predict safety in children. The standard rules for drug dosage that have been used to extrapolate dosage according to age or weight (Clark's, Young's, or Friend's) are not reliable. Using surface area may be more accurate, but it is better to refer to standard pediatric references for specific dosage according to weight. Basic pharmacology and clinical experience are combined to determine safe dosage recommendations. Several aspects of physiologic activity determine drug efficacy, safety, and dosage, including (1) absorption, (2) distribution, (3) metabolism, (4) excretion, and (5) concentration at the site of action. These factors vary significantly with age and are not constant. In addition, dietary and behavior patterns vary throughout childhood and significantly alter drug responses. Water spaces and the ratio of lean mass to total weight also influence distribution. The characteristics of each drug also determine its distribution and function within the body. In general, drug metabolism is not as efficient in the infant and child. Some drugs, such as theophylline, can be measured in the serum and dosages correlated accordingly. Others are administered in fixed dosages based on clinical responses. In children, drug interactions and effects on growth, development, and body chemistry should be appreciated (Table 15–13).

Drug administration in children presents special problems related to flavor; food intake; vomiting; loose stools; relation of absorption of drug to food intake; complexity of dosing; and compliance, both in children who are taking medication and in

Table 15–13. DRUG INTERACTIONS AND EFFECTS ON GROWTH, DEVELOPMENT, AND BODY CHEMISTRY

Erythromycin: inhibits effect of theophylline
Phenobarbital: reduces effect of steroids
Sulfas: results in elevation of bilirubin
Tetracycline: stains teeth
Steroids: inhibit growth

parents who are administering it. A special concern in pediatrics is the use of drugs in pregnancy and their possible effects on the fetus. When one prescribes drugs to sexually active women of child-bearing age, one must consider the possibility they may be pregnant. The administration of a drug to a pregnant woman is also the administration of the drug to the fetus, as is the administration of a drug to a breast-feeding woman the administration of the drug to the infant. As a general rule, one should not give a breast-feeding mother drugs one would not give the child directly. Knowledge of drug crossover into breast milk is somewhat limited.

The proper use and appropriate selection of drugs rest on correct diagnosis in the patient. General principles in evaluating these agents, including physical, biologic, and chemical, relate to:

1. The ability of a substance to cross the placental barrier.

2. The dose of the agent.

3. A reproducible effect.

4. The assumption that all drugs may place the fetus at risk for malformation.

Drugs studied are given a standard relative risk (SRR), the ratio of the observed number to the expected number of defects. From studies, drugs with the greatest risk were (1) aspirin (SRR 6.2), associated with foot abnormalities; (2) boric acid (SRR 13.6), associated with cataracts; (3) diphenhydramine (SRR 29.6), associated with abnormalities of the diaphragm; (4) secobarbital (SRR 15.6), associated with aortic stenosis; and (5) iodides (SRR 11.1), associated with cataracts.

Hypothermia

Hypothermia is a critical concern in the pediatric patient, especially in the infant and small child. Hypothermia increases oxygen consumption and acidosis, depletes glycogen stores, and induces hypoglycemia and hypoxia. Temperature stability should be maintained, and this can be done by appropriate draping, overhead radiant heaters, and circulating warm water mattresses. Continuous temperature monitoring should be done. Malignant hyperpyrexia may follow inhalation anesthesia in children and represents an anesthetic emergency, which is another reason for constant temperature monitoring.

Anesthesia

Balanced local or general anesthesia should be administered by an anesthesiologist experienced with children. All patients should be constantly monitored for temperature, blood pressure by oscillometry, pulse, heart variations by ECG, oxygen by digital oximeter, and heart tones by precordial stethoscope. All patients should be under *constant* visual observation by the anesthesiologist. Podiatric patients are almost always in the first three classes according to the American Society of Anesthesiologists' scale of physical status: class 1, no organic, biochemical, or psychiatric disturbance; class 2, mild to moderate systemic abnormality caused either by the disease to be treated surgically or by another pathophysiologic process; and class 3, severe systemic abnormality of any cause.

Preoperative Psychologic Preparation

Surgery, minor or major, involves significant emotional and psychologic impact for the child or adolescent. One must consider age, developmental stage, personality makeup, and past history of the patient.

Infants, children, and preteen patients should be in a hospital setting with staffing experienced in pediatric care, especially for children with special needs. Children are different, and adult-oriented facilities are not always ideal for their care. Understanding and sympathetic recovery-room personnel are very important in dealing with these children. Hospitalization and surgery can be acutely traumatic to the child and may cause lasting emotional and behavioral problems. Every effort must be made to be sensitive to the needs of the child and adolescent. Properly handled, this experience can lead to an increased maturity for the family and child. The physician should always be honest with all information and should establish a trusting relationship with the child and parent. The child should be encouraged to verbalize concerns and to express emotion. Careful preparation of the family and child may alleviate many emotional stresses. A prehospitalization visit to the hospital may be a great help. It is advisable for parents to be present before and immediately after surgery.

School-Age Children

A child fears separation when removed from home, family, and friends. A child may have unrealistic fears and become very anxious, not realizing what surgery means or what to anticipate. One should allow simple communication and capitalize on interest and curiosity. The physician should always be honest in answering questions. It may be very helpful to have a favorite toy present. Young children are better prepared psychologically for surgery by their parents, after having been instructed by a physician. Timing is important. In a small child, psychologic preparation should be done only hours before surgery, and in the preschool child, hours to days.

Adolescents

An adolescent may show fear, aggression, and irrational behavior. An adolescent may lack self-esteem and have a fragile body image. An adolescent may fear multilation, pain, and talking under anesthesia. One should spend adequate time in discussing the need for the surgery and what the operation entails. Asking what one can do to make the operation easier for the adolescent may help ease him or her. Common fears should be addressed directly. Teens and preteens may be better prepared psychologically by the doctor. Timing is important. In the adolescent, psychologic preparation is appropriate days to weeks prior to surgery.

POSTOPERATIVE MANAGEMENT

Evaluation

Following surgery, vital signs, including temperature, should be monitored until the patient is stable. Urine output should be noted, and the patient should be weighed daily. Constant airway observation is necessary because infants and children are more prone to subglottic edema. If this edema occurs it may be reduced by aerosolized 0.2% racemic epinephrine. Once stable, the child can leave the recovery room, but constant observation is necessary. Atelectasis is a potential problem, and the stimulation to breathe deeply or to cry in the infant, or instruction to blow against resistance using standard apparatus (tri-flow) if the child is old enough, is indicated. Humidity may also be helpful in the patient who is croupy following intubation. Oxygen is seldom necessary and is drying. Humidity reduces water loss; however, significant fluid may be absorbed, causing overhydration, especially if intravenous fluid is being simultaneously administered. Until a child has recovered sufficiently from anesthesia to take oral fluids, intravenous infusion should be maintained, following standard precepts for fluid electrolyte and acid-base balance, which can be found in standard pediatric texts. Most pediatric patients are able to tolerate oral feeding in less than 12 hours, starting with sips of 5% glucose or juices when stable and then half-strength formula to regular formula or milk within 8 hours. If liquids are tolerated the patient may proceed to soft foods, such as rice, applesauce, squash, and soups, and if those are tolerated to regular foods within 24 hours. A major risk to infant and child is postoperative vomiting, hence the need for constant visual observation and immediate availability of suction equipment.

Podiatric Postoperative Medication

The main need of postoperative medication in children is for pain relief or sedation if the patient is agitated (Table 15–14). Routine use of antibiotics postopera-

Table 15–14. COMMON DRUGS USED IN PEDIATRIC PODIATRY

Local Anesthetics (Injectable)*

Lidocaine (Xylocaine) 1%: up to 4.5 mg/kg/
  dose without epinephrine
Mepivacaine 1% (Carbocaine): 5 mg/kg
Procaine: proportional to weight, surface
  area

Barbiturates (Preoperative Sedation)

*Low-Dose Barbiturates (Potentiate All
Depressants)*

Fast-Acting: Secobarbital (Seconal): 2–3
  mg/kg PO (may repeat in 3 hrs)
  Pentobarbital (Nembutal): 4 mg/kg PO
Medium-Acting: Amobarbital: 2–3 mg/kg
  PO (may repeat in 3 hrs)
Long-Acting: Phenobarbital: 2–3 mg/kg
  PO†

Relaxants or Sedatives (for Procedures)

Promethazine (Phenergan): 1 mg/kg up to
  50 mg IM, PO, or suppository
Diphenhydramine (Benadryl): 1–2 mg/kg
  PO or IM
Phenobarbital: 2–3 mg/kg PO
Hydroxyzine (Atarax): 1.5 mg/kg IM or PO
Diazepam (Valium): 0.2 mg/kg PO up to
  10 mg
Secobarbital: 2–3 mg/kg PO
Chloral hydrate (Noctec): 15–25 mg/kg PO
  to 1 g

Analgesics

Mild Pain: Acetaminophen (Tylenol) or
  aspirin: 60–80 mg/yr of age up to 400
  mg
Moderate Pain: Codeine: 0.5 mg/kg q 4 hrs
Severe Pain: Meperidine (Demerol): 1 mg/
  kg q 4–6 hrs PO or IM
  Morphine: 0.2 mg/kg q 4–6 hrs IM or IV
  up to maximum dose of 15 mg

Antipruritics

Mild: Local treatment: Calamine lotion,
  witch hazel
Moderate–Severe: Local plus oral
  treatment:
  Diphenhydramine: 5 mg/kg/day q.i.d.
  Hydroxyzine: <6 yrs old: 20–40 mg/day
  q.i.d.; >6 yrs old: 50–100 mg/day
  q.i.d.
  Cyproheptadine (Periactin): 2–5 yrs old:
  2 mg q 8–12 hrs; 7–14 yrs old: 4–5
  mg q 8 hrs

Antibiotics

Penicillin V potassium: 125–250 mg PO
  q.i.d. 7–10 days
Aqueous Penicillin: 10 mg/kg q 6 hrs IM or
  IV
Erythromycin: 10 mg/kg; up to 250 mg q 6
  hrs or 400 mg b.i.d. PO for 7–10 days
Dicloxacillin: 7.5 mg/kg/day up to 25 mg/
  kg q 6 hrs 1 hr after meals for 10 days
Methicillin: 200 mg/kg/day q 6 hrs IM or
  IV
Vancomycin: 20–40 mg/kg/day q 6 hrs IV

Antihistamines

Promethazine: 0.5 mg to 1 mg/kg up to 50
  mg PO, IM, or by suppository
Diphenhydramine: 1–2 mg/kg PO

Antianxiety Agents‡

Hydroxyzine (Atarax, Vistaril): 1.5 mg/kg
  IM or PO
Diazepam: 0.2 mg/kg PO up to 10 mg
Chloral hydrate: 15–25 mg/kg up to 1 g

Antipyretics

Aspirin: Low Dose: 30 mg/kg/day; Medium
  Dose: 60 mg/kg/day; High Dose: 90
  mg/kg/day§
Acetaminophen (antiinflammatory): Low
  Dose: 30 mg/kg/day; Medium Dose:
  60 mg/kg/day; High Dose: 120 mg/kg/
  day‖

Antiemetics¶

Promethazine: 1 mg/kg up to 50 mg PO,
  IM, or suppository
Dimenhydrinate (Dramamine): 1 mg/kg PO
  or rectally (may repeat in 6 hrs)
Phosphorated carbohydrate solution
  (Emetrol): children, 1–2 tsp q 15 min
  up to 5 doses; adolescents, 1–2 tbls q
  15 min up to 5 doses

---

  * Do not use bupivacaine (Marcaine) in children <12 yrs old.
  † May produce a paradoxic excitement in children.
  ‡ One may use antianxiety agents to decrease narcotic needs.
  § Associated with Reye's syndrome and should not be used in patients with influenza or
chicken pox virus or unknown viral infection.
  ‖ Potential liver toxicity.
  ¶ Prochlorperazine (Compazine) should be used with caution in children.
  b.i.d., Twice a day; IM, intramuscularly; IV, intravenously; PO, by mouth; q.i.d., four times
a day.

tively is not indicated. Antibiotics should be chosen for specific clinical reasons and after suspected infected sites have been appropriately cultured. Tetracycline, which is seldom a first-line drug, stains teeth and may affect bone growth. In infants and young children, the decision to use antibiotics, choice, and dosage would be best reviewed with the child's general physician. The field of antibiotics in children is in constant change.

Drugs Used in Children With Podiatric Problems

When using local anesthesia in children, it is imperative to adhere to safe dosage levels and to use the smallest dose effective in achieving the desired anesthesia. Bupivacaine (Marcaine) should not be used in children under 12 years of age. Relaxant or sedative drugs may be used for local procedures or casting. In most circumstances, however, these drugs are not necessary. In some children, excitation may occur rather than sedation.

Analgesics should be selected with the same precaution one would use with adults. However, there is a tendency to undertreat the child with significant pain because he or she may not verbalize the degree of pain. Careful clinical judgment is required to determine the drug need and potency. Aspirin or acetaminophen (Tylenol) usually suffices. Aspirin is a better anti-inflammatory agent. Aspirin and acetaminophen do not add to each other's toxicity and may be given alternately to achieve greater analgesic effect.

If mild pruritus should occur, local treatment with cool compresses, calamine lotion, or witch hazel (Tucks) may be helpful. Antihistamine-containing lotions, such as Caladryl or Zyradryl, which are potential skin sensitizers, should not be used. Moderate to severe itching can be managed most effectively with local therapy plus oral therapy, such as diphenhydramine (Benadryl), hydroxyzine (Atarax), and cyproheptadine (Periactin), which are all supplied as a syrup.

Preoperative antibiotics are generally not indicated, but any procedure involving an infected surgical site may be treated prophylactically.

General Principles Regarding Pain Management

One should remember that pain is subjective, and one must individualize medications. Children often suffer quietly, and pain may be greater than is apparent. If there is reason to expect pain one may treat even if the child fails to complain. Pain medication should be given prior to the onset of significant pain when possible. Existing pain requires more medication than when the drug is given prior to the onset of pain. Severe pain seldom lasts more than 10 days following surgery. If pain lasts longer than 10 days careful evaluation of the wound site and the patient in general should be done and the need for medication established. One should analyze the problem at hand and use the fewest drugs, the lowest dose, and the shortest duration possible.

Bibliography

Apgar V: A proposal for a new method of evaluation of the newborn infant. Curr Res Anesth 32:360, 1953.

Avery MD, Taeusch HW, Jr: Schaffer's Diseases of the Newborn, 5th ed. Philadelphia, WB Saunders Co, 1984.

Browne D: Congenital deformities of mechanical origin. Arch Dis Child 30:37, 1955.

Committee on Drugs—Section on Anesthesiology Guidelines for the Elective Use of Conscious Sedation, Deep Sedation and General Anesthesia in Pediatric Patients. Pediatrics, 76:317, 1985.

Golbus MS, Holzgreve W, Harrison MR: Direct intrauterine treatment of the fetus. Gynakologe 17:62, 1984.

Heinonen OP, Slone D, Shapiro S: Birth Defects and Drugs in Pregnancy. Littleton, Mass: Publishing Sciences Group, 1976.

Jackson LG: First-trimester diagnosis of fetal genetic disorders. Hosp Pract 20:39, 1985.

Jacob L: Pharmacologic properties of antibacterial agents and their clinical usage. J Am Podiatr Med Assoc 75:132, 1985.

Kaback MM, ed: Medical Genetics. Pediatr Clin North Am 25:3, 1978.

Kaplan EB, et al.: The usefulness of preoperative laboratory screening. JAMA 253:3576, 1985.

Korsch BM, Aley EF: Pediatric interviewing techniques. Curr Probl Pediatr 3:1, 1973.

Kunin CM: Antibiotic accountability (Editorial). N Engl J Med 301:380, 1979.

Levin R: Personal communication.

Pagliaro L, Levin R (eds): Problems in Pediatric Drug Therapy. Hamilton, Ill: Drug Intelligence Publication, Inc, 1979.

Port M, et al.: Prevalence of Dermatologic Problems of the Lower Extremity, Part II. J Am Podiatr Med Assoc, 70:445, 1980.

Root M: Personal communication.

Rosenberg H: Malignant hyperthermia. Hosp Pract 20:139, 1985.

Salter RB, Harris WR: Injuries involving the epiphyseal plate. J Bone Joint Surg 45A:587, 1963.

Sgorlato TE: A Compendium of Podiatric Biomechanics. San Francisco: California College of Podiatric Medicine, 1971.

Shulman ST, et al.: Bacterial endocarditis. AJDC 139:232, 1985.

Stickler GB: Polypharmacy and poisons in pediatrics: The epidemic of overprescribing and ways to control it. Adv Pediatr 27:29, 1980.

Tax HR: Podopediatrics. Baltimore: Williams & Wilkins Co, 1980.

Wilson JG: Misinformation about risks of congenital anomalies. Prog Clin Biol Res 163:165, 1985.

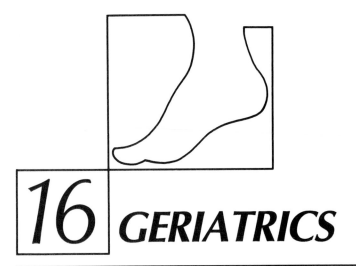

16 GERIATRICS

JAY LUXENBERG

OVERVIEW

An increasing proportion of the population in the United States is elderly, and this trend is expected to continue well into the next century. The oldest segment of the population, those in their 80s and 90s, is the fastest growing. The very old need and receive a disproportionately large amount of health care, and it is incumbent on the podiatric physician to acquire skill in treating this important group.

As we age, we tend to accumulate chronic illnesses. The average 65-year-old has 4 to 6 chronic illnesses, several of which no physician is aware (Table 16–1). Common chronic illnesses in the elderly include degenerative arthritis, hypertension, coronary artery disease, and diabetes mellitus. In addition, as part of normal aging, there are many physical, mental, and physiologic changes that are the inevitable consequence of living a full life span. These changes include decreased

Table 16–1. COMMON CHRONIC
COMPLAINTS* IN THE ELDERLY

Monoarticular and polyarticular pain
Coronary heart disease
Urinary tract infection
Falls
Urinary incontinence
Peripheral edema
Depression
Decreased visual acuity
Obesity
Hypertension
Diabetes mellitus
Confusion
Hearing deficit
Skin disease
Congestive heart failure
Dementia
Hip injuries
Constipation

* 4–6 per 65-year-old.

nerve conduction, decreased cardiac reserve, diminished hearing acuity, loss of muscle mass, and impaired ability to eliminate waste products and drugs from the body. These normal changes of aging combine with the frequent chronic illnesses to produce a state of limited homeostatic reserve. Any new illness or injury, including surgical procedures, must be considered with this altered milieu in mind.

PATHOPHYSIOLOGY

Aging is a universal phenomenon that proceeds at a far from universal rate. Persons of identical chronologic age who physically appear to be decades apart are a common sight. Varied rates of aging cause differences that are exaggerated as time passes; therefore, variability in most physiologic parameters increases with age. A group of 20-year-olds are much more similar to each other than are a group of 80-year-olds. For this reason, far more than chronologic age must be taken into account when evaluating an elderly patient.

Aging has long been a fascination of mankind. Some understanding of the mechanisms of aging has been achieved, but much remains unknown. Gerontology is the study of the aging process, and gerontologists use the tools of epidemiologists as well as those of cellular and molecular biologists.

Maximum Life Span

A useful starting point in attempting to understand the aging process is the concept of maximum life span. Maximum life span is species specific and genetically controlled and often differs dramatically from the average life span. For example, in the 20th century, the average or mean life span has increased by approximately 20 years, but the maximum human life span remains unchanged at about 110 years.

In animals, maximum life span is correlated with body size, fecundity, and sex. Some invertebrates can live only minutes. In mammals, maximum life span ranges from 1 year for a shrew to 70 years for an elephant, 80 for a whale, and more than 110 for a human. Females usually have longer life spans than those of males. Because maximum life span is a fixed characteristic of a given species, the parameter that determines average life span is the rate at which disease and trauma result in premature death. Human average life span has increased because hygiene and medical care have eliminated many childhood and early adulthood deaths. Maximum life span is programmed into the genetic mechanism. A major evolutionary advance was the development of cellular specialization. Germ cells needed the ability to direct the differentiation of multipotent cells into highly specialized cells and tissues. It is thought that this differentiation process forces finite constraints on cellular division and life span. Many well-differentiated, highly specialized cells lose their mitotic ability early in the development of the individual.

Cell Decline

Vital cell lines, such as nerve cells and heart muscle cells, lose their ability to divide. Such cells that are lost to injury or disease cannot be replaced. Evolution tends to conserve features that promote reproductive vigor. Most of the decline that accompanies aging occurs after the reproductive years are over. The same somatic cells and specialized tissues that add reproductive advantage in youth are subject to senescence and decline with age. The very specialization of these cells and tissues ensures their mortality.

The exact mechanism by which the aging process becomes manifest on a cellular and organ level is not known. Several theories have been developed, and it is likely that each will ultimately explain some of the changes that occur with aging (Table 16–2). Accurate transcription of DNA is essential for myriad functions of the postmitotic cell. Efficient mechanisms exist to allow repair of damage to DNA. Radiation, free radical formation, and chemical carcinogens may alter the integrity of DNA molecules. An age-related loss of repair ability could allow multiple genetic injuries to accumulate, leading to production of faulty enzymatic and structural proteins.

DNA is not the only long-lived cellular component subject to oxidative injury and cross-linkage. Cellular lipid components are oxidized to form the age-related pigment lipofuscin. This relatively inert waste product may accumulate to form a substantial fraction of the volume of brain and heart muscle cells, although the contribution of age-related pigments to the functional deterioration of such cells is unknown.

Clinicians have learned to take advantage of the slow nonenzymatic chemical reaction between blood glucose and the protein hemoglobin. This reaction is essentially irreversible, and its rate is proportional to ambient glucose. Because hemoglobin-containing red blood cells (RBCs) have a life span of 120 days, the content of glycohemoglobin reflects the average glucose concentration over that time period. This same nonenzymatic re-

Table 16–2. MAJOR THEORIES ON AGING: DNA "CULPRIT" OR DNA "VICTIM"

Programmed Aging

"Genetic clock"
Decreased DNA synthesis
"Death gene": hormone or enzyme

Extrinsic Damage

Transcription errors
Internal copying error affecting protein and DNA synthesis
Free radicals: cross linking; membrane damage
Immune system deterioration
Biological clock: neurohormonal regulatory clock
Accumulation of age pigment: lipofuscin

---

action, called the browning phenomenon when first described in baked bread, occurs in other long-lived body proteins. Crystallin, the human lens protein, forms cross links when glycosolated. Similar events have been postulated to account for the structural changes that occur in collagen with aging. In short, the nonenzymatically mediated irreversible protein alterations may accumulate, leading to profound structural and functional deterioration.

Organ Function Decline

The age-associated deteriorations observed on a cellular level are mirrored by functional decline of the body's organs and systems. This degeneration progresses at widely varying rates among individuals. Although the magnitude may differ, the changes are universal. Certain of the changes are clinically important, and the practicing podiatrist must be familiar with them.

Special Senses

Aging of the organs of special senses results in significant morbidity. Often awareness of these changes can lead to simple measures that dramatically increase the comfort of the patient.

VISION

The clear parts of the eye, including the cornea, lens, and vitreous humor, all lose transparency with age. The pupil gets smaller and responds less well to light and has less accommodation ability. These changes result in only about one third of the light reaching the retina of an aged eye compared with a young eye. Naturally this means the elderly are more sensitive to poor lighting conditions. The physical properties of the lens change, resulting in loss of accommodation ability with age. The lens continues to grow throughout life, narrowing the depth of the anterior chamber. This narrowing, along with decreased efficiency of intraocular fluid resorption, leads to an increased risk of glaucoma with age.

The aging eye is also subject to external changes. Periorbital fat is lost, lid tissue sags and becomes redundant, and tear secretion decreases. Arcus senilis is the lipid deposit that forms a gray-white ring at the outer edge of the cornea. In the elderly, this phenomenon has not been correlated with advanced atherosclerosis.

Several eye diseases are more common with age. Cataracts, diabetic hypertension retinopathies, and macular degeneration can all lead to visual impairment. These conditions are all alleviated with proper treatment; therefore, early diagnosis is important.

HEARING

Hearing changes with aging, called presbycusis, are inevitable. Presbycusis is predominantly manifested as a loss of high-frequency reception. Unfortunately the frequency of consonants is 2000 Hz and higher. This means that much of the information content of speech is lost in advanced presbycusis. Speech discrimination is more severely affected than pure tone threshold. Often the hearing loss is insidious, and the patient is unaware of its severity. Noise trauma that may have occurred during the patient's working years adds to the impairment.

OTHER SENSES

The senses of smell and taste are also dramatically altered with aging. Diminished taste is compounded by the use of dentures, common in the elderly, which also alters taste. Balance is decreased, with lessened ability to detect deviation from the upright position. It is unclear whether loss of sense of touch is also involved with aging decline.

Cardiovascular System

When considering organ function decline with age, it is important to realize that there are large functional reserves in our vital systems. Age-associated deterioration is often not clinically evident until the system is stressed. In the case of the heart, this functional reserve can be increased with physical training. Functional reserve wanes when physical conditioning is absent. For that reason, it is difficult to separate normal aging changes from changes that occur with inactivity.

The magnitude of conditioning changes may exceed those of aging. For example, an 80-year-old marathon runner may have a greater maximum cardiac output and oxygen consumption than a 30-year-old nonrunner with a desk job. An additional problem in determining age changes is that the changes are superimposed on disease processes. Hypertensive cardiac hypertrophy and atherosclerotic ischemic disease both increase in prevalence with age. When studying the very elderly, it is almost impossible to find subjects unaffected by some cardiac disease. Although carefully performed studies can minimize conditioning and disease as confounders, all data must be interpreted with these potential problems in mind.

As previously mentioned, the clinical manifestation of age changes is often a decline in ability to withstand the stress of exercise. The resting heart fulfills its function as a blood pump equally well in the young and old. With exercise, however, the older heart cannot beat as fast nor pump out as much blood with each heartbeat. Several factors contribute to this change. There is an age-associated loss of sensitivity to sympathetic neurotransmitters. The aged heart must also pump against an increased load because the aorta stiffens and the peripheral vascular resistance increases with age. Although these factors are thought to be quantitatively the most important contributions to diminished cardiac ability with age, there are additional factors. The myocardial cell enzymes that promote energy production have diminished activity in older hearts. Fibrotic and fatty degeneration of cardiac tissue can be observed.

Fibrosis commonly involves the specialized electrical conduction system of the heart, leading to decreased conduction. Often orderly cardiac contraction is impaired. Varying degrees of atrioventricular block are frequently found in older individuals. Spontaneous firing of the pacemaker cells in the sinus node is slowed, contributing to the increased sensitivity of the elderly to bradycardic side effects of many drugs.

The peripheral vasculature also changes with aging. In large arteries and the aorta, the elastic fibrils degenerate, diminishing the resilience of these vessels. Collagen stiffening and calcification also lead to vascular rigidity. On lateral chest radiograph, an uncoiled, dilated, and prominently calcified aorta is a frequent finding in old age. With concomitant vertebral osteoporosis, more calcium may be evident radiographically in the aorta than in the bones. The decreased distensibility raises systolic blood pressure and lowers diastolic pressure at any given systemic resistance, widening the pulse pressure. Total peripheral resistance rises with age and, with the loss in arterial elasticity, results in a disproportionate elevation of systolic pressure.

Respiratory System

The respiratory system also demonstrates physiologic and anatomic changes with aging. The lung tissue itself shows relatively minor changes. Respiratory bronchioles and alveolar ducts enlarge, and the alveoli decrease in absolute number and surface area. These changes resemble a mild case of emphysema. The major changes in pulmonary function result from a loss of lung elasticity and an increase in chest wall stiffness. This loss of elasticity and the accompanying increase in stiffness alter the dynamics of breathing, leading to more air remaining in the lungs at the end of maximal expiration. Total lung capacity does not change, so the vital capacity (total lung volume minus residual volume) also is diminished with aging. Respiratory muscles, similar to the other muscles of the body, weaken with age. Spirometrically measured indicators of ventilatory ability, such as peak flow, reflect this deterioration.

Musculoskeletal System

In evaluating the aging patient, we must recognize that motivation can be the key to health, and a significant factor is maintenance of adequate physical acitivity. In assessing the musculoskeletal system, our focus should be on what the patient can do and what the patient cannot do for himself or herself. This includes such self care activities as dressing, bathing, and safe ambulation.

Osteoporosis is a decrease in skeletal mass that is encountered frequently in women past age 50. Osteoporosis may clinically lead to shortened stature, kyphosis, and skeletal fractures. Many factors are considered in the etiology of postmenopausal and senile osteoporosis, including inactivity, hormonal or calcium deficiency, calcium loss, and inadequate protein nutrition. Smoking, alcohol use, and glucocorticoid steroid use are common contributing factors. Paget's disease is another bone disease of the elderly, more frequently seen in men past 40 than in women. Excess bone resorption and deposition characterize this disease and can result in severe skeletal deformities. Bone pain is the most common symptom. Fractures of the vertebrae and long bones may occur with disease progression.

It is inevitable that the elderly will also have joints with degenerative changes and pain (Table 16–3). The spine and most joints lose a little range of motion, while stretching of the ligaments allows a few other joints to become more mobile. Acute and chronic orthopedic problems are a major force in limiting the mobility of the elderly. The foot and ankle perhaps demonstrate the ravage of time like no other bones or muscles of the musculoskeletal system. Systemic disease frequently attacks the lower extremity (Table 16–4). Morbidity is significant and frequent.

Urinary System

The kidney also changes with age. Blood flow to the kidney lessens, and the number of functioning glomeruli drops. A predictable loss of approximately 1% per year in glomerular filtration rate occurs after age 20. The kidney also loses some of its ability to concentrate and dilute urine and is therefore less able to withstand the stresses of fluid or salt overload and dehydration. One practical manifestation of this change is that drugs eliminated by the kidney are often eliminated much less efficiently in the elderly.

Nervous System

The brain changes as we get older but fortunately only in very minor ways. Thought processes slow, and problem solving may take longer. Some neurons are lost, and other histologic changes are detectable. There is often some short-term memory impairment. No decline of intelligence is detected.

Table 16–3. ETIOLOGY OF MONOARTICULAR AND POLYARTICULAR JOINT PAIN

Monoarticular	Polyarticular
Septic joint	Osteoarthritis
Episodic RA	RA
Mechanical injury	Psoriatic arthritis
Tuberculous arthritis	Gonococcal arthritis
Chondrocalcinosis (pseudogout)	Cervical spondylosis
Gout	Arthritis of rheumatic fever
Serum sickness	Polymyalgia rheumatica
Charcot's joints	Collagen vascular disease
Inflammatory bowel diseae	SLE, ankylosing spondylitis
Occult tumors (lung, prostate)	Hypothyroidism
Osteoporosis	Acute hepatitis-B arthritis
Scleroderma	Polyarticular gout
	Reiter's syndrome

RA, Rheumatoid arthritis; SLE, systemic lupus erythematosus.

Table 16–4. COMMON LOWER-EXTREMITY PROBLEMS IN THE AGING

Corns	Burning	Hallux valgus	Night cramps
Calluses	Dry skin	Onychauxis	Tinea pedis
Onychomycosis	Loss of feeling	Onychocryptosis	Hammer toes
Bunions	Shoe problems	Plantar fasciitis	Mallet toes
Swelling	Ulcers	Metatarsalgia	Hallux rigidus
Varicosities	Equinus	Heel pain	Overlapping digits
Fat pad atrophy	Joint pain	Skin atrophy	

When severe cognitive impairment is present in an older patient, this is the result of a disease process, not normal aging. Alzheimer's disease, a mysterious degeneration of brain tissue, is the most common cause of dementia in the elderly. Incidence of Alzheimer's disease rises with advancing age, but it can occur at any time from early adulthood onward. Long-standing hypertension can result in a memory-destroying series of small strokes, called multi-infarct dementia. Myriad other genetic, toxic, metabolic, neoplastic, and traumatic diseases can result in cognitive impairment in the elderly. For this reason, the presence of mental impairment in an older patient should prompt thorough evaluation. Table 16–5 shows a useful mnemonic for potentially reversible causes of confusion in the elderly.

Table 16–5. CAUSES OF RECENT-ONSET CONFUSIONAL STATES IN THE ELDERLY

D —Drugs (prescription, OTC)
E —Emotional factors (depression)
M —Metabolic (hyponatremia, thyroid disease, hypercalcemia)
E —Eyes and ears (sensory impairment)
N —Nutrition (vitamin deficiency) and Normal pressure hydrocephaly (*rare*)
T —Trauma (subdural hematoma) and Tumors
I —Infection
A —Acute illness (heart attack, pulmonary emboli, stroke, CHF)

CHF, Congestive heart failure; OTC, over the counter.
(Adapted with permission from Lamy PP: Prescribing for the Elderly. Littleton, Mass: PSG Publishing Company, Inc, 1980.)

PRESENTING FEATURES

History

Obtaining a history and performing a physical examination on an elderly person can be a frustrating or a rewarding experience. A knowledge of the aging process and the use of certain techniques can facilitate the examination. Perhaps the most important factor is cultivating the useful but elusive virtue of patience. A frail patient may not tolerate an extensive interrogation and a rigorous physical examination. Fatigue may interfere with obtaining vital information toward the end of the examination. A useful practice when starting an examination of a frail older person is to begin by discussing the active complaint. As one discusses this complaint in detail, one should look for evidence of the patient's tiring. If the patient appears to be developing fatigue, the emphasis of the examination should be shifted to obtaining only the absolutely necessary information, such as medication use, drug allergies, and major diseases, and necessary tests, such as cardiac and pulmonary function tests. It is then imperative that one clearly records what has been learned at the session and obtains the remaining data at subsequent sessions. No one can fault a physician for doing an incomplete initial examination on a very frail person so long as the examination is satisfactorily completed on later visits. An elderly patient has had a longer time to acquire a history, and the physician should be comfortable having the patient recount this history over several sessions.

As previously mentioned, an elderly person may have a loss of ability to hear high frequencies. Speaking louder may only emphasize the lower frequencies and actually decrease the intelligibility of the voice. The secret in speaking to someone with this type of hearing loss is to speak more slowly rather than more loudly. Also one should face the patient when speaking to give visual cues to help the patient understand what is being said. Occasionally the hearing loss is severe enough to interfere with communication in spite of these techniques.

If the patient wears a hearing aid one should make sure the ear piece is clean, the battery is charged, and the aid is functioning and inserted in the ear. In the absence of a hearing aid, an inexpensive pocket-sized amplifier with earphone and microphone can dramatically help with communication. These portable amplifiers are available at most consumer electronic shops and are an excellent investment for professionals with large numbers of elderly patients. In a pinch, using a stethoscope, with the ear pieces in the patient's ears and the physician talking into the stethoscope head, can also be very useful.

The patient's visual impairment may also impede communication. A bright light source should be available to illuminate the physician's face while he or she is talking to the patient. If the patient wears glasses one should make sure the glasses are with the patient and worn when needed.

Because we are a nation of immigrants, in the United States many elderly patients do not speak English as a native language. If any language barrier exists a translator may dramatically improve the physician's ability to obtain a reliable history. An experienced translator may also help overcome cultural or educational factors that contribute to under-reporting of symptoms or otherwise inaccurate histories.

To obtain a useful history, one must be aware of the tendency of many older people to attribute a multitude of symptoms to aging. Forgetfulness, chest pain, shortness of breath, dizziness, and fainting spells are just a sample of the potentially dangerous symptoms that the patient may not volunteer because he or she considers them part of the aging process. Only by carefully inquiring about major symptoms system by system will the careful interviewer get the full clinical picture.

Cognitive impairment can also interfere with obtaining a useful history. Unfortunately evidence of memory impairment becomes more frequent with age. Significant impairment may be present in up to 20% of people over the age of 80. Perhaps nothing is more frustrating than taking the time to obtain a thorough history only to realize that the patient's poor memory makes its value doubtful. A useful technique is to start by asking some general questions to evaluate recent and distant memory. One should ask the patient's date of birth and address, information that can easily be confirmed with the patient's records. An inquiry as to whether the patient follows current events can easily lead to some questions that may reveal quality of recent memory. For a more elderly patient, one can ask, "What was the most recent holiday?" If any doubts arise concerning the patient's cognitive ability the physician should immediately administer any one of the brief mental status tests that have been developed to quantitate mental impairment in the elderly (Table 16–6). One of these tests should be part of the routine neurologic examination in the elderly. Administration of the mental status test can be moved up to the beginning of the history when evidence suggests mem-

Table 16–6. MENTAL STATUS TEST FOR DETECTING COGNITIVE IMPAIRMENT

Introduce self at the beginning of examination.
1. What is your name?
2. What day of the week is it today?
3. What is the year?
4. What is the month?
5. What is the date?
6. What city are we in now?
7. What is my name?
8. If I bought an item for 45 cents, and I gave the clerk a dollar, how much change am I owed?
9. Count backwards from 10.
10. Subtract 3 from 30; keep subtracting from what's left until you are left with zero.
11. Name ten different colors.
12. Remember these 4 items, so you can repeat them to me later: *train, boy, typewriter, orange.*
13. Repeat these items to me now.
14. What is larger, an elephant or a lion?
15. What is the opposite of *hot*?
16. What is the name of the current president of the United States?
17. Who was the president before him?
18. What were the 4 items I asked you to remember?
19. Write a sentence. (Must have a noun and verb.)
20. Read this. (Write: *The boy gave an apple to his teacher.* Remove sentence from view.)
21. What gift did the boy give?
22. To whom did he give it?
23. Spell *world* backwards.

ory impairment to avoid unproductive inquiries. If cognitive impairment is detected history must be obtained from another source. Family, friends, housing managers, and nursing home personnel may all be valuable informants. The patient's primary physician must also be consulted to obtain an accurate medical history.

An elderly patient frequently takes multiple medications. Encouraging the patient to always bring all medications when visiting the physician or coming to the hospital ensures an accurate medication history. In addition to asking about which medicines the patient takes, the physician should specifically ask about compliance.

The frequency of multiple chronic illnesses in the elderly magnifies the importance of obtaining a functional assessment of the patient. Just recording "degenerative arthritis" as a problem adds little information, but noting that the patient is unable to open jars or pill boxes, unable to tie shoes, and unable to walk without severe hip pain can be vitally important. Similarly recording a history of heart disease is useless compared with noting that the

patient cannot walk 20 yards on a level surface without experiencing severe dyspnea. The entire therapeutic approach may differ depending on whether a foot problem prevents walking in a previously fully ambulatory person or is an incidental finding in an otherwise severely impaired individual.

Physical Examination

Physical examination techniques have been presented elsewhere in this text, so the following discussion is limited to factors of particular relevance to the examination of the elderly. Thoroughness is perhaps the most important aspect of the physical examination of the elderly. Unsuspected pathology is very common in the elderly. Podiatrists must realize that prior to considering any surgical treatment of an older patient, a rigorous examination for concurrent problems is needed.

Skin cancers, cardiac valvular lesions, abdominal aneurysms, and endocrine disorders are only a few of the potentially important problems that can be detected by a thorough examination. A disheveled general appearance or poor personal hygiene may be a clue to mental impairment or depression. This possibility must be investigated and certainly may indicate that the patient may have difficulty with outpatient wound care after a podiatric procedure.

A key to successful physical examination in the elderly is to familiarize oneself with normal aging changes (Table 16–7). For example, there are many skin lesions that are so common with aging that they can be considered normal changes. Seborrheic keratoses are raised, greasy-feeling, darkly pigmented lesions that are often found on the trunk and neck and virtually never develop malignant changes. Skin tags are small, flesh-colored fibromas or skin redundancies. Senile lentigines, or liver spots, are flat areas of hyperpigmentation often found on sun-exposed regions. Cherry angiomas are slightly raised, round, red lesions that do not blanch. These benign signs of aging must be differentiated from premalignant actinic keratoses and basal cell, squamous cell, and melanoma skin cancers that require treatment. A good color atlas of dermatology can help one

Table 16–7. COMMON SKIN CHANGES AND CONDITIONS IN THE GERIATRIC PATIENT

Changes

Lentigines (liver spots)	Acrochordons (skin tag)
Senile purpura	Venous stars
Venous lakes	Angiokeratoma
Senile (cherry) angioma	

Conditions

Xerosis	Pruritus ani
Perlèche	Rosacea
Tinea pedis	Verruca
Pruritus vulvae	Cellulitis
Senile seborrheic dermatitis	Hyperkeratosis
Lichen simplex chronicus	
Tinea onychomycosis	

Precancerous Cutaneous Conditions

Seborrheic keratoses	Actinic (solar) keratoses
Keratoacanthoma	Leukoplakia

Cancerous Conditions

Basal cell carcinoma (epithelioma)
Squamous cell carcinoma
Malignant melanoma

Incidental Conditions

Drug eruptions	Psoriasis
Neurodermatoses	Contact dermatitis
Syphilis	Stasis dermatitis
Herpes zoster	

identify these lesions, but when any doubt exists, referral is mandatory.

Because normal aging changes occur in almost every system, these changes must be learned to avoid confusion with more serious pathology. Arcus senilis of the cornea has been mentioned. Soft systolic murmurs of the heart are very common and may reflect age-related fibrosis of the aortic valve region without functional impairment. An S_4 gallop in the elderly may be due to loss of ventricular compliance with age and again may be clinically unimportant. Older women may have atrophic external genitalia from postmenopausal absence of estrogen stimulation. If a so-affected woman is asymptomatic this too may be considered a normal aging change. Degenerative arthritis of the hands is extremely common, and osteophyte formation around the distal interphalangeal joints leads to the deformity called Heberden's nodes. Similar changes of the proximal interphalangeal joints are called Bouchard's

nodes. Neither of these lesions is cause for alarm.

Nerve conduction may diminish with aging, and there is loss of distal vibratory sense. Diminished or absent knee- and ankle-jerk reflexes are common with aging and in the absence of other pathology do not require further evaluation. "Cerebral release" signs, such as extensor plantar, grasp, and glabellar reflexes, may be present without any other evidence of brain disease. As previously mentioned, mental status testing is a must in the elderly. Some allowance of response time can be expected, but any impairment of memory, judgment, alertness, or orientation is abnormal and requires investigation. Confusion is a common manifestation of systemic illness or overmedication in the elderly and is often reversible. One of the many brief mental status screening tests that are available should be memorized and done routinely.

Laboratory and Physiologic Data

Laboratory tests can also help reveal unsuspected illness in the elderly. A frequent error is to attribute abnormalities in common laboratory test results to normal aging. For example, a complete blood count (CBC) is often obtained as a screening test. No abnormality of hemoglobin, hematocrit, white blood cells (WBCs), or platelet count should be discounted in an elderly patient simply because of age. Serum electrolytes, calcium, urea nitrogen, bilirubin, and transaminase levels are similarly unchanged with age. One laboratory value for which slight abnormalities have even more significance in the elderly than in the young is the serum creatinine level. Total body muscle mass decreases, and therefore endogenous creatinine production declines with age. High normal or slightly elevated values may represent markedly reduced renal function.

Normal aging is accompanied by both decreased secretion of insulin after meals and impaired end organ sensitivity to insulin. For this reason, moderately elevated glucose levels after meals should be tolerated in the elderly, although they require further investigation in the young. Diabetes mellitus should be diagnosed only when abnormalities of glucose tolerance exceed this age-related change.

Asymptomatic bacteriuria, often with WBCs, is a common finding on urine analysis and often does not require treatment. Hematuria is often due to prostatic hypertrophy in men but is always to be considered an abnormality that warrants further investigation.

ASSESSMENT OF COMMON PROBLEMS

Pharmacology

The frequency of multiple chronic illnesses in the elderly often leads to the prescription of complicated regimens with multiple drugs given in varied dosage frequencies. It is not unusual to have an elderly patient with poor eyesight and moderate memory impairment bring in a sack of pills, some to be taken every other day, some daily, some two times daily, others after meals, and others "as needed." Not surprisingly, the incidence of both adverse drug reactions and poor compliance rises with advanced age. In addition to understanding the changes in drug metabolism, distribution, and sensitivity that accompany aging, anyone prescribing for the elderly must learn to simplify drug regimens. With careful thought and coordination of efforts with the patient's primary physician, maximum compliance and minimum adverse effects can be achieved.

Pharmacokinetic Changes

Although alterations of gastric emptying and intestinal peristalsis have been documented with aging, most studies suggest no clinically important decline in drug absorption in the elderly. An exception to this principle is in the case of drugs that require gastric acid to dissolve enteric coating. Gastric atrophy with achlorhydria is common with aging and may alter absorption of some extended-action preparations. In contrast to absorption, the distribution of many drugs is dramatically and clinically significantly altered with aging.

Albumin is the major serum protein to which drugs bind. With aging, there is a slight drop in serum albumin level, and in hospitalized elderly patients, this drop is more pronounced. This drop can have a strong influence on the free drug available to act on the tissues after a dose of a strongly protein-bound drug. It can be particularly clinically significant when several protein-bound drugs are given that compete for available albumin-binding sites.

The proportion of body weight that is fat increases with age. Conversely total body water decreases. Roughly these changes result in an increased volume of distribution for fat-soluble drugs, such as diazepam, and diminished volume of distribution for water-soluble drugs, such as antipyrine. Whereas this model is often useful, aging may alter several of the determinants of volume of distribution of a given drug, so that age effects are difficult to predict. Drug half-life is proportionate to volume of distribution, so that any age-related change in volume of distribution influences proper dosing intervals. After a steady-state serum drug level has been achieved, the amount of drug given daily must equal the amount of drug eliminated by the body each day. At a given therapeutic serum drug concentration, total blood clearance of the drug is the sole determinant of appropriate daily dosage.

Drugs are cleared from the body predominantly by two organs, the liver and the kidney. Both hepatic and renal drug metabolism can change with aging. Kidney function predictably deteriorates with aging. By age 70, glomerular filtration rate is only half what it was in youth. Renal blood flow declines proportionally. Many of the drugs commonly prescribed for the elderly are eliminated predominantly by the kidney, and their clearance is decreased with advanced age. Digoxin, penicillin, and aminoglycoside antibiotics are examples of drugs in which diminished clearance may be clinically important. Muscle mass decreases with age, as does total production of creatinine. For this reason, a relatively normal serum creatinine level in an older person may mask a significant loss of renal function.

Drugs that are cleared by the liver have a less predictably altered metabolism in the elderly. Excretion of some drugs is limited by hepatic blood flow, which is approximately 40% lower in the elderly. Such drugs, including lidocaine, have dramatically diminished clearance with aging. Elimination of other drugs is limited by enzymatic activity of the liver, and often these drugs are cleared as well by the elderly as by the young. Warfarin is an example of this type of drug. Unfortunately the age-related changes in hepatic drug metabolism are complicated. Pharmacokinetic studies of each drug are needed to determine whether dose changes are needed.

Pharmacodynamic Changes

Thus far, age changes relating to pharmacokinetics have been discussed. Pharmacokinetics relates to altered serum levels after a given dose of a drug. Pharmacodynamics refers to alterations of drug effects with identical serum levels of a drug. Pharmacodynamic changes of aging are less well studied than pharmacokinetic changes but may be of comparable importance. Examples of this type of age-related change include increased sensitivity to the sedative effects of a given level of diazepam and decreased sensitivity to a given blood level of propranolol. Clearly pharmacodynamic age changes are a fertile field for future research. Unfortunately even a thorough understanding of age changes in the pharmacology of individual drugs is inadequate for safe and effective drug therapy in the elderly.

The number of chronic illnesses per person rises with age and so does the number of medications taken. The risk of adverse side effects dramatically rises as the number of medications taken increases partly because of drug-drug interactions. Compliance is always problematic and drops precipitously as complexity of medication regimens increases. Cost is also often a problem. Medication costs are not always reimbursed by Medicare, and the elderly are one of the poorest segments of society in the United States.

Simple measures can help maximize the benefit elderly patients receive from drug therapy. It is of utmost importance that the indications to start a new drug be clear and treatment goal determined. The physician should attempt to find out all other drugs the patient is taking, preferably having the patient bring all medication to each appointment. It is occasionally necessary to have a public health nurse or family member clean out the patient's medicine cabinet, throwing away all outdated and dis-continued drugs. If the patient is on a complicated regimen and particularly if there are drugs prescribed by multiple physicians the patient's primary care provider should be contacted. A cooperative approach may allow simplification of the medication schedules, and discontinuance of unneeded drugs, thus avoiding drug interaction. If alternative drugs are available the number of daily doses needed, the number of pills taken, the cost, and the potential side effects should be considered. For any drug chosen, the physician should investigate altered metabolism with aging. If possible, one should start with the lowest dose and very gradually raise it until the lowest effective dose is determined.

To facilitate compliance, the physician should carefully instruct the patient and if at all possible relatives and other care givers. The physician should have the pharmacist label drug containers with the purpose of the pills (e.g., "for toe infection"). Containers that are not child proof for situations in which no children can be expected to come in contact with the drugs should be requested. Medication calendars and special pill dispensers can be of help, and in a pinch, an egg carton can serve as a portioned and labeled pill dispenser. On subsequent visits, the physician should review use of the medication and inquire about compliance and side effects.

Surgical Considerations

After age 70, most studies suggest an increased morbidity and mortality in patients related to elective surgery. Proposed reasons include diminished cardiac and pulmonary reserve, coexisting chronic illnesses, and altered presentation and delayed recognition of complications. In spite of this statistical evidence, one of the major advances in modern medicine has been the realization that surgery can be performed on even those of extremely old age with excellent functional results. In podiatry, age alone should not determine whether surgery is performed.

Podiatric problems can have a major role in functional impairment, that is, joint deformities leading to instability or painful bunions or nail disease leading to the patient's "taking to bed." Even in the presence of other chronic illnesses, with care, podiatric procedures can provide dramatic improvement of function and quality of life in the elderly. Older patients are much more likely than younger patients to have diabetes mellitus, heart disease, hypertension, and cognitive impairment. Clearly there is a need for careful cooperation between the podiatrist and the primary physician. Older patients often have problems handling anesthetic agents. Consultation with the anesthesiologist when surgery is first considered may be of great benefit.

A social worker or case manager may need to be contacted prior to scheduling elective surgery to ensure that adequate postoperative home care is provided. Older patients may also benefit from a preoperative visit to the hospital to familiarize themselves with the hospital's routine. Careful instructions as to what to expect preoperatively can do much to allay fears and may minimize postoperative confusion. In patients in whom postoperative confusion is a consideration, familiar items from home, such as pictures of family, can be of great help. Even brief periods of bed rest are a particular danger in the elderly. Stiffening of the joints occurs, and postural reflexes are blunted. Hypostatic pneumonia can develop. Osteoporosis is accelerated. Constipation occurs, and fecal impaction can develop. The elderly are more prone to develop pressure sores. Paget's disease, not uncommon in the elderly, can cause profound and life-threatening hypercalcemia. For these reasons and many more, all efforts must be made to keep the elderly out of bed and if possible ambulating. Judicious use of pain medication is needed, balancing pain relief with the risks of confusion, oversedation, and constipation.

Postoperative Confusion

Postoperative confusion is often a problem in the elderly. As mentioned, drugs are often a culprit. The pain and the stress of surgery may lead to temporary mental impairment. Diminished vision and hearing may cause routine hospital events to acquire a sinister appearance. Hypoxia, fever, electrolyte imbalance, and occult infection can all lead to reversible delirium.

Any cognitive impairment can increase the risk of postoperative complications, such as falls and torn-out intravenous lines. New-onset confusion in an elderly patient mandates a thorough evaluation. A major error is to order a sedative and ignore the underlying cause of confusion. After medical and pharmacologic causes of delirium have been ruled out, confusion may be attributed to the new location and stress of surgery leading to decompensation of a marginally compensated frail older person.

Under these circumstances, recovery is to be expected with time, and the podiatrist's goal should be to minimize the risk of complications. Well-lit rooms with a minimum of distractions should be provided. Restraints should be avoided if at all possible. A patient can be nursed from a mattress on the floor if falls from bed are a problem. All staff should clearly identify themselves and explain what they are going to do during all patient contacts. The patient should wear glasses and hearing aids if needed. Drug use should be minimized, particularly drugs with potential central nervous system effects. If, as a last resort, sedation is deemed necessary very small doses of antipsychotic drugs may be useful (e.g., 25 mg of thioridazine). The extrapyramidal side effects of antipsychotics are of major concern in the elderly. Sedative hypnotic drugs, such as benzodiazepines, can result in paradoxic agitation under circumstances of delirium and should be avoided.

Altered Response to Infection

One manifestation of the aging process that can be confusing to the podiatric physician is an altered response to infection. A localized infection, such as an abscess, pneumonia, or cellulitis, may cause the usual febrile response and elevation of the peripheral WBC count with a shift to the left, i.e., toward an increased percentage of immature cells. This lack of response is not a universal phenomenon but is increasingly common with advanced age. Malnutrition may predispose the patient to this state. Usually some clue to infection is present, such as a WBC count rise in the absence of fever, episode of confusion, development of incontinence, and loss of appetite and general malaise. The clinician must maintain a high degree of suspicion for occult infection in the elderly patient.

Constipation

Another problem in the elderly patient hospitalized for surgery is constipation. Untreated constipation can lead to fecal impaction, the inability to pass large masses of doughy or rock-hard stool. Large masses of hard stool can act as a ball valve, letting liquid stool pass and causing a spurious picture of diarrhea, when the underlying process is really constipation. Fecal impaction may cause abdominal pain or even mental decompensation, confusion, and agitation. Perhaps the most feared complication of fecal impaction is the formation of stercoral ulcerations, pressure ulcerations in the colonic wall from contact with hard stools, which can result in acute abdominal catastrophe.

For constipation, as with so many medical problems, prevention is the key to management. Adequate hydration is needed to prevent overdrying of feces. The patient should be encouraged to drink plenty of water. Inactivity promotes constipation, and early ambulation postoperatively can prevent it. Many patients find a commode or toilet easier to use than a bedpan. Hospital food often lacks bulk, or nondigestible fiber. Poor dentures lead to avoidance of very high bulk foods, which increase stool water content and bowel motility. A hospital dietician can help increase fiber in the patient's diet. Supplemental bulk preparations, such as bran and psyllium, may be useful. Drugs may contribute to the tendency to develop constipation. Opiates, anticholinergics, antidepressants, antipsychotics, antacids, and calcium supplements all can promote constipation. Discontinuing one of these drugs may be more effective than starting another drug to treat constipation.

Occasionally additional treatment is needed. Stool softeners, such as dioctyl sodium sulfosuccinate, are hydrophilic oral agents and may be helpful. Mild laxatives, such as milk of magnesia, should be tried next. Glycerin suppositories are helpful. Stimulant containing bisacodyl or oral senna extracts are used if less aggressive measures have failed. Prepackaged sodium phosphate enemas can clean the rectum and sigmoid colon, and tap water or saline enemas can clean more of the colon. The colon can absorb large volumes of water and electrolytes. If salt retention is a problem tap water is the enema of choice; if hyponatremia is a problem saline is the enema of choice. Soap suds are very irritating and can produce inflammatory colitis. Therefore soap suds enemas should be avoided. For extremely hard stool, rarely an oil enema is useful. Digital disimpaction may be necessary and may provide much appreciated relief.

Urinary Incontinence

Urinary incontinence is another perioperative problem much more common in the elderly than in young adults. This problem is related to the previous two problems discussed in that both confusion and fecal impaction can result in urinary incontinence. The podiatrist must learn to manage both long-established urinary incontinence and the abrupt onset of incontinence during a hospitalization. Chronic urinary incontinence is a frequent problem in the elderly population. This problem can be due to neurologic, mechanical, and functional causes. Incontinence is most certainly not a normal part of the aging process, and it should always be evaluated by the primary care provider.

If no reversible cause is found chronic incontinence must be managed with a maximum of comfort, dignity, and safety for the patient. All too often, management is with a Foley catheter. Bladder stones, infection, and sepsis frequently follow. Although in some cases, catheterization is unavoidable, a trend is to have patients who are living at home or in progressive nursing homes managed with frequent trips to the bathroom. Because bladder capacity decreases with aging and disease states and many incontinent patients have uninhibited bladder emptying when 200 to 300 ml of urine accumulates in the bladder, voiding may need to be as frequent as every 1 to 2 hours. When reminded to void at such intervals, many incontinent patients can be kept dry. Absorbent pads may be used to protect skin and clothes when accidents occur. If such a patient is admitted for a podiatric procedure nurses must be instructed to continue the voiding regimen. Even brief periods of catheterization in these patients may result in bladder shrinkage, interfering with the practicality of returning to the voiding schedule in the future.

In normally continent elderly persons who have been hospitalized, the development of urinary incontinence at some time during the hospital stay is common. It is common for older people to have urgency, or decreased time between first sensing bladder fullness and when they are unable to inhibit bladder emptying. Continence may be maintained in a delicate balance in physically frail older persons. Many factors related to acute illness, surgery, and hospitalization can tip this balance toward incontinence. Acute illness or stress of surgery can precipitate confusion and associated incontinence. The foot problem precipitating hospitalization or the surgical wound can sufficiently interfere with mobility to prevent reaching the toilet in time. Hospital beds, which are high and have side rails, slow the patient. Busy nurses may not reach the patient in adequate time. Bed rest can be a powerful diuretic, compounding the problem.

Certain metabolic abnormalities, such as hyperglycemia and hypercalcemia, can also produce increased urinary volume. Many drugs can contribute to incontinence. Drugs with anticholinergic effects can cause urinary retention with overflow incontinence. As previously mentioned, many drugs lead to confusion in the elderly, often with incontinence. Pain medications and sleeping pills are frequent culprits. Diuretics may increase urinary flow enough to result in incontinence in the frail older patient.

After addressing any reversible factors

Table 16–8. CAUSES OF NEW-ONSET URINARY INCONTINENCE

Urgency

Physical barriers (side rails, restraint, acute podiatric problem, intravenous line)
Slow nursing staff response
Unfamiliar toilet locations

Medical Illnesses

Confusion
Fecal impaction
Urinary tract infection
Hyperglycemia
Hypercalciuria (related to immobility, Paget's disease)
Acute urinary retention (related to immobility, prostatic hypertrophy, drugs)

contributing to incontinence, it may be necessary to manage the newly incontinent patient (Table 16–8). Frequent scheduled voiding can be tried. Bed pads and absorbent underwear combined with excellent nursing care can be used to weather temporary incontinence. In males, condom catheters can be tried. Only if urinary output is monitored or skin breakdown threatens should Foley catheterization, with attendant complications, be risked. In most cases, as the patient recovers, continence is regained.

PODOGERIATRICS

As discussed previously, aging is associated with myriad changes due both to normal aging processes and to the accumulation of chronic illnesses and pathologic damage. The net result is a diminished homeostatic reserve. Homeostatic reserve refers to the ability to return to baseline after some insult, be it physical, psychologic, metabolic, or pharmacologic. Any such insult may lead to a decompensation with loss of function. One function susceptible to loss after a variety of insults is ambulation.

The loss of ambulatory ability can be a major blow to an older person. This loss vastly magnifies dependence; help is needed to shop, cook, bathe, and so forth. The risk of falls increases, along with the risk of deadly hip fractures (Table 16–9). If social support networks, including family and friends, are unable to adequately help, the older individual with impaired walking may be forced into an institutionalized living situation.

It should be obvious that podiatric problems can lead to loss of ambulation in the elderly. The dire consequences of immobility in this age group mandate the goal of excellent foot care for the elderly. Podiatric problems are often preventable or readily treatable. Podiatric care must be seen as a part of the comprehensive approach to the total person. One of the hallmarks of geriatric care is the interdisciplinary team because the problems of an older person are usually interrelated. It is common for the management of a patient's problems to require the input of a primary care physician, a social worker, a case manager, and of course the patient. Additional

Table 16–9. CAUSES OF PATHOLOGIC FRACTURES AND FALLS

| Pathologic Fractures | Falls | | |
	Cardiovascular	Neurologic	Other
Osteoporosis	Postural hypertension	Gait change	Anemia
Paget's disease		Vertigo	Tranquilizers
Osteomalacia	Heart blocks	Muscle weakness	Antihypertensive drugs
Hyperparathyroidism	Stokes-Adams disease	Vestibular problems	
Metastatic cancer			Analgesics
	Silent MI	Motor dysfunctions	
	Atrial fibrillation		Antidepressants
	Aortic stenosis	Neuropathies	
	Ventricular arrhythmias	CVA	
		Dementias	
	Atrial flutter	Uncoordination	
		Seizures	

CVA, Cerebrovascular accident; MI, myocardial infarction.

input is often needed from a physiatrist, physical therapist, occupational therapist, audiologist, psychiatrist, visiting nurse, dentist, lawyer, and any of a host of others. The podiatrist must fit into this team approach, being the patient's advocate for obtaining adequate foot care. From the other disciplines, factors contributing toward the patient's foot problems may become apparent, such as cognitive, visual, and sensory impairment interfering with primary foot care needs. Prescribed periods of foot elevation may be impossible, for example, because of inadequate social supports. It is only by keeping the whole elderly person in mind that maximally effective foot care can be delivered.

Podiatric Problems Related to Aging Changes

Many aging changes combine to promote podiatric problems in the elderly. The connective tissue matrix of the skin changes, leading to thinner and more fragile skin. Vascular impairment leads to loss of hair and sweat glands and markedly inhibited ability to heal. The accumulation of trauma over time leads to onychial dystrophies. Muscular and skeletal changes lead to altered biomechanics of gait and weight bearing. These changes may lead to various hyperkeratotic lesions. Disease processes that occur with increasing frequency in old age include osteoarthritis, stroke, and distal sensory neuropathies.

These processes can all dramatically contribute to foot morbidity. Such disease processes also occur in younger patients, but when they occur in frail elderly persons, the management problems are compounded.

The loss of sweating and subsequent dry skin promote fissures, cracks, and other breaks in the skin barrier. Dry skin also leads to pruritus, with scratching and other self-induced trauma to the foot. Hyperkeratotic lesions may be picked at if painful or unsightly, possibly tearing the skin. Impaired vision, balance, and position sense lead to an increased risk of trauma to the foot. Diminished sensation in neuropathic feet may lead to unawareness of trauma incurred and lack of proper care. If infection develops the elderly are less able to fight it. Impaired circulation contributes to difficulty in healing and in fighting infection. These factors result in an increased risk of loss of life or limb after podiatric problems develop in the elderly.

Decubitus Ulceration of the Lower Extremity

A common podiatric problem that is clearly related to the chronic skin changes in the elderly is decubitus ulceration of the lower extremity. This problem is most often a result of a chronic stasis dermatitis, the long-term consequence of altered venous circulation of the leg, thought to be secondary to prior episodes of deep venous thrombosis. The skin becomes pigmented owing to deposition of breakdown prod-

ucts of blood that leaks from fragile venules. Edema and fibrosis contribute to impaired health of the leg tissue. Recurrent
superficial thrombophlebitis can add an inflammatory component to the clinical picture. Ulcerations, most frequently just
above the medial malleolus, often follow
minor trauma. The poor circulation leads
to impaired healing and suceptibility to superinfection. The ulcer may heal slowly
with scar formation. It is not uncommon to
see evidence of prior ulceration that has
healed when the patient presents with a
new ulcer.

Management of stasis ulcers should be a
concern of both the podiatrist and the primary physician, and team work is often the
key to successful treatment of this problem. Of course, prevention is the best approach, and this is best accomplished by
making all efforts to prevent deep thrombophlebitis. Once a stasis dermatitis exists,
elimination of edema and prevention of its
recurrence are very important. A brief (1-
to 3-day) period of bed rest may be necessary, with elevation of the foot on the
bed. Moist compresses may be used if
weeping is present, applied for 20 minutes
every 3 to 4 hours. A superficial, avascular
ulcer may heal with such conservative
treatment. Topical antibiotics or debriding
agents are rarely indicated. Rapidly growing ulcers may indicate infection is present
and mandate adequate aerobic and anaerobic culture and appropriate antibiotic
treatment.

After relief of edema, compressive support helps to substitute for the incompetent
venous system, preventing further accumulation of edematous fluid. Elastic bandages are preferable unless the patient has
developed a sensitivity to elastic material.
An elastic bandage is best applied prior to
getting out of bed in the morning. If the
patient lacks the ability to fully cooperate
with use of elastic stockings a commercial
paste gelatin boot can be very helpful. This
boot needs to be replaced at least weekly
to allow periodic reinspection. After the
ulcer heals, custom-fitted, pressure-gra-
dient elastic stockings should be worn regularly by the patient. Several pairs may be
necessary to allow frequent washing. If the
ulcer does not heal after these measures
surgical consultation is needed. In certain
patients, skin grafting may allow a successful functional recovery.

Prevention of Podiatric Problems

Clearly preventing podiatric problems is
an attractive alternative to treating them.
Frequently foot disease is related to the patient's personal practices. It is a responsibility of the podiatrist to instruct the elderly patient, the family, and other care
givers in proper foot care. When instruct-
ing an elderly patient on foot care, the simple principles mentioned previously under
History should be applied. Older individuals often have a lower level of formal education than the present generation, and ex-
planations should be simple. Vision and
hearing may be poor, so asking the patient
to repeat instructions is useful. Audiovis-
ual aids are often helpful. Simple terms,
such as "bunion" or "corn," may be mis-
understood and should be explained. The
physician should inquire as to what home
remedies the older patient may be using
and counsel the patient appropriately.
Common concerns of an older patient are
"How much exercise can I do?" and "How
much can I walk?" The patient may assume that because he or she has pedal
problems, he or she should keep off his or
her feet. The importance of maintaining activity must be emphasized. Compliance is
not only a problem with therapeutic modalities but also a problem with preventive
or health maintenance measures. On subsequent visits, the physician should always
inquire about compliance. It may be productive to ask the elderly patient, "What are
you doing to keep your feet healthy?" This
allows the physician to hear the patient in
his or her own words give his or her perception of instructions. Enlisting the help
of family members can also help improve
compliance.

Podiatry in the Nursing Home

With aging, the frequency of functional
impairment increases. Often limitation of
mobility, impairment of cognitive function, and chronic illness prevent older persons from adequately caring for themselves. Fortunately family and friends
often are able to help maintain the older
person in a familiar environment. As age
advances, however, friends and spouses
are likely to die or acquire their own disabilities. The children of the very old are

often old themselves and are unable to care for their parents. When the level of care required to maintain independent living overwhelms the available social supports, some form of alternate living arrangement is needed. If the level of disability is very high nursing homes are often the only available option. If the level of function improves, return to a less restrictive living situation is possible, but often the move to a nursing home is permanent.

Only 5% of all persons 65 and older live in a nursing home at any one time, but approximately one third of those who live to 65 will spend some part of their remaining years in a nursing home. With odds like these, we should all want to improve the quality of life of those living in nursing homes. Nursing home patients are in an extremely dependent situation. By increasing independence of these patients, their enjoyment of life improves. Podiatrists are in a position to improve ambulatory ability and to diminish pain in these patients.

Approximately 50% of nursing home patients are cognitively impaired, and many of the rest are physically unable to care for their feet. The prevalence of foot problems in nursing home patients is high, and the need for adequate treatment is great. The podiatrist can help in two general ways: first, by setting up a comprehensive foot care program within the institution, and second, by teaching nursing staff to provide basic preventative and rehabilitative foot care.

Podiatric Screening

Because of the high prevalence of pedal pathology in the nursing home, one of the most pressing needs is complete podiatric screening after each admission. At that time, the podiatrist can assess whether the patient is capable of adequate self care or whether routine hygienic care needs to be administered by the nursing staff. Treatable lesions can be identified early, when the prognosis for functional improvement is best. This screening is also an opportunity to set up a treatment schedule or to schedule a routine re-evaluation in several months.

Podiatric Care Program

A podiatrist caring for nursing home patients needs adequate room to set up equipment and work. Efficiency can be facilitated by utilizing a nurse's aide to remove shoes and footwear and to help with bedridden patients. A section of the patient's chart should be available for recording podiatric notes. Pertinent medical information must be readily available for each patient. The nurse and aides probably provide the day-to-day foot care for the patients. The staff is also in a position for early detection of pathology if they know what to look for.

The American Podiatry Medical Association has prepared nursing home staff educational materials to help the podiatrist set up a superb in-service program. For those patients cognitively able to benefit from instruction, individual and group instruction on foot care is useful. By projecting an attitude of prevention and early detection of foot problems, the podiatrist can stimulate the enthusiasm of the staff and patients. Through a cooperative effort, excellent foot care can be provided to this needy population.

The Podiatrist and the Aged Patient

The physical, pharmacologic, and physiologic changes that accompany aging justify covering geriatrics separately in a textbook of medicine. Much more important than the differences between young and old, however, are the similarities. The podiatrist will never be able to provide excellent care for elderly patients without connecting with the humanity and personality underneath the aging skin. The dependency that often follows the frailty and physical disabilities of extreme old age makes it all too easy to treat the older patient as a child or an inferior. It is common to hear references to older patients by their first name or as "granny" or "pops." Isolation is a bane of old age, and demeaning treatment only reinforces withdrawal.

Fortunately poverty, which is often the elderly's lot today, need not interfere with adequate podiatric care. Medicare legislation has been rewritten to provide podiatric service for large groups of previously ineligible elderly. Patients with diabetes mellitus, severe peripheral vascular disease, many peripheral neuropathies, and traumatic injuries are now covered. Foot infections, including fungal infections of toenails, are also covered. Diagnostic services are insured for specific foot complaints even if the eventual diagnosis does not qualify for coverage. Because Medicare regulations have frequently changed in the past, the podiatrist must keep informed as new legislation is passed.

Demographic trends indicate that care for the elderly will be an important function of podiatrists in the future. This function is best seen as one of the true challenges in the field. Small interventions can make dramatic improvements in the patient's functional ability and quality of life. The interactions of normal aging changes, chronic disease, and a lifetime of accumulated traumatic injury make the care of the feet of older people very interesting. By developing enthusiasm for geriatric podiatry and keeping abreast of developments in the field of gerontology, podiatrists will be best able to provide truly comprehensive foot care for the elderly as well as the young.

Bibliography

Black JR, Hale WE: Prevalence of foot complaints in the elderly. J Am Podiatr Med Assoc 77:308, 1987.

Cummings JL, Benson DF: Dementia: A Clinical Approach. Boston: Butterworth Publishers, 1983.

Dockery GL (ed): Dermatology of the lower extremities. Clin Podiatr Med Surg 3:3, 1986.

Goroll AH, May LA, Mulley AG: Primary Care Medicine: Office Evaluation and Management of the Adult Patient. Philadelphia: JB Lippincott Co, 1987.

Helfand AE: Clinical Podogeriatrics. Baltimore: Williams & Wilkins Co, 1981.

Helfand AE, Bruno J (eds): Rehabilitation of the foot. Clin Podiatr Med Surg 1:2, 1984.

Kane RL, Ouslander JG, Abrass IB: Essentials of Clinical Geriatrics. New York: McGraw-Hill Book Co, 1984.

Kenney RA: Physiology of Aging: A Synopsis. Chicago: Year Book Medical Publishers, Inc, 1982.

Levy LA (ed): Systemic disease affecting the foot. Clin Podiatr Med Surg 2:4, 1985.

Pearson LJ, Kotthoff ME: Geriatric Clinical Protocols. Philadelphia: JB Lippincott Co, 1979.

Rossman I (ed): Clinical Geriatrics. Philadelphia: JB Lippincott Co, 1971.

Samitz MH, Dana AS Jr: Cutaneous Lesions of the Lower Extremities. Philadelphia: JB Lippincott Co, 1971.

Sculco TP (ed): Orthopedic Care of the Geriatric Patient. St Louis: CV Mosby Co, 1985.

Williams TF (ed): Rehabilitation in the Aging. New York: Raven Press, 1984.

INDEX

Note: Page numbers in *italic* type refer to illustrations; page numbers followed by the letter t refer to tables.

Foot (*Continued*)
  metatarsophalangeal joint of, rheumatoid
      arthritis and, 146–147, *147*
    secondary osteoarthritis and, 142
    synovial fluid analysis of, 140
    urate deposition in, *168*
  plantar fascia of, 160
  polyarticular symmetric arthritis of, 146
  rheumatoid arthritis of, *147, 151*
  subtalar joint of, 138, 140, 146–147, *147*
  synovial fluid analysis of, 140
  talonavicular joint of, 140, 146–147, *147*
Fractures, metabolic bone disease and, 236–
    237
  osteonecrosis caused by, 257
  osteoporosis causing, 237–238, 240–241,
    243, 534
  pseudofractures differentially diagnosed
    from, 248
Freiberg's disease, 512
Friedreich's ataxia, 375
Frostbite, 91–92
Fungal culture, 397
Fungal infections, 411–415, 415t, 492
Furuncles, 394

Gallbladder, 209, *209–210*
Gallstones, 214, 217, 220, 225, 300
Gamma globulin, 292, 299
Gangrene, aortoiliac disease and, 75
  arterial insufficiency and, 74
  arteriogram and, 72
  cold exposure and, 90
  diabetes mellitus and, 190–191
  femoropopliteal disease and, 75
  frostbite and, 92
  ischemia and, 51
  reconstructive surgery and, 84–85
  skin disorders and, 410
  ulceration and, 60, 60t
  vascular diseases as cause of, 60t
  venous thrombosis and, 93
Gastrin, 210
Gastritis, 208t, 217–218
Gastrointestinal bleeding, 217–219, 219t, 504
Gastrointestinal disorders, abdominal pain
    and, 210–211, *211*, 219–220, 230
  acute diarrhea and, 227–231, *228–230*
  bowel habit alterations and, 211–212
  calcium malabsorption and, 236
  gastrointestinal disorders and, 215–217,
    215, 344–345, 345t
  jaundice and, alcoholic liver disease and,
    122
    cirrhosis and, 225–227, 226t
    drug-induced hepatitis and, 224–225
    evaluation of, 220–222, 221, 222t
    extrahepatic obstruction and, 225
    liver disease and, 213, 220–227, *221*,
      222t, *223–224*, 226t
    viral hepatitis A and, 222–223, 222t, *223*
    viral hepatitis B and, 222t, 223–224, *224*
    viral hepatitis non-A, non-B and, 222t,
      224, *224*
  laboratory, physiologic tests of, 214–215
  liver disease and, 213–214, 220–227, *221*,
    222t, *223–224*, 226t
  lower gastrointestinal bleeding and, 219,
    219t

Gastrointestinal disorders (*Continued*)
  medication effects on, 208t
  metabolic, chronic neuropathies and, 365
  osteoporosis and, 238t, 240
  pancreatitis and, 227
  pediatrics and, 502–505
  peritonitis and, 213
  physical examination and, 212–214, 212t–
    213t
  podiatric implications of, 207–208, 208t,
    345
  preoperative assessment and, 449
  upper gastrointestinal bleeding and, 217–
    219
Gastrointestinal system accessory organs of,
    208–209, *209*
  bile function in, 209
  liver function in, 109, *209*
  regulating hormones of, 210
  tubular organs of, 208, *209*
Genetic counseling, 478
Genetic disorders, 476–478
Genetic inheritance, 57
Genital warts, 423t
Genu valgum, 520
Geriatric podiatry, in nursing homes, 545–
    547
  patient history and, 535–537, 537t
  pharmacology and, 539–540
  physical examination and, 537–538, 538t
  physiologic data and, 538–539
  preoperative assessment and, 451
  prevention and, 545
  related to aging, 543–545, 544t
  surgical considerations of, 540–543
German measles, 474, 516
Giant cell arteritis, 81–82, 431
Giant cell tumors, 250, 254, 257–258, 260,
    318
Giantism, 445
Giardiasis, 230
Glomerular filtration, 263–264, *264*
Glomerular proteinuria, 268
Glomerulonephritis, arteriosclerotic
    cardiovascular disease and, 157
  auranofin and, 154
  causes and symptoms of, 270t
  membranous, 154, 274t
  pediatric genitourinary tract disorder and,
    506
  renal disorders caused by, 267, 273, 273t–
    274t
Glomerulonephropathy, 269, 270t
Glomus tumors, 419–420
Glucocorticoids, bone mineral homeostasis
    and, 235
  eosinophils affected by, 292
  fibrous dysplagia caused by, 257
  hypervitaminosis D and, 236
  osteoporosis related to, 241
  postoperative potassium level disorders
    caused by, 458
Glucose levels, albumin excretion affected
    by, 283–284
  diabetic nephropathy affected by, 284
  geriatric podiatry and, 538
  hyperkalemia therapy and, 288
  in normal urinalysis, 265t
  SMA 12 affected by, 444